A Primer in Cartilage Repair and Joint Preservation of the Knee

A Primer in Cartilage Repair and Joint Preservation of the Knee

Edited by

Tom Minas, MD, MS

Associate Professor
Harvard Medical School

Director, Cartilage Repair Center, Brigham and Women's Hospital, Chestnut Hill, Massachusetts

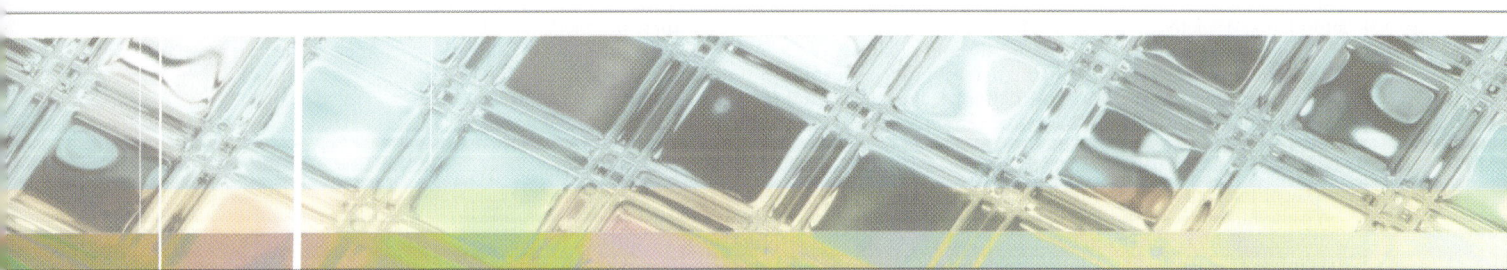

ELSEVIER
SAUNDERS

ELSEVIER
SAUNDERS

1600 John F. Kennedy Blvd.
Ste 1800
Philadelphia, PA 19103-2899

A PRIMER IN CARTILAGE REPAIR AND JOINT
PRESERVATION OF THE KNEE   ISBN: 978-1-4160-6654-5

Copyright © 2011 by Saunders, an imprint of Elsevier Inc.

No part of this publication may be reproduced or transmitted in any form or by any means, electronic or mechanical, including photocopying, recording, or any information storage and retrieval system, without permission in writing from the publisher. Details on how to seek permission, further information about the Publisher's permissions policies and our arrangements with organizations such as the Copyright Clearance Center and the Copyright Licensing Agency, can be found at our website: www.elsevier.com/permissions.

This book and the individual contributions contained in it are protected under copyright by the Publisher (other than as may be noted herein).

Notices

Knowledge and best practice in this field are constantly changing. As new research and experience broaden our understanding, changes in research methods, professional practices, or medical treatment may become necessary.

Practitioners and researchers must always rely on their own experience and knowledge in evaluating and using any information, methods, compounds, or experiments described herein. In using such information or methods they should be mindful of their own safety and the safety of others, including parties for whom they have a professional responsibility.

With respect to any drug or pharmaceutical products identified, readers are advised to check the most current information provided (i) on procedures featured or (ii) by the manufacturer of each product to be administered, to verify the recommended dose or formula, the method and duration of administration, and contraindications. It is the responsibility of practitioners, relying on their own experience and knowledge of their patients, to make diagnoses, to determine dosages and the best treatment for each individual patient, and to take all appropriate safety precautions.

To the fullest extent of the law, neither the Publisher nor the authors, contributors, or editors, assume any liability for any injury and/or damage to persons or property as a matter of products liability, negligence or otherwise, or from any use or operation of any methods, products, instructions, or ideas contained in the material herein.

ISBN: 978-1-4160-6654-5

Acquisitions Editor: Dan Pepper
Developmental Editor: Marla Sussman
Publishing Services Manager: Patricia Tannian
Project Manager: Linda Van Pelt
Design Direction: Lou Forgione

Printed in the United States of America

Last digit is the print number: 9 8 7 6 5 4 3 2 1

Working together to grow libraries in developing countries

www.elsevier.com | www.bookaid.org | www.sabre.org

ELSEVIER   BOOK AID International   Sabre Foundation

Contributors

Julie Glowacki, PhD
Orthopedics Department
Orthopedic Research Laboratory
Medical Research Building
Brigham and Women's Hospital
Boston, Massachusetts

Chapter 2. Cartilage Repair and Regeneration

Andreas H. Gomoll, MD
Cartilage Repair Center
Brigham and Women's Hospital
Harvard Medical School
Chestnut Hill, Massachusetts

Chapter 5. Debridement, Microfracture, and Osteochondral Autograft Transfer for the Treatment of Cartilage Defects
Chapter 12. Meniscal Allograft Transplantation

Dedication

I would like to dedicate this book to Lars Peterson, MD, PhD, Gothenberg, Sweden. The reality of joint preservation in young patients with articular injuries has only become possible because of his vision and courage to persevere with the premise that cultured articular chondrocytes may affect repair. He translated a hypothesis to a preclinical rabbit model in 1982 and then to clinical application in 1987.

He is a pioneer in the field of orthopedics. I thank him and his co-workers Anders Lindahl, MD, PhD, and Mats Brittberg, MD, PhD, for allowing me to be a part of their team. He has been a mentor and great friend over the years as we have tried to promote the field of cartilage repair around the world.

Working and knowing him has been a true honor and privilege.

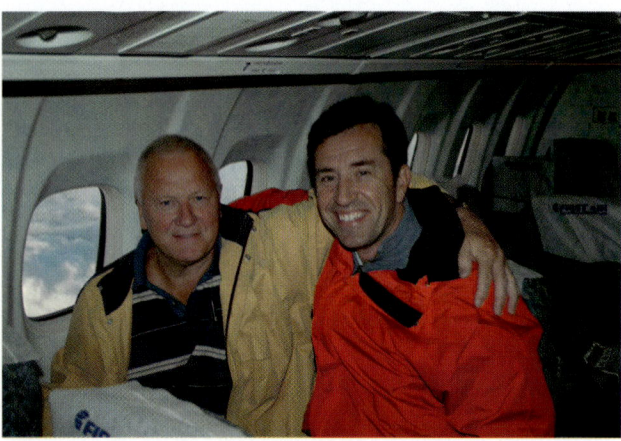

Lars Peterson, MD, PhD, and author – Tom Minas, MD, MS, on their way to Great Slave Lake, NorthWest Territories, Canada, 2005.

Special Thanks

Taking on the task of writing a surgical text, considering the topic was dear to my heart and was what I did every day, at first seemed straightforward. However, it turned out to be quite the opposite and it wouldn't have been possible without my family by my side. I would like to thank my wife Dana for her patience and encouragement and my two beautiful children, Krista and Lucas, who have always been the light in my life. Without their love, enthusiasm, and support, this book would not have come to fruition. For this, I am forever grateful.

I would also like to thank my parents, Mary and Angelo Minas, for their unconditional love and support throughout my life. I have always strived to emulate them in their dedication and commitment to both family and career.

Introduction

The purpose of this book is to provide residents, fellows, and surgeons with a practical approach to the field of cartilage repair. Specialized surgical techniques have been developed combining previous principles of internal fixation, osteotomy, and ligamentous and meniscal surgeries, as well as newly developed cartilage repair techniques. Because joint preservation in young patients is a developing field, it is often confusing to residents, fellows, and experienced surgeons. I will attempt to outline and illustrate my approach using my own experience, rationales, and surgical techniques.

Acknowledgments

My career has been influenced by many people, so I hope that I will not offend any by omission. James Waddell, MD, and Robin Sullivan, MD (deceased), who inspired me to be an orthopedist. Marvin Tile, MD, a great mentor and friend who guided me in critical thinking and the principles of internal fixation. Robert Salter, MD (deceased), my orthopedics professor at University of Toronto, who continued to inspire and encourage me into my clinical path of joint preservation and cartilage repair. Clement Sledge, MD, who introduced me to basic science cartilage repair in Boston. Thomas Thornhill, MD, my chairman, mentor, and friend, who helped me set up the Cartilage Repair Center (CRC) at the Brigham and Women's Hospital and continues to encourage and advise me on new pathways in cartilage repair. Richard Scott, MD, who has taught me so much about knee surgery and gave me the idea to write this book. My basic science collaborators Julie Glowacki, PhD, and Shuichi Mizuno, PhD, who have held me to a high standard of the scientific method and have encouraged me to translate our findings to the bedside and vice-versa.

Over the years as the field of cartilage repair has developed, my residents and clinical fellows have encouraged me to compile a syllabus to guide them as they trained. I hope this book will assist them in their management of patients with this difficult problem. I thank them collectively for their enthusiasm and encouragement.

I would like to thank the members of my team at the CRC. Teamwork has resulted in excellent clinical care of my patients and through outcomes research has advanced the field of cartilage repair. Carl Winalski, MD, Department of Radiology, first started the CRC with me as a collaborator in evaluating cartilage repair by non-invasive methods. His expertise and teamwork has been invaluable. I would like to thank former members, assistant Brenda Surowiec and research assistant Rosa Chiu, and my present team, assistants Jeannette Vannan and Esther Prall. Physician assistant Courtney Van Arsdale has been a great addition to our team. Tim Bryant, RN, BSN, has been involved in my practice since 1993, first as a surgical nurse and then as a research nurse. I thank him for his dedication, loyalty, hard work, and friendship. He is responsible for the excellent data collection and organization of our database and for helping to pass this on to our fellows and co-workers. Finally, Andreas Gomoll, MD, has been an enthusiastic and tireless researcher and partner at the CRC. His addition has brought new energy and ideas for good clinical research and training for our residents and fellows.

Finally, in the light of full disclosure for those who read this book, I am a consultant to Genzyme Biosurgery, which cultures the autologous chondrocytes that are the topic of Chapter 7, and I am on the Scientific Advisory Board and have IP for ConforMIS—with royalties and stock options—which manufactures custom resurfacing implants and is the topic of Chapter 16.

Foreword

This is a timely and unique book by a world pioneer of autologous cartilage transplantation—the first widely successful cell-engineering procedure in surgery.

Tom Minas has compiled an impressive text embracing the whole subject, tracing the etiology of articular cartilage injury, breakdown, and repair and the challenges involved in development of modern treatment. This is combined with his personal contributions to the phenomenal success of this approach in the treatment of acute osteochondral injuries in the knee as well as groundbreaking advances in treatment of early osteoarthritis. His 15-year experience involving over 600 patients with a variety of cartilage injuries has led to his personal philosophy of the optimal applications in a very complex and sometimes controversial clinical field.

It is especially timely because of the considerable confusion concerning the appropriate indications for cell-based and other therapies and the mushrooming of different commercial products entering the market, mostly untried. This is relevant because of the potential to prevent and treat osteoarthritis, which is predicted to affect 20% of the population by 2020.

Beginning in 1995, he stamped his own intellectual rigour and surgical innovative techniques on the management program, taking it from an exciting but relatively simple process to a varied and carefully planned treatment tailored to individual patients with early or late cartilage damage, which now may involve correction of malalignment, ligament and meniscal injuries, advanced bony injury, or even osteoarthritis.

The 16 chapters cover current scientific knowledge of cartilage properties, the etiology of damage and the intrinsic repair and regeneration processes, and a complete account of the systematic approach to diagnosis, patient management, and the details of the surgical techniques and rehabilitation programmes for all types of problems.

This is supplemented by a collection of fascinating and extremely challenging clinical problems and the "Minas touch" required to deal with them.

A constant theme is the need for a scientifically based surgical approach matching the patient's goals with the surgical possibilities, by employing a treatment algorithm based on his 5 'E's—engagement, empathy, education, enlistment, and end solution—which ensure that both patient and surgeon are clear about the realistic outcomes of the treatment. This is combined with a strategy of clinical trials wherever possible. It is notable that in his especially difficult group of osteoarthritic patients, he has achieved an 85% plus patient satisfaction rate

This outstanding book is a scientific treatise and stepwise surgical guide as well as a visionary surgeon's view of this most exciting of musculoskeletal developments of the 21st century. It is beautifully presented and illustrated and a pleasure to read.

It is my privilege to have had a foretaste of a specialist masterpiece.

George Bentley, MB, ChM, DSc, FRCS,
FRCCS (Ed), FMedSc
Emeritus Professor of Orthopaedics
University College, London
Honorary Consultant Orthopaedic Surgeon
Royal National Hospital, London

Contents

PART 1
DECISION MAKING 1

CHAPTER 1
Chondral Injury and Osteoarthritis: The Impact of Articular Cartilage Lesions 2
Tom Minas, MD, MS

CHAPTER 2
Cartilage Repair and Regeneration 8
Tom Minas, MD, MS and Julie Glowacki, PhD

CHAPTER 3
Imaging: The Basis for a Sound Decision in Joint Preservation 22
Tom Minas, MD, MS

CHAPTER 4
Patient Evaluation, Cartilage Defect, and Evidence: Putting It All Together 31
Tom Minas, MD, MS

PART 2
CARTILAGE REPAIR SURGICAL TECHNIQUES 47

CHAPTER 5
Debridement, Microfracture, and Osteochondral Autograft Transfer for Treatment of Cartilage Defects 48
Andreas H. Gomoll, MD and Tom Minas, MD, MS

CHAPTER 6
Use of Fresh Osteochondral Allograft for Chondral and Osteochondral Defects in the Knee 54
Tom Minas, MD, MS

CHAPTER 7
Autologous Chondrocyte Implantation 65
Tom Minas, MD, MS

PART 3
SURGICAL MANAGEMENT OF BACKGROUND FACTORS 121

CHAPTER 8
Tibial Osteotomy 122
Tom Minas, MD, MS

CHAPTER 9
Femoral Varus Osteotomy 146
Tom Minas, MD, MS

CHAPTER 10
Patellofemoral Malalignment, Tibial Tubercle Osteotomy, and Trochleoplasty 160
Tom Minas, MD, MS

CHAPTER 11
Treatment of Deep Osteochondritis Dissecans Lesions, Avascular Necrosis, and Osteochondral Defects of the Knee Using Autologous Bone Grafting 181
Tom Minas, MD, MS

CHAPTER 12
Meniscal Allograft Transplantation 193
Andreas H. Gomoll, MD and Tom Minas, MD, MS

CHAPTER 13
Complex Cases in Cartilage Repair: Tricks and Tips 200
Tom Minas, MD, MS

CHAPTER 14
Emerging Technologies 219
Tom Minas, MD, MS

PART 4
EARLY INTERVENTION IN OSTEOARTHRITIS 251

CHAPTER 15
Patellofemoral Arthroplasty 252
Tom Minas, MD, MS

CHAPTER 16
Patient-Specific Unicompartmental and Bicompartmental Resurfacing Arthroplasty 261
Tom Minas, MD, MS

INDEX 273

PART I

DECISION MAKING

Chapter 1

Chondral Injury and Osteoarthritis: The Impact of Articular Cartilage Lesions

Tom Minas, MD, MS

INTRODUCTION

EFFECT OF RUNNING AND OTHER SPORTS ON OA

ANTERIOR CRUCIATE LIGAMENT INJURY

POSTERIOR CRUCIATE LIGAMENT INJURY

MENISCAL INJURY

ALIGNMENT: TIBIOFEMORAL AND PATELLOFEMORAL

CHONDRAL DEFECT SIZE

EFFECT OF BODY MASS INDEX ON OA

PREVALENCE OF OA

PRESENT VERSUS FUTURE TOTAL KNEE ARTHROPLASTY NUMBERS

ECONOMIC BURDEN

INTRODUCTION

Damage to the articular cartilage comprises a spectrum of disease entities ranging from single, focal chondral defects to more advanced degenerative disease and end-stage osteoarthritis (OA). Focal chondral defects have long been implicated in the subsequent development of OA. Focal chondral defects result from various causative factors that may genetically predispose to early breakdown and wear.

Genetics may predispose to early cartilage wear and OA. In addition, metabolic, inflammatory, and developmental diseases may lead to articular cartilage damage. These may include Gaucher disease, hemophilia, hemachromatosis, ochronosis, Ehlers-Danlos syndrome, Paget disease, acromegaly, avascular necrosis, neuropathic arthropathy, and joint dysplasia.

Patients are approximately evenly split in reporting a traumatic versus an insidious onset of symptoms. Athletic activities are the most common inciting event associated with the diagnosis of chondral lesions.[1] Traumatic events and developmental causative agents such as osteochondritis dissecans predominate in younger age groups. Several large studies have found high-grade chondral lesions (Outerbridge grades III and IV) in 5% to 11% of younger patients (<40 years) and up to 60% of older patients (up to 65 years).[1-3] The most common locations for these defects are the medial femoral condyle (up to 32%) and the patella.[2,3] Most are detected incidentally during meniscectomy or anterior cruciate ligament reconstruction.[1,4] Notably, despite the relatively high incidence, many of these defects are incidental in nature and asymptomatic. Articular cartilage lesions have no spontaneous repair potential and have a propensity to worsen with time. Even though the natural history is not completely understood, those involved in cartilage repair agree on the importance of looking for background factors that predispose to the formation of these defects—malalignment and compartment overload of the tibiofemoral or patellofemoral compartment, joint laxity, contracture, meniscal insufficiency, and, of course, genetic predisposition to OA—for which clinical, biologic, or genetic markers currently are lacking.

EFFECT OF RUNNING AND OTHER SPORTS ON OA

Long-distance running and its relationship to the development of OA is an issue of great interest. Several studies have suggested that recreational long-distance running is not associated with progression of knee OA.[5-8] However, the presence of risk factors such as obesity, muscle weakness, or previous joint injury can make the knee more susceptible to the demands associated with participation in sports or athletics.[9] In contrast to recreational involvement, participation in several athletic and sporting activities at the elite level has been associated with an increased risk of lower-extremity OA.[10–12] These activities include sports involving torsion and impact, such as soccer, weight lifting, and sprinting.[13,14] Ignoring a known cartilage injury and continuing to participate in torsional impact sports, such as soccer, has been shown to cause progression of articular cartilage injuries with development of large areas of delamination.[15] Other studies have demonstrated that known articular injury greater than 1 cm^2 has progressed to OA, with greater than 14-year follow-up in more than half of patients allowed to participate in sports.[16] Even when known cartilage injuries are treated with articular cartilage repair by use of microfracture or autologous chondrocyte implantation, OA may develop in as many as one third of patients[17] as early as 5 years after treatment. This may be due to missed axial alignment versus the severity of the instigating initial injury in producing articular cartilage injury because this has not been found with autologous chondrocyte implantation alone when alignment was carefully assessed and treated.[18,19]

ANTERIOR CRUCIATE LIGAMENT INJURY

Another consideration that often directly relates to participation in athletics is injury to the anterior cruciate ligament (ACL) and subsequent development of knee OA. This severe trauma is generally associated with bone bruising at the time of subluxation of the tibiofemoral joint with tear of the ACL.[20,21] Biopsies of the overlying articular cartilage to the bone bruise have demonstrated that the superficial and middle zones of articular cartilage have greater than 50% cartilage apoptosis in addition to loss of proteoglycans, indicating severe injury to the overlying cartilage surface with a propensity for late articular cartilage loss and delamination and the possibility of progression to OA.[22] Bone bruises in the study have been shown to occur in greater than 80% of ACL-injured knees.[22]

The untreated chronic ACL deficient knee has an increased risk of articular cartilage injury, especially as the time from initial injury increases.[23,24]

Long-term follow-up of ACL-injured patients has consistently demonstrated an association between ACL injury and the development of knee OA. It has been postulated that disruption of the normal mechanics of the knee and continued instability with resultant shear forces to the articular surfaces also predispose to injury to the meniscus, which is the secondary stabilizer of the knee. Loss of the meniscus as a shock absorber is a significant contributor to subsequent OA development. Surgical repair of the ACL aims to restore normal biomechanics to the knee. However, ACL repair has not been shown to reduce the incidence of knee OA compared with nonoperative management.[25] This finding may support the theory that it is the initial trauma and bone bruising with overlying cartilage injury and subsequent ligament failure that eventually lead to OA, which is my belief.

Neuman et al[26] reported that the primary risk factor for development of knee OA after ACL injury was whether a meniscectomy had been performed. This finding seems to support the view that maintenance of knee loading and chondroprotection from the meniscus are important considerations in this issue. More investigation is needed to determine the causative factors responsible for early OA development in this population.

POSTERIOR CRUCIATE LIGAMENT INJURY

The posterior cruciate ligament (PCL) is rarely injured compared to the ACL. Occasionally patients with PCL-injured knees are asymptomatic. When patients are symptomatic, they generally exhibit pain and disability rather than functional instability as seen in patients with ACL-deficient knees. The medial femoral condyle is injured more frequently than the lateral femoral condyle.[27,28] Varus alignment of the limb predisposes to medially based pain in this situation. To prevent further progression of a medial articular injury, PCL reconstruction is recommended. However, valgus tibial osteotomy combined with increased flexion in the sagittal plane decreases posterior translation of the tibia and in itself may unload and add enough stability. Careful assessment of instability, alignment, and cartilage injury is required to determine an appropriate treatment pathway.

MENISCAL INJURY

The role of the meniscus in load distribution and shock absorption has long been understood. The absence of a meniscus has been shown to predictably result in OA of the affected compartment, with characteristic radiographic changes such as flattening of the femoral condyles with peripheral osteophyte formation and sclerosis of the tibial surface.[29–31]

It has been noted that the medial compartment of the knee develops these changes within 10 to 15 years after total meniscectomy; however, the lateral compartment may degenerate within 2 to 5 years after total meniscectomy. These findings led me to consider that the compartments are quite different in their susceptibility to loss of the meniscus. The medial compartment comprises 60% of the weight-bearing surfaces compared to 40% in the lateral compartment. The medial compartment is congruent in that the femoral articular surface is convex and the tibial articular surface is concave. The broad medial collateral ligament in addition to the meniscus stabilizes the medial compartment such that there is a rolling motion of the femur on the tibia without translation and shear, hence the term *medial pivot* with the medial side of the knee being relatively stable and the lateral side exposed to more shear. The medial meniscus does not capture the entire medial femoral condyle because the anterior horn attachment varies and often rolls off the anterior aspect of the tibia, providing less surface to the femoral articular condyle. Therefore, it is less crucial to the medial compartment other than the posterior horn of the medial meniscus, which is loaded continuously during flexion of the knee. The articular surfaces in addition to being congruous have firmer and harder surfaces than the lateral compartment. The increased stability, congruence, and hardness are more protective and in the presence of normal alignment wear are slow to progress. However, varus alignment on the medial compartment usually results in a more rapidly degenerating medial compartment in OA. For this reason, I consider the medial compartment of the knee to be very alignment dependent.

The lateral compartment is very different. The lateral tibial plateau surface is convex, and the articular surface is softer than in the medial compartment. The lateral collateral ligament is thin and posteriorly based. It provides little stability to the lateral compartment itself. However, the meniscus is almost circular and makes up for the lack of congruence of the tibial articulation to the femoral articulation. Loss of the lateral meniscus therefore allows incongruence of the lateral compartment and increased translation and shear with point loading of the femoral condyle on the softer lateral tibial plateau articulation. This predisposes to rapid articular wear, as seen clinically. For this reason, I consider the lateral compartment to be very meniscal dependent as opposed to the medial compartment, which is more alignment dependent.

ALIGNMENT: TIBIOFEMORAL AND PATELLOFEMORAL

The role of alignment in the progression of an articular cartilage injury and OA cannot be underestimated. Sharma et al[32] noted that, in the presence of malalignment of the tibiofemoral joint, the risk of progression of arthritis in the knee was four times in the medial compartment when varus of just 2 degrees and five times in the lateral compartment when only 2 degrees of valgus was present over an 18-month time course. Other studies have shown that malalignment plays a role in articular cartilage degeneration by placing abnormal stresses on the articular cartilage.[33,34] Corrective osteotomy to normalize the forces of the tibiofemoral joint will arrest progression of disease and, in the event of cartilage repair, will improve the environment for optimal reconstitution of the articular surface.

Patellar lateral maltracking, patella baja, and arthrofibrosis of the infrapatellar fat pad all result in abnormal forces across the articulation of the patellofemoral joint. Isolated lateral patellar facet arthritic change may develop with isolated lateral maltracking, and pan patellar articular loss is more common with patella baja and patellar contracture. The underlying causes, which may require soft tissue releases, tibial tubercle osteotomy, vastus medialis obliquus quadriceps advancement, and dysplasia of the trochlea, all must be addressed in order to halt the progression of disease or to allow cartilage repair to pursue without overload and failure.

CHONDRAL DEFECT SIZE

The initiation of an articular cartilage defect frequently is traumatic in more than half of the cases detected; the remainder arise insidiously.[1]

The progression of an articular cartilage lesion to a bipolar articular injury and then to OA is multifactorial, as previously discussed. When considering cartilage repair for such a defect, the size of the defect factors into the choice of repair. The natural history of disease for a known size cartilage defect is not understood. However, even a small defect (e.g., 1 cm^2) may progress if activity is unrestricted.[16] With all other factors being equal after background factors have been corrected, the size of the chondral defect is critical to the treatment being rendered for repair. If the defect is well shouldered when weight-bearing forces are placed across it (Figure 1–1), the shoulders take up the load, protecting the subchondral bone of the defect from stimulation and hence pain. No treatment of this defect may be needed if the defect is asymptomatic and can be observed over time to determine progression of disease. In addition, a treatment that provides a fibrocartilage repair that protects and stabilizes the existing shoulders, thus dispersing the forces throughout the defect, may be adequate over time. However, if the defect is large, the shoulders may not be participating in load bearing, and the subchondral bone of the defect then becomes abrasive to the opposite articular surface, producing bipolar degenerative changes. A repair tissue for this situation would need to bear all of the forces, be sturdy, and have viscoelastic mechanical properties that make it durable and nonabrasive, such as hyaline articular cartilage. These properties will determine treatment options for the patient and are discussed further in Chapter 4 (see Figure 1–1).

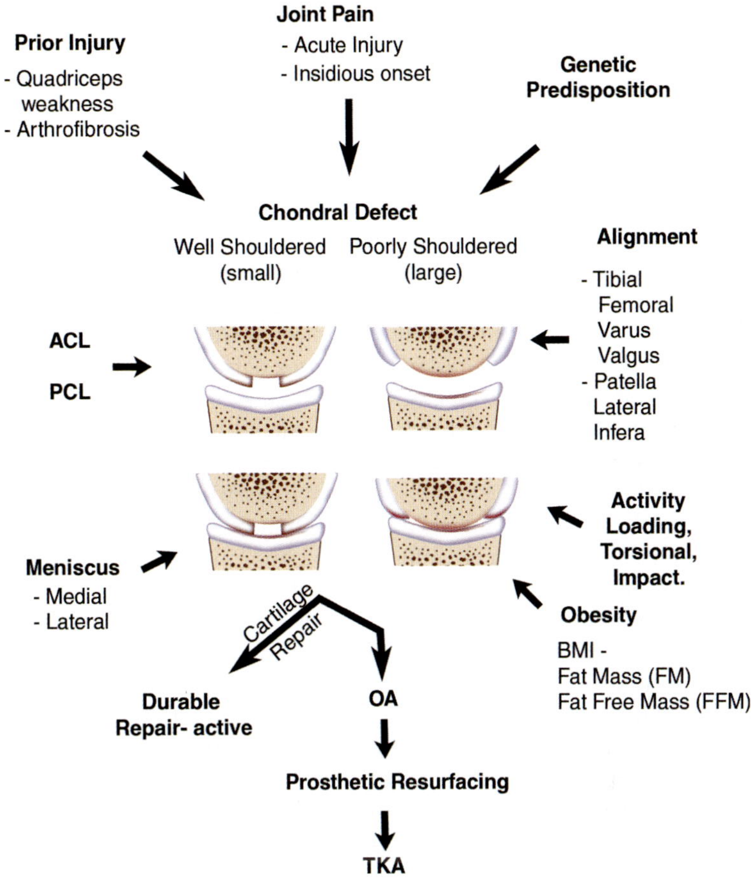

Figure 1-1 Multiple factors influence the progression of cartilage damage to osteoarthritis. Cartilage repair may be successful in halting the progression of disease if these factors can be managed. These factors are frequently referred to as *background factors* when assessing and managing chondral defects with cartilage repair.

EFFECT OF BODY MASS INDEX ON OA

Obesity is a well-documented risk factor for the development of OA of the knee, and weight reduction has been shown to lower the risk of developing OA.[35,36] Body mass index is often used as a measure of obesity. However, these measures do not accurately capture the components of body composition, such as muscle and fat; they only give a measure of total weight or the ratio of weight to height. Wang et al[37] examined the relationship among fat mass, fat free mass, and their effect on tibial cartilage volume. Their analysis showed a positive correlation between increased fat free mass and tibial cartilage volume. Additionally, increased fat mass was correlated with an increased risk for tibial articular cartilage defects. These defects have been shown to be predictive of cartilage loss.[38,39]

PREVALENCE OF OA

OA of the knee is a disease that has a profound presence and impact upon our society. However, accurately estimating the incidence and prevalence of this disease is difficult because of the varied diagnostic criteria available. Estimates of prevalence vary widely based on whether a radiologic, symptomatic, or combination diagnosis is used. Although radiologic methods are more accurately reproducible for longitudinal studies, patient reports of pain and disability give a better picture of the impact of the disease on both society and the health care system.

Perhaps the most well-known study of the prevalence of OA is the Framingham Osteoarthritis Study.[40] This study used a combination of patient responses to a standardized questionnaire, radiographic evidence, and physician assessment. The study demonstrated a clear linear relationship between increasing age and prevalence of OA, with radiographic evidence of disease in 11.5% of patients older than 70 years and in 19.4% of patients 80 years or older. However, by no means did all patients with a radiographic diagnosis report pain. The proportion of patients who reported symptoms rose from 7.6% of patients with no radiographic evidence of disease to 40% of patients with grade 3 or 4 disease. It is interesting that even in the most severe radiographic categories of disease, less than 50% of patients report symptoms of OA. Each year, approximately 25% of adults older than 55 years experience knee pain lasting for at least 1 month. Of this group of patients, about half show radiographic evidence of OA. By using more strict criteria for diagnosis that include both symptoms and radiographic evidence, the prevalence is often estimated at less than 15%.[41] This figure is widely regarded to be a significant underestimate.[40]

PRESENT VERSUS FUTURE TOTAL KNEE ARTHROPLASTY NUMBERS

As our population ages, the number of both primary and revision total knee arthroplasty procedures performed is predicted to rise by over 600%.[42] Between 2005 and 2030, primary total knee arthroplasty demand has been projected to rise by 673%, from 450,000 procedures annually in 2005 to 3,481,000 annually in 2030.[42] The total number of revision knee arthroplasty procedures is projected to rise from 38,300 in 2005 to 268,200 in 2030, an increase of 601%. These numbers have even more impact when compared to the corresponding figures for hip arthroplasty. The numbers of primary and revision total hip arthroplasties are projected to rise by 174% and 137%, respectively. It has been predicted the current supply of orthopedic surgeons will be unable to accommodate such a vast increase in surgical volume.[43]

ECONOMIC BURDEN

In 2003, the cost of arthritis and other rheumatic conditions in the United States was estimated to be 1.2% of gross domestic product.[44] This number is quite significant, especially considering that knee and hip OA have a disproportionate impact on patient disability and health care costs compared to OA in other joints.[45] It is important to consider not only the direct costs associated with OA but also the indirect costs. Gupta et al[46] considered not only direct costs to patients with OA but also wages foregone and costs incurred from informal care given by relatives and others. They reported mean total annual costs to the patient of $12,200 (2002 Canadian dollars, $1.00 CDN ≈ $0.81 US). The majority of costs incurred was attributed to lost wages of the patient and informal caregivers. Similar studies have reported substantial personal costs to OA patients.[47,48]

CONCLUSION

Symptomatic chondral defects represent a difficult clinical treatment pathway. Truly the holy grail when managing knee injury is an injured articular surface. Despite excellent reconstructive measures for associated injuries, an articular cartilage injury is frequently a career-ending injury to an athlete. When managing such an injury, the associated background factors must be assessed and treated either prior to or at the time of articular cartilage injury.

Former athletes frequently develop degenerative arthritis of their joints. They wish to maintain healthy and active lifestyles, as does our society of baby boomers who now are retiring. To do so we must continue striving to preserve the joint while maintaining the option for total knee arthroplasty if necessary. OA of the knee represents a tremendous social and economic burden to our society. Maintaining an enjoyable quality of life through joint preservation has become a reality because of biologic advances in technology and imaging. This book focuses on this possibility by addressing background factors, cartilage repair, and minimally resurfacing prosthetic arthroplasty when necessary.

REFERENCES

1. Aroen A, Loken S, Heir S, et al. Articular cartilage lesions in 993 consecutive knee arthroscopies. *Am J Sports Med*. 2004;32:211–215.
2. Curl WW, Krome J, Gordon ES, et al. Cartilage injuries: a review of 31,516 knee arthroscopies. *Arthroscopy*. 1997;13:456–460.
3. Hjelle K, Solheim E, Strand T, et al. Articular cartilage defects in 1,000 knee arthroscopies. *Arthroscopy*. 2002;18:730–734.
4. Piasecki DP, Spindler KP, Warren TA, et al. Intraarticular injuries associated with anterior cruciate ligament tear: findings at ligament reconstruction in high school and recreational athletes. An analysis of sex-based differences. *Am J Sports Med*. 2003;31:601–605.
5. Chakravarty EF, Hubert HB, Lingala VB, et al. Long distance running and knee osteoarthritis. A prospective study. *Am J Prev Med*. 2008;35:133–138.
6. Cheng Y, Macera CA, Davis DR, et al. Physical activity and self-reported, physician-diagnosed osteoarthritis: is physical activity a risk factor? *J Clin Epidemiol*. 2000;53:315–322.
7. Hannan MT, Felson DT, Anderson JJ, et al. Habitual physical activity is not associated with knee osteoarthritis: the Framingham Study. *J Rheumatol*. 1993;20:704–709.
8. Panush RS, Schmidt C, Caldwell JR, et al. Is running associated with degenerative joint disease? *JAMA*. 1986;255:1152–1154.
9. Felson DT. An update on the pathogenesis and epidemiology of osteoarthritis. *Radiol Clin North Am*. 2004;42:1–9.
10. Kujala UM, Kaprio J, Sarna S. Osteoarthritis of weight bearing joints of lower limbs in former elite male athletes. *BMJ*. 1994;308:231–234.
11. Kujala UM, Kettunen J, Paananen H, et al. Knee osteoarthritis in former runners, soccer players, weight lifters, and shooters. *Arthritis Rheum*. 1995;38:539–546.
12. Teitz CC, Kilcoyne RF. Premature osteoarthrosis in professional dancers. *Clin J Sport Med*. 1998;8:255.
13. Lindberg H, Roos H, Gardsell I. Prevalence of coxarthrosis in former soccer players. *Acta Orthop Scand*. 1993;64:165–167.
14. Kujala U, Ketlunen J, I'aananen H, et al. Knee osteoarthritis in former runners, soccer players, weight lifters, and shooters. *Arthritis Rheum*. 1995;38:539–546.
15. Levy AS, Lohnes J, Sculley S, et al. Chondral delamination of the knee in soccer players. *Am J Sports Med*. 1996;24:634–639.
16. Messner K, Maletius W. The long-term prognosis for severe damage to weight-bearing cartilage in the knee: a 14-year clinical and radiographic follow-up in 28 young athletes. *Acta Orthop Scand*. 1996;67:165.
17. Knutsen G, Engebretsen L, Ludvigsen TC, et al. A randomized trial comparing autologous chondrocyte implantation with microfracture. Findings at 5 years. *J Bone Joint Surg Am*. 2007;89:2105–2112.
18. Peterson L, Brittberg M, Kiviranta I, et al. Autologous chondrocyte transplantation. Biomechanics and long-term durability. *Am J Sports Med*. 2002;30:2–12.

19. Minas T. Autologous chondrocyte implantation for focal chondral defects of the knee. *Clin Orthop Relat Res.* 2001;S349–S361.
20. Rosen M, Jackson D, Berger P. Occult osseous lesions documented by MRI associated with anterior cruciate ligament rupture. *Arthroscopy.* 1991;7:45–51.
21. Spindler K, Schils JP, Bergfield J, et al. Prospective study of osseous articular, and meniscal lesions in recent anterior cruciate ligament tears by magnetic resonance imaging and arthroscopy. *Am J Sports Med.* 1993;21:551–557.
22. Johnson D, Urban W, Carbon D, et al. Articular cartilage changes seen with magnetic resonance imaging: Detected bone bruises associated with acute anterior cruciate ligament rupture. *Am J Sports Med.* 1998;26:409–414.
23. Gillquist J, Messner K. Anterior cruciate ligament reconstruction and the long-term incidence of gonarthrosis. *Sports Med Arthrosc.* 1999;27:143–156.
24. Roos H, Adalberth T, Dahlberg L, et al. Osteoarthritis of the knee after injury to the anterior cruciate ligament or meniscus: The influence of time and age. *Osteoarthritis Cartilage.* 1995;3:261–267.
25. Kessler MA, Behrend H, Henz S, et al. Function, osteoarthritis and activity after ACL-rupture: 11 years follow-up results of conservative versus reconstructive treatment. *Knee Surg Sports Traumatol Arthrosc.* 2008;16:442–448.
26. Neuman P, Englund M, Kostogiannis I, et al. Prevalence of tibiofemoral osteoarthritis 15 years after nonoperative treatment of anterior cruciate ligament injury: a prospective cohort study. *Am J Sports Med.* 2008;36:1717–1725.
27. Geissler V, Whipple T. Intraarticular abnormalities in association with posterior cruciate ligament injuries. *Am J Sports Med.* 1993;21:846–849.
28. Torg J, Barton T, Pavlov H. Natural history of the posterior cruciate ligament-deficient knee. *Clin Orthop Relat Res.* 1989;246:208–216.
29. Fairbank T. Knee joint changes after meniscectomy. *J Bone Joint Surg Br.* 1948;30:664–670.
30. Tapper E, Hoover N. Late results after meniscectomy. *J Bone Joint Surg Am.* 1969;51:517–526.
31. Johnson R, Kettelkamp D, Clark W, et al. Factors affecting late results after meniscectomy. *J Bone Joint Surg Am.* 1974;56:719–729.
32. Sharma L, Song J, Felson DT, et al. The role of knee alignment in disease progression and functional decline in knee osteoarthritis. *JAMA.* 2001;286:188–195.
33. Tetsworth K, Paley D. Malalignment and degenerative arthropathy. *Orthop Clin North Am.* 1994;25:367–377.
34. Wu D, Burr D, Boyd R, et al. Bone and cartilage changes following experimental varus or valgus tibial angulation. *J Orthop Res.* 1990;8:572–585.
35. Felson DT, Anderson JJ, Naimark A, et al. Obesity and knee osteoarthritis. The Framingham Study. *Ann Intern Med.* 1988;109:18–24.
36. Felson DT, Zhang Y, Anthony JM, et al. Weight loss reduces the risk for symptomatic knee osteoarthritis in women. The Framingham Study. *Ann Intern Med.* 1992;116:535–539.
37. Wang Y, Wluka AE, English DR, et al. Body composition and knee cartilage properties in healthy, community-based adults. *Ann Rheum Dis.* 2007;66:1244–1248.
38. Cicuttini F, Ding C, Wluka A, et al. Association of cartilage defects with loss of knee cartilage in healthy, middle-age adults: a prospective study. *Arthritis Rheum.* 2005;52:2033–2039.
39. Ding C, Cicuttini F, Scott F, et al. Association of prevalent and incident knee cartilage defects with loss of tibial and patellar cartilage: a longitudinal study. *Arthritis Rheum.* 2005;52:3918–3927.
40. Felson DT, Naimark A, Anderson J, et al. The prevalence of knee osteoarthritis in the elderly. The Framingham Osteoarthritis Study. *Arthritis Rheum.* 1987;30:914–918.
41. D'Ambrosia RD. Epidemiology of osteoarthritis. *Orthopedics.* 2005;28:s201–s205.
42. Kurtz S, Ong K, Lau E, et al. Projections of primary and revision hip and knee arthroplasty in the United States from 2005 to 2030. *J Bone Joint Surg Am.* 2007;89:780–785.
43. Iorio R, Robb WJ, Healy WL, et al. Orthopaedic surgeon workforce and volume assessment for total hip and knee replacement in the United States: preparing for an epidemic. *J Bone Joint Surg Am.* 2008;90:1598–1605.
44. Centers for Disease Control and Prevention. National and state medical expenditures and lost earnings attributable to arthritis and other rheumatic conditions—United States, 2003. *MMWR Morb Mortal Wkly Rep.* 2007;56:146–149.
45. Burden of Musculoskeletal Diseases in the United States. *Prevalence, Societal and Economic Cost.* 1st ed. Rosemont, Ill: American Academy of Orthopaedic Surgeons; 2008.
46. Gupta S, Hawker GA, Laporte A, et al. The economic burden of disabling hip and knee osteoarthritis (OA) from the perspective of individuals living with this condition. *Rheumatology (Oxford).* 2005;44:1531.
47. Gabriel SE, Crowson CS, Campion ME, et al. Direct medical costs unique to people with arthritis. *J Rheumatol.* 1997;24:719–725.
48. Lapsley HM, March LM, Tribe KL, et al. Living with osteoarthritis: patient expenditures, health status, and social impact. *Arthritis Rheum.* 2001;45:301–306.

Chapter 2

Cartilage Repair and Regeneration

Tom Minas, MD, MS and Julie Glowacki, PhD

CARTILAGE STRUCTURE AND FUNCTION
  The Chondrocyte as an Anabolic/Catabolic Cell

MECHANICAL PROPERTIES OF ARTICULAR CARTILAGE
  Incidence of Cartilage Lesions
  Cartilage Injuries and Repair
  Clinical Repair for Full-Thickness Cartilage Defects

EXPERIMENTAL MODELS AND USEFULNESS

TRANSLATIONAL RESEARCH
  State of the Art
  Tissue Engineering
    Engineered Cartilage Implantation
  Cell Based

  Gene Therapy
  Materials
  Future Directions

CARTILAGE STRUCTURE AND FUNCTION

The Chondrocyte as an Anabolic/Catabolic Cell

Chondrocytes are highly specialized cells that differentiate from clusters of mesenchymal cells during skeletal embryogenesis. The chondrocyte synthesizes and secretes the components of the extracellular matrix, primarily proteoglycans and type II collagen. Most of the immature cartilage is temporary and is replaced by bone during epiphyseal development, whereas the regions nearest the synovial cavity remain as the permanent articular cartilage of the adult. During growth and development, immature cartilage undergoes cellular replication in both the superficial and deep zones. However, as skeletal maturity approaches, replication occurs only in the deep zone. Cell replication after skeletal maturity is rare. The cell content of articular cartilage is low, occupying no more than 10% of the tissue volume in humans. Cell density has been estimated as 10^5 cells per cubic millimeter in newborns and $1/10$ of that in adult cartilage. Values are higher in the superficial than in the deeper zone. Experimental animals have far greater cellularity. For example, adult rabbits have nearly 10-fold greater cell density than human cartilage, and mice have 25-fold greater cell density.[1] The general cellular morphology ranges from flattened and discoidal in the most superficial zones to ovoid in the deeper regions. The ovoid cells display enlarged Golgi bodies, a characteristic of cells actively secreting proteins, and cellular processes that extend into the adjacent pericellular matrix.

Chondrocytes are normally long-lived cells. They are not replaced by new cells as occurs in the turnover of other tissues. However, the capacity for cell division is manifest when the integrity of the matrix is compromised, as in osteoarthritis. Cartilage fibrillation is associated with necrosis in the superficial zone and with clusters of cells in deep zones. Metabolic studies show increased sulfate incorporation by the cells in the clusters surrounded by proteoglycan-poor matrix. If viewed as an attempt to repair, the cells in clusters are active in matrix synthesis but are not capable of matrix replacement at distances from the clusters. Thus, the overall content of proteoglycan is low in fibrillated cartilage.

Chondrocytes are embedded in an avascular matrix in which nutrients and waste products must diffuse. Oxygen tension is approximately $1/3$ that measured between capillaries in soft tissues. On a per cell basis, oxygen uptake is $1/50$ that of kidney, but the rates of glycolysis between chondrocytes and kidney are comparable. Thus, chondrocytes engage in relatively anaerobic metabolism.

Chondrocytes are dynamic cells with anabolic and catabolic activity; they mediate both synthesis and degradation of the matrix. Proteoglycan metabolism has been studied extensively. As is typical for other cells, the protein components are synthesized in the cytoplasmic rough endoplasmic reticulum, and sulfation of the polysaccharides occurs in the Golgi bodies. Ex vivo studies with radioactive tracer isotope of ^{35}S-sulfate show incorporation into glycosaminoglycans by intermediate and deep cells and subsequent movement into the matrix. Type II collagen is synthesized and secreted as separate procollagen chains with extensions on its ends, converted to tropocollagen, and organized into fibrils with small amounts of type IX and type XI collagen. In contrast to the dense, thick, highly oriented collagen fibers of bone, cartilage fibrils are thin and cross-linked into an open meshwork. The fibrils contain variable amounts of noncollagenous macromolecules, notably decorin. The half-life of type II collagen is more than 200 years in humans. Thus, the major component of the native fibrils does not appear to be renewed or reparable in the normal setting. The collagen fibrillar network is under tension and serves to contain the glycosaminoglycans in a compressed state. It is difficult to imagine how that network could be turned over without compromising the mechanical integrity of the tissue or how denatured foci could be mended. Evidence shows damage to the fibrillar network in osteoarthritis. Osteoarthritis drastically affects the mechanical properties of cartilage. Excessive swelling of osteoarthritic samples in dilute salt solution is taken as evidence of the loss of resistance afforded by the fibrillar net to absorption of water by the polysaccharides. Although there appears to be little turnover of the fibrillar network, the entrapped proteoglycans undergo turnover that can be accelerated by local cytokines. Chondrocytes are responsible for maintaining the matrix environment in which they are encased and hence ensure the tissue's mechanical characteristics.[2] They are protected from osmotic and mechanical damage by the rigid pericellular matrix, called the *chondron*. Maintenance of the matrix involves degradation by proteinases and free radicals generated by the chondrocyte. Matrix metalloproteinases and aggrecanase catalyze the turnover of cartilage matrix in normal as well as in diseased cartilage. Because many of the matrix components in cartilage are specific to that tissue, there is great interest in developing and validating assays for their degradation products in plasma or synovial fluid as markers for turnover.[3]

In the modern view, osteoarthritis is considered to result from an imbalance between dynamic anabolic and catabolic activities that are normally well balanced. The chondrocyte functions as the agent of these two processes. This is in contrast to bone tissue, for example, in which anabolic activities are ascribed to the osteoblast and catabolic or osteolytic activities to the osteoclast. Although normally interaction between the two cell types maintains skeletal mass constant within the remodeling process, imbalance occurs with aging, osteoporosis, and infection. The situation in cartilage is distinct. Evidence suggests that the earliest stages of osteoarthritis are balanced by an up-regulation of the biosynthetic processes. Synovial fluid collects a byproduct of procollagen II processing, called *chondrocalcin* or *C-propeptide*, whose levels are elevated in traumatic and primary osteoarthritis.

Previously, cartilage was regarded to be immunologically privileged because of either the absence of transplantation antigens or the protective effect of the matrix. These states were invoked to explain the endurance of allografts in heterotopic sites. It is now appreciated that chondrocytes do display major transplantation antigens and that components of the matrix are weakly antigenic. In healthy intact cartilage, these determinants are probably shielded from antibodies because of steric hindrance due to the proteoglycans in the matrix. Preservation of matrix integrity appears to be essential to prevent exposure of the cells and rejection of the tissue.

The heterogeneous group of inflammatory joint diseases involve underlying disturbances in immune regulation. In rheumatoid arthritis, the synovial lining is the initial target of inflammatory pathology. Proliferation of synovial lining cells and infiltration by lymphocytes and activated macrophages produce a tissue mass called the *pannus*. The pannus can invade and destroy the integrity of articular cartilage. Products of the pannus act as cytokine mediators of both chondrolysis and osteolysis. The major agents are interleukin-1 (IL-1) and tumor necrosis factor-α. These agents signal the cascade of release of IL-6, IL-8, IL-17, cyclooxygenase-2, and nitric oxide, all of which are actual or potential targets of pharmacologic management. In vitro models have been useful to describe the mechanisms by which these immunomodulatory cytokines change gene expression in chondrocytes, thus promoting chondrolysis.

MECHANICAL PROPERTIES OF ARTICULAR CARTILAGE

Articular cartilage is a hypocellular, viscoelastic tissue that lines synovial joints, providing them with a nearby frictionless environment. Synovial cartilage articulations provide a coefficient of friction for joint motion that is less than 1/5 that of ice on ice.[4] The mechanical properties of articular cartilage depend upon its composition and its architecture. Normally, the hydrophilic proteoglycans and collagen constitute 30% of the tissue mass; the remainder is water. Cartilage matrix can be viewed as a biphasic material in which the fluid phase flows upon mechanical deformation of its solid phase. Although the water is constrained by the proteoglycan molecules, the fluid phase can also be called the *porosity* of the cartilage. The high water content of the tissue also generates its high viscoelasticity. Its elastic modules is low at slow rates of loading but is two orders greater at physiologic rates.

The surface cartilage layer or "skin" is resistant to compressive loads or penetration. The vertically arranged collagen fibers of the radial and calcified zones are resistant to shear. Upon application of pressure to articular cartilage through weight bearing, the water contained within the cartilage exudes upon pressure. With diminished pressure, water is drawn back to the aggrecan. The surface protein dermatan sulfate also acts as an anti-adhesion substance. The fine filaments of the superficial zone combine with water so that articulation with the opposite joint surface also occurs with combined water and superficial zone filaments.[2] Therefore, the lubricating barrier between joint surfaces is mostly water. Water is released during weight-bearing pressure from hyperhydrated negatively charged proteoglycans in articular cartilage. With damage or degeneration, loss of proteoglycans and water results in impaired mechanical properties and joint function.

Incidence of Cartilage Lesions

The true incidence of cartilage lesions and their natural history are unknown. It has been proposed that between 5% and 10% of acute knee hemarthroses after a work-related or sports injury is associated with an acute chondral injury.[5] In a retrospective review of 31,516 knee arthroscopies, the prevalence of chondral lesions was 63%. However, isolated unipolar chondral defects in patients younger than 40 years were rare, occurring in only 5% of this patient population.[6] Both clinical and experimental evidence showed that with time focal cartilage injuries will enlarge and progress to osteoarthritis.[7]

Mechanical injury to articular cartilage during sporting injuries may occur with shearing forces secondary to disruption of the anterior cruciate ligament. Shearing osteochondral fractures occurring at the time of ligament disruption have been noted. Blunt injury to the joint surfaces may cause injury to and death of articular chondrocytes. If the articular chondrocyte cannot continue to synthesize and remodel its matrix macromolecules, the pericellular matrix eventually will degenerate. This may account for the high incidence of osteoarthritis encountered with anterior cruciate ligament injuries. Acutely the incidence of chondral injuries is approximately 2% but may approach 20% in the long run.[8]

In a study performed by Repo and Finlay,[9] blunt force to articular chondrocytes in excess of 25 MPa reproducibly resulted in death of articular chondrocytes. Hence there appears to be a threshold to which articular chondrocytes can withstand blunt trauma. This may be an important factor in understanding articular cartilage degeneration after injury and may be an important technical factor during new repair techniques, such as osteochondral graft transfers. Large impaction forces needed to introduce osteochondral grafts to recipient sites may result in injury and cell death to the cartilage cap of the osteochondral grafts, leading to failed long-term results.

Magnetic resonance imaging scans demonstrated bone bruises after blunt injuries sustained during work-related and sporting activities. Arthroscopic biopsy studies of cartilage overlying bone bruises demonstrated superficial chondrocyte death and matrix dehydration.[10] Cartilage cell death is proposed to arise directly from the blunt trauma exceeding this threshold.

The natural history of osteoarthritis itself is unknown. A Swedish longitudinal study notes radiographic progression of osteoarthritis in the knee occurs over a 20-year time course when greater than 50% joint space narrowing is present at initial evaluation (Ahlback stages 2–4).[11] However, only 60% of patients with Ahlback stage 0 (peripheral osteophytes and a normal joint space) or Ahlback stage 1 (<50% joint space narrowing) at initial presentation will progress radiographically. Not all radiographic osteoarthritis will progress.

In the United States, more than 450,000 total knee replacements are performed annually. The disability and economic hardship encountered by osteoarthritis are substantial. This is especially true if a cartilage injury occurs at a young age when socioeconomic productivity and recreational activities are especially affected. The problem arises from the unique structure, function, and repair mechanisms of articular cartilage.

Cartilage Injuries and Repair

Articular cartilage is devoid of a nerve supply. Cartilage covers and protects the richly innervated subchondral bone plate from stimulation. Once articular cartilage is damaged, pain can result from contact of the subchondral bone plate. If a healing response does not develop, load will be borne by the shoulders of the chondral defects in addition to the exposed subchondral bone. This situation will result in overload and breakdown of the shoulders of the defect, with progressive enlargement of the defect. The opposing articulation would be exposed to a bare bone surface with resultant erosive degradation of its cartilage surface. The resultant bone-on-bone articulation is by definition osteoarthritis. Symptoms from direct stimulation of the subchondral bone plate or from indirect stimulation to the bone via an attached cartilage flap may occur. Breakdown products from the cartilage along with liberated enzymes may cause effusions in the joint, capsular distention, or synovitis as other mechanisms of pain. As the subchondral bone plate hardens, secondary vascular venous congestion in the medullary cavity results and may cause deep aching pain.

Cartilage repair would be beneficial in the short term to alleviate symptoms and in the long term to prevent progressive breakdown of the articulations of the joint and the development of osteoarthritis. Thus, the goal of cartilage repair is to produce a tissue that will fill the defect, integrate with the adjacent articular cartilage and subchondral bone plate, have the same viscoelastic mechanical properties, and maintain its matrix over time without breakdown. That is, the goal is to restore the osteochondral functional unit with a repair tissue that approaches regeneration.

Clinical and experimental evidence shows that damage involving the articular cartilage surface and confined to the cartilage undergoes little restoration. Cartilage has little intrinsic ability to heal. Chondrocytes in mature articular cartilage rarely divide, and their density declines with age. In contrast, lesions that extend to the subchondral marrow may heal clinically.[12] Therefore, a cell source for cartilage regeneration or repair must arise from the underlying subchondral bone marrow, the adjacent synovial tissue, or an exogenous source.

Absence of blood supply and endogenous source of new cells contribute to cartilage's incapacity for repair. The typical wound healing response of hemorrhage, fibrin clot formation, and mobilization of cells and growth factors is absent. The only spontaneous repair reaction may occur at the edge of superficial articular cartilage lesions. Articular cartilage is isolated from the subchondral bone marrow cells by the dense subchondral bone and cartilage matrix.

Cartilage repair is dependent on the mobilization of cells derived from the subchondral bone marrow, which include multipotential cells, osteoblasts, chondroblasts, fibroblasts, and hematoprogenitor cells.[13] Therefore, the repair tissue that results may be variable dependent based on the predominant cell line that proliferates and its modulation by local growth factors, cytokines, and the local mechanical environment.

Clinical Repair for Full-Thickness Cartilage Defects

The spectrum of repair tissue clinically is variable, depending on the clinical technique used as well as intrinsic and local factors. Repair tissue may be fibrous tissue, transitional tissue, fibrocartilage, hyaline cartilage, articular cartilage, bone, or a mixture of these tissues.[14] Fibrous tissue consists of fibrocytes and a type I collagen fibrous matrix. Transitional tissue consists of ovoid cells that may produce proteoglycans as well as a fibrous matrix. The matrix may stain positively with safranin O for proteoglycan production. Fibrocartilage consists of round chondrocyte-appearing cells with a type I collagen fibrous matrix. Hyaline cartilage consists of chondrocytes in a matrix of type II collagen and proteoglycans, with a hyaline, ground-glass appearance by light microscopy. The cellular and matrix organization may be different than normal articular cartilage. Articular cartilage resembles normal articular cartilage. Articular cartilage is essentially a regenerating tissue with articular chondrocytes, arranged in the usual palisading columns found in normal articular cartilage, with markers of normal articular cartilage matrix including type II collagen, proteoglycans, etc. A mixture of all these components may be present at a single repair site. The predominant repair tissue type will determine the long-term outcome of the patient. If the majority of the repair tissue is hyaline or articular cartilage, then the viscoelastic properties found with a type II collagen framework and proteoglycans will give a durable repair and usually a superior clinical result. Fibrocartilage and fibrous repairs consist of type I collagen, which is usually not as strong as type II collagen and often contains short-chain proteoglycans. Fibrocartilage and fibrous repairs do not maintain a high negative charge density, are soft, and break down (Figure 2–1).

Factors that may influence the quality of repair tissue noted clinically include acuteness of injury, age, size of defect, ligament stability, axial alignment, and presence or absence of the meniscus.[12,15] In a study conducted by Nehrer and associates[14] (Table 2–1), failed repair tissues were analyzed after three techniques of marrow stimulation: drilling, abrasion, and microfracture. The repair tissues retrieved were composed predominantly of fibrous and fibrocartilaginous tissues. The tissues were soft and degenerating. They had poor mechanical viscoelastic properties even though they filled the defects. The repair tissues clinically failed by 2.5 years after treatment, with an average defect size greater than 3 cm^2. Cartilage defects that were treated by perichondrial grafting had an excellent clinical result early postoperatively. By 4 to 5 years postoperatively, however, the repair tissue had undergone enchondral ossification. The perichondrial chondrocytes had features of hypertrophic chondrocytes, notably type X collagen, a precursor to mineralization (Figure 2–2). Although those grafts had a high percentage of hyaline cartilage, they also contained bone. The autologous chondrocyte implantation grafts that failed did so early (<6 months after implantation) due to trauma as the grafts were growing. At this early stage of repair, a high percentage of the repair tissue was fibrous or transitional in nature. Mature autologous chondrocyte implant grafts (>2 years after implantation) may have excellent clinical outcomes, with hyaline cartilage repair having firm viscoelastic properties (Figure 2–3).

Intrinsic repair in the acute situation is possible by marrow stimulation repair if chondral injury involves the underlying subchondral bone. However, appropriate rehabilitation after injury is critical (Table 2–2). The factors previously described delineating the possibility of a successful repair are important. Rehabilitation after such an injury is also important. However, there may be a critical size of subchondral bone involvement that will result in cystic degeneration rather than repair. This occurs specifically in osteochondritis dissecans or when lesions are deep. A study with experimental osteochondral defects greater than 8 mm in diameter and deep in adult goats demonstrated cystic enlargement of the defects rather than repair.[16] Therefore, repair of osteochondral defects is more complex. A staged reconstruction using autogenous tissues is required. Other options include allogeneic osteochondral reconstruction or autologous-derived tissue engineering solutions (Figure 2–4).

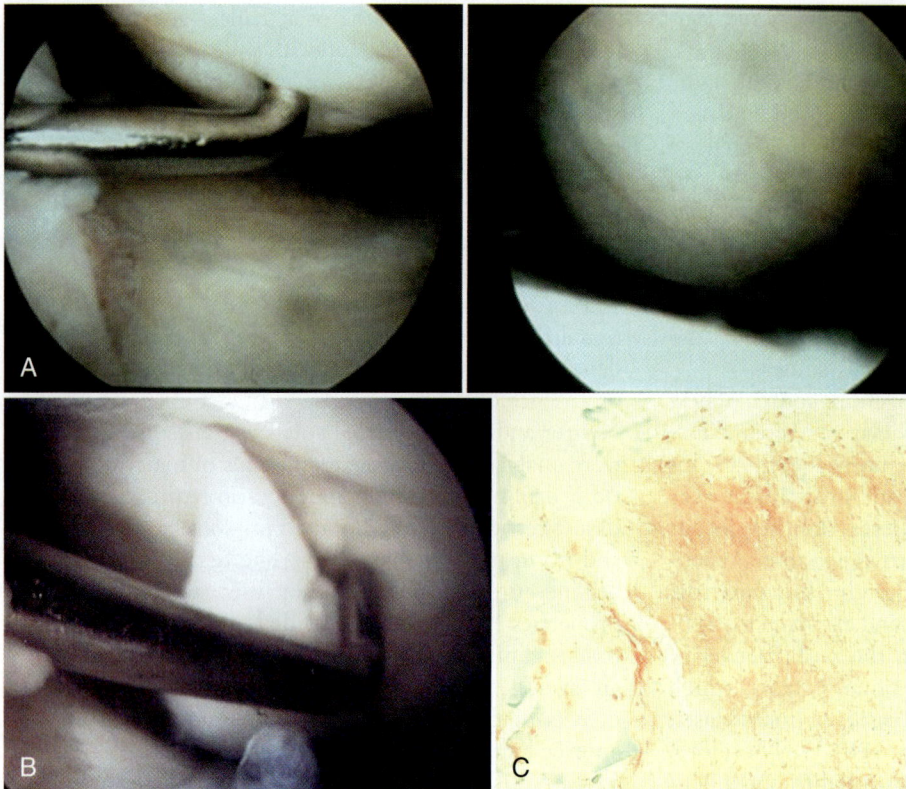

Figure 2-1 *A*, Arthroscopic appearance of a symptomatic fibrocartilage repair after drilling. Repair tissue is evident from native articular cartilage. Complete fill of defect with white repair tissue is evident. However, its mechanical properties are insufficient and soft, with resultant symptoms. *B*, Arthroscopic appearance of a symptomatic fibrocartilage flap after drilling. Poor integration as well as mechanically soft tissue have resulted in a poor clinical result. *C*, Low-power photomicrograph of retrieved fibrocartilage repair stained for proteoglycans with safranin O. Alternating layers of fibrous and fibrocartilage repair tissue have a porous appearance and a degenerating surface. This human retrieval resulted from a failed arthroscopic abrasion arthroplasty with resultant filled defect and soft repair tissue as shown in panel A.

Table 2-1 Evaluation of Tissue Retrieved after Failed Articular Cartilage Repair Procedures: Histologic and Immunohistochemical Comparative Analysis

	Treatment			P value
	Arthroscopic abrasion arthroplasty (n = 12)	Perichondrial rib grafting (n = 4)	Autologous chondrocyte implantation (n = 6)	$P < .05$ (ANOVA)
Follow-up (mo)	21 ± 4	31 ± 8	3 ± 1	
Tissue Type (%)				
Articular cartilage	2 ± 1	3 ± 2	0	NS
Hyaline cartilage	30 ± 10	47 ± 7	2 ± 1	Sig.
Fibrocartilage	28 ± 7	15 ± 4	6 ± 2	NS
Transition tissue	18 ± 2	12 ± 3	31 ± 7	NS
Fibrous tissue	22 ± 9	4 ± 2	61 ± 9	Sig.
Bone	0	19 ± 6	0	Sig.

Quantities of tissue types for failed cartilage repair procedures (arthroscopic abrasion arthroplasty, perichondrial rib grafting, and autologous chondrocyte implantation) in a human series at various time intervals after treatment are listed.
NS, not significant.
From Nehrer S, Spector M, Minas T: Histologic analysis of failed cartilage repair procedures. Clin Orthop Relat Res. 1999;365:149–162.

EXPERIMENTAL MODELS AND USEFULNESS

Selection of an appropriate animal model to assess the mechanisms and outcomes of procedures for cartilage repair has been problematic. The ideal is a skeletally mature animal with anatomic and morphologic similarities to the human clinical situation. Inclusion of multiple control groups is essential to assess the hypothesis that a certain treatment is superior. In this way the relative value of a therapy can be assessed but with limited translation to humans. However, this is not always feasible

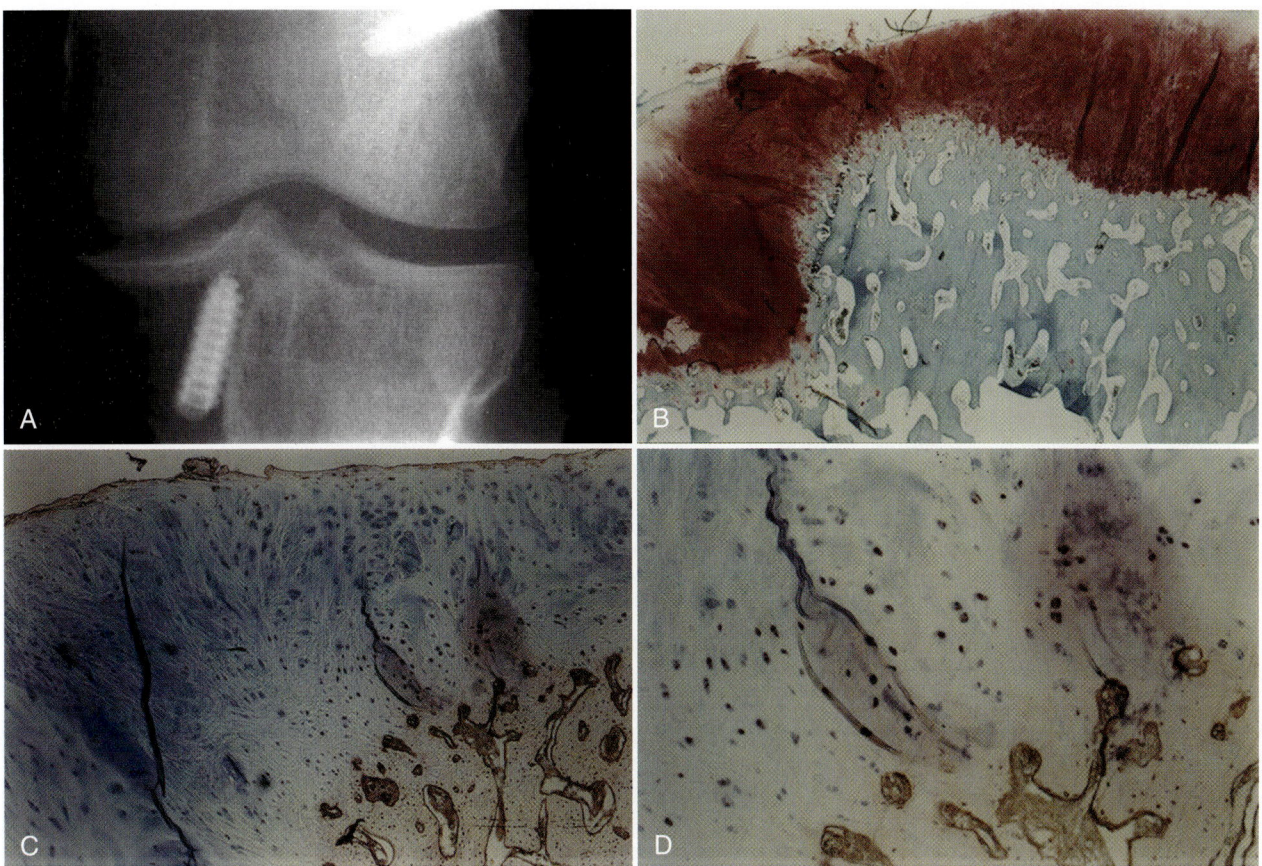

Figure 2-2 *A,* X-ray appearance of medial femoral condyle autologous perichondrial graft undergoing ossification. Ossification developed 3 years after cartilage repair, with initial excellent clinical result. Revision cartilage repair with autologous chondrocyte implantation graft resulted in successful clinical outcome. Retrieval of failed perichondrial graft specimen allowed histologic analysis. *B,* Low-power photomicrograph of retrieved perichondrial autograft undergoing enchondral ossification stained with safranin O. Notice excellent proteoglycan production as demonstrated by *red staining.* However, an advancing front of bone formation *(blue stain)* will eventually ossify the entire cartilage graft without stabilization with a tidemark. *C,* Low-power photomicrograph of antibody staining *(brown)* to type X collagen demonstrating intracellular production of type X collagen as expressed by hypertrophic chondrocytes undergoing enchondral ossification. *D,* High-power photomicrograph demonstrating intracellular antibody staining to type X collagen of hypertrophic chondrocytes. This is a common mechanism of failure of perichondrial autografts seen clinically.

because bilateral simultaneous treatments may not be ethically or physiologically sound for the repair model. The duration of the experiment needed to confirm endurance of cartilage repair and prevention of osteoarthritis usually is cost prohibitive.

Use of periosteum to treat full-thickness chondral defects under the influence of continuous passive motion has been investigated in a rabbit model.[17] An elegant experiment demonstrated that periosteum was capable of undergoing neochondrogenesis and that, under the influence of continuous passive motion, the quality of the repair tissue was similar to hyaline cartilage.

The translation of this model to demonstrate proof of principle in humans has not been fully realized.[18,19] Whether the rabbit is capable of an unusually robust healing response and whether technical differences in the experimental methodology account for unpredictable results in patients are not known.

The technique of autologous chondrocyte implantation has been controversial.[20–23] Much of the controversy apparently has been due to the conflicting results with two different animal models. The Swedish model was based on a pilot study performed in patellar chondral defects in rabbits.[24] The rabbit model showed that the implanted in vitro–labeled chondrocytes were largely responsible for the repair tissue that developed to fill chondral defects. The repair tissue was superior to that of periosteum alone.

The quality and quantity of repair tissues remained consistently higher in the rabbit model when compared to empty defects, periosteum, periosteum plus autologous chondrocytes, and carbon fiber pads plus autologous chondrocytes.[25] A similar study was performed in a rabbit model with bilateral patellar chondral defects, unlike the human situation in which defects are most commonly found on the femoral condyles.

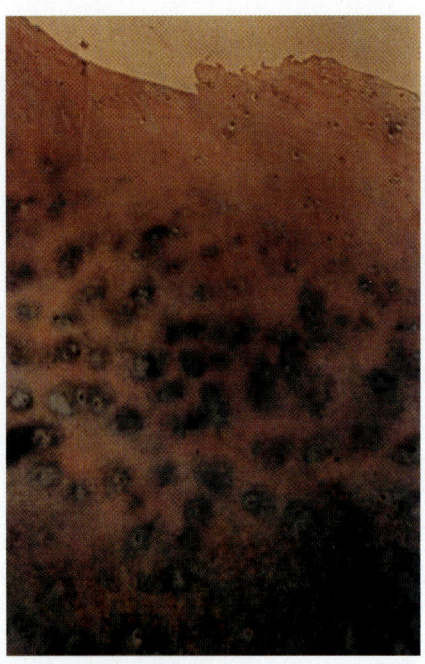

Figure 2-3 High-power photomicrograph of biopsy stained with safranin O of autologous chondrocyte implantation in a human. Note homogeneous ground-glass appearance of matrix and abundant chondrocyte formation.

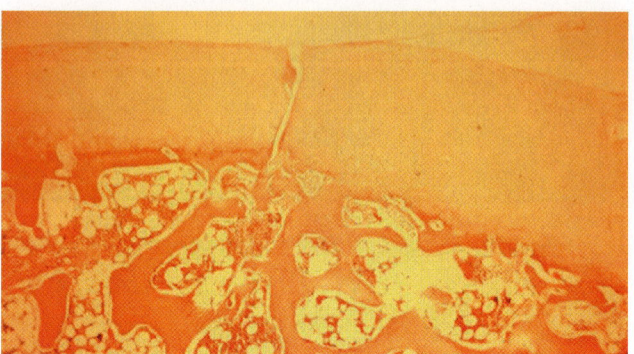

Figure 2-4 Low-power photomicrograph of canine biopsy specimen at the junction of the osteochondral graft transfer and native cartilage margin. Note the persistent cleft without integration at the cartilage junctures and the various thicknesses of articular cartilage with the different tidemark junctures. Excellent bony remodeling is noted in the subchondral bone marrow. *(Courtesy Laszlo Hangody, MD, Budapest, Hungary.)*

When the experiment was completed in a canine model using the femoral sulcus, the results comparing empty defects, periosteum, and periosteum plus autologous chondrocytes were similar in the early postoperative period (<6 months) but were uniformly osteoarthritic in the long term (12–18 months).[13,26] No treatment difference could be detected. A clear species difference between rabbit and dog was seen at 12 months (Figures 2–5 through 2–12).

Table 2-2 Clinical Recommendations for Careful Rehabilitation after Autologous Chondrocyte Implantation

	Time		
	0–6 Weeks	7–12 Weeks	>13 Weeks–3 Years
Stage	Proliferation	Transition	Remodeling and maturation
Histology	Rapid proliferation of spindle shaped cells with defect fill. Mostly type I collagen with early formation of colonies of chondrocytes forming type II collagen	Matrix formation, mostly chondrocytes producing type II collagen and proteoglycans Poor integration to underlying bone and cartilage	Ongoing remodeling of matrix with reorganization and quantity of type II collagen, and integration to bone (arcades of Benninghoff) and adjacent host cartilage Large-chain aggregates of proteoglycans, with increased water content of cartilage
Viscoelastic arthroscopic appearance	Filled, soft, white tissue	Jelly-like firmness, with "wave-like" motion when probed, not yet firm and integrated to underlying bone	Firm "indentable" but not "wave-like" when probed 4–6 mo after autologous chondrocyte transplantation Graft whiter than host cartilage and may demonstrate periosteal hypertrophy (20%) Equal firmness to host cartilage 9–18 mo after autologous chondrocyte transplantation
Activity level	• CPM starts 6 hr after surgery for 6–8 hr/day × 6 wk • Touch WB • Isometric muscle exercises and ROM	• Discontinue CPM • Active ROM • Partial graduated WB to full WB by 12 wk • Functional muscle usage, stationary bicycle, treadmill	• Discontinue assistive devices 4–5 mo postoperatively if free of pain, catching, swelling • Distance walking, resistance walking • Nonpivoting running at 9–12 mo • Pivoting allowed at 14–18 mo

Clinical recommendations made for careful rehabilitation after autologous chondrocyte implantation based on correlative observations on the basic science repair process learned from a canine model and arthroscopic evaluations in humans (with biopsies) at various stages of repair to determine viscoelastic mechanical maturation over time and prevent prematurely overloading of healing grafts.
CPM, continuous passive motion; ROM, range of motion; WB, weight bearing.

From Minas T, Peterson LL: Autologous chondrocyte transplantation. Oper Tech Sports Med. 2000;8:144–157.

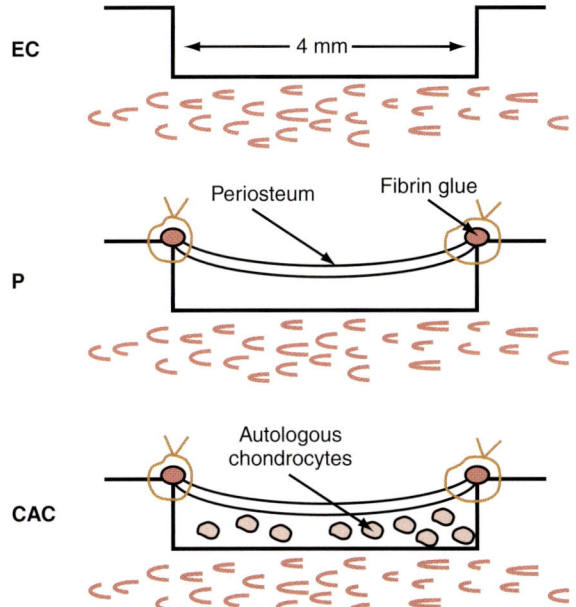

Figure 2-5 Schematic representation of canine experiment evaluating the effect of autologous chondrocyte implantation using cultured articular chondrocytes (CAC), versus periosteal resurfacing alone (P), versus empty control (EC), 4-mm defect. The periosteum was microsutured using absorbable suture to the native articular margins with the cambium layer of periosteum facing the bony surface. The margins were then sealed with autologous fibrin glue. The animal was protected with an external fixation device for 10 days and then allowed to bear weight as tolerated. Two chondral defects were made per knee, in the femoral sulcus or the trochlea (see Figure 2–6).

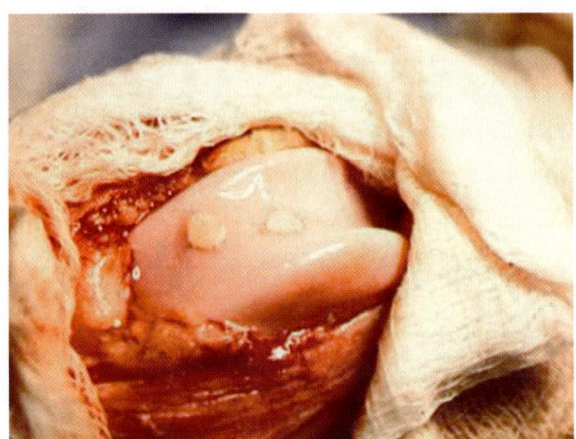

Figure 2-6 Gross appearance of periosteal patches sutured to chondral defects undergoing autologous chondrocyte implantation on the femoral sulcus in a canine model. The chondral defects measured 4 mm in diameter.

TRANSLATIONAL RESEARCH

It may be that there is no perfect animal model with repair characteristics similar to the human species. However, new technologies and treatment options may be evaluated in an animal model with control groups. In this way, the efficacy of repair may be assessed. In general, proof of

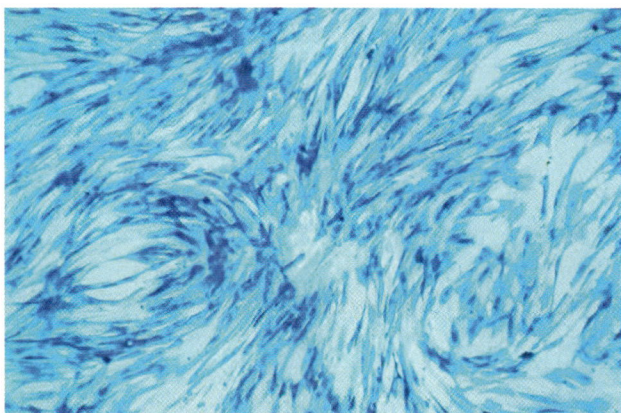

Figure 2-7 High-power photomicrograph of beta-galactosidase–labeled reporter gene *(blue)* in chondrocyte culture in monolayer approaching confluence. The reporter gene allows tracking of implanted chondrocytes over time. The label was no longer effective after 3 months in vivo.

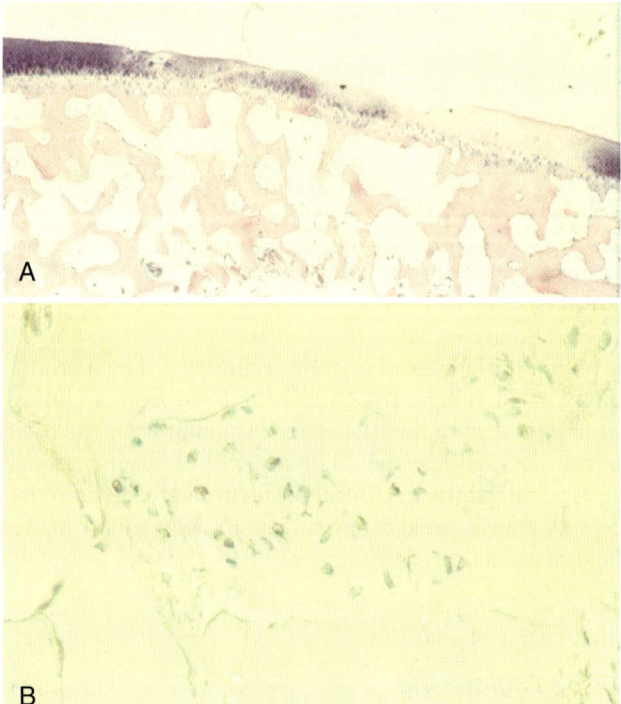

Figure 2-8 *A*, Low-power histologic section with hematoxylin and eosin staining of canine defect treated by autologous chondrocyte implantation at 3 months. The defect appears filled but has poor staining characteristics, although the repair tissue appears to consist predominantly of cellular chondrocytes. *B*, High-power photomicrograph of area that is poorly staining in panel A, demonstrating the persistence of beta-galactosidase reporter gene labeling of implanted chondrocytes 3 months after implantation. This image demonstrates that the implanted chondrocytes are responsible for the repair tissue and not local cellular repair.

principle involves the progression of scientific methodology from in vitro methods to small animal experimentation to larger animal validation prior to human clinical trials and is the desired scientific method. The hypotheses for the scientific methods are derived from clinical

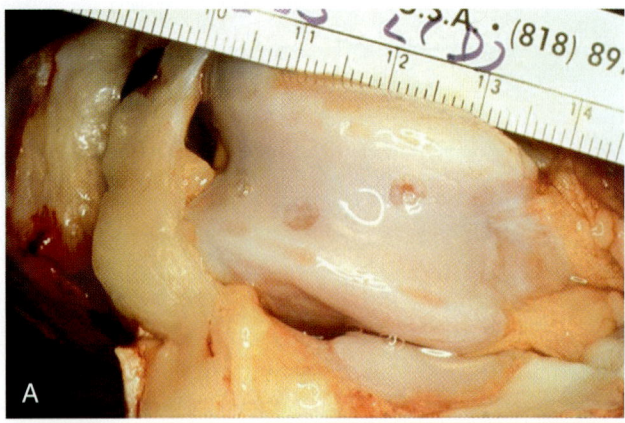

Figure 2-9 *A*, Gross appearance of empty canine defects 6 months after treatment. Minimal repair tissue is seen around the margins. *B*, Low-power histologic section with hematoxylin and eosin staining of canine defect as control defect at 6 months. Note lack of repair tissue fill except around the margins.

problems or failures of existing techniques. The methodology of pursuing a hypothesis rendered from a clinical situation taken to the basic science laboratory is the basis of translational research. The topic of cartilage repair is an especially difficult clinical problem and field. The concept of translational research is especially suited in the field of cartilage repair.

State of the Art

Tissue Engineering

Because cartilage is a relatively simple tissue because of its cellular homogeneity and avascularity, it has been a model for research of in vitro engineered tissues.[27] Progress has been slow and obstructed on several levels. The adult chondrocyte has limited capacity for proliferation and has both catabolic and anabolic functions. These metabolic features must be optimized and controlled for engineered tissue to endure. The motivation for tissue engineering is to promote biologic repair or regeneration. Conceptual approaches include implantation of inert substitutes for discontinuities or missing parts, drug or matrix treatments to stimulate tissue regeneration, autogenous cell or tissue transfer, and in vitro production of tissues or tissue equivalents for implantation. Three considerations when designing a

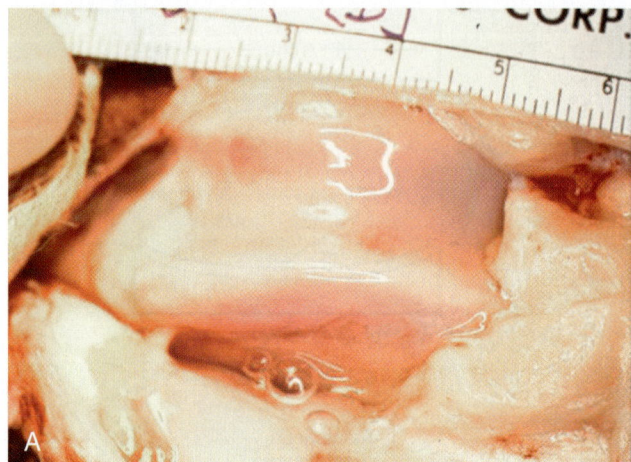
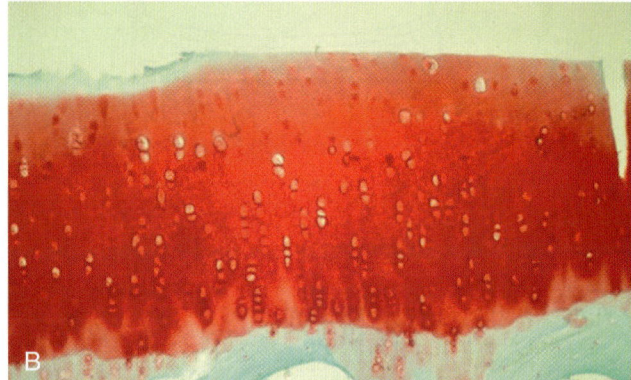
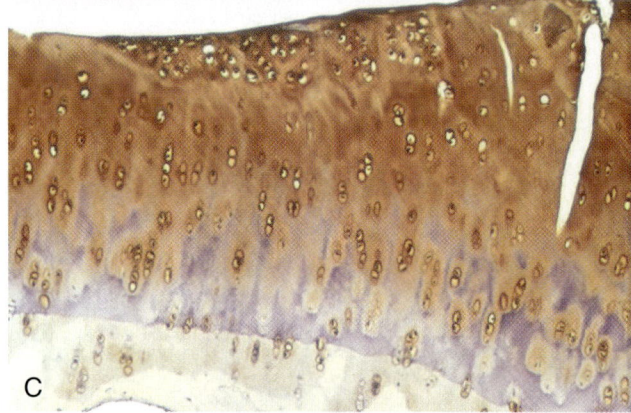

Figure 2-10 *A*, Gross appearance of defects in a canine model 6 months after treatment with autologous chondrocytes. Note the complete fill and smoothness of the surface. *B*, High-power photomicrograph with safranin O staining of retrieved tissue shown in panel A. Hyaline cartilage repair tissue with deep proteoglycan staining, palisading chondrocyte arrangement, and excellent subchondral bone integration with tidemark formation are seen. However, note the cleft to the far right of the cartilage integration. This is a common finding early after treatment with autologous chondrocyte implantation grafting. *C*, Same specimen stained with antibody to type II collagen *(brown)*. Note uniform density of staining.

construct for engineered tissue are (1) the source of cells, if any; (2) the nature of the carrier or scaffold; and (3) the use, if any, of genes, factors, or adjuvants.

Interestingly, cultured chondrocytes under the influence of constant hydrostatic pressure perfusion versus

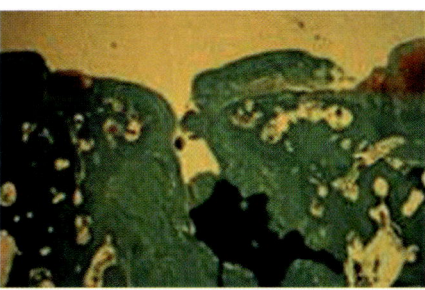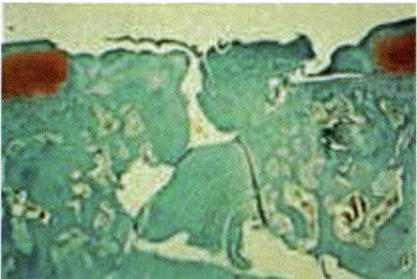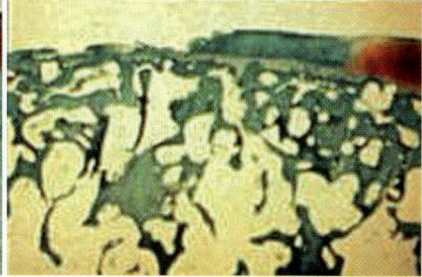

Figure 2–11 Low-power photomicrographs of empty defect *(left)*, periosteum alone *(center)*, and autologous chondrocyte implantation *(right)* in canine experiment 12 months postimplantation. The worst-case scenario demonstrates collapse of the subchondral bone plate with fibrous tissue formation in an empty defect in both the empty control and periosteum alone groups. The autologous chondrocyte implantation treatment group similarly has a poor repair tissue that is delaminating, but the subchondral bone is intact. Difference between the three treatments could not be graded by independent observation by a histologist.

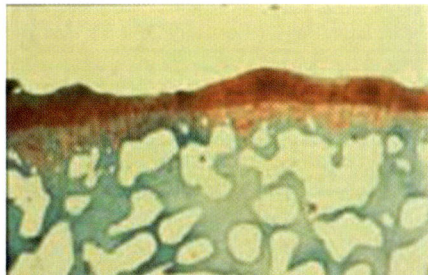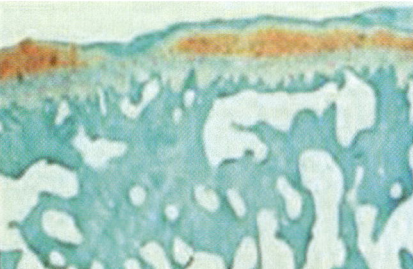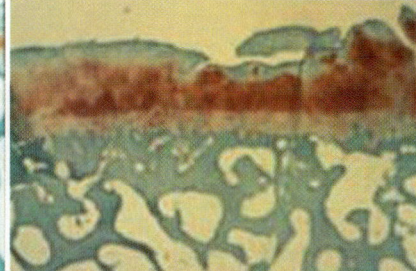

Figure 2–12 Low-power photomicrographs of the same treatments shown in Figure 2–11. In the best-case scenario, repair tissue in all three treatment arms could not be graded as different. No difference in treatment effect was apparent. The canine model for cartilage repair for periods of time greater than 12 months demonstrated spontaneous repair or degeneration to a similar treatment and point. However, autologous chondrocyte implantation for less than 6 months demonstrated a superior repair.

intermittent perfusion demonstrate improved cartilage matrix production (Figure 2–13). Experimental work was performed at our laboratory (Tom Minas, MD, Julie Glowaki, PhD, Shahram Solhpour, MD, and Shuichi Mizuno, PhD, Skeletal Biology Laboratory, Orthopedic Research, Cartilage Repair Center, Brigham and Women's Hospital and Harvard Medical School, Boston, MA) to assess this effect in an in vivo evaluation of cartilage repair in an animal model (Autologous Cartilage Repair in Rabbits with Chondrocytes in 3D Collagen Sponges Precultured with Hydrostatic Pressure, unpublished data).

The goal of our study was to assess a collagen sponge seeded with autologous cultured chondrocytes under the influence of hydrostatic pressure as a tissue-engineered construct, versus the gold standard of autologous cultured chondrocyte implantation under a periosteal flap, versus control groups of empty defect, empty sponge, periosteum without cells. Information on the treatment groups is given in Table 2–3.

Seven-month-old New Zealand white male rabbits were used in the study. After a medial parapatellar incision was made, the patella was dislocated laterally, and a 3-mm-diameter defect was created in the center of the patella using a circular stainless-steel punch. Cartilage tissue was harvested using a beaver blade, and a sharp edge of host cartilage was created using a curette. The defects were cylindrical in shape and extended over the tide mark. The knee was closed.

Chondrocyte Isolation: The cartilage slices were harvested and digested. The isolated chondrocytes were seeded to T-25 culture flasks and incubated for 6 days. The chondrocytes were harvested using trypsin, and 300,000 cells in 25 µl of medium were injected into collagen sponges. The sponges were incubated using a pressure/perfusion culture system at 0.7 MPa, 0.015 Hz, and 0.3 ml/min for 7 days (Figure 2–13*A*).

Engineered Cartilage Implantation

The second operation was performed after 2 weeks of in vitro monolayer culture and pressure/perfusion culture. A full-thickness defect (3-mm diameter and over the tidemark) through the articular cartilage was created in the femoral weight-bearing condyle using a circular stainless steel punch. The lesion produced was a deep defect that extended through all chondral layers into the calcified zone. It was termed a *full-thickness lesion* to distinguish it from an osteochondral bone plate.

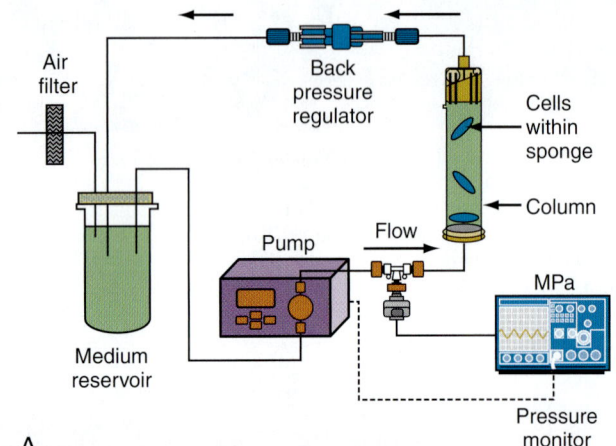

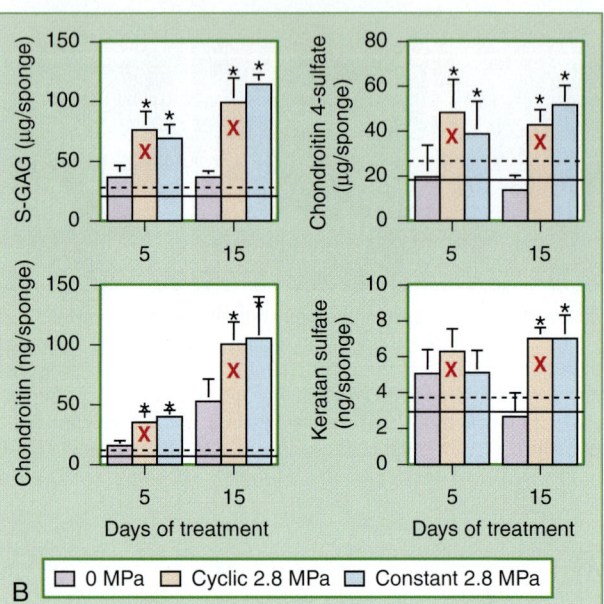

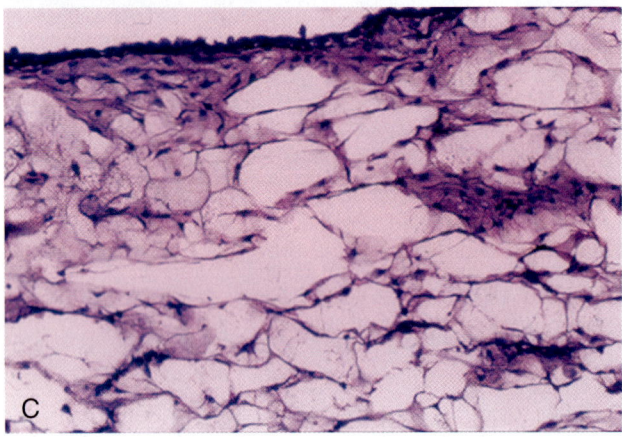

Figure 2–13 *A*, Illustration of hydrostatic pressure culture system used for the experimentation described in text to produce a tissue-engineered cartilage implant evaluated in the New Zealand rabbit model (Mizuno et al. Mat Sci Eng C, 1998.) *B*, Graphs which demonstrate the production of proteoglycan macromolecules found in articular cartilage increase with time under pressure perfusion which is improved with constant perfusion versus intermittent perfusion or no pressure. (Mizuno S, Tateishi T, Ushida T, Glowacki J: Hydrostatic fluid pressure enhances matrix synthesis and accumulation by bovine chondrocytes in three-dimensional culture. *J Cell Physiol* 2002;193: 319–327.) *C*, Photomicrograph of type I collagen sponge seated with autologous rabbit chondrocytes under the influence of 0.7-MPa constant pressure perfusion (magnification ×50). Note distribution of cells throughout the sponge producing early matrix 7 days after onset of perfusion.

Under aseptic conditions, the autologous cartilage was trimmed using a 4-mm punch and directly sutured into the defect. The knee was closed in separate layers.

Rabbits from each treatment group (see Table 2–3) were euthanized at time points of 4 weeks and 12 weeks. The tissue around the defect was harvested for histologic analysis.

Histologic Evaluation: The sections were graded as poor, fair, good, or excellent by three blinded individuals.

Results: Sponges with chondrocytes that were cultured for 5 days with hydrostatic pressure accumulated more metachromatic matrix than did those cultured without hydrostatic pressure.

Clinically, some of the control empty defects and those with cell-free collagen sponges were partially filled, but the collagen sponge + cells scored consistently higher than the other treatment groups.

Histologically, most of the empty controls showed poor repair (Figure 2–14). Collagen sponge + cells showed better repair than did collagen sponge alone. Collagen sponge + cells were similar to the autologous chondrocyte implantation group.

We concluded that tissue-engineered cartilage demonstrated histologic repair superior or similar to that of autologous chondrocyte implantation and was better than the controls of empty defect, periosteum alone, or empty sponge. However, some of the empty sponge defects did demonstrate a reasonable repair tissue migration into the sponge and partial repair.

From an experimental translational research model, this work was continued and was the basis for the formation of a clinically relevant human cartilage repair trial (see the NeoCart system in Chapter 14).

Cell Based

Theoretically, cartilage tissue appears well suited for transplantation because it lacks a blood supply, is nourished by diffusion, and has a low cell-to-matrix ratio. It

Table 2-3 Treatment Groups

Group	Left Knee	Right Knee
1	Periosteum + autologous cultured chondrocytes	Periosteum
2	Periosteum + autologous cultured chondrocytes	Empty defect
3	Engineered cartilage	Periosteum + autologous cultured chondrocytes
4	Engineered cartilage	Collagen sponge control
5	Allo-engineered cartilage	Periosteum + allo-autologous cultured chondrocytes

has sites for donor tissue, especially for pediatric patients. Transplanted autogenous cartilage has been used successfully for construction of ears in children having congenital microtia or atresia, with excellent long-term maintenance. Long-term results of osteochondral shell allograft resurfacing of knees indicate better function in unipolar than bipolar cases. However, segments of cartilage are less suitable for repair of articular surfaces or intracartilaginous defects where bonding to the tissue bed is important. Autogenous cells, often expanded in vitro, have been useful for cartilage tissue engineering. Precursor/progenitor cells derived from marrow, perichondrium, periosteum, and other sources also have potential for cartilage repair. Human dermal fibroblasts can be induced to differentiate to chondrocytes and to produce cartilage matrix by culture in the presence of demineralized bone powder.[28] Whether chondrocytes that are differentiated in vitro will maintain the articular phenotype or will develop into hypertrophic chondrocytes may depend upon the site into which they are implanted or the mediators in their microenvironment. More information about the plasticity of chondrocytes and their potential for developing endochondral bone will be needed prior to clinical applications.

Gene Therapy

Advances in gene transfer technology have been translated to clinical applications. Proof of principle has been demonstrated for in vivo and ex vivo transfection of genes into articular chondrocytes. Efficient transfection requires vectors, materials, or methods to promote uptake and expression of the gene of interest. In principle, different methods may result in transient or more enduring expression of the gene product. For chondrocytes, some of the useful genes include insulin-like growth factor-I, transforming growth factor-α, and IL-1 receptor antagonist.

Materials

Delivery of simple cell suspensions is of limited value in musculoskeletal applications because of the requirement for cells to be retained at the desired site. Isolated chondrocytes lack adherence to lesion sites, and suspensions may produce fibrocartilage or small foci of cartilage. Fluid carriers or three-dimensional scaffolds can be used for delivery and retention of cells. Popular natural hydrogels such as alginates, fibrin, denatured collagen gels, hyaluronan, and admixtures are useful for containing or immobilizing cell suspensions. In addition to their important function as a carrier of cells, three-dimensional scaffolds are useful for defining the space for new tissue and potentially for enhancing the maturation and function of regenerated tissue. Candidate scaffolds include natural polymeric materials such as collagen lattices, synthetic polymers, biodegradable polymers, and polymers with adsorbed proteins or immobilized functional groups.

The key requirements of bioresorbable materials are that (1) their rates of degradation must be compatible with the intended use and (2) the products of their degradation must be nontoxic. Of the synthetic materials, polyglycolic acid, polylactic acid, and their copolymers are most widely studied.

Future Directions

Widespread discourse about the early experiments on tissue and organ engineering has generated public demand and expectations for the availability of engineered tissues in the near future. However, critical hurdles need to be overcome. In the case of engineered cartilage, it would be desirable to avoid harvesting normal tissue and to have a single operation for implantation of engineered tissue. Mature chondrocytes are exceptional in their ability to serve catabolic as well as anabolic functions. Control in inhibiting the chondrolytic activities of chondrocytes seems important for maintaining engineered tissues. Consideration of the limited proliferative and regenerative capacity of adult chondrocytes and the potential for dedifferentiation upon expansion also leads to the goal of alternate sources of cells. Use of xenogeneic or allogeneic cells requires selective shattering of the immunogenicity barrier in transplantation. Difficulties remain in incorporating neocartilage into adjacent healthy tissue.

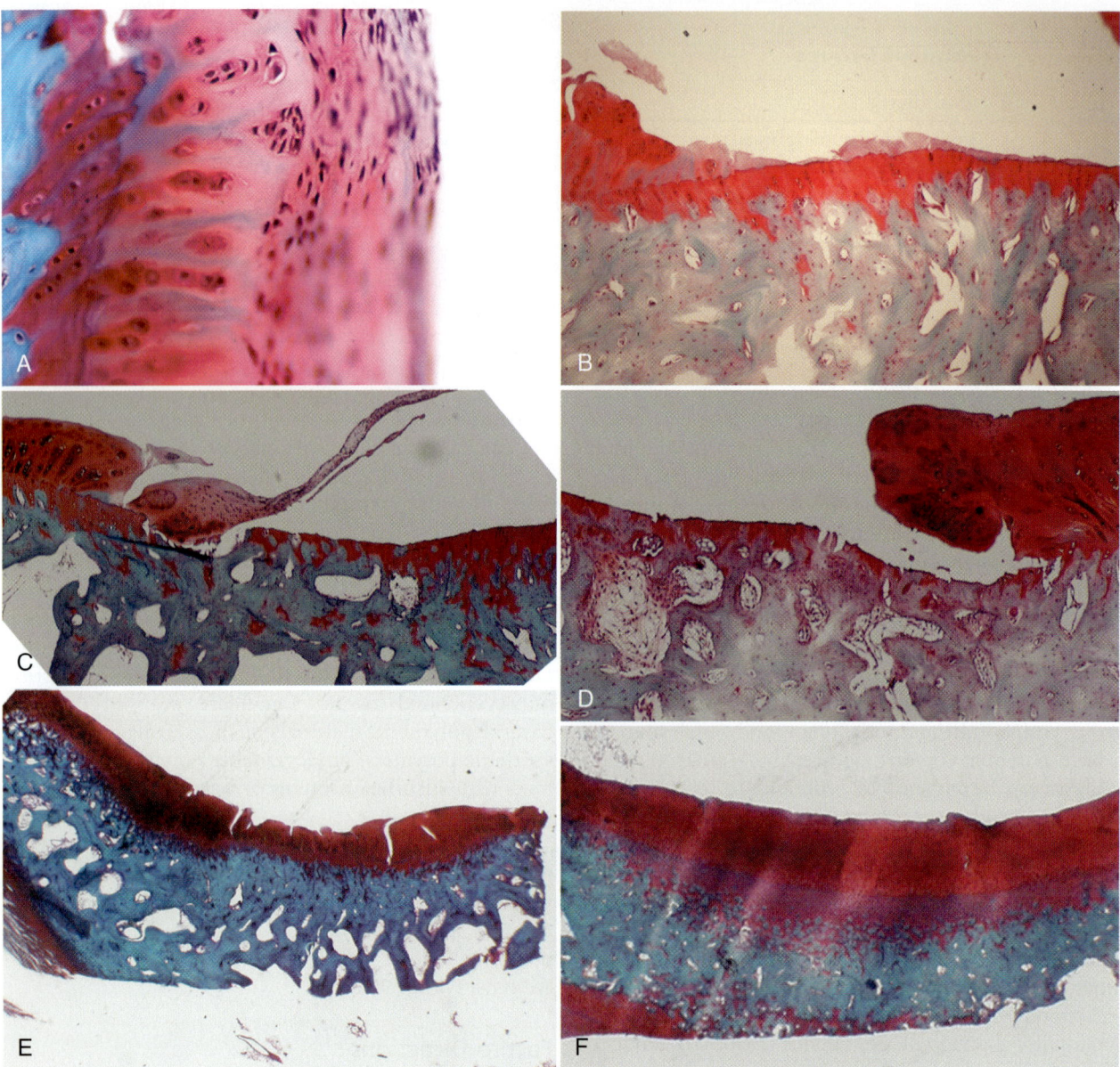

Figure 2–14 *A*, One-month patellar defect of tissue-engineered implant in a New Zealand rabbit (safranin O staining, magnification ×100). Note excellent integration, fill, and cellular proliferation within the defect. *B*, Three-month patellar empty defect (magnification ×25). Note complete absence of repair tissue in the defect except for the margins. *C*, Three-month patellar defect repaired with an empty sponge. Poor filling and only marginal repair are seen. *D*, Three-month patellar defect repaired with periosteum alone without cells. No tissue repair is seen except for the margins of the defect. *E*, Three-month patellar defect repaired with autologous chondrocyte implantation under a periosteal patch. Excellent cellular response in the defect with fill and subchondral bone integration are seen. Some minor fissuring at the edges of the defect has occurred. *F*, Tissue-engineered cartilage implant produced under the influence of constant hydrostatic pressure perfusion of a collagen sponge implanted into a 4-mm-diameter chondral defect. Excellent fill, integration, and proteoglycan staining with cellular proliferation and organization are seen.

Our understanding of the relationship between cartilage and vascular response to wounding is incomplete. Engineered cartilage needs to attach to the implantation site without evoking an angiogenic response. It is conceivable that genetically modified cells could be grown on a biocompatible scaffold with internal signals for programmed histogenesis. Advances in materials design may generate "smart" scaffolds that control tissue topology and have surface modifications to stimulate cell attachment, differentiation, and growth.

REFERENCES

1. Stockwell RA, Meachim G. The chondrocytes. In: Freeman MAR, ed. *Adult Articular Cartilage*. Kent: Pitman Medical; 1979:69–144.
2. Mankin HJ, Mos VW, Buckwalter JA, Iannotti JP, Ratcliffe A. Articular cartilage structure, composition and function. In: Buckwalter JA, Einhorn TA, Simon SR, eds. *Orthopaedic Basic Science*. Rosemont, IL: American Academy of Orthopaedic Surgeons; 2000.
3. Seibel MJ, Robbins SP, Bilezikian JP, eds. *Dynamics of Bone and Cartilage Metabolism*. San Diego: Academic Press; 1999.
4. Mow VC, Ratcliffe A. Structure and function of articular cartilage and meniscus. In: Mow VC, Hayes WC, eds. *Basic Orthopaedic Biomechanics*. Philadelphia: Lippincott Raven; 1997.
5. Noyes FR, Bassett RW, et al. Arthroscopy in acute traumatic hemarthrosis of the knee: Incidence of anterior cruciate tears and other injuries. *J Bone Joint Surg Am*. 1980;62:687–695.
6. Curl W, Krome J, et al. Cartilage injuries: A review of 31,516 knee arthroscopies. *Arthroscopy*. 1997;13:456–460.
7. Messner K, Maletius W. The long-term prognosis for severe damage to weight-bearing cartilage in the knee. A 14-year clinical and radiographic follow-up in 28 young athletes. *Acta Orthop Scand*. 1996;67:165–168.
8. Minas T, Nehrer S. Current concepts in the treatment of cartilage defects. *Orthopedics*. 1997;20:525–538.
9. Repo RU, Finlay J. Survival of articular cartilage after controlled impact. *J Bone Joint Surg Am*. 1977;59:1068–1076.
10. Johnson DL, Urban WP, Caborn NNM, Carlson C, Van Arthros W. *Articular cartilage pathology associated with MRI detected "bone bruises" after ACL rupture*. Atlanta: American Academy of Orthopaedic Surgeons Society for Sports Med Specialty Day; February 25, 1996.
11. Sahlström A, Johnell O, Redlund-Johnell I. The natural course of arthrosis of the knee. *Clin Orthop Relat Res*. 1997;40:152–157.
12. Dzioba RB. The classification and treatment of acute articular cartilage lesions. *Arthroscopy*. 1988;4:72–80.
13. Breinan H, Minas T, Hsu HP, et al. Effect of cultured articular chondrocytes on repair of chondral defects in a canine model. *J Bone Joint Surg Am*. 1997;79:1439–1451.
14. Nehrer S, Spector M, Minas T. Histologic analysis of failed cartilage repair procedures. *Clin Orthop Relat Res*. 1999;365:149–162.
15. Friedman MJ, Berasi CC, Fox JM, et al. Preliminary results with abrasion arthroplasty in the osteoarthritic knee. *Clin Orthop Relat Res*. 1984;182:200–205.
16. Jackson DW, Lalor PA, Aberman HM, Simon TM. Spontaneous repair of full-thickness defects of articular cartilage in a goat model: a preliminary study. *J Bone Joint Surg Am*. 2001;83:53–64.
17. O'Driscoll SW, Salter R. The induction of neochondrogenesis in free intra-articular periosteal autografts under the influence of continuous passive motion. *J Bone Joint Surg Am*. 1984;66:1248–1257.
18. Angermann P, Riegels-Nielsen P, Pedersen H. Osteochondritis dissecans of the femoral condyle treated with periosteal transplantation. Poor outcome in 14 patients followed for 6–9 years. *Acta Orthop Scand*. 1998;69:595–597.
19. Madsen BL, Noer HH, Carstensen JP, Normark F. Longterm results of periosteal transplantation in osteochondritis dissecans of the knee. *Orthopedics*. 2000;23:223–226.
20. Brittberg M, Lindahl A, Nilsson A, Ohlsson C, et al. Treatment of full-thickness cartilage defects in the human knee with cultured autologous chondrocytes. *N Engl J Med*. 1984;331:889–895.
21. Messner K, Gillquist J. Cartilage repair: A critical review. *Acta Orthop Scand*. 1996;67:523–529.
22. Brittberg M. A critical analysis of cartilage repair. *Acta Orthop Scand*. 1999;88:186–191.
23. Jackson DW, Simon T. Current concepts. Chondrocyte transplantation. *Arthroscopy*. 1996;12:732–738.
24. Grande DA, Pitman ML, et al. The repair of experimentally produced defects in the rabbit articular cartilage by autologous chondrocyte transplantation. *J Orthop Res*. 1989;7:208–218.
25. Brittberg M, Nilsson A, Lindahl A, et al. Rabbit articular cartilage defects treated with autologous cultured chondrocyte. *Clin Orthop Relat Res*. 1995;326:270–283.
26. Breinan H, Minas T, Barone L, et al. Histological evaluation of the course of healing of canine articular cartilage defects treated with cultured chondrocytes. *Tissue Eng*. 1998;4:101–114.
27. Glowacki J. In vitro engineering of cartilage. *J Rehabil Res Dev*. 2000;37:171–177.
28. Mizuno S, Glowacki J. Chondroinduction of human dermal fibroblasts by demineralized bone in three-dimensional culture. *Exp Cell Res*. 1996;227:89–97.

Chapter 3

Imaging: The Basis for a Sound Decision in Joint Preservation

Tom Minas, MD, MS

INTRODUCTION

RADIOLOGIC PATTERNS
OF OSTEOARTHRITIS

Medial Osteoarthritis
Lateral Tibiofemoral Osteoarthritis
Dysplasia and Degenerative Osteoarthritis of the
  Patellofemoral Joint

MAGNETIC RESONANCE IMAGING
OF ARTICULAR CARTILAGE

INTRODUCTION

Radiologic assessment of the knee may provide a tremendous amount of information when proper radiographs are performed and patterns of wear are recognized. A standard series of digital radiographs that we perform at our center include a 54-inch anteroposterior (AP) axial alignment x-ray (with radiographic markers for magnification), standing bilateral AP, 45-degree bent standing posteroanterior (PA; Rosenberg views[1]), and a tangential patellar skyline view at 45 degrees supine. *Supine AP radiographs of the knee should not be performed* because they are not useful for determining the cartilage joint space and hence the potential for joint preserving-surgery.

Patients with articular cartilage injuries referred to us for treatment frequently have high-resolution MRI scans and arthroscopy photographs available. However, they do not have standing x-ray films, which would demonstrate whether they have preexisting bone-on-bone osteoarthritis. Simple radiographs would inform us that these patients are not suitable for cartilage repair based on their bone-on-bone changes but still may be suitable for osteotomy or possibly unicompartmental replacement.

RADIOLOGIC PATTERNS
OF OSTEOARTHRITIS

Advanced tricompartmental osteoarthritis is exceedingly rare except in the presence of advanced unicompartmental disease with tibiofemoral subluxation. Ahlback[2] reviewed a Swedish population in the region of Stockholm and published his report in 1968. He reviewed weight-bearing radiographs of 1,800 knees from approximately 1,200 patients. A series examining arthrosis reviewed 281 patients comprising 370 knees with joint space narrowing. Standing AP projections (but not PA projections) were taken: loading 20 degrees bent axial patellofemoral views and supine lateral views. The Venn diagrams shown in Figure 3–1 were constructed depicting the wear patterns noted.

The predominant arthritic wear patterns in the medial and patellofemoral articulations occur in 80% patients. The lateral compartment usually wears posteriorly.[1] These numbers may change slightly if standing PA views are included. In any case, the Venn diagrams demonstrate that unicompartmental and bicompartmental wear are more common than tricompartmental wear. Therefore, total knee arthroplasty may be an overly aggressive solution to osteoarthritis in a younger patient population. Cartilage repair, possibly combined with osteotomy, or unicompartmental or bicompartmental resurfacing arthroplasty when bone-on-bone changes are present may be more suitable in an attempt to preserve the joint for as long as possible.

Medial Osteoarthritis

Standing AP x-ray films generally demonstrate early joint space narrowing for the medial wear pattern of osteoarthritis (Figure 3–2). With medial osteoarthritis, a standing

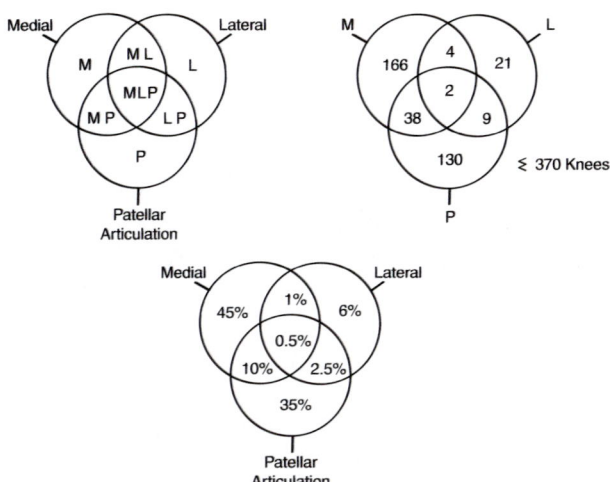

Figure 3-1 Venn diagrams demonstrating the predominance of osteoarthritic joint space narrowing in the medial and patellar articulations of the knee. In this classic study, which was the basis for the classification proposed by Ahlback,[2] tricompartmental arthritis was exceedingly rare in a Swedish cohort of 370 knees examined in the 1960s in the Stockholm region.

PA x-ray film may demonstrate increased posterior joint space unless anterior cruciate ligament (ACL) deficiency is present, in which case tibial translation anteriorly permits a posterior wear pattern on the medial side (Figure 3–3).[3]

Lateral Tibiofemoral Osteoarthritis

Lateral osteoarthritic changes usually occur in the central to posterior aspect of the lateral tibial plateau, regardless of whether the changes are due to valgus malalignment or ACL deficiency or occur after meniscectomy. Early joint space narrowing with peripheral osteophyte formation may be noted in a standing AP x-ray film; however, the standing 45-degree Rosenberg PA x-ray film usually demonstrates loss of articular space and always should be included (Figure 3–4).[1]

Dysplasia and Degenerative Osteoarthritis of the Patellofemoral Joint

Just as dysplasia of the hip joint results in early osteoarthritis secondary to abnormal contact forces in patients in their early 40s and 50s, a similar condition exists in the patellofemoral joint. Dysplasia of the trochlea has been discussed in Europe, especially France, since the 1970s but has just started being recognized in the United States in the last decade. Dejour[4] has done much work demonstrating the radiographic abnormalities present in a patient with dysplasia of the trochlea (Figure 3–5). Dysplasia may present as a poorly formed or flattened sulcus or a convex trochlea (see Chapter 10). The lateral x-ray film does not demonstrate the "crossing sign," which is characteristic of a patient with dysplasia, because a poorly formed sulcus does not show a double dip on lateral x-ray film. These patients frequently present with an adolescent dislocation of the patella, anterior knee pain, or both. The pain may persist through young adulthood and by the fourth or fifth decades presents with end-stage patellofemoral isolated osteoarthritis (see Figure 3–5).

MAGNETIC RESONANCE IMAGING OF ARTICULAR CARTILAGE

The clinical suspicion of an articular cartilage defect may be confirmed by magnetic resonance imaging (MRI) or at arthroscopic surgery. Although arthroscopy is the

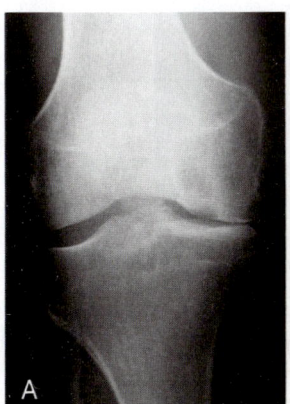 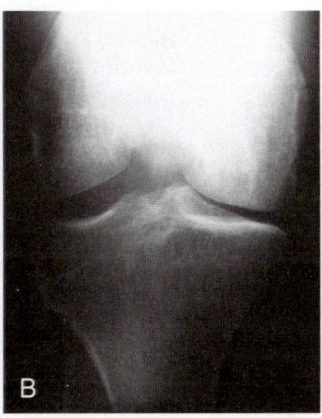 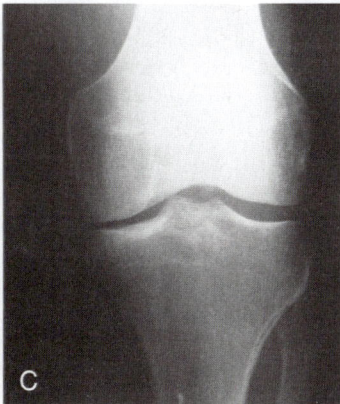 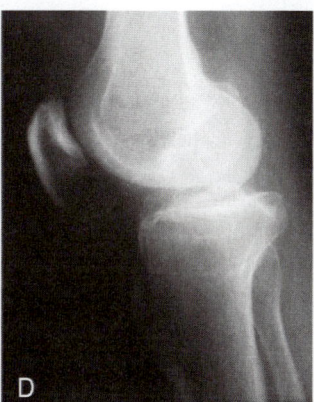

Figure 3-2 A 40-year-old man with bilateral varus knees has a classic anterior medial wear pattern of osteoarthritis. *A*, Standing anteroposterior (AP) view demonstrating loss of joint space in full extension. *B*, Standing 45-degree bent PA view demonstrating a preserved posterior medial joint space. The patient had childhood medial femoral condyle osteochondritis dissecans. *C, D,* Left knee in the same patient demonstrating loss of joint space in extension on anteroposterior x-ray film *(C)* and an anterior wear pattern on lateral x-ray film *(D)*.

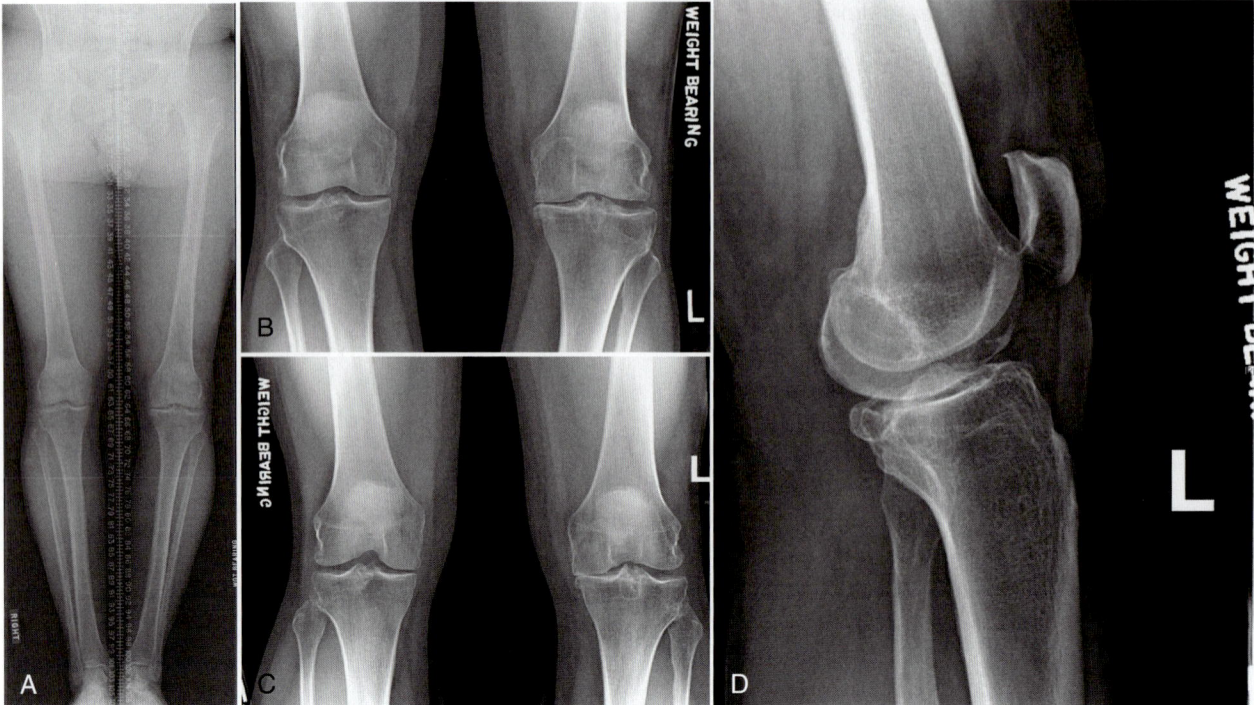

Figure 3–3 Effect of anterior cruciate ligament (ACL) deficiency in a 40-year-old man. *A*, Long standing alignment x-ray film demonstrates varus alignment of the lower extremities. *B*, Standing anteroposterior x-ray film demonstrates medial joint space loss with peripheral osteophyte formation and residual joint space remaining. *C*, Standing posteroanterior x-ray film demonstrates complete obliteration of the posterior medial joint space. This is typical of a chronic ACL-deficient knee, with tibial wear translating further posterior as the tibia subluxes anteriorly secondary to ACL deficiency. *D*, Lateral x-ray film demonstrates atypical "cupola" or cupped appearance of the tibia.

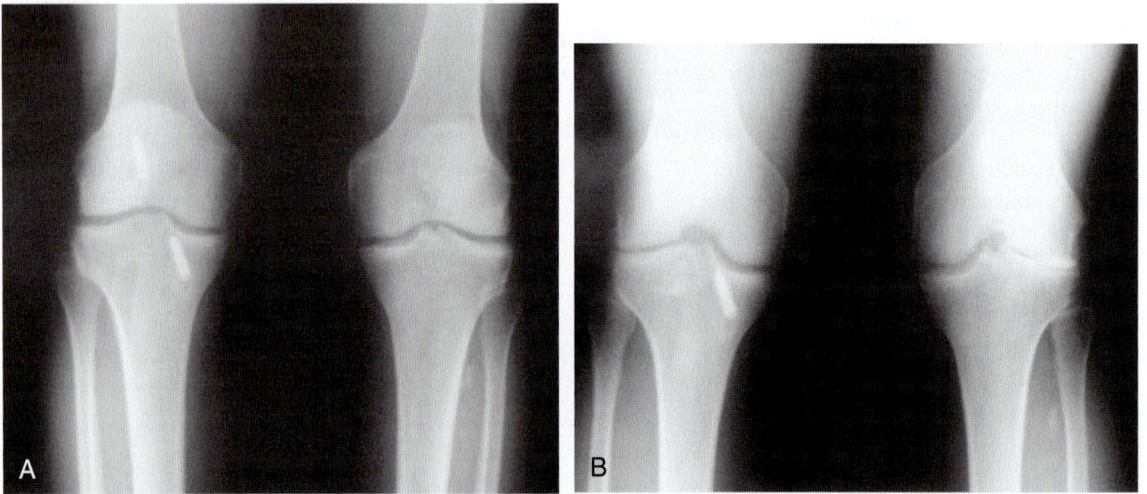

Figure 3–4 A 50-year-old patient with a previous anterior cruciate ligament–injured knee, mild varus alignment of the lower limb, and lateral joint pain. *A*, Standing anteroposterior (AP) x-ray film shows the joint space is intact. *B*, Rosenberg posteroanterior view demonstrates the bone-on-bone changes that would otherwise be missed on a standard AP x-ray film.

gold standard for evaluation of articular surface lesions, MRI is currently considered the best noninvasive means of diagnosis.[5] We have found that sequences obtained with a standard 1.5–T magnet at thinner slice thicknesses and longer acquisition times have provided excellent imaging of the articular surfaces.[6] Our standard series have been published and are outlined in Tables 3–1 and 3–2.

Setting up slice sequences that are orthogonal to the articular surfaces to be imaged is important for obtaining

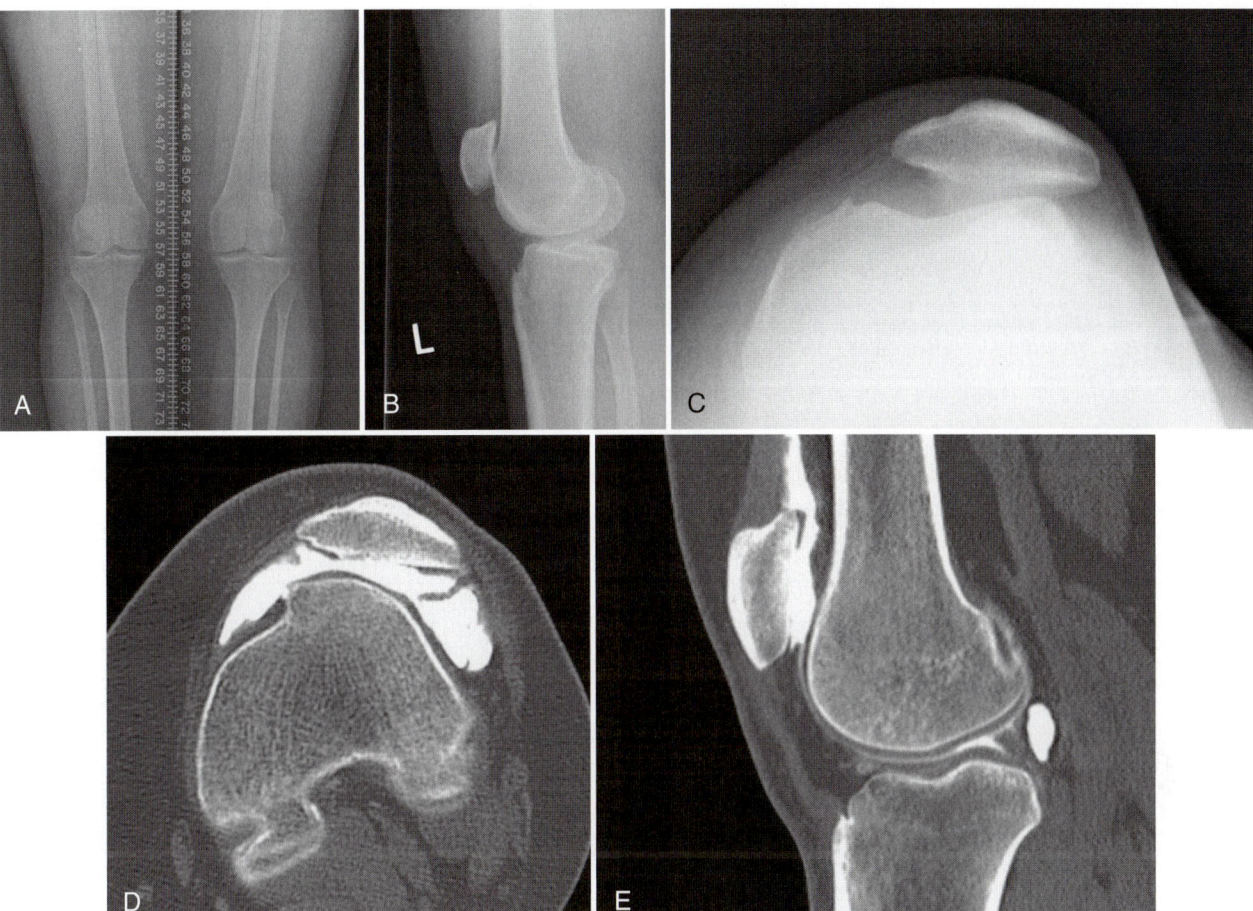

Figure 3–5 *A,* Cropped image of long alignment x-ray film in a 19-year-old woman with severe anterior knee pain and recurrent dislocations. The left knee is most symptomatic. Axial alignment is neutral to slight varus. *B,* Lateral x-ray film demonstrates lack of a "crossing sign" of Dejour[4] of the proximal trochlea as the patella engages the sulcus. The trochlea is either barrel shaped or convex at its entry site. *C,* Skyline x-ray film demonstrates both tilt and subluxation of the patella. Computed tomographic (CT) arthrography very clearly demonstrates dysplasia of the trochlea and loss of articular cartilage on the patella. CT arthrogram is my preferred imaging study for assessment of patellofemoral dysplasia and damage to the articular surfaces. *D,* Axial image of CT arthrogram clearly demonstrates the dysplastic nature of the trochlea with a very prominent and convex proximal lateral facet and cartilage loss to the central and lateral facets of the patella. *E,* Sagittal image of the CT arthrogram demonstrates that the articular surface of the trochlea remains intact; however, the inferior two thirds of the articular cartilage on the patella is completely lost (centrally). Note excellent visualization of the tibiofemoral cartilage and the meniscus on this spiral CT arthrogram. However, a CT arthrogram does not demonstrate the subtle nature of subchondral changes, such as bone marrow edema, or cartilage fluid update, which may indicate softening and early degeneration; these are better visualized with magnetic resonance imaging scan. Hence, both studies occasionally are required to obtain the complete picture of the clinical situation.

accurate full-thickness assessments of articular cartilage (Figure 3–6), otherwise tangential cartilage volume defect artifact may occur.

The literature reports that MRI is 50% to 96% sensitive in detecting articular cartilage lesions.[7] Fat-suppressed T1-weighted gradient echo (e.g., spoiled gradient-recalled echo) and intermediate-weighted fast spin echo (FSE) are among the most commonly used sequences for cartilage imaging. Improved sensitivity to edema-like signal in the subchondral bone marrow may be achieved by the addition of fat suppression to FSE sequences, either with a fat-selective presaturation pulse or a short tau inversion recovery (STIR) sequence.[5,8–10]

The presence of focal edema-like signal in the subchondral marrow may indicate the presence of an overlying cartilage defect, and may, in fact, be easier to detect than the cartilage defect itself (Figure 3–7).[11]

MR arthrography with enhancement of the joint fluid by a contrast agent, performed by either direct injection of a dilute gadolinium-based contrast agent (direct MR arthrography) or intravenous (IV) injection of contrast followed by joint motion (IV or indirect MR arthrography) (Figure 3–8), can be used to provide additional image contrast for evaluation of cartilage defects.[12,13]

Direct MR arthrography has proved useful in evaluating the stability of osteochondral lesions.[14] More recent work

Table 3-1 Standard Knee Protocol for ACI Imaging without Intravenous Contrast Enhancement[6]

Plane	Sequence	TR (ms)	TE (ms)	TI (ms)	ETL	Slice (thickness/gap in mm)	Matrix	Fat Saturation
Coronal	T1W	500–800	20			3.5/0.5	512 × 256	No
Coronal	IRFSE	2,000–3,000	8	160	8	4/1	256 × 192	No
Sagittal	FSE	3,000–4,000	25		8	3.5/0.5	512 × 256	Yes
Sagittal	FSE	3,000–4,000	38		8	3.5/0.5	512 × 256	No
Axial	FSE	3,000–4,000	25 and 130		12	4/1	256 × 256	No
Oblique*	FSE	3,000–4,000	25		8	3.5/0.5	512 × 256	Yes

Note: All scans are performed with a field of view between 14 and 16 cm. Field of view and matrix size are adjusted to patient size and signal-to-noise ratio of the magnetic resonance imaging system.
*Oblique scan is oriented orthogonal to the autologous chondrocyte implantation (ACI) site (e.g., for ACI in the inferior part of the trochlea, an oblique coronal plane parallel to the roof of the intercondylar notch is chosen).
ETL, echo train length; FSE, fast spin echo; IRFSE, inversion recovery fast spin echo; T1W, T1 weighted.

Table 3-2 IV (Indirect) Arthrography Knee Protocol for ACI Imaging[6]

Plane	Sequence	TR (ms)	TE (ms)	TI (ms)	ETL	Slice (thickness/gap in mm)	Matrix	Fat Saturation
Coronal	T1W	500–800	20			3.5/0.5	512 × 256	No
Coronal	IRFSE	2,000–3,000	8	160	8	4/1	256 × 192	No
Sagittal	FSE	3,000–4,000	25		8	3.5/0.5	512 × 256	Yes
Sagittal	FSE	3,000–4,000	38		8	3.5/0.5	512 × 256	No
Axial	FSE	3,000–4,000	25 and 130		12	4/1	256 × 256	No
Sagittal	T1W	500–800	14			3.5/0.5	512 × 256	Yes
Oblique*	T1W	500–800	14			3.5/0.5	512 × 256	Yes

Note: All scans are performed with a field of view between 14 and 16 cm. Field of view and matrix size are adjusted to patient size and signal-to-noise ratio of the magnetic resonance imaging (MRI) system.
Before imaging, 0.1 mmol/kg of intravenous (IV) gadolinium-DTPA is administered. The patient is then asked to perform 15 minutes of motion exercise within the limits of their rehabilitation protocol, usually walking, to promote uniform joint fluid enhancement. MRI can begin any time after the exercise period. Because joint fluid enhancement persists for over 1 hour, the start of imaging can be delayed for up to 45 minutes without severe loss of joint fluid enhancement.
*Oblique scan is oriented orthogonal to the autologous chondrocyte implantation (ACI) site (e.g., for ACI in the inferior part of the trochlea, an oblique coronal plane parallel to the roof of the intercondylar notch, or for a patellar ACI, a true axial image plane is chosen).
ETL, echo train length; FSE, fast spin echo; IRFSE, inversion recovery fast spin echo; T1W, T1 weighted.

From Alparslan L, Minas T, Winalski CS: Magnetic resonance imaging of autologous chondrocyte implantation. Semin Ultrasound CT MR. 2001;22:341–351.

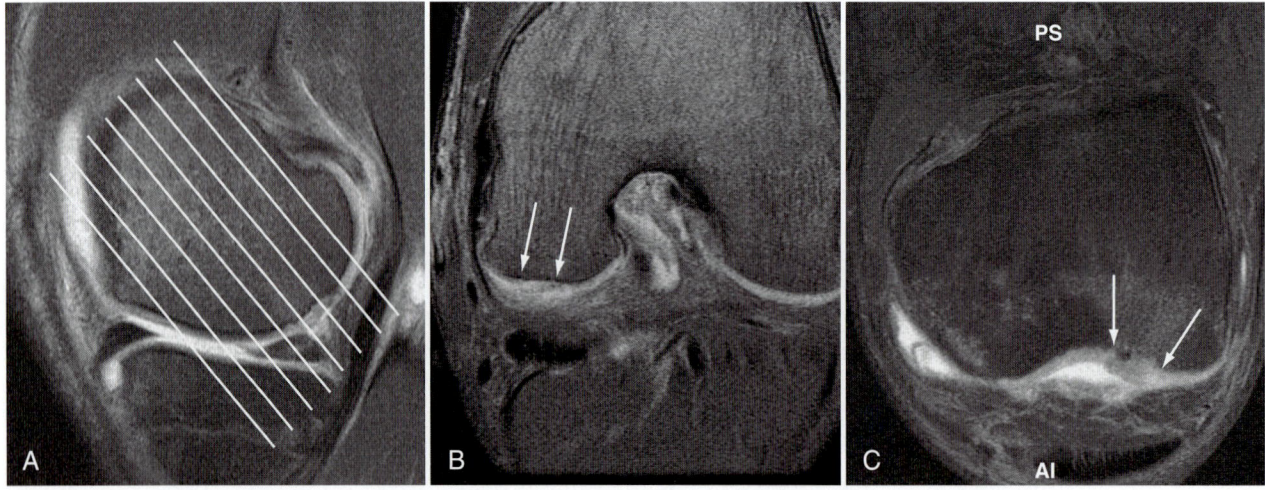

Figure 3-6 Example of an oblique scan being taken to demonstrate *(arrows)* posterior medial femoral condyle autologous chondrocyte implantation (ACI) graft *(B)* and lateral trochlea facet ACI graft *(C)*. The scan must be positioned orthogonal to the graft sites *(A)* to ensure appropriate image acquisition. This underlines the importance of a good relationship between the orthopedist and the musculoskeletal radiologist who is performing the images in order to maximize the information gained from the evaluation. *(Courtesy Dr. Carl Winalski.)*

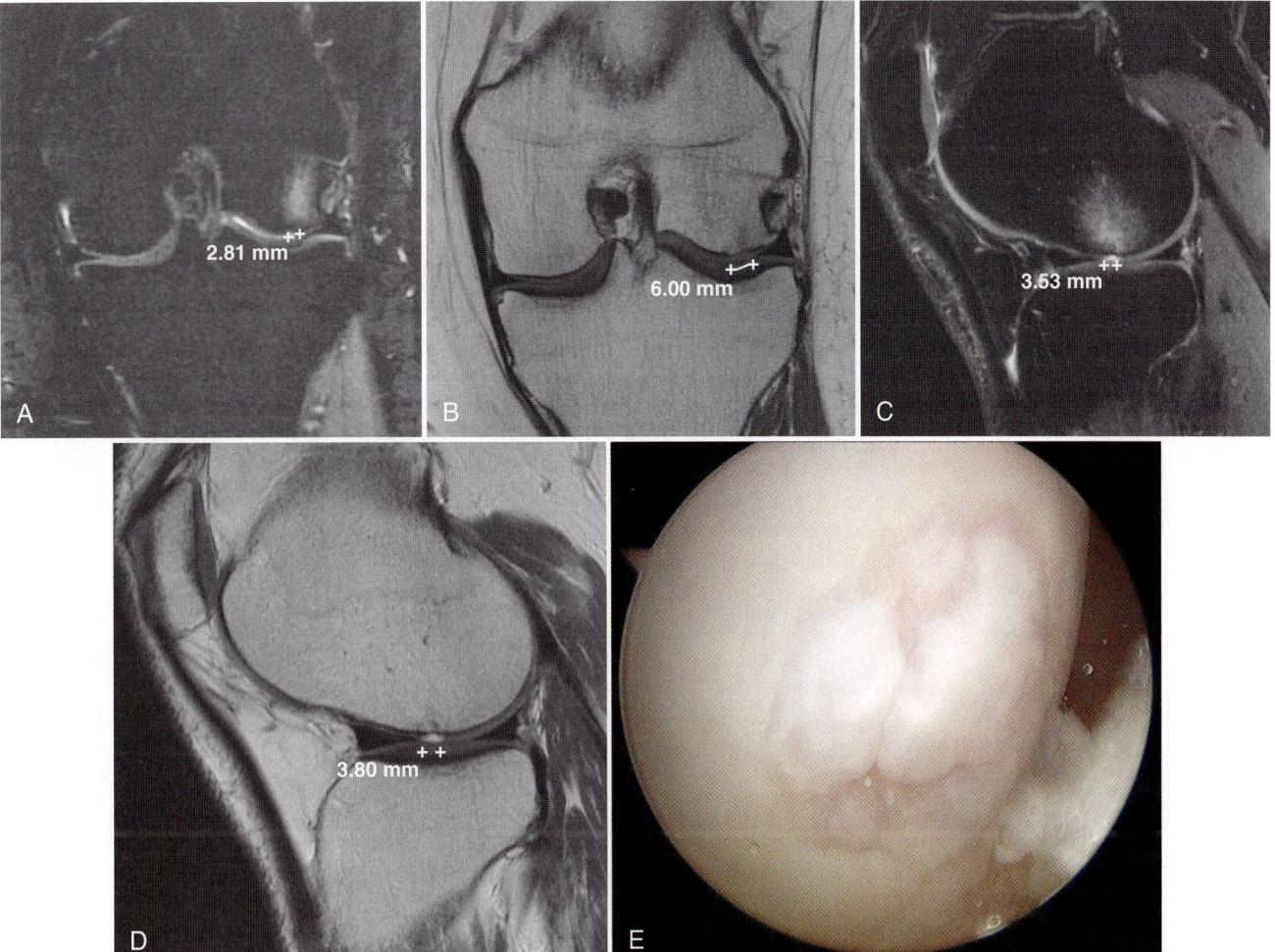

Figure 3-7 Coronal magnetic resonance imaging (MRI) with fat suppression (A) and without fat suppression (B). Bone marrow edema on the fat-suppression image brings attention to the overlying articular cartilage injury, which occurred 2 years after microfracture to the lateral femoral condyle. The defect might have otherwise been missed on the proton density image alone (B). Sagittal MRI fat-suppressed (C) and non–fat-suppressed (D) images of the same patient demonstrating bone marrow edema that brings attention to the small overlying articular cartilage defect. E, Arthroscopic appearance of cartilage defect shown by MRI 2 years after microfracture. This patient had a bony repair tissue with large intralesional osteophyte formation and a thin fibrous film covering it.

has shown the ability to determine the relative proteoglycan concentration of articular cartilage in vivo using an IV MR arthrography technique called *delayed gadolinium-enhanced magnetic resonance imaging of cartilage* (dGEMRIC) (Figure 3–9).[15] This technique holds great promise not only for following the progression or regression of a cartilage lesion but also for noninvasively evaluating the success of a cartilage repair by assessing the progression of glycosaminoglycan synthesis (Figure 3–10).[16]

Although MRI has proved very sensitive for detecting defects, it has limitations with regard to accurately defining the depth (grade) and size of articular cartilage lesions. The accuracy of MRI in detecting, grading, and sizing defects is very sensitive to the acquisition parameters used. Because most diagnostic difficulties arise from partial volume artifacts caused by a combination of the curved surfaces of the joint surfaces and the relatively large voxel dimensions of MR images, close attention should be paid to obtaining the highest-resolution images possible. In our experience, we have found that MR images tend to underestimate the size and depth of cartilage lesions, that significant lesions may exhibit very subtle findings on MR images, and that lesions may be visualized accurately on only one slice plane (Figure 3–11).[17]

Despite these limitations, the sensitivity of MRI for articular cartilage defects is valuable not only for the diagnosis of a cartilage lesions but also for planning treatment, particularly of the knee. For example, when considering a valgus-producing high tibial osteotomy or unicompartmental arthroplasty for a knee with varus alignment due to severe medial compartment cartilage loss, it is important to assess the status of the articular cartilage in the joint compartments. If significant cartilage lesions are present

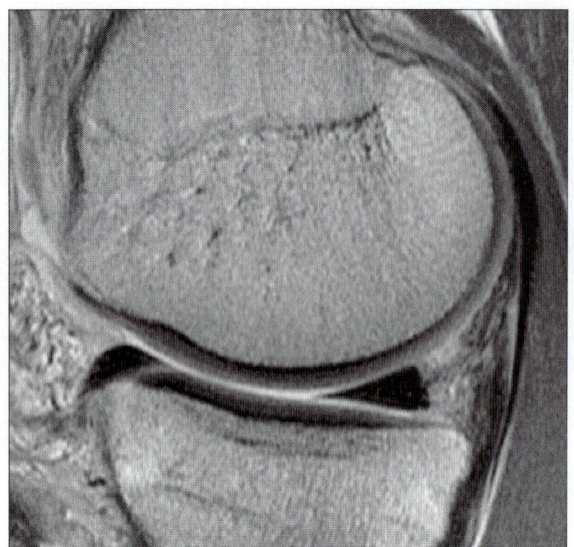

Figure 3-8 Enhancement of the articular surface with intravenous magnetic resonance arthrography demonstrates an excellent interface between cartilage and joint space on the sagittal image of the medial femoral condyle. *(Courtesy Dr. Carl Winalski).*

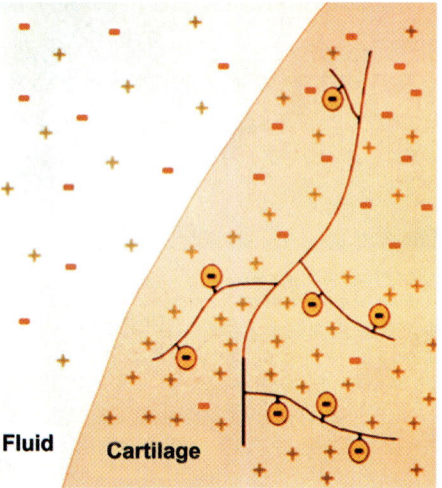

Figure 3-9 Schematic delayed gadolinium-enhanced magnetic resonance imaging of cartilage (dGEMRIC) works on the premise that proteoglycans found in articular cartilage are negatively charged molecules. When the gadolinium-DTPA^{2-} intraarticular contrast agent is allowed to set and equilibrate over time, the distribution of gadolinium-DTPA in the articular cartilage will be inversely proportional to the proteoglycan content of the articular cartilage. Abnormal areas will have a lower T1 signal, so T1 maps will quantify abnormal areas in the articular cartilage. A clinical example is given in Figure 3-10.

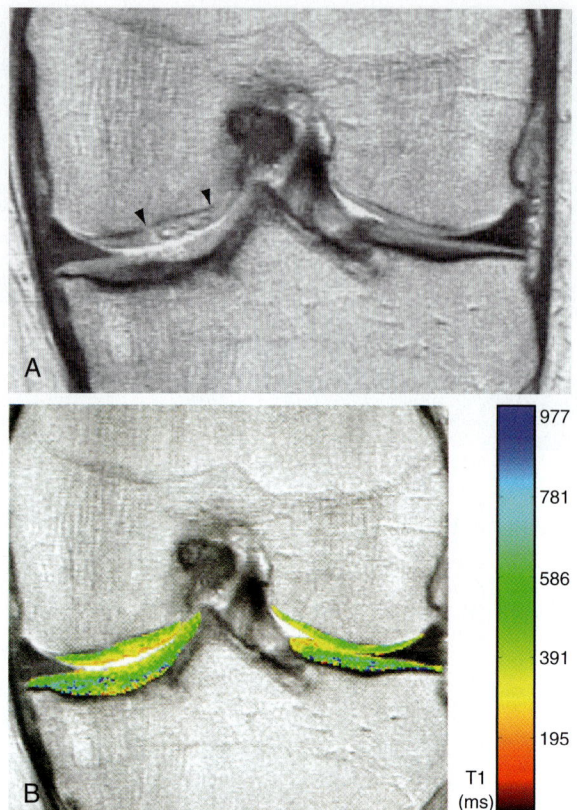

Figure 3-10 *A,* Non-delayed gadolinium-enhanced magnetic resonance imaging of cartilage (dGEMRIC). *Arrows* indicate autologous chondrocyte implantation (ACI) on the medial femoral condyle (MFC). The patient is doing well and is clinically symptom free. The highest numbers on the dGEMRIC scale represent high proteoglycan content and are *blue-green* in color. The lowest numbers in *yellow-red* represent lessened proteoglycan content. The highest proteoglycan content is generally in the deep and middle layers of the articular cartilage, as is seen in this image. *Yellow* represents the fibrous surface of the periosteum on the MFC of this ACI repair or the fibrous lamina splendens of the native articular cartilage. *(Courtesy Dr. Carl Winalski.)*

in the other lateral and patellofemoral joint compartments, the osteotomy or unicompartmental arthroplasty may fail to relieve symptoms because of the increased load on this diseased cartilage produced by the change in the mechanical axis. Prior to surgery, the overall assessment of the cartilage is traditionally done arthroscopically. This arthroscopy is not required for performance of the surgery and potentially adds morbidity and expense. However, preoperative MRI that can accurately assess the status of the articular cartilage in all compartments can alert the surgeon to the presence of cartilage abnormalities in other portions of the joint and help determine the feasibility of reconstructive procedures that address only specific compartments of the knee. Furthermore, such an assessment can help physicians better prepare their patients for the treatment most likely to be performed than the standard combination of diagnostic arthroscopy followed by either a unicompartmental treatment approach or total arthroplasty. Currently we use global assessment of knee cartilage by MRI to exclude patients from unicompartmental therapy when cartilage lesions are found in other compartments.[17]

A similar approach has been suggested for preoperative assessment of the knee prior to meniscal allograft surgery.[18]

MRI is also valuable in assessing the status of articular cartilage repair tissue after reconstructive efforts.[19,20]

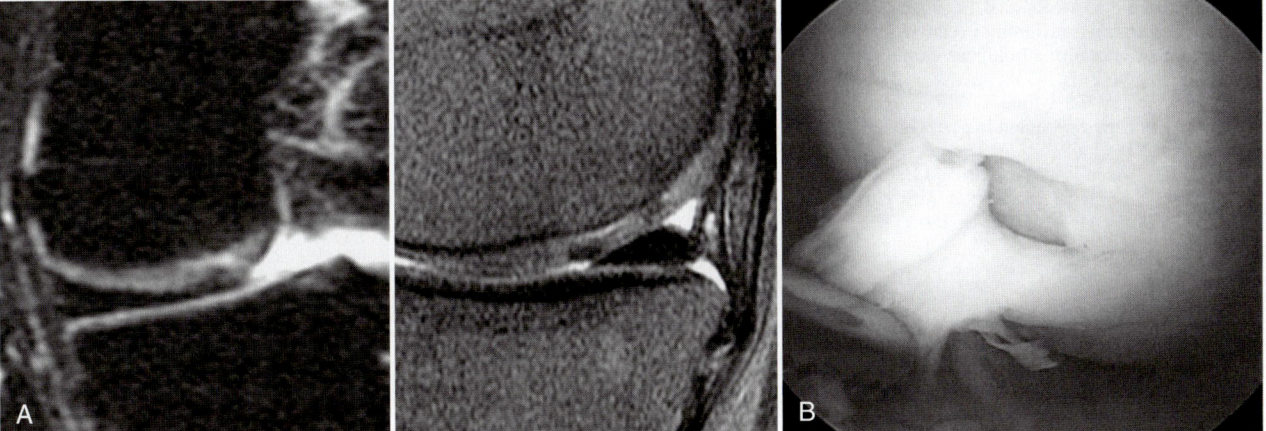

Figure 3–11 *A,* Magnetic resonance imaging (MRI) of fast spin echo with fat-suppressed and non–fat-suppressed sequences demonstrating subtle fluid signal under articular cartilage. This chondral flap was confirmed by arthroscopy. *(Courtesy Dr. Carl Winalski.) B,* Undermined articular cartilage at the time of arthroscopy noted by MRI scan.

It can assess repair site surface congruity and incorporation following many repair techniques as well as identify many of the complications that may occur following cartilage repair. Presently, the application of carefully performed MRI studies may preclude the need for invasive arthroscopic evaluation of articular cartilage lesions and reconstructions.

In summary, knowledge of existing radiographic patterns of wear for medial and lateral tibiofemoral disease, patellofemoral dysplasia, and ACL deficiency assists in subtle diagnoses that are critical for understanding a patient's disease pattern. In addition to a careful history, physical examination, and high-quality digital x-rays and long alignment x-rays, the surgeon should have a good idea of the diagnosis of the patient's clinical disability. High-resolution MRI scan using a standard 1.5-T magnet, set with the appropriate sequences, slice orientation, and image acquisition time with the possibility of image contrast, will give excellent quality assessment of the articular cartilage surfaces of the knee joint. As a result of the high-quality software available that limits artifact from prostheses, computed tomographic scan with image contrast may complement and supplement the images obtained with MRI scan to specifically help address bony deficiencies with osteoarticular fragments, maltracking of the patella and trochlea dysplasia, and articular, meniscal, or ligamentous injury associated with unicompartmental knee replacements.

Because of the excellent quality of MRI and computed tomography imaging now available, I have found that arthroscopy is rarely needed for diagnosing articular cartilage injury and treatment planning. The key to high-quality imaging is a team approach with a dedicated musculoskeletal radiologist who understands the needs of the orthopedist and sets the parameters for the images needed.

REFERENCES

1. Rosenberg T, Paulos L, Parker RD, et al. The forty-five-degree posteroanterior flexion weight bearing radiograph of the knee. *J Bone Joint Surg Am.* 1988;70(10):1479–1483.
2. Ahlback S. Osteoarthrosis of the knee: a radiographic investigation. *Acta Radiol Suppl.* 1968;277:7–72.
3. Harmon MK, Marcovich GD, Banks SA, Hodge W. Wear patterns on tibial plateaus from varus and valgus osteoarthritic knees. *Clin Orthop Relat Res.* 1998;352:149–158.
4. Dejour H, Walch G, Nove-Josserand L, Guier C. Factors of patellar instability: an anatomic radiographic study. *Knee Surg Sports Traumatol Arthrosc.* 1994;2:19–26.
5. Recht M, Bobic V, Burstein D, et al. Magnetic resonance imaging of articular cartilage. *Clin Orthop Relat Res.* 2001;391:S379–S396.
6. Alparslan L, Minas T, Winalski CS. Magnetic resonance imaging of autologous chondrocyte implantation. *Semin Ultrasound CT MR.* 2001;22(4):341–351.
7. Winalski CS, Minas T. Evaluation of chondral injuries by magnetic resonance imaging: repair assessments. *Oper Tech Sports Med.* 2000;8(2):108–119.
8. Disler DG, Peters TL, Muscoreil SJ, et al. Fat-suppressed spoiled GRASS imaging of knee hyaline cartilage: technique optimization and comparison with conventional MR imaging. *AJR Am J Radiol.* 1994;163(4):887–892.
9. Potter HG, Linklater JM, Allen AA, Hannafin JA, Haas SB. Magnetic resonance imaging of articular cartilage in the knee. An evaluation with use of fast-spin-echo imaging. *J Bone Joint Surg Am.* 1998;80(9):1276–1284.
10. Recht MP, Kramer J, Marcelis S, et al. Abnormalities of articular cartilage in the knee: analysis of available MR techniques. *Radiology.* 1993;187(2):473–478.
11. Rubin DA, Harner CD, Costello JM. Treatable chondral injuries in the knee: frequency of associated focal subchondral edema. *AJR Am J Radiol.* 2000;174(4):1099–1106.
12. Kramer J, Recht MP, Imhof H, Stiglbauer R, Engel A. Postcontrast MR arthrography in assessment of cartilage lesions. *J Comput Assist Tomogr.* 1994;18(2):218–224.
13. Winalski CS, Aliabadi P, Wright RJ, et al. Enhancement of joint fluid with intravenously administered gadopentetate dimeglumine: technique, rationale, and implications. *Radiology.* 1993;187(1):179–185.
14. Kramer J, Stiglbauer R, Engel A, Prayer L, Imhof H. MR contrast arthrography (MRA) in osteochondrosis dissecans. *J Comput Assist Tomogr.* 1992;16(2):254–260.
15. Bashir A, Gray ML, Boutin RD, Burstein D. Glycosaminoglycan in articular cartilage: in vivo assessment with delayed Gd(DTPA)(2-)-enhanced MR imaging. *Radiology.* 1997;205(2):551–558.

16. Gillis A, Bashir A, McKeon B, Scheller A, Gray ML, Burstein D. Magnetic resonance imaging of relative glycosaminoglycan distribution in patients with autologous chondrocyte transplants. *Invest Radiol*. 2001;36(12):743–748.
17. Azer N, Winalski CS, Minas T. MR imaging for surgical planning and postoperative assessment in early osteoarthritis. *Arthritis Imaging*. 2004;42(1):43–60.
18. Potter HG, Rodeo SA, Wickiewicz TL, Warren RF. MR imaging of meniscal allografts: correlation with clinical and arthroscopic outcomes. *Radiology*. 1996;198(2):509–514.
19. Alparslan L, Winalski CS, Boutin RD, Minas T. Postoperative magnetic resonance imaging of articular cartilage repair. *Semin Musculoskelet Radiol*. 2001;5(4):345–363.
20. Gold GE, Bergman AG, Pauly JM, et al. Magnetic resonance imaging of knee cartilage repair. *Top Magn Reson Imaging*. 1998;9(6):377–392.

Chapter 4

Patient Evaluation, Cartilage Defect, and Evidence: Putting It All Together

Tom Minas, MD, MS

THE DECISION TO PROCEED WITH JOINT PRESERVATION
   The History
   Patient Characteristics

INJURED KNEE
   Critical Cartilage Defect Size
      Prevalence of Articular Cartilage Injury

   The Asymptomatic Defect

TREATMENT OF SYMPTOMATIC DEFECTS
   Options

EVIDENCE
   Microfracture
   Autologous Chondrocyte Implantation

   Osteochondral Autograft Transplantation
   Osteochondral Allograft Transplantation

AREAS OF UNCERTAINTY
   Study Design and Indications
   Background Factors
   Guidelines
   Recommendations

THE DECISION TO PROCEED WITH JOINT PRESERVATION

The History

In order for a surgeon to have a successful relationship with a patient, the desires, needs, and expectations of the patient must be balanced with what is possible. The surgeon must use his or her best judgment and draw upon the best available evidence and his or her own experience and skills to match these goals. If this is not possible, then the patient should be referred to an expert on the condition. Patients often present with pain and limitation of function. They are often anxious and have different reasons for the appointment. Determining the pathology and considering surgical options may not necessarily be the patient's goal.

An opening questions such as "What is your goal in coming to see me today?" usually helps to direct the surgeon's line of questioning and the treatment options offered to the patient. The patient may respond as follows:

"I have knee pain. I want to know what is causing it and if it can be treated with physical therapy."

"I have knee pain and a family history of osteoarthritis, and I want to avoid knee replacement surgery."

"I have been referred to see you by Dr. X for a specific knee reconstructive procedure."

"I have no pain, but I was sent here because I have a cartilage defect."

Alternatively, the patient may be self-referred based on his or her own ambitions. This is becoming more commonplace in the modern age of the Internet because patients are often well informed and wish to take matters into their own hands ("empowerment of the patient"). Figure 4–1 illustrates this concept. A useful tool for developing a healthy relationship with the patient is the five *E*s (Figure 4–2).

Cartilage repair and joint preservation are relatively new topics in the orthopedic management of young patients, as no large cohorts of patients have received treatment or been followed for the long term. Information obtained from the Internet is not always reliable, is not peer reviewed, and may be market driven; therefore, it is up to the orthopedic surgeon to know the existing evidence and to present it to the patient as an educator, patient advocate, and doctor.

Patient Characteristics

The surgeon's recommendation of treatment options may well depend on patient characteristics. A patient who has a

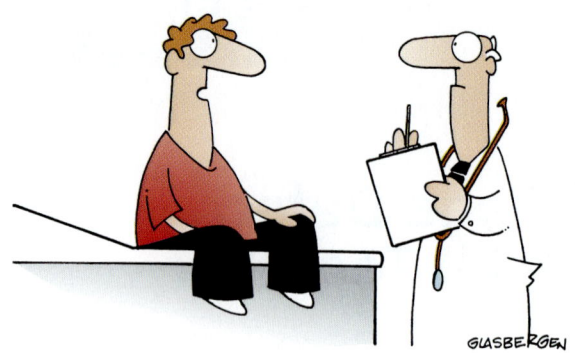

Figure 4–1 Empowerment of the patient. Copyright 2005 by Randy Glasbergen.

high sense of vitality and an optimistic outlook with strong social supports has demonstrated a good clinical outcome with almost any surgical procedure. We reviewed our clinical outcome data using the Medical Outcomes Study 36-Item Health Survey (SF-36)[1] and noted that vitality and social supports played strong into a positive clinical outcome with regard to physical pain relief and well-being (presented at the International Cartilage Repair Society 2002). I have also found that patients who are athletic at baseline and had a relatively acute injury less than 1 year do better clinically after surgery.[2–4] It is suspected that as the athlete becomes deconditioned, the injury becomes chronic, with thickened subchondral bone and expanding margins such that both the patient and the lesion require more extensive rehabilitation. Obesity is another factor that surgeons encounter. It is approaching epidemic proportions in the United States, with approximately 30% of the population being considered obese. The osteotomy literature had demonstrated that body weight greater than 1.32 times normal adversely affects the outcome and survivorship of osteotomy surgery.[5] Obesity has also been shown to correlate with an increased incidence of osteoarthritis, which presumably corresponds to enlargement of an existing cartilage defect, or factors adversely toward a cartilage repair procedure because of the force across the regenerative tissue. Counseling the patient regarding weight loss prior to a biologic repair procedure may actually prevent the need for the procedure based on symptom relief with weight loss. For the morbidly obese with body mass index (BMI) greater than 40, surgical gastric bypass surgery may be necessary. Some insurance carriers in the United States will not allow cartilage repair for patients with BMI greater than 30; for other carriers the cutoff is BMI of 35. Further research on the correlation between weight and progression of cartilage damage is necessary.

Patients who are taking medications for depression or anxiety and who have addictive baseline behavior patterns, such as alcohol consumption, smoking, or narcotic usage for pain outside of the postoperative setting, tend to demonstrate difficult postoperative patient management patterns. These factors must be delineated preoperatively and addressed individually. Providing preoperative counseling and maximizing medications for patients who have depression and anxiety in order to improve their postoperative sense of well-being and compliance is important. I do not operate on patients who are taking narcotics for baseline pain management of chondral defect or osteoarthritis until they are weaned off to a minimum baseline amount of narcotics that will allow good postoperative pain management. Smoking has demonstrated an adverse effect on bone healing and spinal fusions, long bone fractures, and trauma and on proteoglycan formation during cartilage healing. For this reason, we do not offer biologic repair to smokers until they have completed a smoking cessation program. If patients are unwilling or unable to stop smoking and they are at the transition age for a prosthetic reconstruction, then a unicompartmental, bicompartmental, or total knee arthroplasty is recommended.

INJURED KNEE

As discussed in Chapter 1 on the characteristics that predispose to progression of cartilage injuries to osteoarthritis, a thorough evaluation that assesses the background factors of cartilage loss is critical to the potential success of a biologic preserving procedure. Radiographic studies to delineate long axial alignment of the limb relative to the knee joint and weight-bearing x-ray films in extension and flexion to assess joint space narrowing or complete obliteration (a good screening tool to rule out the possibility of cartilage repair and recommend osteotomy or arthroplasty in isolation) must be performed.

A careful physical examination will note the patient's gait pattern, varus or valgus thrust of the leg, atrophy of the musculature, range of motion of the tibiofemoral joint, effusion in the knee, status of the patellofemoral joint with regard to quadriceps angle, presence or absence of a J-sign from extension into flexion, mobility of the patella (medial, lateral, proximal or distal), possible contracture of the patellofemoral articulation, crepitus in the patellofemoral or tibiofemoral joint, and instability of the collaterals and cruciates. The physical examination also is important for determining the localization of the pain, that is, whether medial tibiofemoral, lateral tibiofemoral, patellofemoral, or a combination.

At this juncture, a tentative diagnosis is made based on the patient's history, x-ray studies, and physical examination. Magnetic resonance imaging (MRI) scan at this time is helpful for making an accurate diagnosis without proceeding to arthroscopy.

If a cartilage injury is suspected, a high-resolution MRI scan with intraarticular dye enhancement (either

PATIENT FIRST TIP

To consistently provide excellent customer service always remember to use the **5 E's** in interactions with every patient or family member, whether in person on the phone

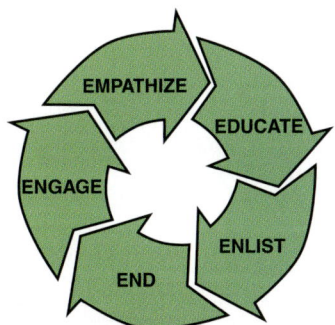

Step 1: ENGAGE

Build a relationship with the patient!
- Sit/stand straight keep your body relaxed
- Make eye contact
- Give the patient your attention
- Have an appropriate rate and volume of speech
- Speak clearly and pronunciate

Step 2: EMPATHIZE

Assure the patient feels seen, heard and accepted!
- Step into the patient's shoes to view their situation and try to understand their feelings
- Refrain from attaching your own judgment or feelings to the situation
- Offer a gesture of empathy (provide a tissue, nod your head to show you are listening, offer a blameless apology)

Step 3: EDUCATE

Inform the patient and answer questions/concerns!
- Define the problem, separating it from its emotional content try to understand their feelings
- Check continually for understanding so that you remain on the same page
- Describe what you can do and what your limitations are (use positive language)

Step 4: ENLIST

Invite the patient to collaborate as a decision maker on their plan of care!
- Invite the patient to discuss their situation
- Explain the available options
- Let the patient choose what they think/feel is best
- Support two-way conversations to empower the patient
- Agree on a solution

Step 5: END

Insure you have made a positive connection with the patient!
- Summarize the key points and what has been agreed upon
- Review next steps (ensure you follow-up on what it is promised)
- Ask if the patient has any remaining questions
- End with your own personal touch and 'goodbye and thank you'

Adapted from Carroll, J. & Keller, V., 'E4 Model'
Bayer Institute of Healthcare Communication, 1992

Figure 4–2 The five *E*s is a useful tool for developing a healthy relationship with the patient.

indirect intravenous gadolinium arthrogram[6] or direct intraarticular arthrogram) will maximize the information obtained prior to making any recommendations for surgery. In this way, leg alignment and normal cartilage space are assessed, cartilage defect(s) is delineated, underlying bone marrow edema or cysts are identified, volume and status of the menisci are determined, and preservation of the anterior and posterior cruciate ligaments is noted. Contracture of the Hoffa fat pad as well as intra-articular adhesions, loose bodies, synovitis, and effusion may be identified.

If the patient was referred from another orthopedist, then prior arthroscopic photographs and operative notes may be valuable for accurately making a diagnosis and treatment plan. At this stage, the diagnosis usually is made based on the background factors responsible for the pain and articular cartilage loss and possibly the size of the defects present.

Critical Cartilage Defect Size

Cartilage defects may be present and minimally symptomatic if the defect is small or the activity level is insufficient to cause progression of disease. Previous studies have reported that 2-cm^2 lesions coexist without degenerative changes in the knee up to 4 years after onset of symptoms.[7,8] More recent studies have shown no difference in clinical outcomes in anterior cruciate ligament–injured and stabilized knees with 2.1-cm^2 chondral defects at 15 years compared with controls in 36 knees.[9] This finding supports the idea that progression of lesions smaller than 2 cm^2 is unlikely and that 2 cm^2 may represent a critical defect size. Based on these studies, early algorithms delineated 2 cm^2 as a small defect.[10–12]

A critical size defect is considered a defect that shoulders the subchondral bone well from stimulus, thus lessening the symptoms from subchondral bone nerve stimulation and the abrasive effects of subchondral bone on the opposing articular cartilage and therefore the development of bipolar changes. A larger defect that is poorly shouldered will damage the opposing articular surface, resulting in progressive joint space cartilage loss, will remain symptomatic, and will enlarge quickly because of the excessive force on the edges of the defect. Figure 4–3 demonstrates this principle, which we described previously.[12]

A relatively small defect that is symptomatic may be either treated by arthroscopic debridement of the unstable margins and then left alone, or stabilized with a repair tissue of fibrocartilaginous or hyaline cartilage. However, a larger poorly shouldered chondral defect will require a repair tissue with the same or nearly the same viscoelastic and mechanical properties as normal hyaline cartilage (Figure 4–4). Procedures that may

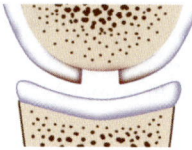 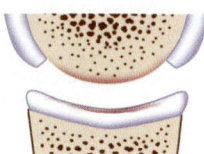

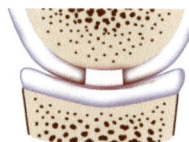 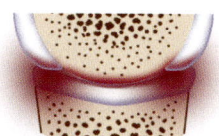

Figure 4–3 A small well-shouldered chondral defect on the *left* prevents damage to the opposing surface because the shoulders of the defect support the subchondral bone. However, the defect on the *right* excessively overloads the shoulders, leading to premature breakdown of the supporting surface with abrasive changes developing on the opposing tibial surface. Persistent symptoms and degenerative changes are likely in this situation. A repair tissue that stabilizes the small defect usually is adequate. A repair tissue that simulates the normal viscoelastic mechanical properties of hyaline cartilage in the larger defect is necessary if the repair is to allow high-demand activities and be durable.

produce hyaline-like cartilage for this situation are discussed in the remainder of this chapter (Figure 4–5).

Prevalence of Articular Cartilage Injury

In making recommendations to the patient, it is important to recognize the defects that are causing symptoms.

The spectrum of disease entities that cause damage to the articular cartilage ranges from single, focal chondral defects to more advanced degenerative disease. Focal chondral defects result from various etiologies. An approximately even number of patients have reported a traumatic versus an insidious onset of symptoms. Athletic activities are the most common inciting event associated with the diagnosis of chondral lesions.[13] Traumatic events and developmental etiologies such as osteochondritis dissecans predominate in younger age groups. Several large studies have found high-grade chondral lesions (Outerbridge grades III and IV; Figure 4–6) in 5% to 11% of younger patients (<40 years) and in up to 60% of older patients.[13–15] The most common locations for these defects are the medial femoral condyle (up to 32%) and the patella.[14,15] Most are detected incidentally during meniscectomy or anterior cruciate ligament reconstruction.[13,16] Many of these defects are incidental in nature and asymptomatic.

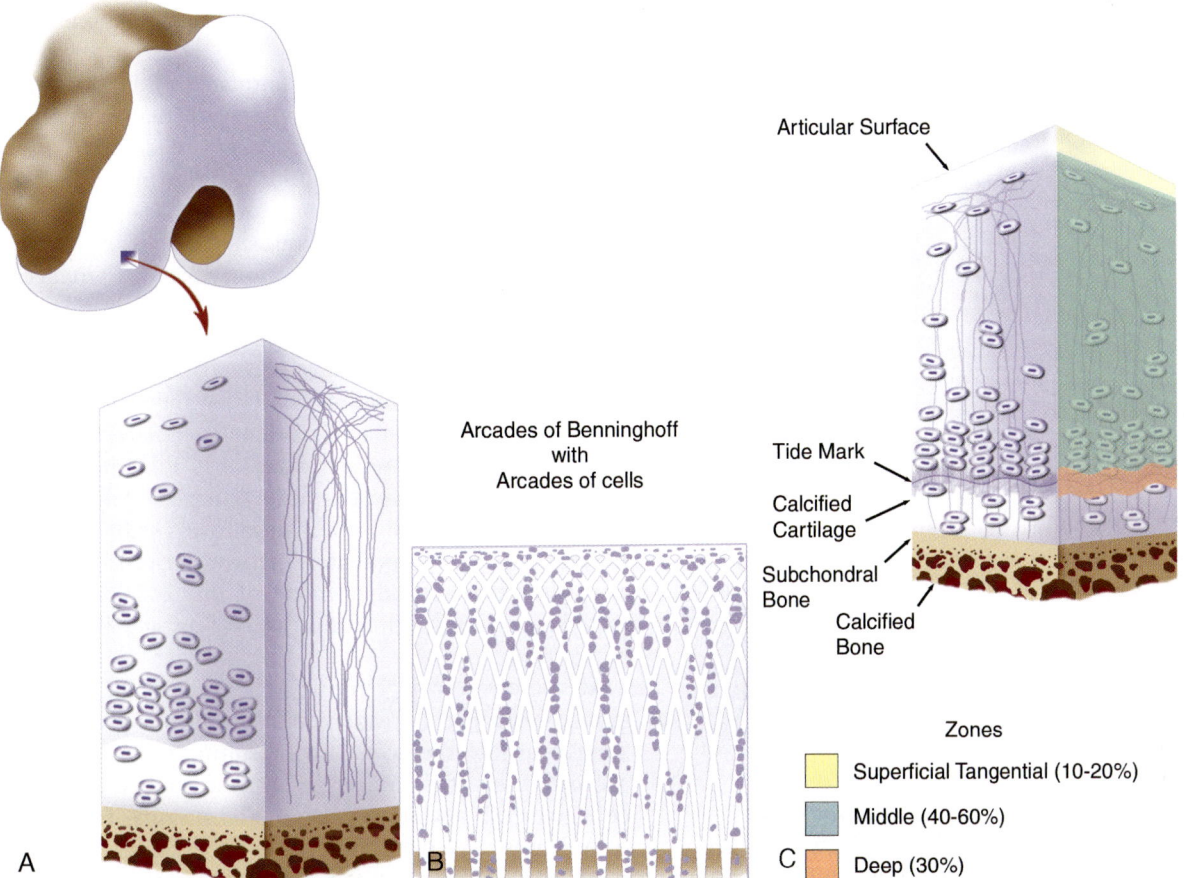

Figure 4-4 *A,* Articular cartilage can be thought of as a viscoelastic mechanical tissue that integrates into the subchondral bone, allowing force transmission through an "osteochondral unit." Restoration of the osteochondral unit via cartilage repair is the goal. *B,* Type II collagen, unique to articular cartilage, is arranged vertically. It then is anchored to the subchondral bone at the level of the tidemark of articular cartilage, running parallel to the articular surface and forming a regularly arranged scaffold that is well bonded to the bone and produces the framework for articular cartilage (arcades of Benninghoff). Characteristic deep middle and superficial layers of cartilage cells with their distinct behavioral properties are shown on the *right.* *C,* Schematic diagram of cartilage layers.

The Asymptomatic Defect

The patient may have a known cartilage defect that is relatively asymptomatic. The question then becomes, "Will the lesion progress over time?" I have counseled patients in this situation to modify their activities to avoid impact and torsional sports and to cross-train with activities such as cycling, swimming, elliptical trainer, and upper-body weight training. These patients are followed-up with annual high-resolution MRI scans to determine whether the defect size is enlarging (Figure 4–7). If no enlargement is seen, annual weight-bearing x-ray films are obtained to determine joint space loss or the onset of symptoms, which include activity-related effusions of the knee despite an absence of pain, which indicates a degenerative response of the joint. If the disease has progressed or the patient is concerned about losing the opportunity for cartilage repair and preservation of the joint, a treatment-based discussion ensues. The discussion is based on the defect size, existing background factors, and the treatment options available surgically versus nonoperative intervention and the possibility of a prosthesis.

TREATMENT OF SYMPTOMATIC DEFECTS

The field of cartilage repair is a recent development within orthopedic surgery, with techniques that continue to evolve. Although no formal treatment algorithms have been agreed upon and validated by prospective comparative trials of emerging techniques, practice-based algorithms have been recommended based upon existing evidence and matching of patient characteristics to treatment efficacy and risks. High-quality outcomes research is needed to provide a better understanding of the efficacy of these procedures and to enable physicians to properly indicate treatment.

An overview of the existing techniques and supporting data is given here to guide surgeons in the

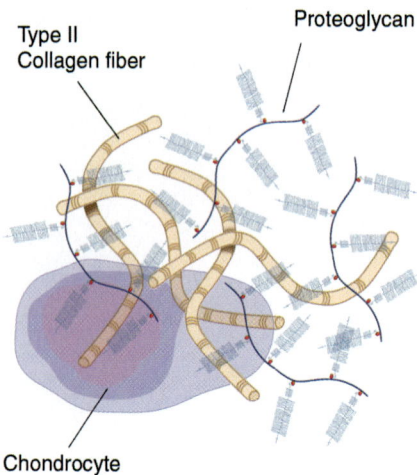

Figure 4-5 Proteoglycans produced by articular chondrocytes are highly negatively charged, attracting and binding to positively charged water molecules and forming a very resilient and unique viscoelastic mechanical tissue. In order for a tissue to withstand large mechanical compressive, torsional, and shearing forces, a reparative tissue that is hyaline-like is required. This is the goal of cartilage repair for large lesions.

indications for treatment of cartilage defects of the knee. In the end, however, practical realities prevail. Surgeons will use the techniques with which they are comfortable and which are available to them and will consider the costs associated with the treatment and the health care system in which they practice.

Options

Until the 1990s, orthopedists were restricted to procedures that aimed to palliate the effects of chondral lesions or attempted to stimulate a healing response initiated from the subchondral bone, resulting in the formation of fibrocartilage to fill the defect. Simple arthroscopic lavage and debridement of lesions has been used since the 1940s in an effort to reduce symptoms resulting from loose bodies and cartilage flaps and is a common first-line treatment, especially for coincidental defects. Arthroscopic debridement on its own has been demonstrated to produce measurable symptomatic improvement. Hubbard[17] noted that grade IV femoral condyle defects randomized to arthroscopic lavage versus debridement did better when they were debrided. Without defect repair, the Lysholm score increased 28 points at 1 year and 21 points at 5 years in more than 50% of patients. Defect size was not measured and radiographic evidence of progression or follow-up arthroscopy was not obtained in that study.

Levy et al[18] noted that debridement for acute small lesions (average 42 mm^2) in 15 young soccer players allowed all players to return to soccer at 10.8 weeks postoperatively, with 6 excellent and 9 good results. One player developed extensive continued delamination. Follow-up was short (1 year).

The natural history of an untreated chondral injury is not yet known, although most agree that even small lesions (<1 cm^2) likely will progress very slowly,[19] with greater than 50% developing osteoarthritis over a 14-year follow-up.

Marrow stimulation techniques, such as drilling, abrasion arthroplasty, and microfracture, attempt to induce a reparative response by perforating the subchondral bone after radical debridement of damaged cartilage and removing the tidemark "calcified" zone to enhance integration of repair tissue. The resultant blood clot and the primitive mesenchymal cells contained within may differentiate into a fibrocartilaginous repair tissue that fills the defect. Unlike hyaline cartilage, this fibrocartilage largely consists of type I collagen and is mechanically less stable and less durable.[20] The pluripotential marrow-derived cells may also form bone, another mode of marrow stimulation technique–related failure that is increasingly becoming recognized.[21]

Restorative cartilage repair techniques such as autologous chondrocyte implantation (ACI) introduce chondrogenic cells into the defect area, resulting in formation of a repair tissue that more closely resembles the type II collagen–rich hyaline cartilage. The original technique of ACI was developed more than 20 years ago[7] and has been used in the United States to treat more than 10,000 patients since its approval by the U.S. Food and Drug Administration (FDA) in 1997. ACI is indicated for the treatment of medium- to large-size chondral defects with no or shallow associated osseous deficits. It originally received FDA approval for application in the femoral condyle (medial, lateral, and trochlea), but it also has been used successfully to treat patellar defects. ACI in its current form is a two-stage procedure consisting of an initial arthroscopic cartilage biopsy followed by a staged reimplantation through an arthrotomy. The next-generation technique, ACI-C (collagen-covered), was developed to reduce the reoperation rate due to hypertrophy of the periosteal patch used to cover the defect. This was achieved by substituting periosteum with a collagen membrane that frequently consists of a porcine type I/III collagen bilayer membrane. The latest generation of ACI, *MACI* (membrane-associated), cultures the chondrocytes directly on the bilayer collagen membrane, which is then implanted arthroscopically or through a mini-open approach with fibrin glue or limited suturing.

Cartilage replacement techniques include osteochondral autograft and allograft transfers, such as the osteochondral autograft transfer system (OATS; Arthrex, Naples, FL), mosaicplasty (Smith & Nephew, Andover, MA), and mega-OATS techniques. Osteochondral autograft transplantation is used to address small- to medium-size defects (1–4 cm^2), often with associated

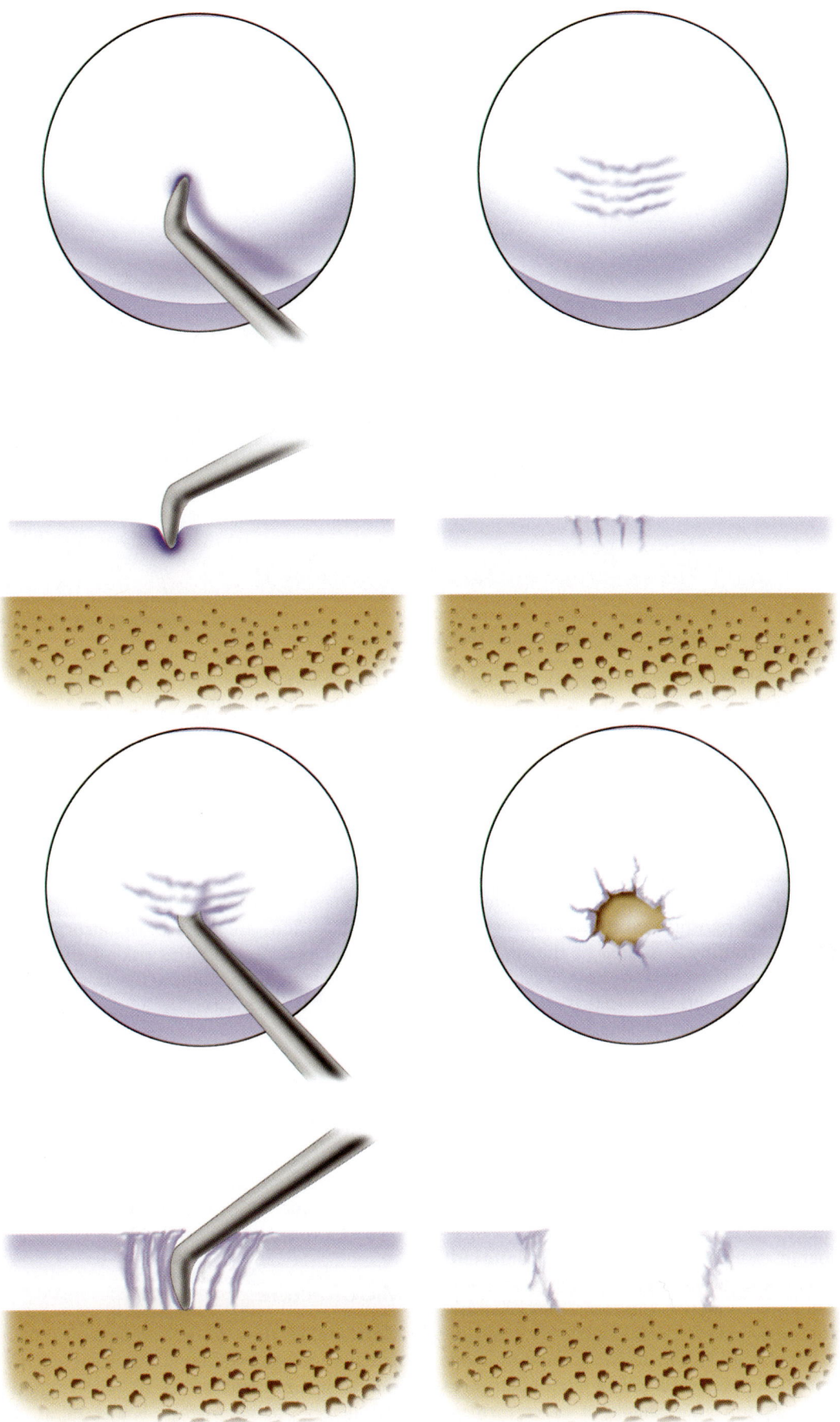

Figure 4-6 Modified Outerbridge classification. Grade 1: intact articular cartilage with softening of the surface. Grade 2: fissuring of the surface up to 50% of the thickness of the articular cartilage. Grade 3: fissuring to the subchondral bone. Grade 4: exposed bone with undermining of cartilaginous tissue. *(From Ref. 40.)*

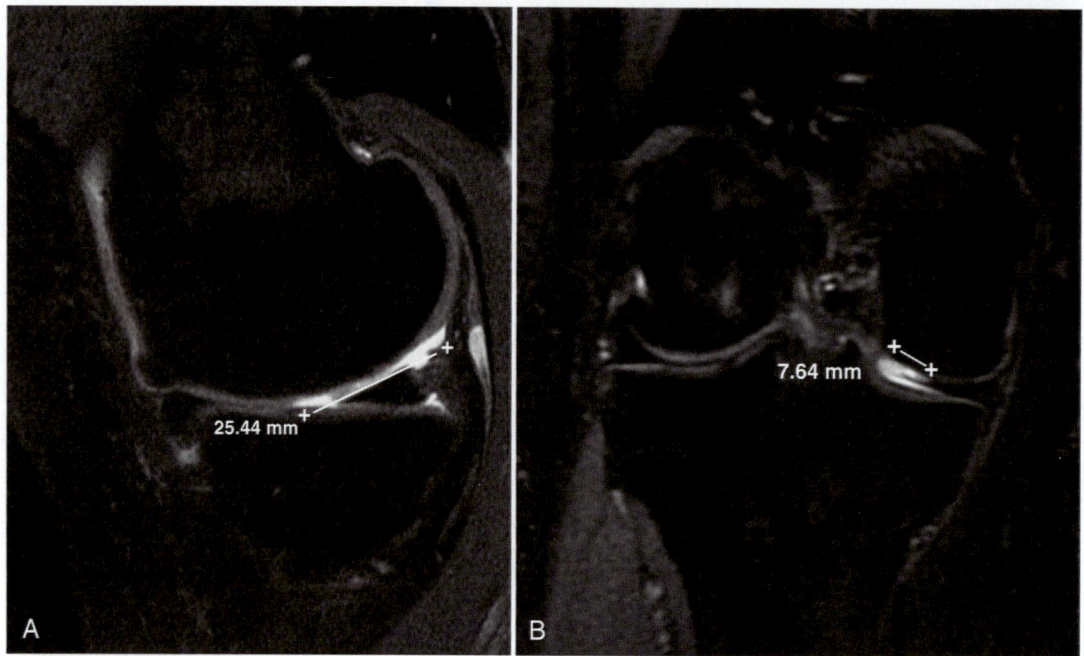

Figure 4-7 High-resolution magnetic resonance (MRI) scan with 20 cc of intravenous gadolinium in a 32-year-old woman who has an asymptomatic medial femoral condyle, Outerbridge grade IV cartilage defect. The patient had been followed for 3 years with consecutive MRI scans to assess articular cartilage degeneration and progression of disease. *Left,* Contrast-enhanced fat-suppressed sagittal image shows the defect is 25 mm long. *Right,* Coronal image shows the defect is 8 mm wide. This long and narrow lesion, which is present in a slim patient with slight valgus to her knee, can be followed nonoperatively. If she were to develop symptoms, effusions, or progression of an enlarging cartilage defect, a discussion regarding cartilage repair would ensue.

bone loss. Osteochondral cylinders are harvested from lesser marginal weight-bearing areas of the knee joint and press fitted into the prepared defect. Commonly, multiple cylinders are transplanted to fill larger defects. Osteochondral autografting is limited by the amount of cartilage that can be harvested without violating the weight-bearing articular surface,[22] that is, "taking from Peter to pay Paul." The main advantage lies in its autogeneity, avoidance of disease transmission, immediate graft availability through harvesting of the patient's own tissue, and decreased cost of this single-stage procedure.

The treatment of chondral defects with fresh osteochondral allografts has garnered significant attention because of its potential to restore and resurface even extensive areas of damaged cartilage and bone. Osteochondral allograft transplantation is used predominantly for the treatment of large and deep osteochondral lesions resulting from osteochondritis dissecans, osteonecrosis, and traumatic osteochondral fractures, but it can also be used to treat peripherally uncontained cartilage and bone defects. Furthermore, osteochondral allografting presents a viable salvage option after failure of other cartilage resurfacing procedures. The main advantages over autograft transplantation are the ability to very closely match the curvature of the articular surface by harvesting the graft from a corresponding location in the donor condyle, the ability to transplant large grafts, and the avoidance of donor site morbidity. The main concerns with allograft transplantation are failure to incorporate with subchondral collapse and the risk of disease transmission (estimated at 1:1.6 million for transmission of human immunodeficiency virus[23]).

EVIDENCE

Following is a review of the published reports on techniques for cartilage repair, evaluating the indications, defect size, locations within the joint, and efficacy of the technique with the levels of evidence of the studies reviewed (summarized in Table 4–1[24]).

Microfracture

Most studies show good outcomes in 60% to 80% of patients. Several studies have attempted to define the indications for microfracture with regard to patient and defect characteristics. Kreuz et al demonstrated improved results in patients younger than 40 years with regard to both validated scores and MRI findings of better fill and quality. They also demonstrated a worsening

Table 4-1 Summary of Published Reports on Techniques for Cartilage Repair

Study	Design (Level of Evidence)	Follow-up Interval (No. of Patients)	Patient Population	Patient Age (Defect Size)	Treatment Group	Results
Kreuz[41]	Prospective (LoE 2)	3 yr (70 patients)	Grade 3 and 4 chondral defects treated with microfracture	30 and 39 yr (average 2.2 cm^2)	Patient age: <40 yr, >40 yr	All groups improved significantly; younger patients improved more. Older patients and patellofemoral lesions in younger patients worsened between 18 and 36 mo.
Kreuz[42]	Prospective (LoE 2)	3 yr (70 patients)	Grade 3 and 4 chondral defects treated with microfracture	40 yr (average 2.2 cm^2)	Defect locations: Femoral condyle, trochlea, tibia, patella	All groups improved significantly, mostly in the femoral condyle group. Results decreased between 18 and 36 mo.
Mithoefer[21]	Case series (LoE 4)	41 mo (48 patients)	Grade 3 and 4 chondral defects treated with microfracture	41 yr (median 2.8 cm^2)	N/A	Significant improvement until 24 mo postoperatively, then deterioration. Poor fill on magnetic resonance imaging correlated with poor outcome. Body mass index >30 associated with poor fill and outcome.
Blevins[26]	Case series (LoE 4)	3.7 yr (140 patients)	Grade 3 and 4 chondral defects treated with microfracture	26 and 38 yr (average 2.2 cm^2)	Activity status: High-level vs recreational athletes	Both groups showed significant improvement. Second-look arthroscopy revealed no improvement of lesion grade in 8% of high-level and 35% of recreational athletes.
Bartlett[31]	RCT (LoE 1)	12 mo (91 patients)	Grade 3 and 4 chondral defects	34 yr (average 6 cm^2)	ACI technique: ACI-C, MACI	No statistically significant differences between groups. Better outcomes in patients younger than 35 yr and with symptoms for <50 mo. Reoperation rate for graft hypertrophy was 9% of ACI-C and 6% of MACI.
Gooding[30]	RCT (LoE 1)	24 mo (68 patients)	Grade 3 and 4 chondral defects	31 yr (average 4.5 cm^2)	ACI technique: ACI-P, ACI-C	Good and excellent results (Cincinnati score) in 74% of ACI-C and 67% of ACI-P, but dissimilar defect locations: 61% of lesions treated with ACI-P were patellar, whereas only 20% of those treated with ACI-C were in this location. Reoperation rate for graft hypertrophy was 36% for ACI-C and 0% for ACI-C.

Continued

Table 4-1 Summary of Published Reports on Techniques for Cartilage Repair—cont'd

Study	Design (Level of Evidence)	Follow-up Interval (No. of Patients)	Patient Population	Patient Age (Defect Size)	Treatment Group	Results
Bentley[28]	RCT (LoE 1)	19 mo (100 patients)	Grade 3 and 4 chondral defects	31 yr (average 4.7 cm^2)	Cartilage repair technique: ACI-C, mosaicplasty	Good and excellent results (Cincinnati score) in 88% of ACI and 69% of mosaicplasty patients. All five patellar mosaicplasties failed. No graft hypertrophy in ACI patients (collagen membrane used).
Knutsen[32]	RCT (LoE 1)	2 yr (80 patients)	Grade 3 and 4 chondral defects	33 yr (average 5 cm^2)	Cartilage repair technique: ACI, microfracture	No statistically significant differences between groups at 2 yr, except SF-36, which was better in the microfracture group. Patients younger than 30 yr and more active (Tegner score >4) did better, regardless of treatment. Defects >4 cm^2 fared worse with microfracture; no similar effect was seen with ACI
Gudas[34]	RCT (LoE 1)	37 mo (57 patients)	Grade 3 and 4 chondral defects	24 yr (average 2.8 cm^2)	Cartilage repair technique: Microfracture, OATS	Good and excellent results in 96% of OATS and 52% of microfracture patients. Return to sports in 93% of OATS and 52% of microfracture patients. Microfracture significantly worse in lesions >2 cm^2, and results deteriorated after 12 mo. Both groups showed better results in patients <30 yr.
Gross[35]	Case series (LoE 4)	10 yr (127 patients)	Osteochondral defects of femur and tibia	27 yr (femur) 43 yrs (tibia)	N/A	Survivorship of 95% at 5 years, 80-85% at 10 years and 65-74% at 15 years
Gortz[36]	Case series (LoE 4)	4.5 yr (43 patients)	Osteochondral defects of femur	35 yr (average 5.9 cm^2)	N/A	Good and excellent results in 88%.

ACI-C, autologous chondrocyte implantation collagen-covered; ACI-P, autologous chondrocyte implantation periosteal-covered; LoE, level of evidence; MACI, autologous chondrocyte implantation membrane–associated; N/A, not applicable; OATS, osteochondral autograft transfer system; RCT, randomized controlled trial; SF-36, Medical Outcomes Study 36-Item Health Survey.

between the 18- and 36-month follow-up scores for all patients in the older age group and for younger patients with patellofemoral defects.[25] In another study, the same authors reported on the association between outcomes and defect locations and found the best outcomes in femoral condyle lesions, whereas those in the patella fared worst.[15] Other authors have described better results in smaller lesions, patients with body mass index less than 30, and shorter duration between onset of symptoms and treatment.[21,26,27]

Autologous Chondrocyte Implantation

Several long-term case series have reported good to excellent results in 70% to 90% of patients after ACI in the knee, depending on the location (patella and femoral condyle) or the clinical series.[4,10] Bentley et al[28] compared ACI-C with mosaicplasty in a prospective randomized controlled trial (RCT) and showed good and excellent results (Cincinnati score) in 88% of ACI patients but in only 69% of mosaicplasty patients. All five patellar mosaicplasties were considered failures. In a similar study by Horas et al,[29] mosaicplasty performed significantly better than ACI. Biopsies obtained from a subgroup of patients uniformly revealed fibrous tissue in all defects treated with ACI. However, that study was limited by the use of nonstandard cell culturing facilities.

In a prospective RCT comparing ACI-P (periosteal-covered) with ACI-C, Gooding et al[30] found no statistically significant differences in clinical outcome, but the reoperation rate for symptomatic graft hypertrophy was 36% in the periosteal covered group versus 0% in the collagen membrane group. Bartlett et al[31] presented a prospective RCT comparing the advanced techniques ACI-C and MACI, and reported no statistically significant differences between the groups. They also found improved outcomes in patients who were younger than 35 years and had preoperative symptoms for less than 50 months. Knutsen et al[32] compared ACI to microfracture and found no significant differences. The SF-36 improved more in the microfracture group, and the authors hypothesized whether this result could be due to the more invasive nature of ACI. Furthermore, they observed better results in younger (<30 years) and more active patients (Tegner score >4). Defects larger than 4 cm^2 fared worse than did smaller lesions after microfracture treatment; no such effect was seen after ACI.

Graft hypertrophy resulting in mechanical symptoms (e.g., clicking, popping) occurs in up to 25% to 30% of patients, typically 7 to 9 months after the procedure[33] and can be addressed with arthroscopic debridement of the hypertrophic tissue. Newer techniques such as ACI-C and MACI have decreased the rate of symptomatic graft hypertrophy to less than 10%.[31]

Osteochondral Autograft Transplantation

Patients treated with osteochondral autograft transplantation experienced good to excellent results for approximately 90% of condylar lesions, 80% of tibial defects, and 70% of trochlear lesions.[25] The technique is technically demanding arthroscopically and is more reproducible by open or mini-open techniques. The treatment of patellar defects remains controversial, with some groups reporting almost universal failure in this location.[28] Gudas et al[34] compared OATS with microfracture in a group of athletes and demonstrated good and excellent results in 96% of patients treated with OATS versus 52% of those treated with microfracture. Return to sports was 93% with OATS and 52% with microfracture. Microfracture performed significantly worse for lesions larger than 2 cm^2, and results started to deteriorate after the 12-month follow-up examination. Both groups showed better results in patients younger than 30 years.[34]

Osteochondral Allograft Transplantation

Gross et al[35] reported on a large series of fresh osteochondral allografts for the treatment of predominately traumatic distal femoral and proximal tibial defects. Survivorship analysis demonstrated intact and well-functioning grafts (Hospital for Special Surgery [HSS] score >70) in 95% of patients at 5 years, which decreased to 80% to 85% at 10 years and 65% to 74% at 15 years. Gortz and Bugbee[36] reported good and excellent results in 88% of 43 fresh osteochondral allografts of the distal femur at average follow-up of 4.5 years.

AREAS OF UNCERTAINTY

Study Design and Indications

Symptomatic chondral defects are rarely seen in clinical practice; therefore, a surgeon must have a large tertiary referral practice in order to develop clinical expertise in this area. Comparing treatments for a rare problem such as a chondral defect requires a large difference in treatment outcomes in order to have a study with adequate statistical power. However, the time endpoints must be established in this field because any fibrocartilage repair may do well in the first 3 years but then the tissue and the clinical results may deteriorate. Therefore, not only an adequately powered study but an appropriate length of follow-up are needed to determine the durability of repair and the prevention of degenerative joint disease. A multicenter prospective randomized study is necessary in order to recruit adequately.

Several authors have conducted studies comparing different repair techniques, such as microfracture, mosaicplasty, and ACI, with conflicting results. These studies are often compromised by the nature of the procedures they were designed to investigate; for example, ACI as a cell-based therapy is dependent on a sophisticated cell culturing process. The cell culturing process requires phenotypic validation, cell viability assessment, and sterility process validation according to the FDA, GLP (Good Laboratory Practices), and GMP (Good Manufacturing Practices) to ensure sterile, safe, phenotypically stable cell implantation; however, not all authors use standardized and approved laboratory facilities.

The technical skill factor and "learning curve" for the ACI procedure and multiple osteochondral grafting technique are crucial. These procedures are challenging. Some studies have used multiple surgeons performing few surgeries, which may compromise the clinical outcomes. This is another appealing facet of the microfracture technique—its technical ease of performance in most parts of the knee joint, which may bias against a comparative study using ACI or mosaicplasty in which technical perfection is a must in order to obtain a good clinical result.

Every chondral defect likely is not amenable to every available treatment; rather, the differences in results will depend on the exact defect size and location. Therefore, even well-designed prospective RCTs attempting to compare treatment options for a wide range of defects are bound to yield conflicting results.

In order to formulate better treatment guidelines, each treatment option will first have to be investigated on its own to ascertain the type of defect for which it is most efficacious. The success rates and clinical outcomes can be established from well-performed prospective clinical cohorts, and a range of patient characteristics, defect locations, and sizes can be established. Each defect will have one or several associated treatment options. We then will be able to conduct well-designed, adequately powered, ethically sound, comparative studies. These will be true level 1 evidence-based outcome studies that will help guide treatments for our patients and provide data for evidence-based treatment algorithms. Only then will we be able to properly design trials that compare the efficacy of treatment options for the same type of defect.

Jakobsen and Engebretsen[37] evaluated the quality of cartilage repair studies in a update to a previous publication[38] and commented on this subject as follows: "The increased focus on methodology in major journals by marking original articles with a level-of-evidence is highly appreciated. However, we would like to emphasize the fact that randomized controlled trials can have serious design flaws (i.e., not using independent reviewers, no statistical power analysis, not using an adequate randomization procedure, not accounting for eligible subjects not included in study), and therefore be rated as level-of-evidence II. We would also like to draw the reader's attention to the fact that several well performed case series (level-IV evidence) score very well on the CMS. These studies largely take into consideration multiple aspects of good methodological quality such as independent investigator, sufficient number of patients, well-described rehabilitation protocol, validated outcome measures and so forth, and are mainly lacking in not having a control group. We therefore recommend the reader to not entirely dismiss articles marked level-IV evidence, yet themselves assess the methodological quality of the paper when interpreting the results (for example using a grading system like the CMS)." I agree with their recommendation that inclusion and exclusion criteria should be well established, that validated outcome measures for cartilage injuries should be used, and that outcome assessment should be performed by an independent investigator, ideally by the patient without assistance.

Background Factors

The presence of associated abnormalities introduces an additional layer of variability into studies because the reproducibility of assessing background factors between surgeons and treating these abnormalities prior to or concomitantly with treatment of the chondral defect varies. To date, this correlation has not been firmly established. The disappointing early results of cartilage repair have been explained by the failure to properly diagnose and correct associated bony and ligamentous abnormalities. For example, in early studies of patellar defects treated with ACI alone, good and excellent results were found in only one third of patients.[7] However, later studies identified patellar maltracking as an important associated abnormality, and concurrent use of a corrective osteotomy led to 71% good or excellent results[39] and improved the initial poor results in the series by Peterson et al[4] to 79%, excluding the early cohort when tracking of the patella was also treated. These reports emphasize the importance of a thorough patient evaluation to correctly identify and treat all associated abnormalities to ensure the long-term success of chondral repair.

Guidelines

No established societal (International Cartilage Repair Society [ICRS], American Academy of Orthopedic Surgeons [AAOS], Arthroscopy Association of north America [AANA], International Society of Arthroscopy, Knee Surgery, and Orthopedic Sports Medicine [ISAKOS], etc.) guidelines based on comparative trials for the treatment of articular cartilage exist. An evidence-based treatment algorithm that I have previously published[10] is shown in Figures 4–8 and 4–9. My personal treatment preferences are given in the Recommendations section.

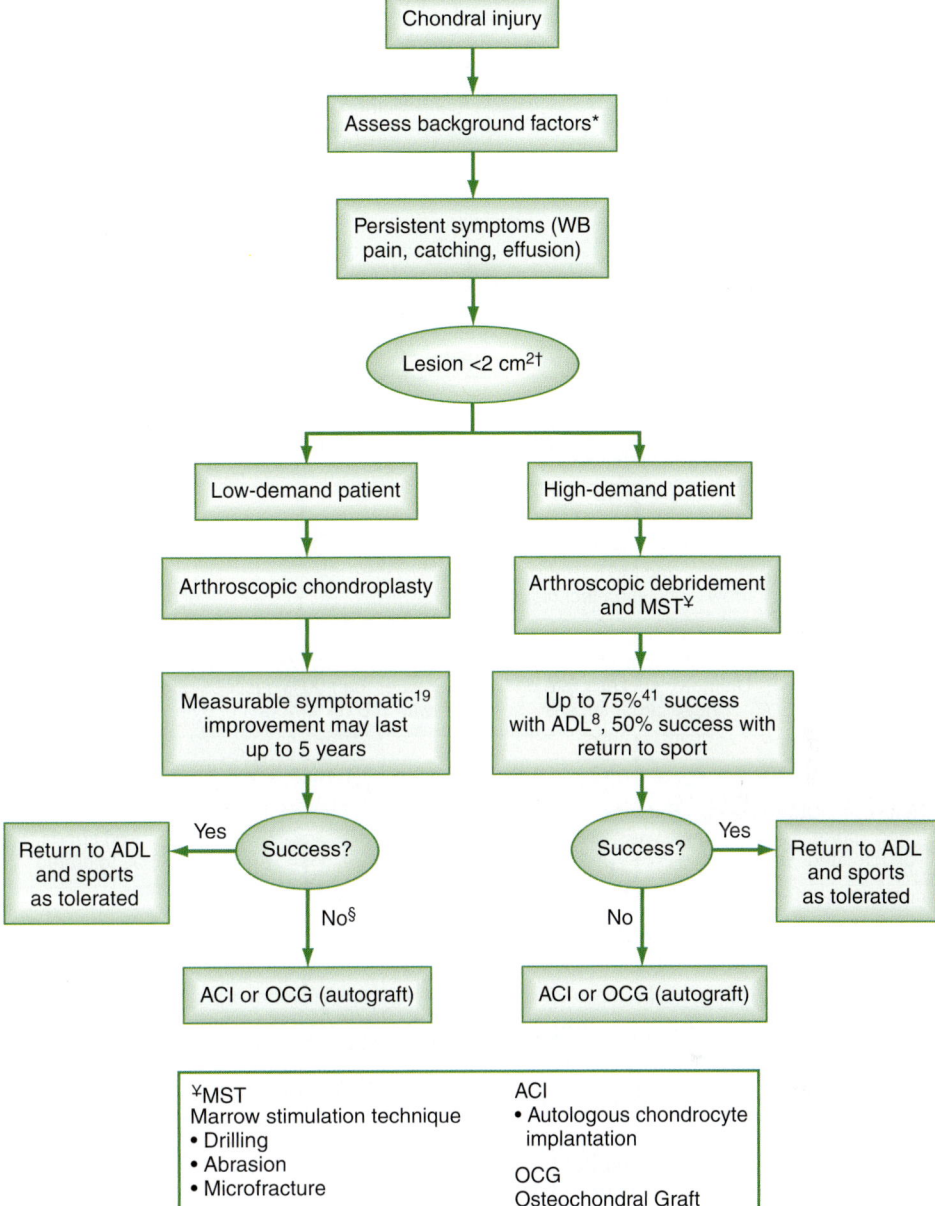

Figure 4-8 Modified and updated clinical algorithm for management of symptomatic cartilage defects of the femoral condyle when the defect is small (<2 cm²), based on patient activity level and after assessment of background factors.

Recommendations

My preferred treatment algorithm is outlined in the following section (Table 4-2). I do not treat asymptomatic chondral defects at this time because of the possibility of worsening the patient's condition. Existing techniques presently do not report excellent results greater than 90%, and the natural history and progression of a chondral defect remain unknown for a given individual. Careful longitudinal follow-up in this situation is recommended to the patient, with annual clinical evaluation by physical examination for progressive crepitus and effusion. High-resolution MRI scan is also performed to measure whether the defect size has progressed, and standing anteroposterior and flexion posteroanterior radiographs are obtained to help assess the overall cartilage space. Counseling regarding weight gain and avoidance of impact loading sports is recommended. If the patient becomes symptomatic or defect size progresses, then surgery is recommended after the risks and benefits are discussed with the patient and informed consent is obtained. This is based on the most appropriate treatment from the guidelines that follow.

The background factors for the cartilage defect are evaluated by clinical examination and long alignment radiographs. We perform corrective osteotomy to mechanical neutral, without overcorrection, for defects

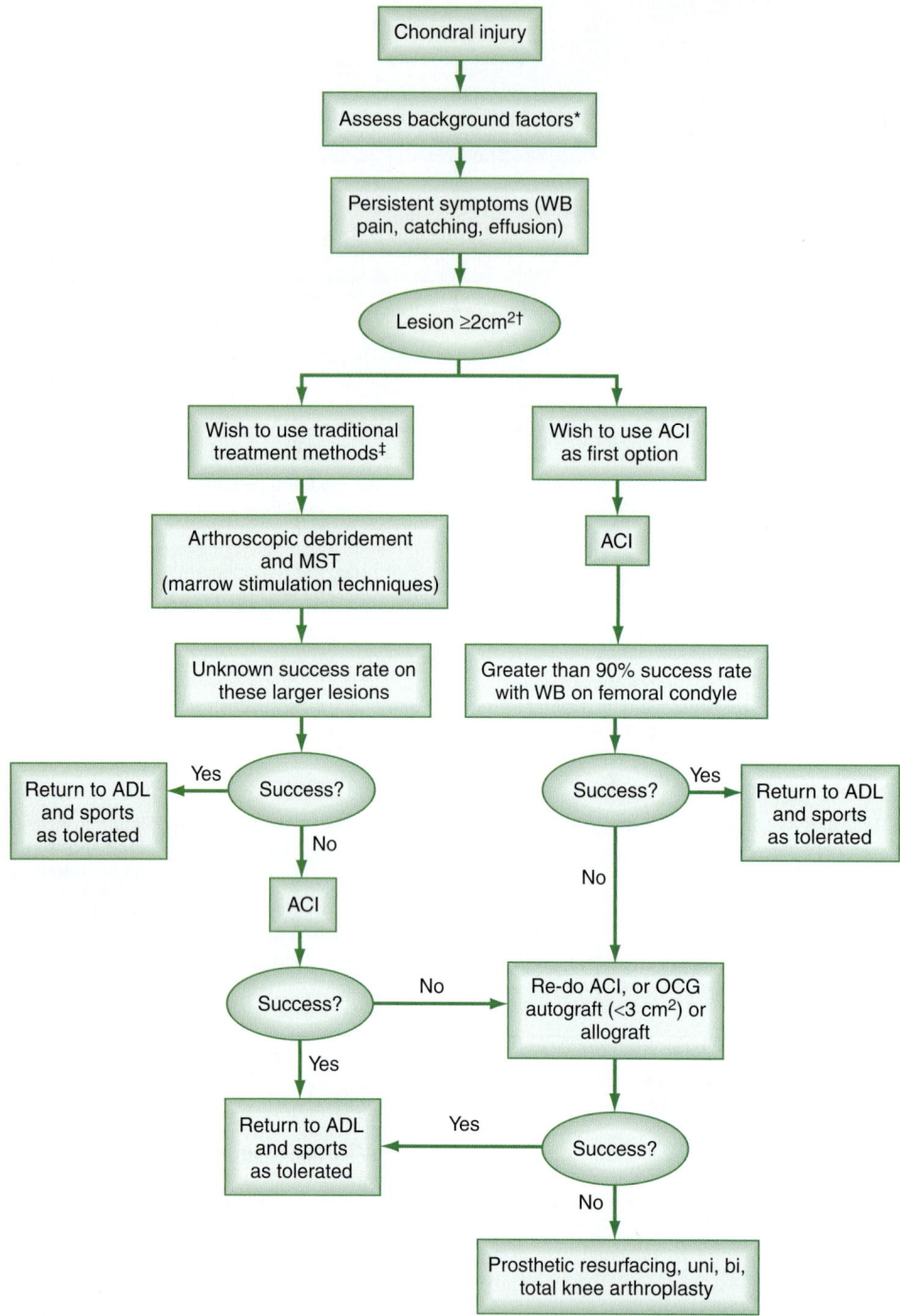

Figure 4-9 Modified and updated clinical algorithm for management of symptomatic cartilage defects of the femoral condyle when the defect is large (>2 cm²), based on patient activity level and after assessment of background factors.

Table 4-2 Treatment Recommendations and Respective Level of Evidence

Level of Evidence*	Recommendation
B	Microfracture treatment shows better results in smaller defects (<2–4 cm^2)
B	Microfracture treatment shows best results in femoral condyle lesions
B	Microfracture treatment results in better outcomes in younger patients (<30–40 yr)
C	Microfracture treatment results in better outcomes in patients with body mass index <30
I	ACI, microfracture, or mosaicplasty result in outcomes superior to each other
B	Shorter duration of symptoms prior to cartilage repair results in better outcomes
A	Use of collagen membrane in place of periosteal patch for ACI reduces reoperation rate for graft hypertrophy
A	ACI-C and MACI have comparable outcomes
B	Osteochondral defects are amenable to osteochondral allograft transplantation

*A, good evidence (level I studies with consistent finding) for or against recommending intervention; B, fair evidence (level II or III studies with consistent findings) for or against recommending intervention; C, poor-quality evidence (level IV or V with consistent findings) for or against recommending intervention; I, insufficient or conflicting evidence not allowing a recommendation for or against intervention.

ACI, autologous chondrocyte implantation; ACI-C, autologous chondrocyte implantation collagen-covered; MACI, autologous chondrocyte implantation membrane-associated.

larger than 2 cm^2 at the time of cartilage repair if there is 2 or more degrees of mechanical varus or valgus and any patellar maltracking through an anteromedialization of the tibial tubercle.

Single full-thickness chondral defects of the weight-bearing femoral condyles and trochlea of less than 10 mm in diameter are amenable to osteochondral autograft transfer procedures (OATS or mosaicplasty). Occasionally in a large knee two plugs are used to repair a lesion 15 mm in diameter. The advantages of this technique are that it is a single-stage procedure, it involves transfer of mature hyaline cartilage into the defect, and it has a comparatively uncomplicated postsurgical recovery. Donor site morbidity is acceptable when a single plug is used. The donor sites are frequently "backfilled" with synthetic calcium sulfate–PLA/PGA copolymer (OBI TruFit plugs, Smith & Nephew). Drains are used after surgery to prevent hemarthrosis and arthrofibrosis. Defects of the patella and tibial plateau should not be managed with this technique because the cartilage thickness mismatch between donor site (average 2 mm) and patella (average 5–7 mm) results in incongruities, resorption, and failure. Osteochondral autograft transfer can be performed arthroscopically but must be a precise fit—flush to the surface and orthogonally placed—so miniarthrotomy for accurate placement should be considered if there is any concern for graft placement by arthroscopy.

Defects of the weight-bearing condyles, tibia, trochlea, and patella 1 to 2 cm^2 in size are amenable to microfracture with acceptable long-term results. The recovery and return to sports are longer than with osteochondral autografting; the success rate is less. However, microfracture is easier for all locations within the knee. Long-term follow-up is necessary because the durability is less predictable, and recurrent symptoms are common 2.5 to 5 years after surgery.

We prefer to treat defects larger than 2 cm^2 with ACI because of the good and predictable long-term results of the technique. Associated osseous defects deeper than 6 to 8 mm must be addressed with a bony procedure, either in a staged fashion with bone grafting followed by ACI 9 to 12 months later or with single-stage osteochondral allograft transplantation (mega-OATS).

We prefer allograft for a large peripherally bony uncontained defect or for an ACI that has failed fibrous repair. Otherwise, bone deficiency is not a contraindication for ACI if the defect is first bone grafted. Because the long-term results of ACI are superior to those of allograft, our preference for a young person is a staged bone–cartilage repair with ACI.

The field of cartilage repair is evolving. The relative efficacies of the differing techniques and their limitations are being elucidated by carefully performed prospective cohorts that are not at the highest levels of evidence to determine the best cartilage technique per defect. However, these studies will afford us success and failure rates that can be used in designing comparative, statistically well powered, ethically just RCTs that will answer the question, "What is the best repair technique for this defect?" At that time, we will be able to advocate an evidence-based algorithm for treatment based on patient and defect characteristics that will be cost effective and sound.

REFERENCES

1. Ware Jr JE, Sherbourne CD. The MOS 36-item short-form health survey (SF-36). I. Conceptual framework and item selection. *Med Care.* 1992;30(6):473–483.
2. Mithofer K, Minas T, Peterson L, Yeon H, Micheli LJ. Functional outcome of knee articular cartilage repair in adolescent athletes. *Am J Sports Med.* 2005;33(8):1147–1153.
3. Mithofer K, Peterson L, Mandelbaum BR, Minas T. Articular cartilage repair in soccer players with autologous chondrocyte transplantation: functional outcome and return to competition. *Am J Sports Med.* 2005;33(11):1639–1646.
4. Peterson L, Minas T, Brittberg M, et al. Two- to 9-year outcome after autologous chondrocyte transplantation of the knee. *Clin Orthop Relat Res.* 2000;(374):212–234.
5. Coventry MB, Ilstrup DM, Wallrichs SL. Proximal tibial osteotomy. A critical long-term study of eighty-seven cases. *J Bone Joint Surg Am.* 1993;75(2):196–201.
6. Winalski C, Aliabadi P, Wright R, et al. Enhancement of joint fluid with intravenously administered gadopentetate dimeglumine: technique, rationale, and implications. *Radiology.* 1993;187:179–185.
7. Brittberg M, Lindahl A, Nilsson A, et al. Treatment of deep cartilage defects in the knee with autologous chondrocyte transplantation. *N Engl J Med.* 1994;331(14):889–895.
8. Homminga GN, Bulstra SK, Bouwmeester PSM, et al. Perichondral grafting for cartilage lesions of the knee. *J Bone Joint Surg Br.* 1990;72:1003–1007.
9. Widuchowski W, Widuchowski J, Koczy B, Szyluk K. Untreated asymptomatic deep cartilage lesions associated with anterior cruciate ligament injury. *Am J Sports Med.* 2009;37(4): 688–692.
10. Minas T. The role of cartilage repair techniques, including chondrocyte transplantation, in focal chondral knee damage. *Instr Course Lect.* 1999;48:629–643.
11. Minas T. Treatment of chondral defects in the knee. *Orthop Spec Ed.* 1997;Summer/Fall:69–74.
12. Minas T, Nehrer S. Current concepts in the treatment of articular cartilage defects. *Orthopedics.* 1997;20(6):525–538.
13. Aroen A, Loken S, Heir S, et al. Articular cartilage lesions in 993 consecutive knee arthroscopies. *Am J Sports Med.* 2004;32(1):211–215.
14. Curl WW, Krome J, Gordon ES, et al. Cartilage injuries: a review of 31,516 knee arthroscopies. *Arthroscopy.* 1997;13(4):456–460.
15. Hjelle K, Solheim E, Strand T, Muri R, Brittberg M. Articular cartilage defects in 1,000 knee arthroscopies. *Arthroscopy.* 2002;18(7):730–734.
16. Piasecki DP, Spindler KP, Warren TA, Andrish JT, Parker RD. Intraarticular injuries associated with anterior cruciate ligament tear: findings at ligament reconstruction in high school and recreational athletes. An analysis of sex-based differences. *Am J Sports Med.* 2003;31(4):601–605.
17. Hubbard MJ. Articular debridement versus washout for degeneration of the medial femoral condyle. A five-year study. *J Bone Joint Surg Br.* 1996;78(2):217–219.
18. Levy AS, Lohnes J, Sculley S, et al. Chondral delamination of the knee in soccer players. *Am J Sports Med.* 1996;24:634–639.
19. Messner K, Maletius W. The long-term prognosis for severe damage to weight-bearing cartilage in the knee: a 14-year clinical and radiographic follow-up in 28 young athletes. *Acta Orthop Scand.* 1996;67(2):165–168.
20. Nehrer S, Spector M, Minas T. Histologic analysis of tissue after failed cartilage repair procedures. *Clin Orthop Relat Res.* 1999;(365):149–162.
21. Mithoefer K, Williams 3rd RJ, Warren RF, et al. The microfracture technique for the treatment of articular cartilage lesions in the knee. A prospective cohort study. *J Bone Joint Surg Am.* 2005;87(9):1911–1920.
22. Garretson 3rd RB, Katolik LI, Verma N, et al. Contact pressure at osteochondral donor sites in the patellofemoral joint. *Am J Sports Med.* 2004;32(4):967–974.
23. Gitelis S, Cole BJ. The use of allografts in orthopaedic surgery. *Instr Course Lect.* 2002;51:507–520.
24. Minas T, Gomoll A. What is the best treatment for chondral defects in the knee. In: Wright JG, ed. *Evidence-based Orthopaedics.* Philadelphia: Saunders/Elsevier; 2009:638–645.
25. Hangody L, Fules P. Autologous osteochondral mosaicplasty for the treatment of full-thickness defects of weight-bearing joints: ten years of experimental and clinical experience. *J Bone Joint Surg Am.* 2003;85-A(Suppl 2):25–32.
26. Blevins FT, Steadman JR, Rodrigo JJ, Silliman J. Treatment of articular cartilage defects in athletes: an analysis of functional outcome and lesion appearance. *Orthopedics.* 1998;21(7):761–767 discussion 767–8.
27. Steadman JR, Briggs KK, Rodrigo JJ, et al. Outcomes of microfracture for traumatic chondral defects of the knee: average 11-year follow-up. *Arthroscopy.* 2003;19(5):477–484.
28. Bentley G, Biant LC, Carrington RW, et al. A prospective, randomised comparison of autologous chondrocyte implantation versus mosaicplasty for osteochondral defects in the knee. *J Bone Joint Surg Br.* 2003;85(2):223–230.
29. Horas U, Pelinkovic D, Herr G, Aigner T, Schnettler R. Autologous chondrocyte implantation and osteochondral cylinder transplantation in cartilage repair of the knee joint. A prospective, comparative trial. *J Bone Joint Surg Am.* 2003;85-A(2):185–192.
30. Gooding CR, Bartlett W, Bentley G, et al. A prospective, randomised study comparing two techniques of autologous chondrocyte implantation for osteochondral defects in the knee: Periosteum covered versus type I/III collagen covered. *Knee.* 2006;13(3):203–210.
31. Bartlett W, Skinner JA, Gooding CR, et al. Autologous chondrocyte implantation versus matrix-induced autologous chondrocyte implantation for osteochondral defects of the knee: a prospective, randomised study. *J Bone Joint Surg Br.* 2005;87(5):640–645.
32. Knutsen G, Engebretsen L, Ludvigsen TC, et al. Autologous chondrocyte implantation compared with microfracture in the knee. A randomized trial. *J Bone Joint Surg Am.* 2004;86-A(3):455–464.
33. Micheli LJ, Browne JE, Erggelet C, et al. Autologous chondrocyte implantation of the knee: multicenter experience and minimum 3-year follow-up. *Clin J Sport Med.* 2001;11(4):223–228.
34. Gudas R, Kalesinskas RJ, Kimtys V, et al. A prospective randomized clinical study of mosaic osteochondral autologous transplantation versus microfracture for the treatment of osteochondral defects in the knee joint in young athletes. *Arthroscopy.* 2005;21(9):1066–1075.
35. Gross AE, Shasha N, Aubin P. Long-term followup of the use of fresh osteochondral allografts for posttraumatic knee defects. *Clin Orthop Relat Res.* 2005;(435):79–87.
36. Gortz S, Bugbee WD. Allografts in articular cartilage repair. *Instr Course Lect.* 2007;56:469–481.
37. Jakobsen RB, Engebretsen L. An analysis of the quality of cartilage repair studies - an update. In: *ISAKOS Current Concepts Winter 2007.* 2007.
38. Jakobsen RB, Engebretsen L, Slauterbeck JR. An analysis of the quality of cartilage repair studies. *J Bone Joint Surg Am.* 2005;87(10):2232–2239.
39. Minas T, Bryant T. The role of autologous chondrocyte implantation in the patellofemoral joint. *Clin Orthop Relat Res.* 2005;(436):30–39.
40. Outerbridge RE. The etiology of chondromalacia patellae. *J Bone Joint Surg Br.* 1961;43-B:752–757.
41. Kreuz PC, Erggelet C, Steinwachs MR, et al. Is microfracture of chondral defects in the knee associated with different results in patients aged 40 years or younger? *Arthroscopy.* 2006;22(11):1180–1186.
42. Kreuz PC, Steinwachs MR, Erggelet C, et al. Results after microfracture of full-thickness chondral defects in different compartments in the knee. *Osteoarthr Cartil.* 2006;14(11):1119–1125.

PART 2

CARTILAGE REPAIR SURGICAL TECHNIQUES

Chapter 5

Debridement, Microfracture, and Osteochondral Autograft Transfer for Treatment of Cartilage Defects

Andreas H. Gomoll, MD and Tom Minas, MD, MS

INTRODUCTION

PLANNING

SURGICAL TECHNIQUE
Debridement and Chondroplasty

Microfracture
Osteochondral Autograft Transfer

INTRODUCTION

All three techniques discussed in this chapter are considered first-line treatment options for articular cartilage defects, predominately because of their low invasiveness. Debridement is mostly indicated for treatment of (1) incidental lesions discovered during surgery directed at other joint pathology, such as meniscectomy and anterior cruciate ligament reconstruction, and (2) lesions in lower-demand patients who are reluctant to undergo other cartilage repair procedures that are more invasive and/or require long rehabilitation. Debridement is also a good initial treatment option for lesions that are deemed borderline or too large for microfracture or osteochondral autograft transfer (OAT) because it does not appear to compromise later treatment with autologous chondrocyte implantation.

Microfracture is a minimally invasive option whose indications have been refined in the last few years through multiple investigations. It has a high success rate when used appropriately for the treatment of small ($<2-4$ cm^2) defects in the femoral condyles of younger ($<35-40$ years) patients with acute defects.[1] Larger defects and those located in the patellofemoral joint deteriorate after 24 to 36 months.[2]

OAT is generally indicated for treatment of small ($<2-4$ cm^2) defects in the femoral condyles and trochlea but not in the patella.[3] The recommendation for size is based on the limited availability of cartilage elsewhere in the knee (donor site morbidity) and on the ability to minimize the complication of plug necrosis, which is seen more frequently in central plugs that are completely surrounded by other plugs and therefore have no direct contact to native bone for integration. Although lesions up to 4 cm^2 have been indicated for OAT, it is our preference to use this technique as first-line treatment for active, fit individuals with lesions 1 to 1.5 cm^2 because OAT does not cause donor site symptoms in patients with these small lesions and results in a rapid return to sport (4–8 months) with a mature hyaline cartilage repair.

PLANNING

Standard radiographic and magnetic resonance imaging should be performed preoperatively to determine the size and number of lesions to be treated because both microfracture and OAT have upper size limitations. Similar to the more invasive cartilage repair techniques, long-leg films are crucial to determine alignment. Any significant malalignment should be corrected through neutralization osteotomy to maximize the success rate of cartilage repair.

SURGICAL TECHNIQUE

Debridement and Chondroplasty

Debridement is performed arthroscopically, largely for the treatment of incidental lesions found during treatment of other issues in the joint. Although removal of loose flaps with the motorized shaver is considered debridement, which is our preference, true chondroplasty requires a more thorough treatment of the defect, with removal of degenerated tissue and creation of stable vertical shoulders, similar to the process outlined later for microfracture. It generally requires the use of sharp curettes in addition to a shaver. The purpose of chondroplasty is to alleviate mechanical symptoms but not effect repair.

Postoperatively, patients return to activities as tolerated with no specific precautions or restrictions.

Microfracture

Microfracture is performed arthroscopically in the vast majority of cases. Setup and patient positioning follow that of routine knee arthroscopy. However, especially for very posterior defects, the leg should be positioned so that knee hyperflexion can be achieved.

After routine diagnostic arthroscopy to evaluate the defect (Figure 5–1) and the rest of the joint for potential other comorbidities, loose flaps and degenerated tissue are debrided using a motorized shaver. Subsequently, a curette is used to trim back any soft and fissured cartilage along the rim to create stable vertical shoulders (Figure 5–2). The debridement includes the calcified

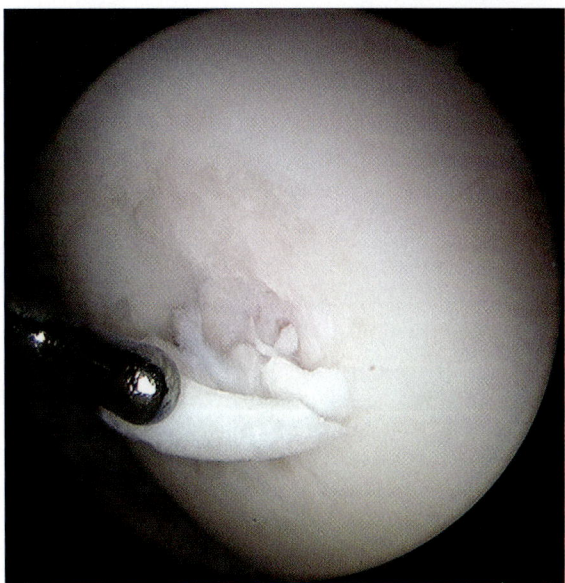

Figure 5-1 Arthroscopic probe demonstrating a loose flap in a chondral defect of the femoral condyle.

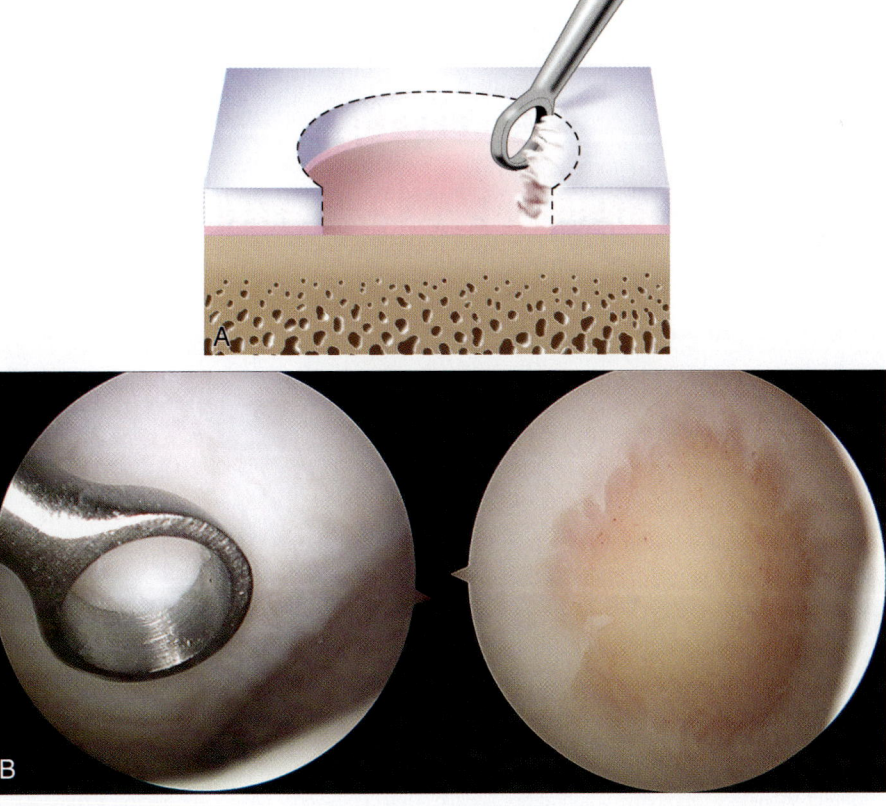

Figure 5-2 Defect preparation. Drawing *(A)* and arthroscopic images *(B)*. *Left,* Sharp ring curette for debridement of cartilage. *Right,* Defect after thorough debridement of degenerated tissue and creation of stable shoulders.

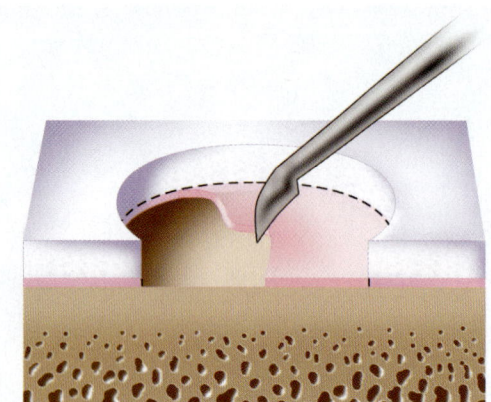

Figure 5-3 Debridement of zone of calcified cartilage.

cartilage layer (Figure 5–3) but should not violate the subchondral plate. Rarely, accessory portals have to be created depending on the exact defect size and location.

After thorough debridement, multiple holes are created in the subchondral plate using a microfracture awl (Figure 5–4). This step should be performed last if multiple procedures are planned in the same setting, such as concomitant meniscal debridement or anterior cruciate ligament reconstruction; otherwise the marrow elements are washed away by the prolonged arthroscopy irrigation. When placing the microfracture holes, attention should be turned toward not destabilizing the subchondral plate when holes become confluent or break into each other. This can occur when holes are placed too closely; ideally, the microfracture holes are spaced approximately 3 to 4 mm apart, resulting in three to four holes per square centimeter. Also, if the microfracture awl is placed at low angles to the bone, there is a tendency to skive off or create a hole that is not round but oblong, further destabilizing the bone. In an effort to remain perpendicular to the chondral surface, it may be necessary to flex and extend the knee to rotate the articular surface in line with the awl or create accessory portals. Stability of the transition zone between surrounding cartilage and regenerate fibrocartilage can be improved by placing holes as closely as possible to the surrounding cartilage. After completion of the microfracture, the tourniquet (if used) is deflated and pump pressure is lowered. Bleeding should be observed from all holes, eventually filling the defect with a clot (Figure 5–5).

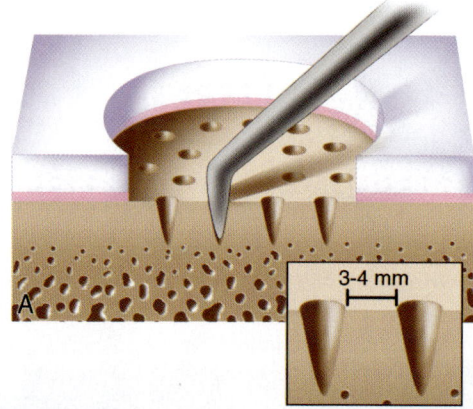

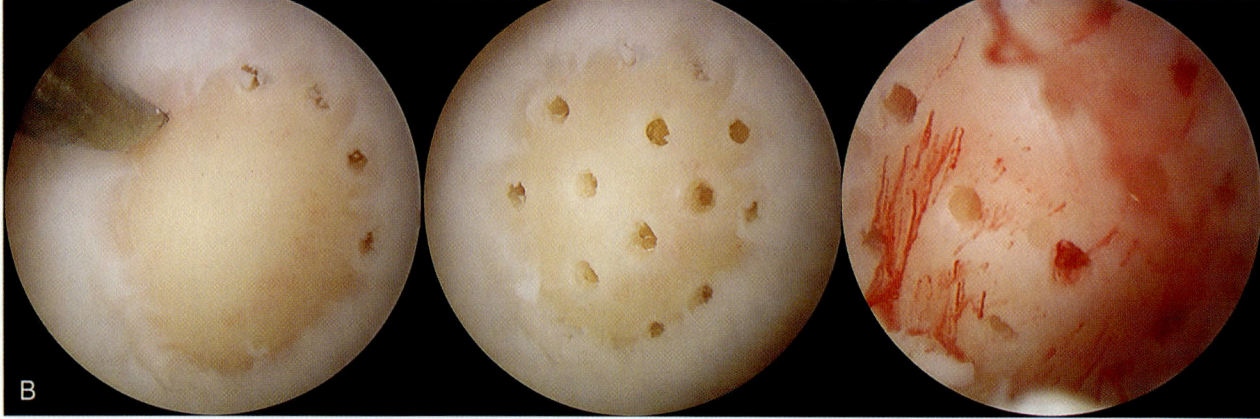

Figure 5-4 Microfracture. Drawing (A) and arthroscopic images (B). Left, Multiple microfracture holes are placed directly adjacent to the defect shoulders to improve integration. Middle, Defect is evenly filled with microfracture holes. Right, After release of cartilage tourniquet, bleeding is observed from the microfracture holes.

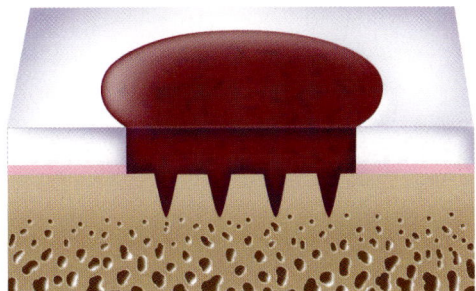

Figure 5–5 Blood clot fills the defect, eventually forming a fibrocartilaginous repair tissue.

Postoperatively, patients are placed on touch-down weight-bearing restrictions for 6 weeks and start a continuous passive motion (CPM) machine on postoperative day 1 for 6 weeks, 6 to 8 hours per day. Return to athletic activities is based on the size of the defect but should be delayed 6 to 9 months to allow for tissue maturation.

Osteochondral Autograft Transfer

OAT can be performed either arthroscopically or through an open approach, based on the exact defect size and location and the surgeon's preference.

The lesion is evaluated arthroscopically, and accessory portals are created through spinal needle localization to allow perpendicular orientation of the instrumentation to the articular surface, both for the donor and recipient sites. Horizontal skin portals are preferred for an arthroscopic approach because it allows transverse enlargement of a portal to ensure orthogonal placement of the grafts. Occasionally, a central, transpatellar tendon approach is required. In this case, the patellar tendon should be split in line with its fibers and repaired at the end of the procedure. First, sizing guides are used to determine the size and number of grafts required to fill the defect (Figure 5–6). Subsequently, an appropriately sized harvesting tube is selected and an osteochondral plug is obtained, usually approximately 10-mm long, being mindful to introduce the harvester perpendicular to the articular surface (Figure 5–7). Several sites in the knee joint have been identified as being suitable for osteochondral plug harvest. Although the superior lateral trochlear ridge (Figure 5–8A) is considered a lesser weight-bearing area of the knee, it is an important load-bearing portion of the patellofemoral joint in 40 to 70 degrees of flexion and may cause significant symptoms if harvested. We prefer to harvest two to three plugs from the area of the sulcus terminalis on the lateral femoral condyle, the transition zone between the tibiofemoral and patellofemoral weight-bearing areas (Figure 5–8B), or the lateral intercondylar notch. After a plug has been obtained, the length and any potential angulation are noted (Figure 5–9). A defect harvesting tube is now used to remove an appropriately sized and angled plug from the defect, and the depth is checked with a sizing rod to ensure that the defect is approximately 1 mm deeper than the length of the graft. The graft is then advanced within the harvesting tube so that the end is just visible. The harvester is introduced into the joint, oriented perpendicularly to the articular surface, and the graft is slowly advanced into the recipient site (Figure 5–10). The harvester then is removed (Figure 5–11), and the graft is fully seated and made flush by gentle pressure using an oversized tamp (Figure 5–12). Slightly recessing the graft is preferable to leaving it proud in order to reduce contact forces. The process is then repeated until the defect is filled.

Postoperatively, patients are placed on touch-down weightbearing restrictions for 6 weeks but do not routinely require the use of a CPM machine because the mature hyaline cartilage was transferred. If there are

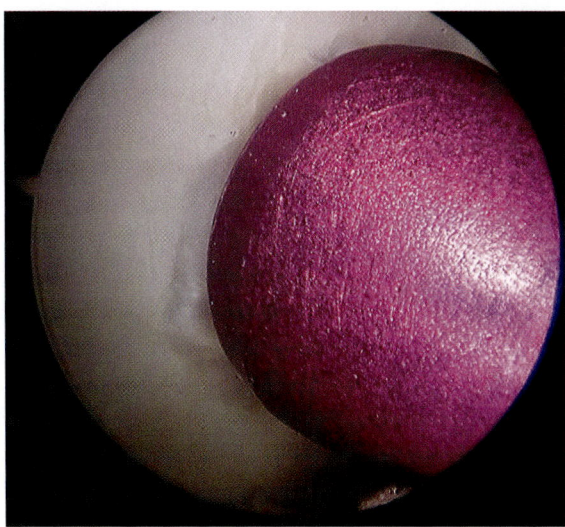

Figure 5–6 Defect is measured using sizing rods to estimate the size and number of plugs required to fill the area.

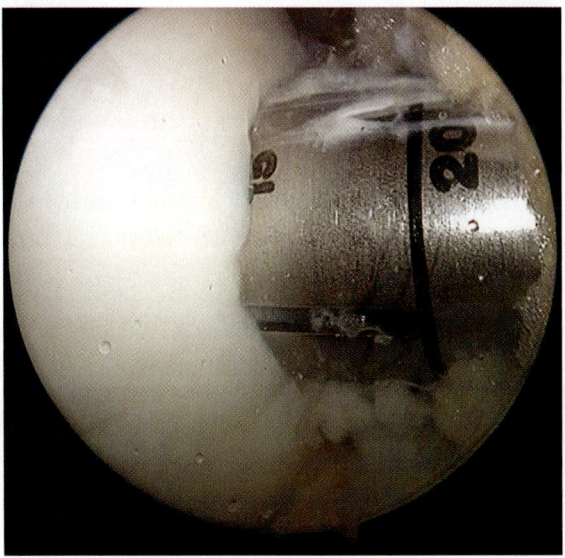

Figure 5–7 Osteochondral plug is retrieved using a harvesting tube.

PART 2 CARTILAGE REPAIR SURGICAL TECHNIQUES

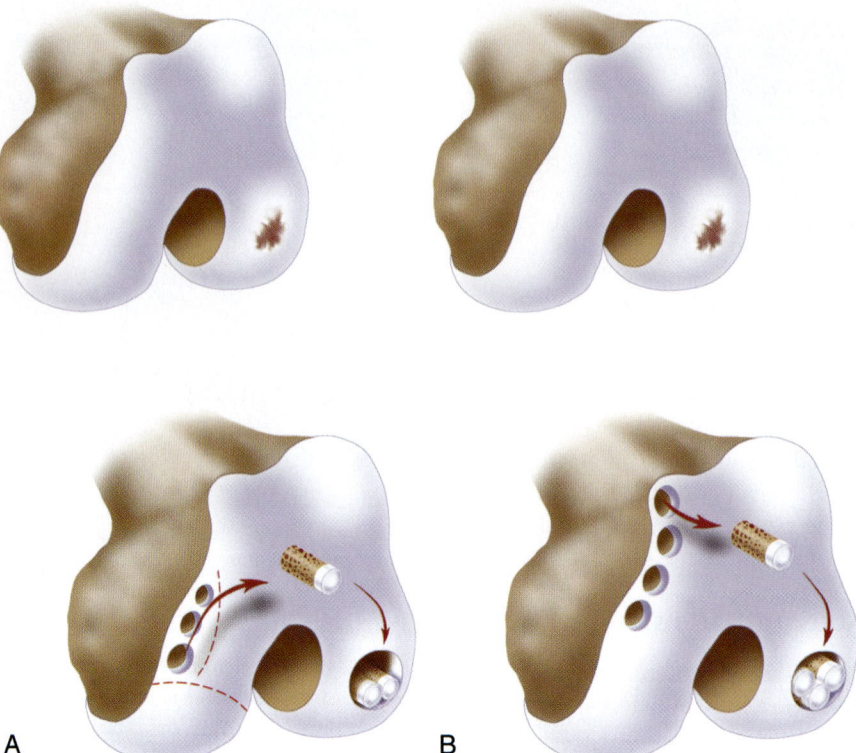

Figure 5-8 *A,* Plug harvest from trochlear ridge. Although the superior lateral trochlear ridge is considered a lesser weight-bearing area of the knee, it is an important load-bearing portion of the patellofemoral joint in 40 to 70 degrees of flexion and may cause significant symptoms if harvested. *B,* Plug harvest from area of sulcus terminalis on lateral femoral condyle is the preferred harvest site. Lateral intercondylar notch proximal to sulcus terminalis is another suitable site.

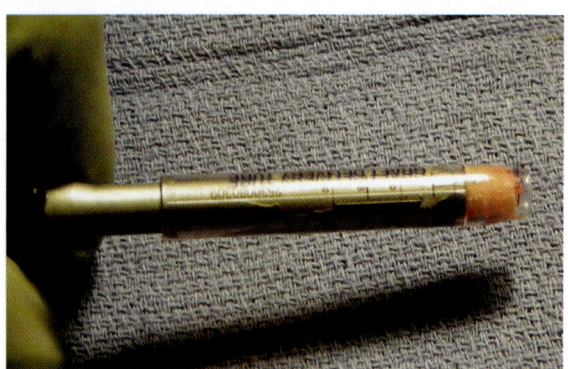

Figure 5-9 Harvesting tube with osteochondral plug ready for deployment.

concerns for postoperative stiffness, CPM can be used for 2 to 3 weeks as needed. Return to athletic activities is based on the size and location of the defect but should be delayed for 4 to 6 months to allow for return of quadriceps strength and proprioception.

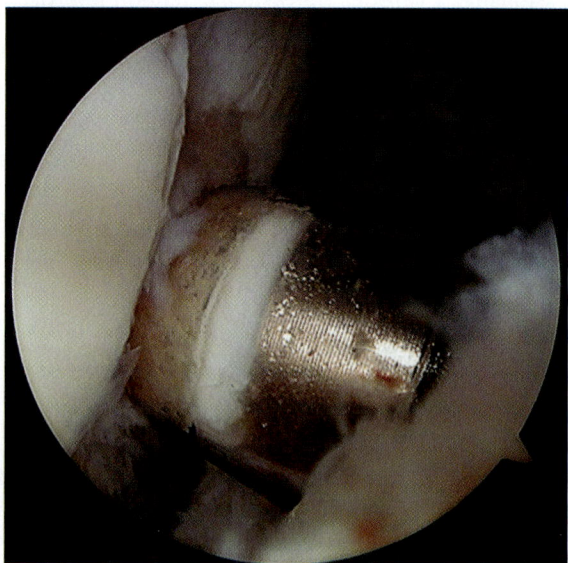

Figure 5-10 Introduction of plug into recipient defect using gentle pressure.

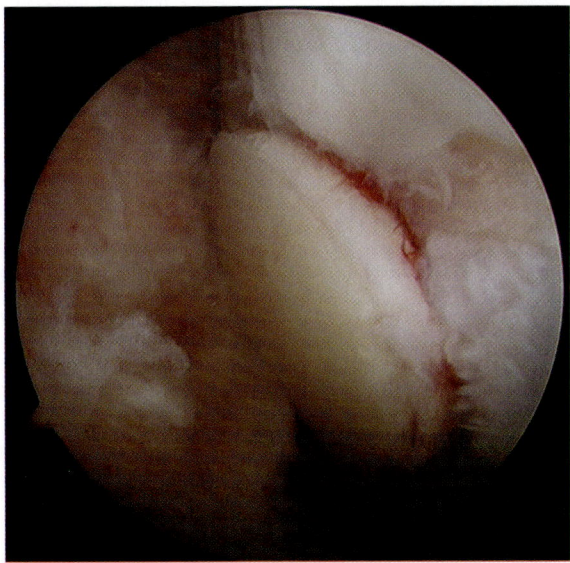

Figure 5–11 Plug slightly proud prior to final seating.

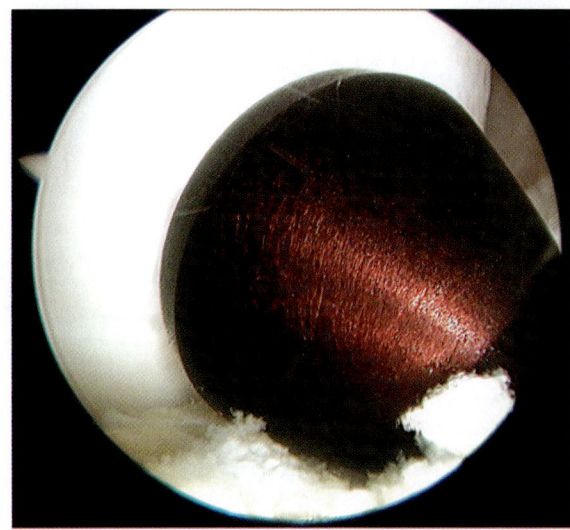

Figure 5–12 Seating of plug using an oversized tamp.

REFERENCES

1. Mithoefer K, McAdams T, Williams RJ, Kreuz PC, Mandelbaum BR. Clinical efficacy of the microfracture technique for articular cartilage repair in the knee: an evidence-based systematic analysis. *Am J Sports Med.* 2009;37(10):2053–2063.
2. Kreuz PC, Steinwachs MR, Erggelet C, et al. Results after microfracture of full-thickness chondral defects in different compartments in the knee. *Osteoarthr Cartil.* 2006;14(11):1119–1125.
3. Bentley G, Biant LC, Carrington RW, et al. A prospective, randomised comparison of autologous chondrocyte implantation versus mosaicplasty for osteochondral defects in the knee. *J Bone Joint Surg Br.* 2003;85(2):223–230.

Use of Fresh Osteochondral Allograft for Chondral and Osteochondral Defects in the Knee

Tom Minas, MD, MS

INTRODUCTION

GRAFT PROCUREMENT AND STORAGE

SAFETY AND RISK OF DISEASE TRANSMISSION

IMMUNOLOGY

INDICATIONS

SURGICAL TECHNIQUES

RESULTS AND CONCLUSIONS

INTRODUCTION

Fresh osteochondral allografts are composite grafts consisting of a living mature hyaline cartilage portion anchored to a nonliving subchondral bone portion, forming an intact osteochondral functional unit that replaces a damaged corresponding tissue in the recipient joint.

Increasing demand for allografts has been met with advancements in tissue procurement and increased availability of fresh donor tissue from commercial entities as opposed to university-based specialized transplantation centers, which in the past had limited availability to orthopedists in the community.[1–3]

The advantage of fresh osteochondral allografting is the transplantation of mature hyaline cartilage with viable chondrocytes,[4] which survive hypothermic storage and transplantation while maintaining their metabolic activity and sustaining the surrounding collagen matrix.[5] Investigations have focused on extending the storage interval of fresh human osteochondral allograft tissue. Ball et al[6] compared the effects of different storage media on human osteochondral allograft tissue when stored hypothermically in either lactated Ringer's solution or a standard culture media containing amino acids, glucose, and inorganic salts. The standard culture media demonstrated superior storage properties as measured by chondrocyte density, viability, and metabolic activity.

Biomechanical properties of the matrix remained relatively intact in both media. Chondrocyte viability essentially remained unchanged from baseline for as many as 14 days in the standard media, at which time viability was 90.5% in standard media versus 80% in lactated Ringer's solution.

GRAFT PROCUREMENT AND STORAGE

Availability of suitable graft tissue remains the limiting factor. Fresh osteochondral allografting is associated with inherent challenges related to tissue recovery, storage, and timely delivery for treatment.

Recovery, processing, and testing of donor tissue follow guidelines established by the American Association of Tissue Banks (AATB)[7,8] and is under the authority of the U.S. Food and Drug Administration (FDA).[9] Most tissue banks have a 24-hour time limit for retrieval of tissue from refrigerated cadaveric donors in a sterile operating room environment following strict sterile technique. Donors between the ages of 15 and 40 years are generally considered for inclusion in the donor pool if their articular surfaces pass direct inspection for cartilage quality.

It is the policy of tissue banks to hold transplants for a minimum of 14 days to allow completion of microbiologic and serologic testing prior to release. Hence the actual surgical implantation is delayed by 3 and to 6 weeks after procurement compared to university center clinical practice of implanting allografts usually within 1 week of harvest. Although results using this traditional fresh tissue protocol have been good even in mid-term follow-up,[10] the effects of prolonged allograft storage on clinical outcomes have not yet been determined.

Use of fresh-frozen grafts improves graft availability, reduces immunogenicity, and may be appropriate for bulk allografting in major osseous reconstruction as encountered in musculoskeletal tumor cases. However, deep freezing of chondrocytes within their extracellular matrix (usually at −80° C) practically eliminates all viable chondrocytes in the articular cartilage portion of osteochondral grafts. Furthermore, clinical experience indicates that the articular matrix in frozen allografts deteriorates over time, presumably because insufficient surviving cells are present within the matrix to maintain tissue equilibrium.[11,12] However, retrieval studies have demonstrated that with fresh, cold-stored osteochondral allografts, viable chondrocytes are present and mechanical properties of the matrix are maintained many years after transplantation.[13,14]

SAFETY AND RISK OF DISEASE TRANSMISSION

Osteochondral allografts are aseptically procured, which reduces but does not eliminate the risk of graft contamination during recovery via postmortem invasion by gastrointestinal flora or occult infection in the donor. Any transplantation of allogeneic organs or tissue is associated with a residual risk of transmission of infectious disease, despite donor screening and testing, and rare allograft-associated bacterial infections have been reported. Advances in serologic testing for human immunodeficiency virus, hepatitis, and other diseases have improved safety, but a measurable risk does remain. The surgeon and the patient should be well aware of the possibility of risk for transmission of serious diseases when fresh allograft tissue is used, making the discussion of the risk of bacterial or viral disease transmission part of the informed consent.[15]

IMMUNOLOGY

Small-fragment allografts are not human leukocyte antigen (HLA) or blood-type matched between the donor and recipient. Although hyaline cartilage appears to be relatively immunoprivileged,[16] fresh unmatched osteochondral allografts elicited a variable immune response in one study of fresh osteochondral allografts, and 50% of individuals generated serum anti-HLA antibodies.[17] The presence of anti-HLA antibodies correlated with an inferior appearance of the graft–host interface on magnetic resonance imaging (MRI) studies. Poor MRI incorporation also has been correlated with inferior clinical results[10] and may be a result of immunologic mechanisms. The issue of immune behavior ultimately may become clinically relevant, and it is clearly an area where more knowledge is necessary in order to improve outcomes of the use of fresh osteochondral allografts.

INDICATIONS

As per other cartilage repair procedures, successful reconstruction is dependent upon careful evaluation of background factors and their treatment at the time of or prior to fresh osteochondral allografting. These factors include tibial femoral and patellofemoral malalignment, joint stability, and meniscal deficiency.

Specific conditions that are most amenable to allografting in clinical practice include osteochondritis dissecans,[18] osteonecrosis,[19,20] and posttraumatic defects, such as those occurring after periarticular fractures about the knee.[21] A particularly troublesome condition to manage is posttraumatic tibial plateau fracture, which is especially suitable to management by fresh osteochondral allograft.[22] Allografts have also proved valuable for the salvage of knees for which other cartilage resurfacing procedures, such as microfracture, autologous chondrocyte implantation (ACI), and transfer of autologous osteochondral plugs.

Contraindications include inflammatory arthritis, chondrocalcinosis involving the cartilage articular surface, generalized osteoarthrosis of the joint, patients who are obese or noncompliant with postoperative rehabilitation, and those who are smokers or narcotic dependent.

Common to all allografting procedures is matching donor with recipient on the basis of size.[23] In the knee, an anteroposterior radiograph with a standardized magnification marker is used, and the mediolateral dimension of the tibia, just below and parallel to the joint surface, is measured. The measurement is accurately adjusted for magnification, and the tissue bank makes a direct measurement on the donor tibial plateau. Alternatively, a measurement of the affected condyle can be performed. A match is considered acceptable within 2 mm.

SURGICAL TECHNIQUES

Surgical transplantation of a fresh osteochondral allograft requires a medial or lateral arthrotomy. Occasional meniscal takedown for very posterior lesions with possible patellar eversion may be necessary. The lesion then is inspected and palpated with a probe to determine its extent, margins, and maximum size. Two techniques commonly used for preparation and implantation of osteochondral allografts are the press-fit plug (dowel) technique (Figure 6–1) and the shell graft technique (Figure 6–2). Each technique has advantages and disadvantages. The press-fit plug technique is similar in principle to autologous osteochondral transfer systems. It is optimal for contained condylar lesions between 15 and 35 mm in diameter. Fixation is generally not required because of the stability achieved with the press fit. Disadvantages include the fact that many lesions,

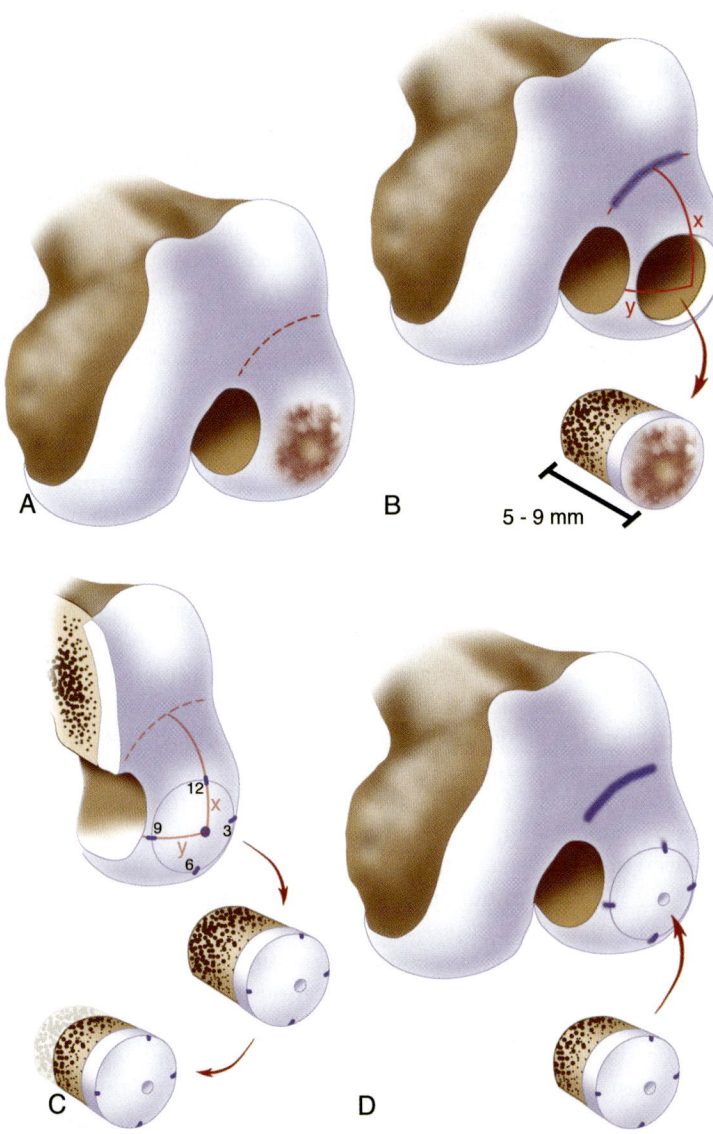

Figure 6-1 Diagrammatic representation of modern-day osteochondral allograft procedure by the dowel technique. *A,* Large focal chondral defect on the medial femoral condyle and its position relative to the sulcus terminalis (leading weight-bearing surface in full extension of the medial or lateral femoral condyles) is identified. *B,* Chondral defect is sized and removed as an osteochondral dowel for a total depth, including cartilage, of 5 to 9 mm. The position of the osteochondral defect is measured and referenced relative to the sulcus terminalis and the intercondylar notch in order to harvest a similar healthy osteochondral dowel from the donor allograft tissue. A donor osteochondral dowel will be oversized by 1 mm to provide a press fit at the time of implantation. Some systems require the recipient site to be conically dilated in order to allow ease of implantation, press fit, and no need for internal fixation. *C,* The donor osteochondral dowel is harvested relative to the position of the sulcus terminalis and intercondylar notch for its central coring reamer guidewire. The orientation of the dowel is marked with a sterile marking pen at the four quadrants of 12, 3, 6, and 9 o'clock in order to facilitate accurate placement at the recipient socket. The larger the diameter of the donor dowel, the more important it is to ensure that the quadrant marking depths are absolutely precise in order to have a flush transplant that is neither proud nor recessed below the articular surface. *D,* The deep surface of the donor dowel is measured and cut to depth precisely at all four quadrants. The recipient socket is usually dilated with a conical dilator prior to a press fit of the donor osteochondral allograft dowel. Implantation is performed with hand pressure or a gel-covered impaction device so as not to injure the fresh preserved cartilage cap.

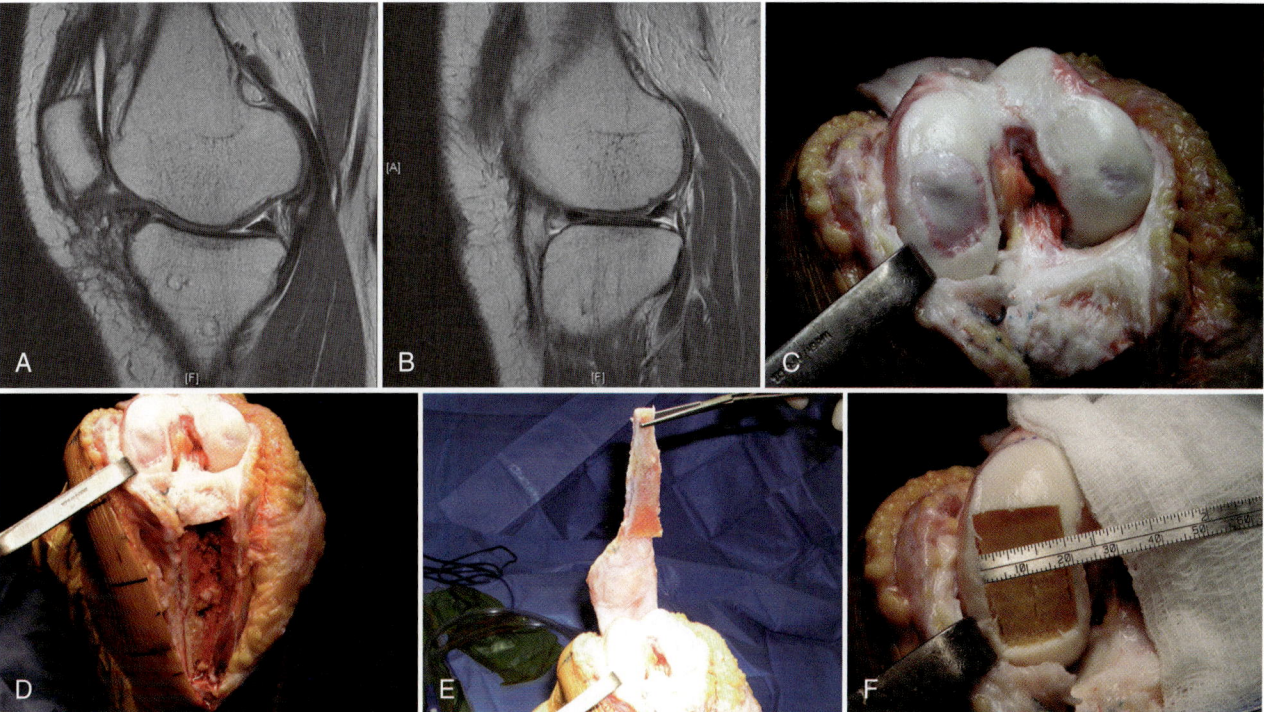

Figure 6-2 A young woman in her late 20s sustains a severe tibial plateau fracture to the left knee when she is kicked by a horse. Open reduction internal fixation is performed, and the fracture goes on to union. However, the patient is left with disabling, medially based pain following a large articular injury to the medial femoral condyle. The patient has developed patella infera with limited range of motion of the knee after the fracture. This was treated by autologous chondrocyte implantation (ACI) to medial femoral and lateral femoral condyles with lysis of adhesions by open technique. Despite early improved motion, she develops recurrent stiffness and continued weight-bearing pain. Her patella infera worsens. This case demonstrates the use of fresh shell osteoarticular allograft with an inlay technique to the medial femoral condyle and a dowel technique to the lateral femoral condyle as well as proximalization of the extensor mechanism with an extended tibial tubercle osteotomy. *A*, Sagittal magnetic resonance imaging (MRI) scan demonstrates patella infera, flattening of posterior medial femoral condyles at ACI transplant site, and old screw holes in the proximal tibia from the previous fracture. *B*, Sagittal MRI scan demonstrates a small lateral femoral condyle at ACI transplant site that is also somewhat flattened and incompletely filled. *C*, Open appearance of left knee with large medial femoral condyle and small lateral femoral condyle incompletely filled at ACI graft sites. Extended tibial tubercle osteotomy is performed to provide excellent exposure and allow proximalization of extensor mechanism to restore motion. *D*, Proximal tibia appearance after extended tibial tubercle osteotomy. *E*, Tibial tubercle osteotomy with medial and lateral subvastus arthrotomies maintaining quadriceps mechanism intact. *F*, Preparation of recipient bed on patient's medial femoral condyle to accept a fresh shell osteochondral allograft.

Continued

such as very posterior femoral, tibial, patellar, and trochlear lesions, are not accessible to a circular coring system. In addition, the more ovoid the lesion, the more normal cartilage must be sacrificed at the recipient site in order to accommodate a circular donor plug. Shell grafts are technically more difficult to perform and typically require fixation. However, depending on the technique used, less normal cartilage may need to be sacrificed. Also, certain lesions are more amenable to shell allografts because of their location.

Several proprietary instrumentation systems are available for the preparation and implantation of press-fit dowel allografts up to 35 mm in diameter. Presently this technique is the most commonly used. The lesion is identified, and the proposed graft is outlined and a template made using sizing dowels. After a size determination is made, a guidewire is driven into the center of the lesion, perpendicular to the curvature of the articular surface. If more than one dowel is required to treat the defect, one proximal to the other, then a "snowman" technique can be used or a cut can be made into the graft in order to maximize the treated surface. The remaining articular cartilage is scored, and a core reamer is used to remove that piece of cartilage and at least 3 to 4 mm of subchondral bone. When a patient has a deeper lesion, fibrous and sclerotic bone is removed up to a healthy, bleeding osseous base. When a lesion is very deep, coring should not exceed 10 mm in depth, and packed morselized autologous bone graft should be used to fill any deeper or more extensive osseous defects. The

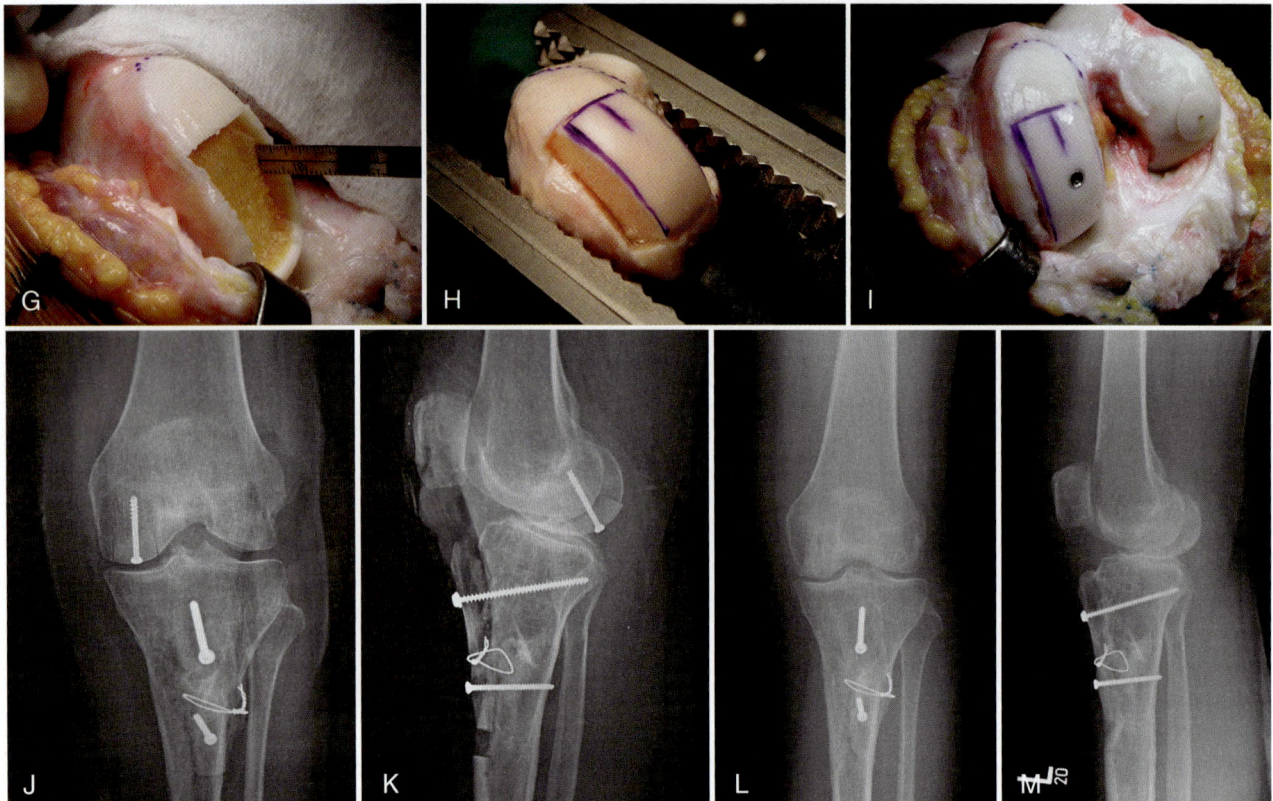

Figure 6-2—cont'd *G,* Exact measurements that include length, width, and depth are necessary. *H,* Preparation of shell allograft on back table. *I,* Final appearance of medial femoral condyle shell allograft after fixation with cannulated screw (buried screwhead). Lateral femoral condyle restoration with a dowel technique fresh osteochondral allograft. *J,* Anteroposterior radiograph after allograft implantation and proximalization of tibial tubercle osteotomy. *K,* Immediate postoperative lateral radiograph. *L, M,* Four-year postoperative radiographs demonstrate maintenance of joint space after allograft transplantation and proper patella height. The patient has maintained full range of motion of the knee, no extensor lag, good quadriceps strength, and pain-free function.

guidewire then is removed, and circumferential depth measurements of the prepared recipient site are made so the donor can be matched exactly.

The corresponding anatomic location of the recipient site then is identified on the graft, which is placed into a graft holder or is held with bone-holding forceps. A saw guide is placed in the appropriate position, again perpendicular to the articular surface, and an appropriately sized tube saw is used to core out the graft. Before the graft is removed from the condyle, an identifying mark is made to ensure proper orientation. Once the graft has been removed, the depth measurements determined from the recipient are transferred to the graft. This graft then is cut with an oscillating saw and trimmed with a rasp to the appropriate thickness in all four quadrants. The donor is then copiously pulse lavaged with bacitracin and saline to remove marrow elements from the donor. The donor is orientated appropriately and gently press fit so that it is flush to the host articular surface. Figure 6-3 shows the technique for a failed ACI procedure left in mechanical varus that requires fresh osteoarticular allograft with high tibial valgus-producing osteotomy. Figure 6-4 shows the technique for a patient with osteonecrosis.

The troublesome condition of posttraumatic collapse of the lateral tibial plateau with valgus deformity is ideally treated with fresh osteochondral allograft. My preference is to incorporate the meniscus with the allograft osteoarticular surface because its quality and its integration to the tibial plateau are perfect. The important thing to recognize after obtaining a perfect size match is that the valgus deformity cannot be corrected by the tibial plateau "stuffing the joint." This inevitably leads to premature wear and collapse of the allograft. A staged femoral osteotomy with tibial plateau allograft or simultaneous procedure, which is my preference, is appropriate. I have used an external tibial alignment guide, which is used for total knee replacement surgery, to make my sagittal and axial bone cuts to remove the damaged proximal lateral tibial plateau, leaving a perfect recipient site for the fresh osteoarticular allograft. The posterior capsule is dissected out first in preparation for passage of sutures through the capsule to anchor the posterior horn of the lateral meniscus. The anterolateral

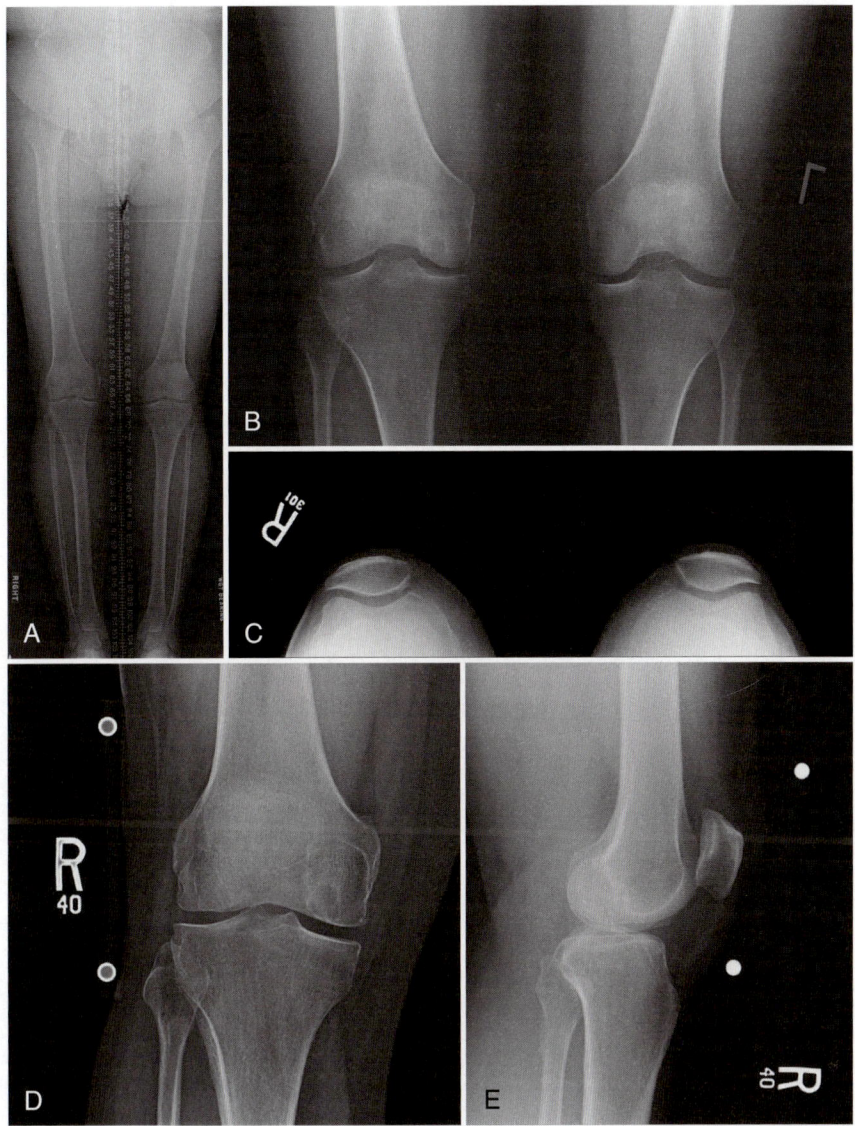

Figure 6-3 Case of a 42-year-old man who has failed autologous chondrocyte implantation (ACI) to the medial femoral condyles in a knee that remains in mechanical varus. Arthroscopic evaluation of the knee demonstrated a failed fibrous repair tissue. The decision was made to treat the defects (medial femoral condyles and trochlea) and to find an alternative cartilage repair technique that did not require cellular repair (i.e., fresh osteoarticular allograft with correction of mechanical overload). *A,* Long alignment radiographs demonstrate mechanical varus alignment of the right knee. *B,* Flexed 45-degree posteroanterior Rosenberg views demonstrate a characteristic medial femoral condyle lesion of osteochondritis dissecans. *C,* Skyline radiographs demonstrate well-preserved patellofemoral articulations. *D,* In preparation for fresh osteoarticular allograft, magnification markers for radiographic sizing are performed. A 10-cm radiographic marker is noted on anteroposterior (AP) x-ray film. *E,* The same procedure is performed on a lateral radiograph. The radiographic marker is measured, as is the AP and lateral dimensions of the tibia. In this way, a size match for a fresh osteoarticular allograft within 2 mm may be found.

Continued

arthrotomy takes down the capsule from the diseased proximal lateral tibial plateau to the posterior lateral corner at the level of the popliteus tendon. The donor allograft is measured to the recipient prepared bed, cut slightly oversized, and then trimmed as needed until a perfect fit is obtained. Fixation is generally achieved with just one or two lag screws to apply compression to the allograft, with large cancellous bony surfaces ensuring rapid osseous union (Figure 6–5). The bony thickness of the lateral tibial plateau should be the minimal amount to allow osseous union and creeping substitution without resorption and collapse of the allograft. From 5 to 10 mm of bone is usually adequate in addition to the 4 or 5 mm of cartilage that is present on the lateral tibial plateau surface.

A new technique of transplantation of allograft articular cartilage has been devised. Figure 6–6 illustrates the case of a young woman with advanced patellofemoral articular cartilage loss with maltracking. Minced juvenile human articular cartilage, when placed in a well-prepared articular

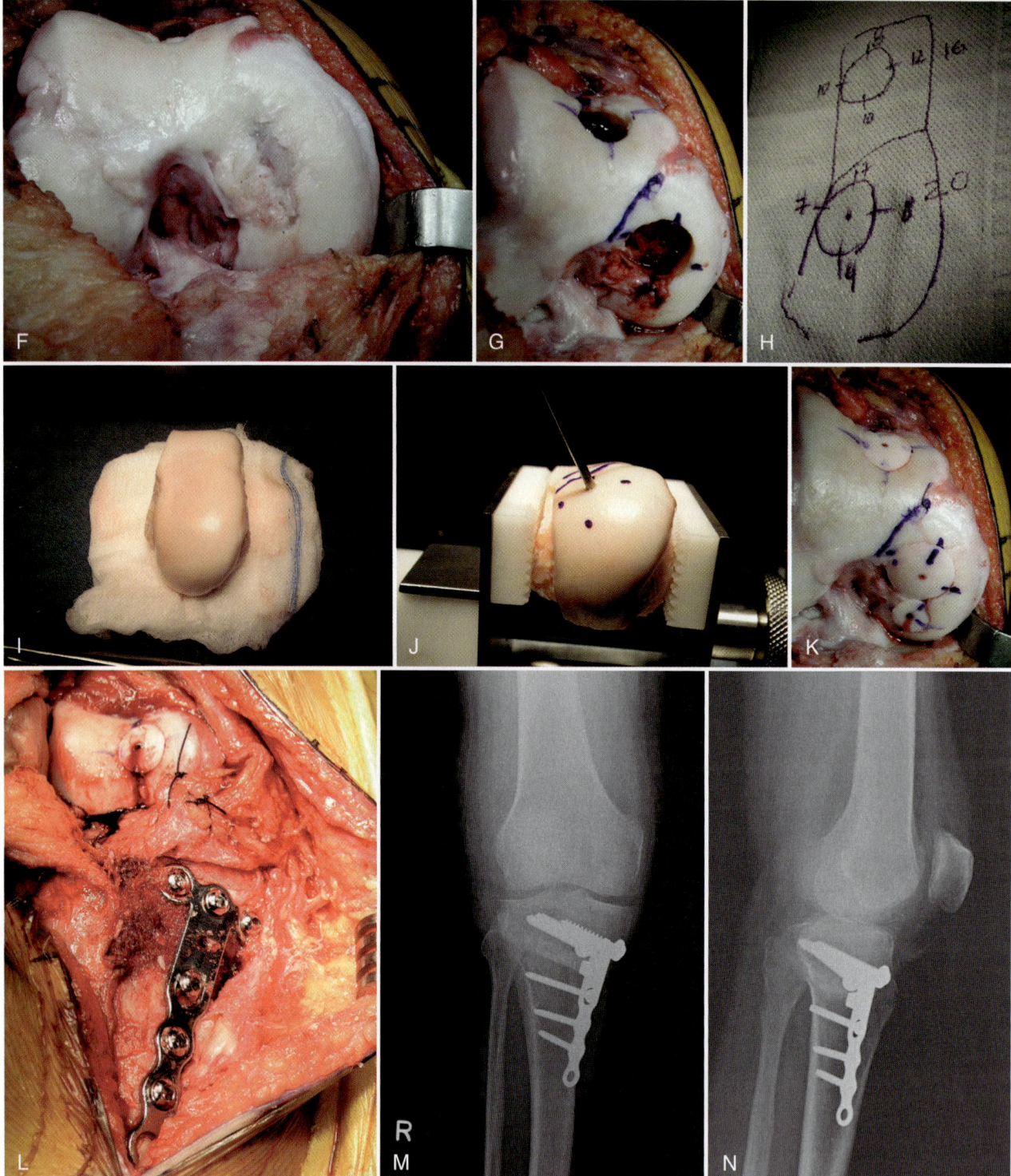

Figure 6-3—cont'd *F*, Open appearance of the failed ACI to the medial femoral condyle and trochlea. *G*, Sulcus terminalis of the medial femoral condyle is marked in terminal extension with a purple marking pen shown. Circular reamers are used over a guidewire perpendicular to the articular surface to ream out the articular defects until healthy subchondral bone is noted, which is usually a total depth of 5 to 9 mm from the articular surface. Markings are then used at all four quadrants of each defect. *H*, The depth of the defects are measured and noted. *I*, Fresh size-matched medial femoral condyle osteoarticular allograft is taken out of its preservative. The sulcus terminalis is noted, as is the top of the intercondylar notch. *J*, The central guidewire is positioned identically to the patient's defects, and a coring reamer 1 mm larger than the recipient site is used. Once the osteochondral dowel is extracted from the donor allograft, the quadrant depths at all four positions are measured on the allograft and cut precisely over a clamp. The recipient site is dilated 1 mm, and a donor allograft is carefully hand fit and pressed flush with the articular surface using a gel-covered impaction device. *K*, In this case, a second smaller more posterior dowel is added to cover the defect entirely, frequently resembling a snowman (i.e., the snowman technique). *L*, Opening wedge tibial valgus-producing osteotomy to normalize the mechanical axis to the center of the knee is performed simultaneously with the osteochondral allografts to the medial femoral condyles and trochlea. This is performed through a single midline incision. *M, N,* AP and lateral radiographs, respectively, 1 year postoperatively demonstrate well-preserved tibiofemoral and patellofemoral joint spaces with neutral mechanical alignment. The patient's painful mechanical and weight-bearing symptoms are completely resolved.

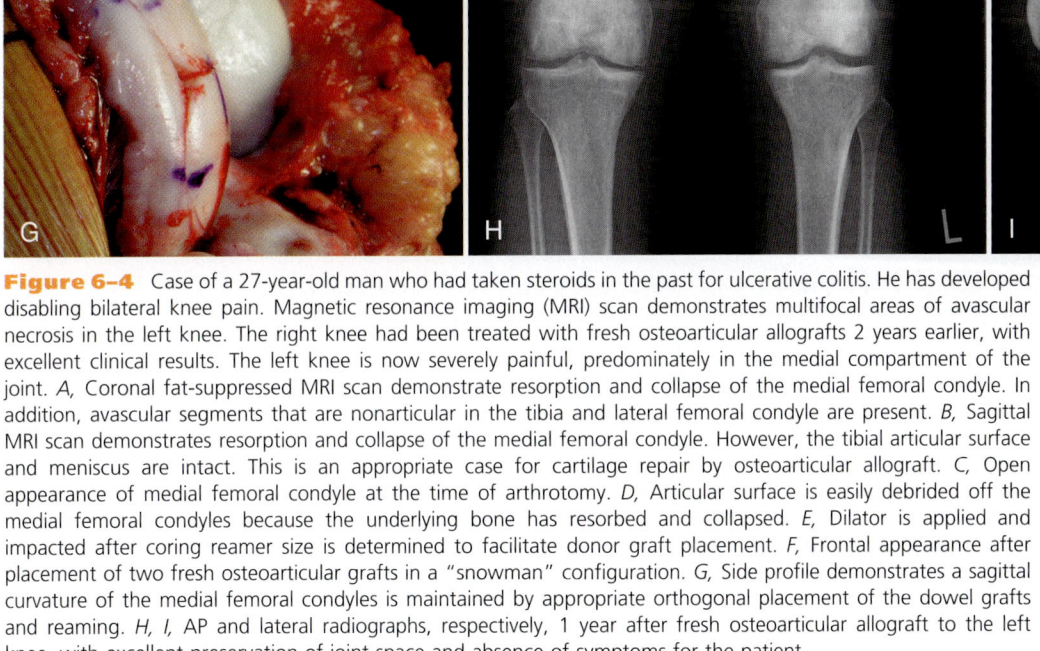

Figure 6-4 Case of a 27-year-old man who had taken steroids in the past for ulcerative colitis. He has developed disabling bilateral knee pain. Magnetic resonance imaging (MRI) scan demonstrates multifocal areas of avascular necrosis in the left knee. The right knee had been treated with fresh osteoarticular allografts 2 years earlier, with excellent clinical results. The left knee is now severely painful, predominately in the medial compartment of the joint. *A,* Coronal fat-suppressed MRI scan demonstrate resorption and collapse of the medial femoral condyle. In addition, avascular segments that are nonarticular in the tibia and lateral femoral condyle are present. *B,* Sagittal MRI scan demonstrates resorption and collapse of the medial femoral condyle. However, the tibial articular surface and meniscus are intact. This is an appropriate case for cartilage repair by osteoarticular allograft. *C,* Open appearance of medial femoral condyle at the time of arthrotomy. *D,* Articular surface is easily debrided off the medial femoral condyles because the underlying bone has resorbed and collapsed. *E,* Dilator is applied and impacted after coring reamer size is determined to facilitate donor graft placement. *F,* Frontal appearance after placement of two fresh osteoarticular grafts in a "snowman" configuration. *G,* Side profile demonstrates a sagittal curvature of the medial femoral condyles is maintained by appropriate orthogonal placement of the dowel grafts and reaming. *H, I,* AP and lateral radiographs, respectively, 1 year after fresh osteoarticular allograft to the left knee, with excellent preservation of joint space and absence of symptoms for the patient.

chondral defect as per ACI, may repair the defect through migration of the juvenile chondrocytes out of the matrix into the recipient bed, forming a chondral repair. This technology is new and represents a new paradigm of treatment. Equine research has demonstrated that this technique is effective even with xenograft species transplants. Human adolescent cartilage transplanted into horse chondral defects has demonstrated effective repair tissue originating from the human cartilage transplant. Unfortunately, the data are not yet published. Clinical human transplants at this time are demonstrating efficacy (see Chapter 14).

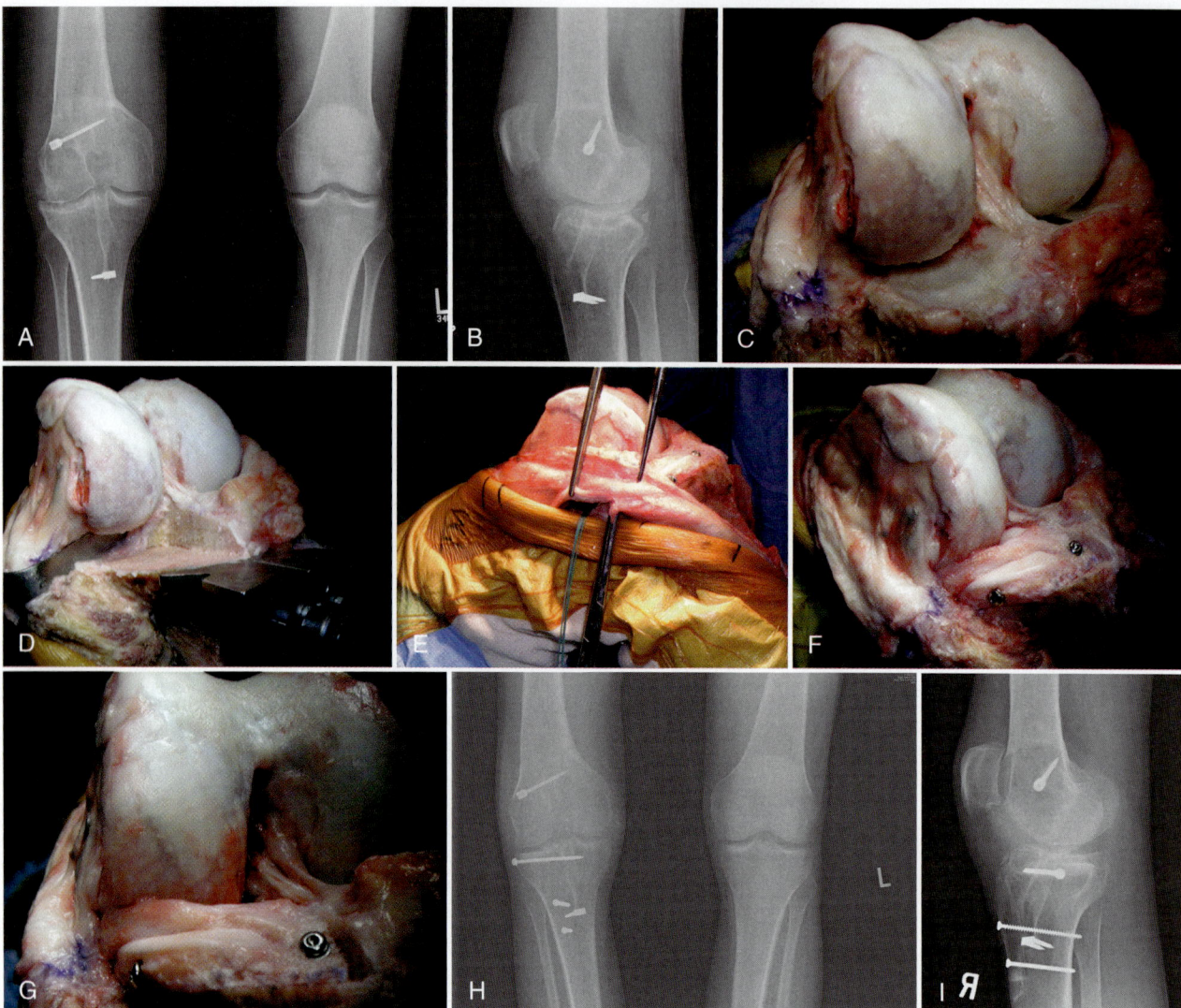

Figure 6–5 Case of a 21-year-old man who sustained a lateral tibial plateau fracture with collapse and valgus deformity. It was treated by varus femoral osteotomy and debridement of the lateral tibial plateau. The patient has persistent lateral-based pain and requires the use of narcotics and single crutch ambulation in order to get around. At the time of arthroscopic assessment, grade 4 changes throughout the lateral tibial plateau and an absent meniscus were noted. The lateral femoral condyle was intact. The plan was to perform a fresh combined osteoarticular and meniscal allograft transplantation. Because of delay in approval of the transplantation and graft match availability, at the time of open transplantation, grade 4 changes to the lateral femoral condyle had also developed. The lateral tibial plateau and meniscus were transplanted, followed 3 months later by transplantation to the lateral femoral condyle by autologous chondrocyte implantation (ACI). *A,* Anteroposterior (AP) radiograph demonstrates widening and irregularity, with early joint space narrowing and collapse of the lateral tibial plateau. *B,* Lateral radiograph demonstrates lateral tibial plateau depression. *C,* Tibial tubercle osteotomy and lateral subvastus exposure to the lateral compartment demonstrates depressed and widened lateral tibial plateau with grade 4 changes now evident on the lateral femoral condyle. *D,* External tibial alignment guide used for a total knee replacement for resection of damaged lateral tibial plateau. *E,* Posterior aspect of the knee has been dissected through the anterior flap for suture passage of the posterior horn of the lateral meniscal allograft through the capsule, deep to the lateral head of the gastrocnemius muscle. *F,* Side view of lateral tibial plateau with internal fixation. *G,* Frontal view. *H, I,* AP and lateral radiographs, respectively, 1 year after reconstruction with lateral tibial plateau and meniscal allograft transplantation combined with ACI to the lateral femoral condyle. The arthritic lateral compartment has been salvaged in this young man in his early 20s. The patient has pain-free function with activities of daily living.

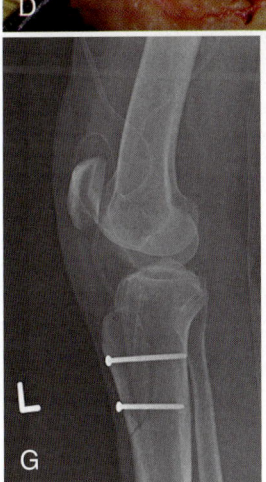

Figure 6-6 Case of a 40-year-old woman with chronic patellofemoral instability, crepitus A. nature knee pain. She is treated with morselized juvenile articular cartilage reconstruction of the patella with realignment tibial tubercle osteotomy. *A,* Axial computed tomographic (CT) arthrogram demonstrates patellar subluxation and near-pan patellar cartilage loss across the median ridge. *B,* Sagittal CT arthrogram demonstrates loss of articular cartilage to the patella on the distal half of the patellar surface. *C,* Open appearance of the patella after radical debridement of damaged articular cartilage. *D,* Using an aluminum template of the defect, the white allogeneic morselized juvenile articular cartilage fragments are evenly spread out and admixed with fibrin glue sealant. The entire slurry is then placed into the chondral defect and a type I-III collagen membrane is sutured overtop the injured region. *E,* Final appearance of transplanted morselized juvenile allograft cartilage. *F, G,* AP and lateral radiographs after transplantation with tibial tubercle osteotomy.

RESULTS AND CONCLUSIONS

Fresh osteochondral allografts demonstrate results similar to those of ACI in the short to mid term. When allografts fail, they do so by the process of incomplete incorporation of the osseous segment of the allograft or by creeping substitution with resorption and collapse of the allograft. For this reason, it is my opinion that when defects are large, it is prudent to treat surface defects that are truly isolated articular injuries by a surface repair with ACI. It is best to reserve osteoarticular allograft for failed ACI treatments or for their ideal indications of osteochondral defects, such as osteochondritis dissecans, osteonecrosis, posttraumatic osteochondral defects, and peripheral uncontained defects.

Gross et al[21] reported Kaplan-Meier survivorship scores of 95% at 5 years and 85% at 10 years for femoral allografts. When the defects failed, it was due to resorption and collapse necessitating prosthetic reconstruction. The graft survivorship observed by Williams et al[10] (84% at 4 years) was lower than that reported by Gross et al at mid-term follow-up with cold-stored commercial allografts. Nevertheless, allografts provide an excellent treatment option for osteochondral deficient lesions, which represent the ideal indication for allograft use to preserve the joint.

REFERENCES

1. Gross AE, Silverstein EA, Falk J, Falk R, Langer F. The allotransplantation of partial joints in the treatment of osteoarthritis of the knee. *Clin Orthop Relat Res.* 1975;108:7–14.
2. Gross AE, McKee NH, Pritzker KP, Langer F. Reconstruction of skeletal deficits at the knee. A comprehensive osteochondral transplant program. *Clin Orthop Relat Res.* 1983;174:96–106.
3. Convery FR, Meyers MH, Akeson WH. Fresh osteochondral allografting of the femoral condyle. *Clin Orthop Relat Res.* 1991;273:139–145.
4. Czitrom AA, Keating S, Gross AE. The viability of articular cartilage in fresh osteochondral allografts after clinical transplantation. *J Bone Joint Surg Am.* 1990;72:574–581.
5. Williams SK, Amiel D, Ball ST, et al. Prolonged storage effects on the articular cartilage of fresh human osteochondral allografts. *J Bone Joint Surg Am.* 2003;85:2111–2120.
6. Ball ST, Amiel D, Williams SK, et al. The effects of storage on fresh human osteochondral allografts. *Clin Orthop Relat Res.* 2004;418:246–252.
7. *Standards for tissue banking.* Arlington, VA: American Association of Tissue Banks; 1987.
8. American Association of Tissue Banks. *Standards for Tissue Banking.* Updated November 4, 2003. Available at http://www.aatb.org/standards-and-regulatory. Accessed 11/8/2010.
9. Food and Drug Administration. *Guidance for Industry: Screening and Testing of Donors of Human Tissues Intended for Transplantation.* Available at http://www.fda.gov/BiologicsBloodVaccines/TissueTissueProducts/Regulation-ofTissues/ucm1.
10. Williams RJ, Ranawat AS, Potter HS, Carter T, Warren RF. Fresh stored allografts for the treatment of osteochondral defects of the knee. *J Bone Joint Surg Am.* 2007;89(4):718–726.
11. Ohlendorf C, Tomford WW, Mankin HJ. Chondrocyte survival in cryopreserved osteochondral articular cartilage. *J Orthop Res.* 1996;143:413–416.
12. Enneking WF, Campanacci DA. Retrieved human allografts: a clinicopathological study. *J Bone Joint Surg Am.* 2001;83:971–986.
13. McGoveran BM, Pritzker KP, Shasha N, Price J, Gross AE. Long-term chondrocyte viability in a fresh osteochondral allograft. *J Knee Surg.* 2002;15:97–100.
14. Convery FR, Akeson WH, Amiel D, Meyers MH, Monosov A. Long-term survival of chondrocytes in an osteochondral articular cartilage allograft. A case report. *J Bone Joint Surg Am.* 1996;78:1082–1088.
15. Friedlaender GE. Appropriate screening for prevention of infection transmission by musculoskeletal allografts. *Instr Course Lect.* 2000;49:615–619.
16. Langer F, Gross AE, West M, Urovitz EP. The immunogenicity of allograft knee joint transplants. *Clin Orthop Relat Res.* 1978;132:155–162.
17. Sirlin CB, Brossmann J, Boutin RD, et al. Shell osteochondral allografts of the knee: comparison of MR imaging findings and immunologic responses. *Radiology.* 2001;219:35–43.
18. Garrett JC. Fresh osteochondral allografts for treatment of articular defects in osteochondritis dissecans of the lateral femoral condyle in adults. *Clin Orthop Relat Res.* 1994;303:33–37.
19. Bugbee W, Khadavi B. *Fresh osteochondral allografting in the treatment of osteonecrosis of the knee.* Presented at: American Academy of Orthopaedic Surgeons 71st Annual Meeting; March 10–14. San Francisco, Calif; 2004.
20. Gortz S, Bugbee WD. Allografts in articular cartilage repair. *J Bone Joint Surg Am.* 2006;88(6):1374–1384.
21. Gross AE, Shasha N, Aubin P. Long-term followup of the use of fresh osteochondral allografts for posttraumatic knee defects. *Clin Orthop Relat Res.* 2005;435:79–87.
22. Locht RC, Gross AE, Langer F. Late osteochondral allograft resurfacing for tibial plateau fractures. *J Bone Joint Surg Am.* 1984;66:328–335.
23. Highgenboten CL, Jackson A, Aschliman M, Meske NB. The estimation of femoral condyle size. An important component in osteochondral allografts. *Clin Orthop Relat Res.* 1989;246:225–233.

Chapter 7

Autologous Chondrocyte Implantation

Tom Minas, MD, MS

INTRODUCTION
  Historical Perspective
  Indications

ARTHROSCOPIC ASSESSMENT AND CARTILAGE BIOPSY FOR CELL CULTURING

SURGICAL CORRECTION OF BACKGROUND FACTORS PREDISPOSING TO CHONDRAL INJURY

SURGICAL IMPLANTATION OF AUTOLOGOUS CHONDROCYTES

ADVANCED TECHNIQUES FOR SURGICAL TRANSPLANTATION OF AUTOLOGOUS CHONDROCYTES
  Exposures
    Posterior Femoral Lesions and Tibial Plateaus
    ACI plus High Tibial Osteotomy, High Tibial Osteotomy plus Tibial Tubercle Osteotomy, Distal Femoral Varus Osteotomy
    ACI plus Tibial Tubercle Osteotomy for Posterior Exposure/with Patella/Trochlea ACI
    ACI with Osteochondritis Dissecans, Prior Bone Grafting, or Single-Stage Sandwich Technique ACI
    ACI plus ACL
    ACI plus Meniscal Allograft
    ACI after Marrow Stimulation Techniques
    ACI in Osteoarthritis, Uncontained Defects, and Sclerotic Subchondral Bone

AFTER CARE/REHABILITATION

COMPLICATIONS

CLINICAL OUTCOMES USING ACI
  ACI in Adolescents
  ACI in Soccer Players
  ACI in the Patellofemoral Joint
    Update on 130 Patients with Patellofemoral ACI
  ACI in Patients Older than 45 Years
    Conclusion
  ACI for Joint Preservation in Patients with Early Osteoarthritis: 2- to 11-Year Follow-up
    Autologous Chondrocyte Implantation
    Outcome Measures
    Results
      Patient and Defect Characteristics
      Treatment Failures and Revision Surgery
      Outcome Measures
      Additional Analyses
  ACI in Patients after Marrow Stimulation Techniques
    Increased Failure Rate of ACI after Previous Treatment with Marrow Stimulation Techniques
  Use of Type I–III Collagen Membrane for ACI Compared to Periosteum

CLINICAL COST EFFECTIVENESS OF ACI

SUMMARY

INTRODUCTION

Historical Perspective

Autologous chondrocyte transplantation is known as *autologous chondrocyte implantation* (ACI) in North America. After several visits to Sweden in the early 1990s, I adapted the technique described by Peterson and coworkers[1] (Figure 7–1). After institutional review board approval was given in 1994, the technique of ACI has been used to manage large acute and chronic focal articular cartilage injuries in the knee since March 1995. As of 2010, more than 600 treatments have been performed at our institution. More than 15,000 patients have been treated with ACI in North America and another 20,000 have been treated worldwide, for a total of 35,000 patients.

Use of autologous chondrocytes for patient care in the United States has been carefully regulated by the U.S. Food and Drug Administration (FDA, Biologics Division) and has required both Good Laboratory Practices (GLP standards) and Good Manufacturing Practices (GMP standards) since its introduction in the United States. This practice has been cost prohibitive to private and academic institutions with regard to patient care and therefore has been performed by industry (Genzyme Biosurgery, Cambridge, MA). As of August 22, 1997, the FDA formally approved ACI (FDA Biologics License 1233) for the management of focal chondral defects of femoral articular surfaces. This approval was based on the early data of 159 patients evaluated in Sweden as of 1997. Because early

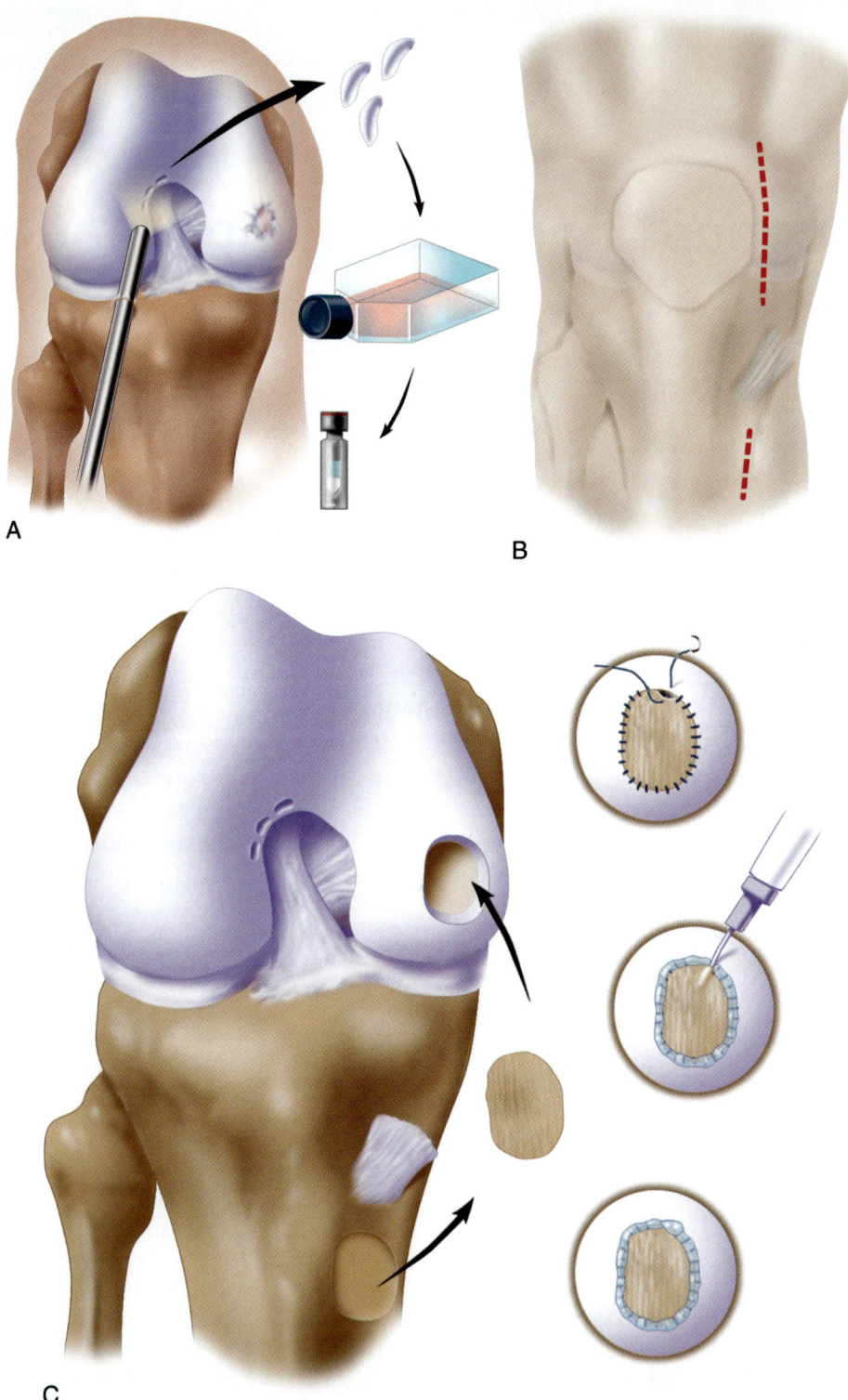

Figure 7-1 Classic technique for autologous chondrocyte implantation (ACI). *A,* Arthroscopic evaluation of the knee joint and identification of a full-thickness medial femoral condyle injury. A cartilage biopsy is taken from the superior intercondylar notch, digested, and cultured. Autologous chondrocyte transplantation will occur when the cells have reached a volume that can fill the articular cartilage defect. *B,* A two-incision approach is made to the knee. The first is a medial arthrotomy to expose the full-thickness medial femoral condyle defect. The second is an incision distal to the pes anserinus tendon insertion to harvest periosteum templated exactly to the defect after it is debrided. *C,* The technique of ACI. A periosteal patch is harvested distal to the pes anserinus tendons. It is microsutured with interrupted 6.0 Vicryl sutures flush to the articular surface and tested for water integrity tightness. It is then sealed with fibrin glue to maintain water tightness. The autologous chondrocyte suspension is injected deep to the periosteal cover to fill the defect, and the opening is sutured over and sealed with fibrin glue. The knee joint is closed. The patient undergoes careful rehabilitation to restore motion and allow the graft to mature uneventfully.

results were not favorable for management of the patella or tibia or for cases involving early bipolar or arthritic lesions, these defects have been considered "off label." However, prior to the FDA approval, I had gained considerable experience in the treatment of these off-label uses based upon experience with patients who had been referred for management of these troublesome lesions.

In my experience, the patient who is highly motivated, is realistic about the rehabilitation protocol, is a nonsmoker, and is not using narcotics for pain management is desirable. A strong social support system and a sense of vitality as measured by the Medical Outcomes Study 36-Item Short-Form Health Survey (SF-36) proved to be high statistical predictors of a good physical outcome in a study conducted at our institution and presented at the International Cartilage Repair Society in Toronto Canada 2001.[2] Patients younger than 18 years also have an excellent chance of returning to full activities.[3]

This chapter discusses the role of ACI for the treatment of full-thickness cartilage injuries of the knee. Since the initial publication on this topic,[1] there has been a renewed interest in the treatment and research of this clinical problem. The earlier published study indicated good and excellent results in 14 of 16 patients treated on the weight-bearing femoral condyles. Only 2 of 7 patients with patellar lesions who were treated had similar results.

Indications

The initial early indication for ACI was a symptomatic full-thickness weight-bearing chondral injury of the femoral articular surface in a physiologically young patient who was compliant with the rehabilitation protocol. The results of chondral injuries for the patellofemoral joint were not as consistently high as the results of femoral weight-bearing condyles. Cases of osteochondritis dissecans have also done well.[4] The ideal indication for ACI is treatment of a symptomatic unipolar Outerbridge grade III or IV injury, with no more than the reciprocal articular surface having Outerbridge grade I to II chondromalacia.

However, these injuries are uncommon. In a classic review of 31,516 knee arthroscopies, Curl et al[5] found that the incidence of an isolated femoral condyle defect in patients younger than 40 years was less than 5%. However, the incidence of articular cartilage injuries throughout the knee was almost 60%. This has also been my experience.

Because of the heterogeneous nature of articular cartilage defects found in knee arthroscopies that are symptomatic yet focal in nature, early on I elected to classify the treatments into relatively homogeneous groups: simple, complex, and salvage.[6,7]

Simple: Isolated Outerbridge grade III or IV weight-bearing femoral condyle defect is in a neutrally aligned knee that is stable with an intact meniscus.

Complex: Isolated or multiple Outerbridge grade III or IV chondral defect(s) is(are) on any surface within the knee joint. As unipolar lesions, background factors may require correction either before or at the time of cartilage surgery.

Salvage: Patients have early osteoarthritic lesions. Radiographically, early joint space narrowing and intralesional or peripheral osteophyte formation may be seen. Arthroscopically, bipolar lesions may be present in the patella–trochlea or tibia–femur, and generalized chondromalacia may be present. The lesions may be peripherally uncontained.

As of June 2009, 550 transplants (simple 35, complex 221, salvage 294) have been performed in 500 patients. In my series, simple cases accounted for only 35 (6.4%) of 550 treatments.

Management of the larger group of patients in the complex and salvage treatment categories has resulted in excellent clinical outcomes despite the heterogeneous nature of the cartilage injuries.[7] For this reason, my approach to treating young patients who are disabled with pain and poor function involves careful assessment of long-leg alignment x-ray films, a well-preserved weight-bearing joint space or early joint space narrowing, magnetic resonance imaging (MRI) scan, or arthroscopic evidence of focal acute or chronic articular cartilage injury. If the lesions are focal in nature when assessed arthroscopically and have identifiable borders and reasonable cartilage thickness, I consider the patient for ACI if the patient's symptoms appear to be referrable to the areas of chondral damage. A cartilage biopsy is then performed, and the cells are cultured, cryopreserved, and stored for second-stage implantation.

At the first postoperative visit, a careful discussion with the patient covers the proposed reconstructive surgery and addresses the background factors that require correction as well as the transplantation to the focal articular cartilage defects. The individualized surgery, hospitalization, and rehabilitation are discussed. The potential postoperative risks of stiffness and periosteal hypertrophy and how they will be managed if they occur are addressed. The patient's proposed goals for the final clinical outcome are assessed at this visit. If the goals are unrealistic, then other goals are discussed with the patient and realistic expectations are set. We do not proceed with surgery if the patient remains on baseline narcotics or is a smoker, or there is concern about the patient's emotional well-being. When these issues are addressed and resolved, we can proceed with the recommended reconstruction.

ARTHROSCOPIC ASSESSMENT AND CARTILAGE BIOPSY FOR CELL CULTURING

Arthroscopic assessment of the joint and possible biopsy for articular cartilage culturing require careful and systematic evaluation of the articular surfaces with an arthroscopic probe to demonstrate and determine the extent of grade III and IV chondromalacia of the symptomatic lesion. The opposing tibial articular surface must be probed throughout to ensure that the meniscus is intact, the articular surface is healthy, and the chondromalacia is no greater than grade II (superficial fissuring) ideally, otherwise it may also be considered for repair if the radiographic joint space is intact and the defect rim is healthy (Figure 7–2). The femoral condyle lesion should be assessed for its anterior to posterior length and whether it is a contained or an uncontained lesion. The quality and thickness of the surrounding articular cartilage should be assessed. This will determine whether healthy cartilage will be available for periosteum or colagen membrane suturing or whether an uncontained chondral injury will require suturing through synovium or small drill holes through the bone. The posterior extent of the lesion is critical because it must be accessed at the time of open arthrotomy for periosteal suturing.

If a lesion is considered appropriate for treatment, then a biopsy site for cartilage procurement must be selected (Figure 7–3). In Europe, the site most commonly chosen for biopsy is the superior medial edge of the trochlea, adjacent to the medial patella (odd) facet (Figure 7–4). The biopsy site will not produce a reciprocal symptomatic injury because there will be no opposing articular surface to make its contact. The patellofemoral joint must be assessed carefully. If a patellar facet is overhanging on the medial side, often the superior lateral facet may be

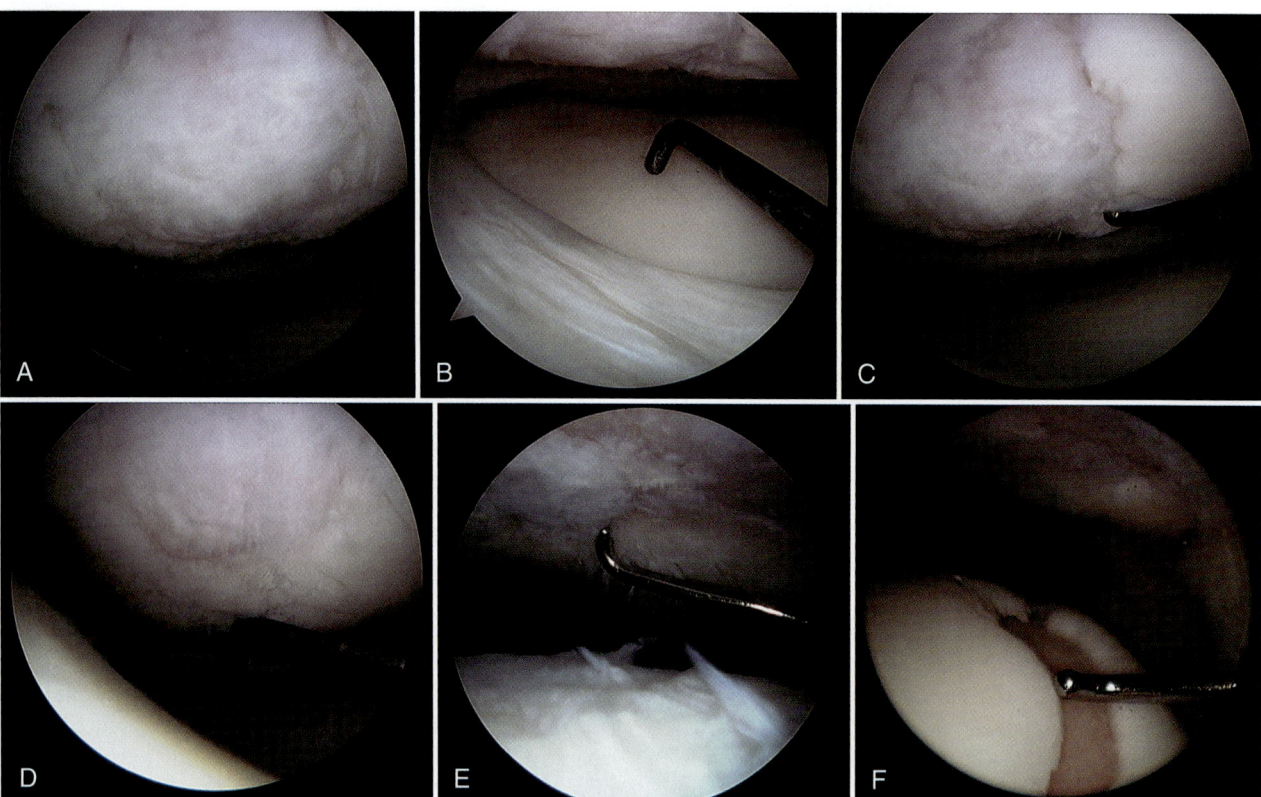

Figure 7–2 Arthroscopic knee joint evaluation. *A,* A focal area of cartilage damage is identified on the lateral femoral condyle. *B,* The tibial plateau is carefully probed to ensure that it is intact. *C,* The meniscus is also probed to ensure that it is intact. Some superficial Outerbridge grade II changes to the lateral tibial plateau are seen but are of no consequence. *D,* The chondral injury is carefully probed to identify that there is only a superficial fibrous tissue cover over a large intralesional osteophyte that has developed following a previous microfracture to the lateral femoral condyle. This patient is a candidate for autologous chondrocyte implantation (ACI). *E,* Another patient with arthroscopic evaluation of the patellofemoral joint. A large grade 4 defect of the patella is noted with intact margins. The trochlea has Outerbridge grade II superficial changes. Various lateral maltracking of the patella. The patient is a good candidate for ACI to the patella with tibial tubercle anteromedialization. *F,* A long focal grade 4 defect of the trochlea is 4 cm long and 1 cm wide. This patient also is a candidate for ACI.

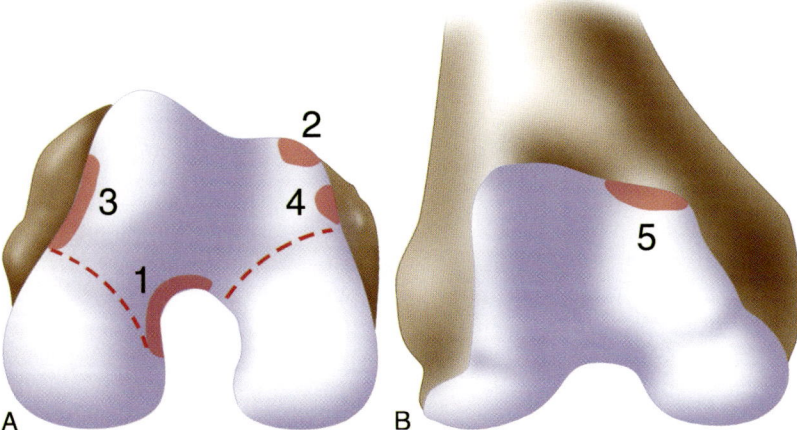

Figure 7-3 Arthroscopic biopsy sites for autologous chondrocyte implantation (ACI). *A*, Possible locations for biopsy performed for ACI. *Dotted lines* represent the leading weight-bearing surfaces of the femoral condyles, the sulcus terminalis both medial and lateral. Cartilage biopsies taken from the margins of the trochlea should be taken just proximal to the weight-bearing surfaces. When the intercondylar notch is harvested, the biopsy is taken from the superior surface to the sulcus terminalis on the lateral wall. *B*, Another location that can be used is the superior portion of the trochlea on the medial corner when all other sites are not appropriate.

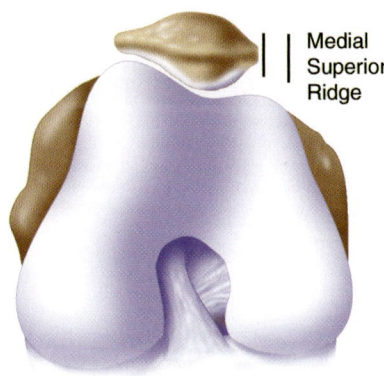

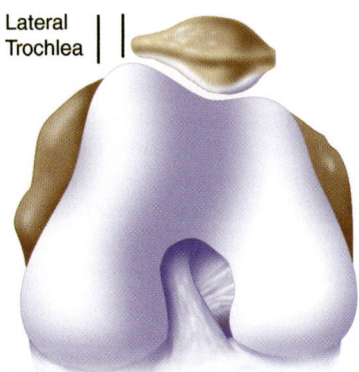

Figure 7-4 Classic location for harvest of cartilage for autologous chondrocyte implantation is the superior medial corner of the trochlea adjacent to the odd facet of the patella in a nonarticulating margin. However, when the medial patellar facet overhangs this margin, another location with no engagement of the patella should be found. Frequently the distal lateral trochlea proximal to the sulcus terminalis can be used.

harvested. My preferred location is the superior and the lateral intercondylar notch because it is convenient and is known to not create problems when removed, as in anterior cruciate ligament (ACL) reconstruction (Figure 7-5). Finally, the superior transverse trochlea margin adjacent to the supracondylar synovium, which may be biopsied through a separate superior portal, or the distal lateral trochlea at the sulcus terminalis as per harvesting an osteochondral autograft transfer system graft. At the time of open implantation, the synovium may be advanced over the biopsy site via sutures through the articular cartilage.

Approximately 200 to 300 mg of articular cartilage is required for enzymatic digestion for cell culturing. This is approximately a cartilage surface of 5 mm wide by 1 cm long. This piece will contain approximately 200,000 to 300,000 cells, which may be enzymatically digested and grown to approximately 12 million cells per 0.4 ml of culture media per implantation vial.

Biopsy instruments may include ring curette or sharp gouges. It is often helpful to incise and score the area of biopsy before attempting to remove it. A whittling, side-to-side motion of the gouge or curette will more accurately remove the desired cartilage without an unwanted slip. Full-thickness cartilage down to bone should be biopsied. It is helpful to leave an end of the articular biopsy attached so that it can be grasped with an arthroscopic grasper and torn off. This avoids an unwanted loose body in the joint, which then must be captured. Following in vitro expansion of cells 3 to 5 weeks later, a suitable number and volume of cells will be grown to accommodate the required defect size. At this time, second-stage open implantation may occur.

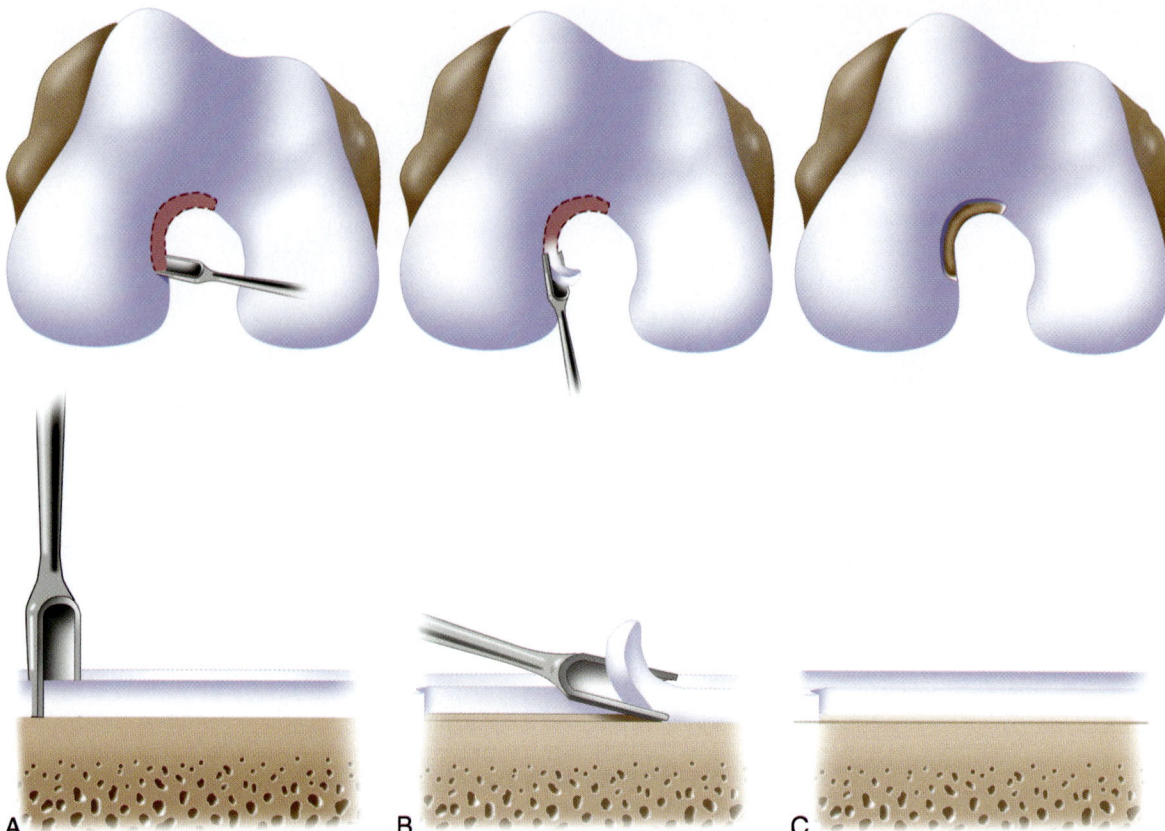

Figure 7-5 Surgical technique for harvesting articular cartilage from the intercondylar notch. *A*, Diagrammatic representation of the use of a sharp small gouge for scoring the articular cartilage from the superior intercondylar notch to the sulcus terminalis on the lateral wall. *B*, All layers of cartilage down to bone should be harvested to take representative articular cartilage layers using a side-to-side whittling motion. *C*, The defect left behind measures approximately 5 mm wide by 1 to 1.5 cm long. The full-thickness articular cartilage (usually 200–300 mg) is adequate for cell culture and expansion. It represents a non–weight-bearing portion when the knee is brought into full extension and visualized.

Continued

SURGICAL CORRECTION OF BACKGROUND FACTORS PREDISPOSING TO CHONDRAL INJURY

Several factors predisposing to chondral injury must be assessed so that they can be corrected in a staged or concomitant fashion with ACI. Tibial femoral malalignment, patellofemoral malalignment, and ligamentous, meniscal, or bone insufficiency must be assessed prior to definitive cartilage cell reimplantation.

Long-leg alignment is evaluated in all patients (see Chapter 3) with double leg stance long alignment digital radiographs that include the hip, knee, and ankle for varus and valgus mechanical alignment assessment. Clinical examination is notoriously unreliable for long-leg alignment.

Patellofemoral alignment is assessed by clinical examination with localization of the tibial tubercle, determining the quadriceps angle measured with the patella in the reduced position in the trochlea, the presence of a J-sign as the patella relocates from the extended into the flexed position, and the absence or presence of crepitus of the patella with active extension of the knee. If the patient is overweight and the clinical examination is difficult, a computed tomographic (CT) scan can be performed with the knee in extension, first with the quadriceps in the relaxed and then in the contracted position to assess patellofemoral subluxation (see Chapter 10). Dye can be added within the joint to localize and measure the chondral defect(s) in the patella, trochlea, or both.

A clinical examination is best for ligamentous instability unless the patient is very muscular or obese, in which case an MRI scan or an examination under anesthesia may be necessary.

Meniscal insufficiency is difficult to quantify with MRI scan unless the meniscus is completely absent. Arthroscopic assessment is best performed to assess the status of the meniscus and the residual hoop stress capability at the time of arthroscopy for cartilage biopsy for cell transplantation.

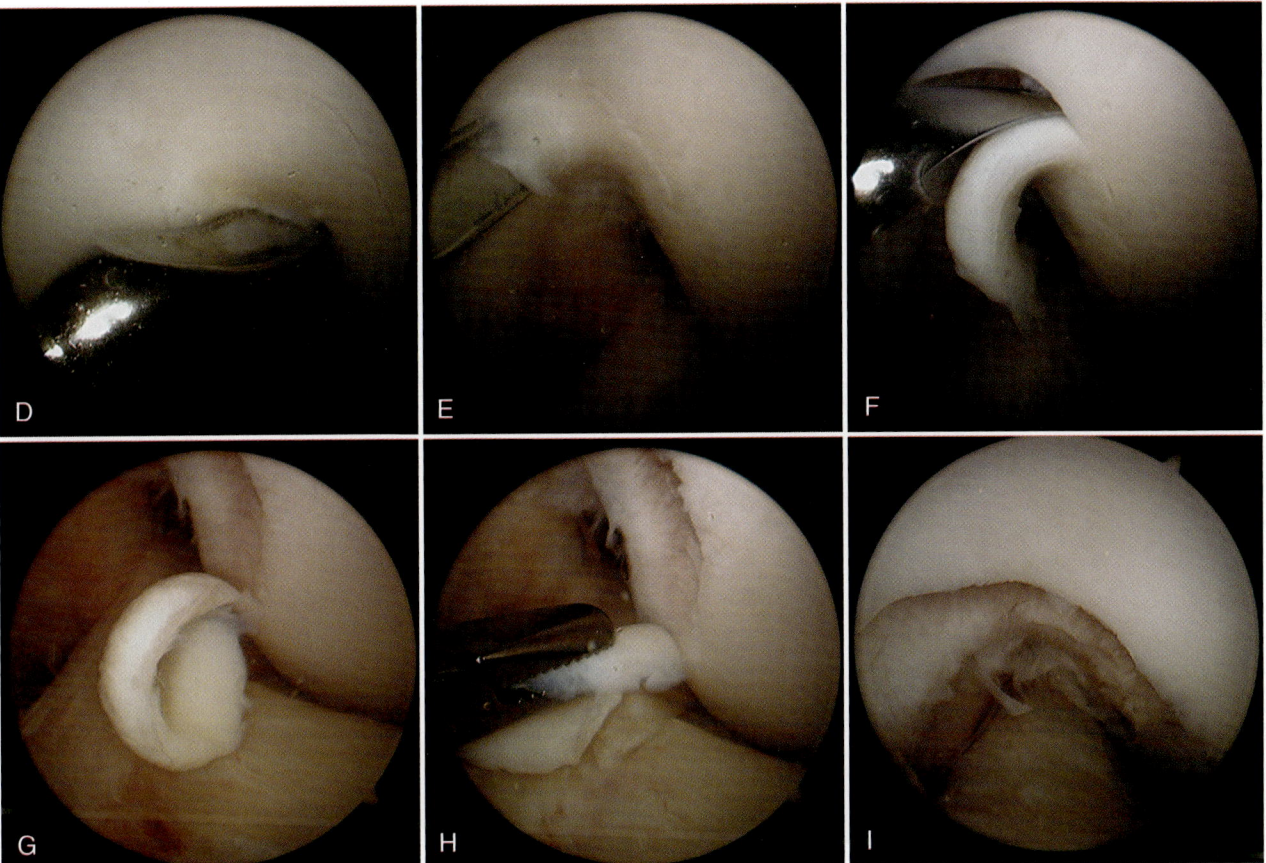

Figure 7-5—cont'd *D,* Arthroscopic appearance of the intercondylar notch at the time of biopsy in the left knee. Scoring of the articular cartilage to ensure that the gouge does not stray when pressure is applied to harvest cartilage. *E,* The gouge is started at the 11 o'clock position in a whittling manner. Full-thickness cartilage is engaged down to bone. *F,* The cartilage is left intact as it is brought to the lateral side of the intercondylar notch. *G,* The cartilage is left attached at its distal-most attachment site at the sulcus terminalis of the lateral femoral condyle. *H,* It is then grasped with a grasper and brought out of the medial arthroscopic portal as one piece. *I,* In full extension, no impingement of the cartilage on the tibial spines or the weight-bearing surfaces is seen.

Although arthroscopy is helpful in assessing the depth and character of an osteochondral defect, CT scan generally is more useful in determining the presence of subchondral bony cysts that cannot be visualized at the time of arthroscopy. This will help in addressing whether isolated ACI can be performed for an osteochondritis dissecans lesion or whether autologous bone grafting is necessary into a staged or single-step sandwich technique ACI. These techniques are discussed after open surgical transplantation of autologous chondrocytes is reviewed, in the case of an ideal lesion suitable for transplantation.

SURGICAL IMPLANTATION OF AUTOLOGOUS CHONDROCYTES

The steps in open implantation include arthrotomy, defect preparation, periosteum procurement, periosteum fixation, periosteum watertight integrity testing, autologous fibrin glue sealant, chondrocyte implantation, wound closure, and rehabilitation.

For a unicondylar injury, a medial or lateral parapatellar arthrotomy is used. This is usually accomplished through a midline skin incision or a longitudinal parapatellar incision. Adequate exposure is crucial to good suturing of periosteum, and several retractors are often required in order to obtain this goal. Posterior lesions on the femur will often require hyperflexion of the knee and occasional takedown of the meniscus in subperiosteal fashion with intermeniscal ligament takedown and coronary ligament release off the tibia as the meniscus is peeled back with the entire sleeve of tissue (Figure 7-6). A repair of these at the end is then undertaken during closure. For multiple lesions, a traditional medial parapatellar arthrotomy is often required with subluxation or dislocation and eversion of the patella with hyperflexion.

If the chondral defect is lateral, obtaining access to a posterior lesion frequently is difficult if the tibial tubercle is positioned laterally on the tibia. In this case, a tibial tubercle osteotomy (TTO) and elevation are helpful for exposing the lesion and realigning the extensor mechanism centrally (see section on ACI plus Tibial

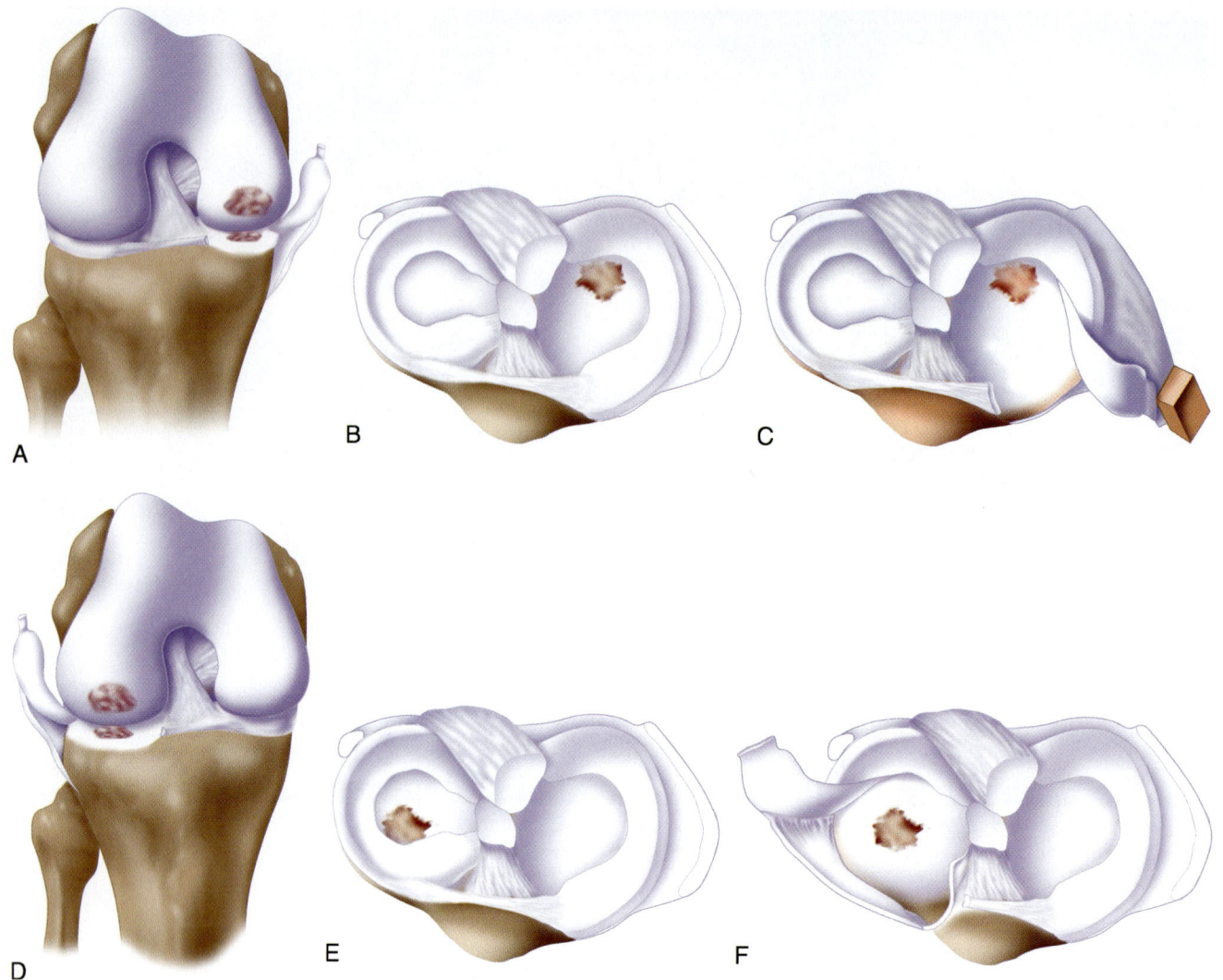

Figures 7–6 Deep dissection of a medial or lateral arthrotomy to obtain exposure to the posterior medial femoral condyle or tibial plateau, or a lateral femoral condyles and lateral tibial plateau. *A,* Frontal view demonstrating a medial femoral condyle defect that is posterior or a central or posterior medial tibial plateau defect. The intermeniscal ligament is taken down, as is the coronary meniscal attachment on the tibia down to the medial meniscus. The entire soft tissue sleeve is dissected posteriorly so that it is continuous and deep to the superficial medial collateral ligaments. By hyperflexing and externally rotating the tibia, the tibial plateau can be delivered almost entirely or the medial femoral condyle posteriorly. *B,* Superior view of a posterior tibial plateau chondral defect in relation to the intermeniscal ligament and the meniscus and superficial and deep medial collateral ligaments. *C,* As the medial sleeve is taken down in a posterior direction off the tibia to expose the posterior tibial plateau but is still too tight, then a bone block attachment to the femoral condyles origin of the medial collateral ligament will allow the entire medial side of the knee to be opened quite easily. It is then reattached with a screw and washer fixation at the end of the procedure. I have found this is rarely required. *D,* Frontal view of the lateral femoral condyle and lateral tibial plateau after dissection of a lateral sleeve of meniscus, coronary ligament, and portion of the iliotibial band insertion to gain exposure to the posterior lateral femoral condyles or lateral tibial plateau. *E,* View of the lateral tibial plateau cartilage defect from above, with structures intact. *F,* Superior view after release of the intermeniscal ligament and coronary ligament with lateral meniscus takedown of a lateral soft tissue subperiosteal sleeve. Upon completion of autologous chondrocyte implantation, the origins of the anterior horns of the medial or lateral menisci are reattached to their native positions using transosseous Ethibond sutures.

Tubercle Osteotomy for Posterior Exposure/with Patella/Trochlea ACI). This method will often allow a very posterior exposure to the femoral condyles without taking down the intermeniscal ligament with the meniscus and coronary ligament off the tibia.

Defect preparation is critical. Radical debridement of all fissured and undermined articular cartilage surrounding the full-thickness chondral injury to healthy contained cartilage is desirable. Early failures occurred due to inadequate debridement with poor integration to adjacent cartilage, leading to progression of disease in the adjacent nondebrided fissured cartilage or delamination of the repair tissue from the damaged native tissue. Oval or curvilinear excisions are made using a no. 15 blade to incise the articular cartilage vertically down to the subchondral bone plate without penetrating the bone. Small ring or closed curettes and periosteal elevators are used to debride the degenerating articular cartilage back to healthy host cartilage. Maintaining an intact subchondral bone plate without subchondral bone bleeding is important. It is essential not to perforate the subchondral bone plate so that a mixed marrow cell population does not populate the chondral defect in addition to the end-differentiated chondrocytes that have been grown in vitro. A contained lesion is desired, and it is better to leave a minimally chondromalacic cartilage border than to remove the border and leave an uncontained lesion that would require suturing to synovium or microholes through bone drills (Figure 7–7). Once a healthy defect bed is prepared, its length and width are measured. If the bed is irregularly shaped, then a template can be made with sterile tracing paper (sterile glove packaging paper works well). A sterile marker can be used to make a template of the defect, which can be cut out to fit the defect perfectly. This template then can be oversized by approximately 2 mm in both length and width on the periosteal site when it is prepared (the periosteum shrinks as it is procured). Alternatively, this can be measured and marked with a marker pen directly onto the periosteum if it is an uncomplicated shape and then cut directly (Figure 7–8).

Any subchondral thickening, sclerosis, or intralesional osteophyte formation at the base of the chondral defect as a result of a prior marrow stimulation technique (drilling, abrasion, microfracture) should be taken down to the level of native subchondral bone. This can be performed with a rongeur and a high-speed bur (usually 5-mm diameter) to the level of native subchondral bone (Figure 7–9). This will provide a cavity for the cell suspension, which is injected underneath the membrane cover and will lessen the stiffness of the subchondral bone so that newly forming cartilage repair tissue will integrate and form a new osteochondral unit with a viscoelastic cartilage surface, a subchondral bone plate that is not overly stiff to cause premature degeneration of the tissue and a normal subchondral cancellous bone. Surprisingly, this thickened and calloused bone does not bleed when a tourniquet is let down. Bleeding, if it occurs, usually is scant and easily managed with a neural patty soaked with thrombin and epinephrine or with a drop of fibrin glue. Occasionally a fine-tip electrocautery is used.

Thickening and sclerosis of the subchondral down is also found in patients having early osteoarthritis with chronic articular chondral defects. In these cases, the surrounding cartilage is often thinned out, and the periphery of the defect is marginally uncontained. A contained

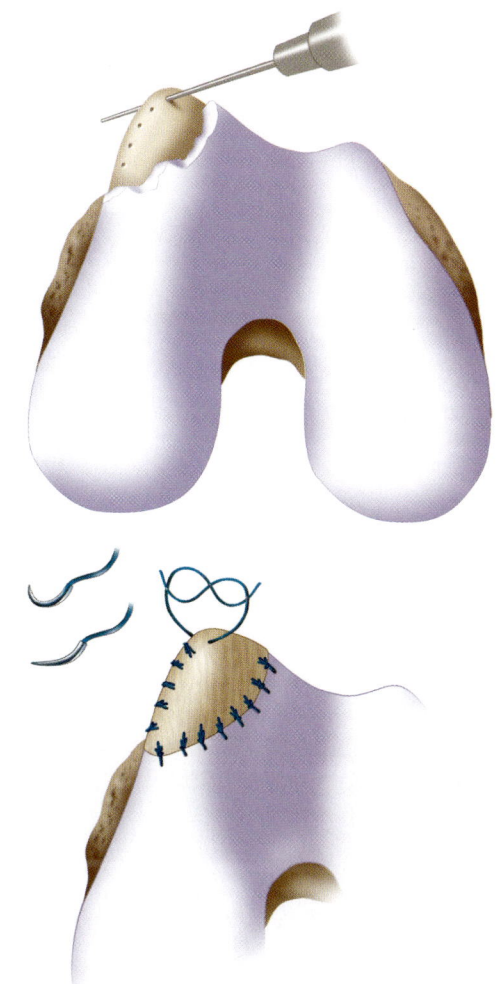

Figure 7-7 Transosseous drill hole fixation for uncontained cartilage defects. A large uncontained lateral trochlea defect is demonstrated. Radical debridement of the cartilage is performed. Any sclerotic bone is removed with a sharp ring curette and possibly deepened with a high-speed bur if the bone is very sclerotic, leaving a prominent peripheral margin intact. Transosseous drill holes through the margin then allow a cavity to be formed. A small P1 cutting needle is straightened out with two heavy needle drivers. The sutures are transfixed through the membrane and the drill holes to maintain a peripheral seal to the defect. This is reinforced with fibrin glue sealant around the uncontained margins, checked for water tightness, and then injected with autologous cultured chondrocytes once the defect margins are secured and watertight.

defect can be made using a high-speed bur to deepen the area of bony exposure to a level of more normal-appearing subchondral bone and using transosseous drill holes around the periphery to anchor the membrane and provide a cavity for the cartilaginous tissue repair. Frequently this has been my method of repair for patients in the salvage category of treatment.

The easiest and most suitable location for periosteum procurement is the proximal medial tibia, distal to the pes anserinus insertion on the subcutaneous border.

74 PART 2 CARTILAGE REPAIR SURGICAL TECHNIQUES

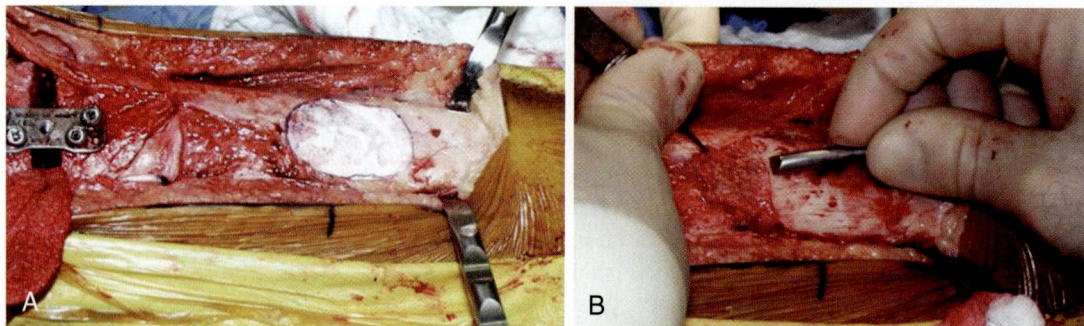

Figure 7-8 Periosteal harvest. *A,* Paper template is applied distal to pes anserinus tendons on the subcutaneous medial border of the tibia onto the periosteum directly. It is sharply oversized by 1 mm circumferentially using a no. 15 blade. *B,* A small sharp periosteal elevator is used to remove the entire periosteal membrane off the bone, maintaining the deep cambium layer orientation. The superficial fibrous layer is marked with a sterile marking pen to ensure this orientation.

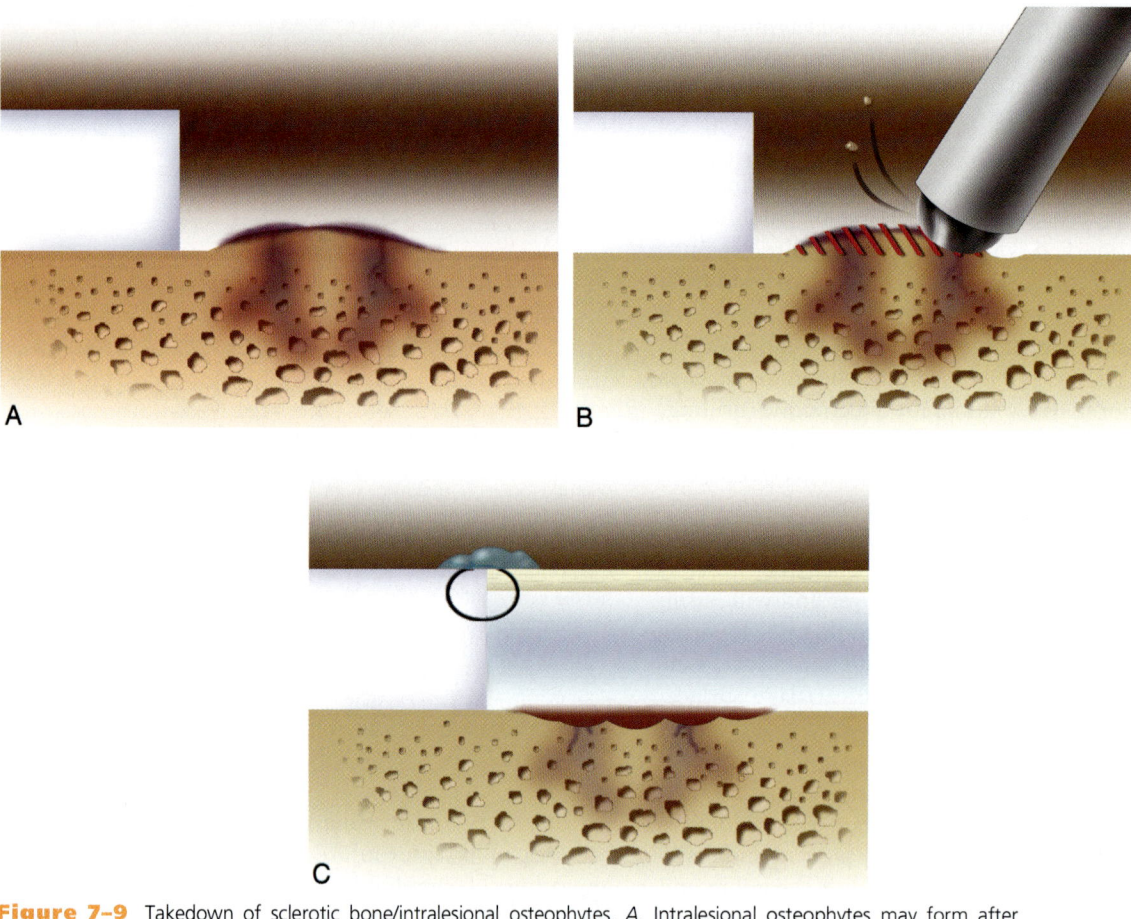

Figure 7-9 Takedown of sclerotic bone/intralesional osteophytes. *A,* Intralesional osteophytes may form after marrow stimulation techniques (abrasion, drilling, microfracture) as well as from idiopathic osteoarthritis. *B,* A 5-mm high-speed bur is used to gently under irrigation may be been used to take down this sclerotic cortical type bone to the level of the adjacent native subchondral bone. *C,* When the tourniquet is let down, little bleeding occurs from these sites. Autologous chondrocyte implantation (ACI) may then be performed safely on a chondral defect whose depth has not been taken up by bone. Whether this technique will improve the results of ACI after marrow stimulation techniques is unknown.

This site has subcutaneous fat, a very thin fascial layer, and easy access to the periosteum. Once defect size has been assessed and a template made, a second incision is made approximately a finger's breadth distal to the pes anserinus insertion, in the center of the medial subcutaneus border of the tibia. Subcutaneous fat is incised initially, and then scissor dissection will reveal the shiny white proximal tibial periosteum. A wet sponge can be sued to sweep away loose areolar tissue. Electric cautery should not be used around periosteum because it will necrose the periosteum with the very sensitive cambium layer of cells on its deep surface.

The template is placed on the periosteum; alternatively it is marked with a ruler and a sterile marking pen. A sharp no. 15 blade is used to incise sharply, oversizing the periosteum 1 mm in all directions down to bone. A small sharp periosteal elevator is useful for very gently advancing the periosteum from its bony bed and preventing it from under-rolling so that it does not rip. Nontoothed forceps will aid in pulling the periosteum upward as it is gently removed from the tibia. A gentle push–pull type of motion of the periosteal elevator from side to side across the periosteum will help with its removal. The outside of the periosteum should be marked as the superficial surface so that it is not inadvertently placed on upside down.

At this time the defect site is inspected, the tourniquet can be either let down to assess bleeding of the subchondral bone plate or let down at the end of the procedure if the surgeon is confident that the bone bed does not appear to be violated. Any bleeding of the bony bed can usually be stopped using a combination of thrombin and epinephrine soaked in a neural patty, which is applied to the defect and gently pressed for several minutes. If some bleeding continues after the neural patty is removed, a small drop of fibrin glue will usually suffice to dry the defect.

The goals of periosteum or collagen membrane fixation are threefold: (1) to provide a watertight membrane that acts as a mechanical seal, (2) to act as a semipermeable membrane for intraarticular synovial nutrition to chondrocytes, and (3) to maintain a viable periosteal cambium layer of cells so that interactive growth factors between chondrocytes and periosteum can enhance chondrocyte growth. These factors include transforming growth factor-β, insulin-like growth factor, interleukin-2 (IL-2), and IL-6. They have been found to enhance chondrocyte colony formation when they are separated from periosteum and delivered directly to chondrocytes in suspension. To this end, it is important to handle the periosteum delicately so that it is not perforated and to keep it moist so that it does not undergo shrinkage or cambium cell death. Its orientation is always maintained so that a cambium layer is facing in toward the subchondral bone plate as noted by a pen mark on the superficial aspect.

Periosteum may then be placed gently onto the defect in the appropriate orientation. Nontoothed forceps are used to handle the periosteum by its edges only. Suturing is usually done with 6.0 Vicryl suture on a P-1 cutting needle, which has been immersed in sterile mineral oil or glycerin. An 8-inch length usually is adequate; the remainder of the suture is cut off and discarded. Suturing is done in an interrupted and alternating fashion. Sutures are placed through the periosteum and then the articular surface. The knots are tied on the side of the periosteum so that they remain below the level of the adjacent cartilage. In this way, they will not unravel with motion and evert the periosteal edge; rather, they act as a washer seal on the edge of the vertical articular cartilage defect (Figure 7–10). Hence, a watertight seal can be obtained by suture technique alone in most cases. When alternately suturing

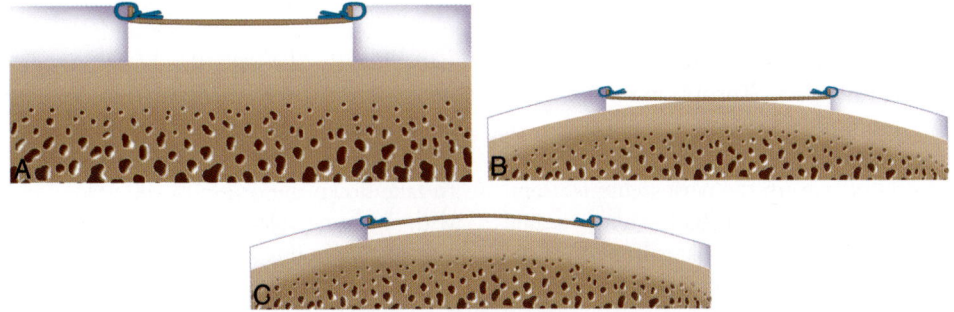

Figure 7–10 Suturing techniques for large femoral condylar defects. *A,* Example of good suturing technique for a cartilage defect. The suture is placed through the periosteum and then the cartilage to obtain a good purchase of both tissues. The knot is tied on the side of the periosteum so as to evert the periosteum flush to the cartilage side wall and make it watertight, like a washer. In this way, the suture is also below the level of the articular cartilage and is less likely to unravel once the knee starts to undergo motion. The membrane is flush with the articular surface and forms a cavity or bioactive chamber for the cells to grow to the limiting surface membrane. *B,* Four long femoral condylar defects in the anterior to posterior direction suturing technique is important to maintain a uniform cavity throughout the length of the defect. If medial to lateral suturing is not performed through the length of the defect from anterior to posterior, the membrane may bottom out on the center aspect of the length of the curve. This site is more likely to undergo premature breakdown. *C,* If the periosteal or collagen membrane is oversized in the anterior to posterior length direction, suturing is started at the center of the defect in a medial to lateral direction, and then anterior to posterior. The chamber cavity will maintain a uniform depth and more likely will undergo full, even cartilage fill for the length of the defect.

corners, the analogy of tightening up a drum skin alternately is followed. In this way the patch is tensioned adequately throughout the entire defect, and the most superior aspect of the periosteal patch is left open to accept saline to check edge integrity and then chondrocytes. Interval sutures of approximately 3 to 6 mm are made and protrude through the articular surface by at least 3mm.

Periosteum watertight integrity testing is assessed using a plastic 18-gauge 2-inch angiocath with a tuberculin syringe filled with saline. This step is usually avoided when a collagen membrane cover has been used because it tends to displace the cell suspension and prevents it from being absorbed to the collagen membrane, which is the desired effect. The angiocath is placed deep to the periosteum into the defect, and the defect is gently filled with saline. A meniscus should rise to the opening if the defect is watertight. Any leakage can easily be seen around the perimeter of the repair site. An additional suture may be required to achieve water integrity. The saline then is aspirated out of the defect. If water integrity cannot be obtained by suture technique alone, then a fibrin sealant is also used.

For autologous fibrin sealant, the patient must donate 1 unit of whole blood preoperatively. The whole blood is spun off for a pack of red blood cells as well as a supernatant, which is concentrated to produce cryoprecipitate by a double-spin freeze–thaw technique. This process takes 14 days of preparation prior to surgery. Following the double-spin freeze–thaw technique, a concentration of approximately 80 to 100 mg/dl fibrinogen can be obtained. The fibrinogen or cryoprecipitate is activated with bovine thrombin and calcium. A double-barreled syringe is required. One barrel contains the cryoprecipitate; the other barrel contains a 50/50 admixture of 10% calcium chloride and a superconcentrated bovine thrombin. Fibrinogen is cleaved into active fibrin, which is deposited along the margins of the defect, sealing them. Commercially available Tisseel (Baxter Biosurgery, Deerfield, IL) is made from pooled human serum and is available in Europe and the United States.

After the defect is sealed, water integrity is tested again. The angiocath underneath the periosteum is useful to ensure that the periosteum is not inadvertently sealed to the subchondral bone. The saline is aspirated out of the defect bed, and the defect is now ready to accept chondrocyte implantation. The chondrocyte suspension is sterilely aspirated in a tuberculin syringe through an 18-gauge or larger needle (smaller gauges will damage the cells), and the needle is removed and switched to a flexible 18-gauge 2-inch angiocath. The cells are very gently delivered through the superior opening of the periosteal defect margin down to the base of the defect as the angiocath is withdrawn cues are injected until a meniscus comes to the surface. After the defect is filled with cells, it is covered with several sutures and then sealed with fibrin glue.

The procedure is now complete. Drains generally are not used within the joint so as not to damage the periosteal patch or suck out the cells from the defect but should be used without suction if needed. The wound is closed in layers, and a soft dressing is applied to the knee.

ADVANCED TECHNIQUES FOR SURGICAL TRANSPLANTATION OF AUTOLOGOUS CHONDROCYTES

Exposures

Posterior Femoral Lesions and Tibial Plateaus

When attempting to approach a femoral condyle lesion that is very posterior or a tibial plateau lesion, and a takedown of a soft tissue envelope to varying degrees may be necessary. This involves incising the intermeniscal ligament followed by the coronary ligament attachment to the tibial plateau with a subperiosteal peel off the tibia in a posterior direction. It is easier to perform on the medial side with a long sleeve of medial retinaculum to the deep portion of the medial collateral ligament in the midcoronal plane. This usually is enough to get to a posterior medial femoral condyle. Two options are available to get to the midportion of the medial tibial plateau or the posterior portion. The deep medial collateral ligament may be further taken off in a continuous sleeve with the anterior portion until the entire tibial plateau is delivered anteriorly by externally rotating the tibia and hyperflexing the knee. Transosseous sutures with no. 2 Ethibond can be used to reattach the sleeve of tissue back to its native position at the time of closure. This process is relatively easy when the sutures are passed almost at the level of the joint where the metaphyseal bone is softer and the suture needle can pass directly through the bone in one easy step. The anterior horn of the medial meniscus is reattached through transosseous sutures back to its native origin. The intermeniscal ligament is repaired. The other option is to take down the origin of the medial collateral ligament with a bone block off the femoral condyle, which completely opens up the medial side of the knee. I have found that this is rarely necessary and that the first option is preferable unless a very posterior medial tibial plateau requires suturing (Figure 7–11).

Approaching the lateral tibial plateau or posterior lateral condyles is often more difficult. A lateral parapatellar arthrotomy is performed. The intrameniscal ligament is released and the coronary ligament with the anterior horn of the lateral meniscus peeled subperiosteally with the sleeve, which will often include some of the

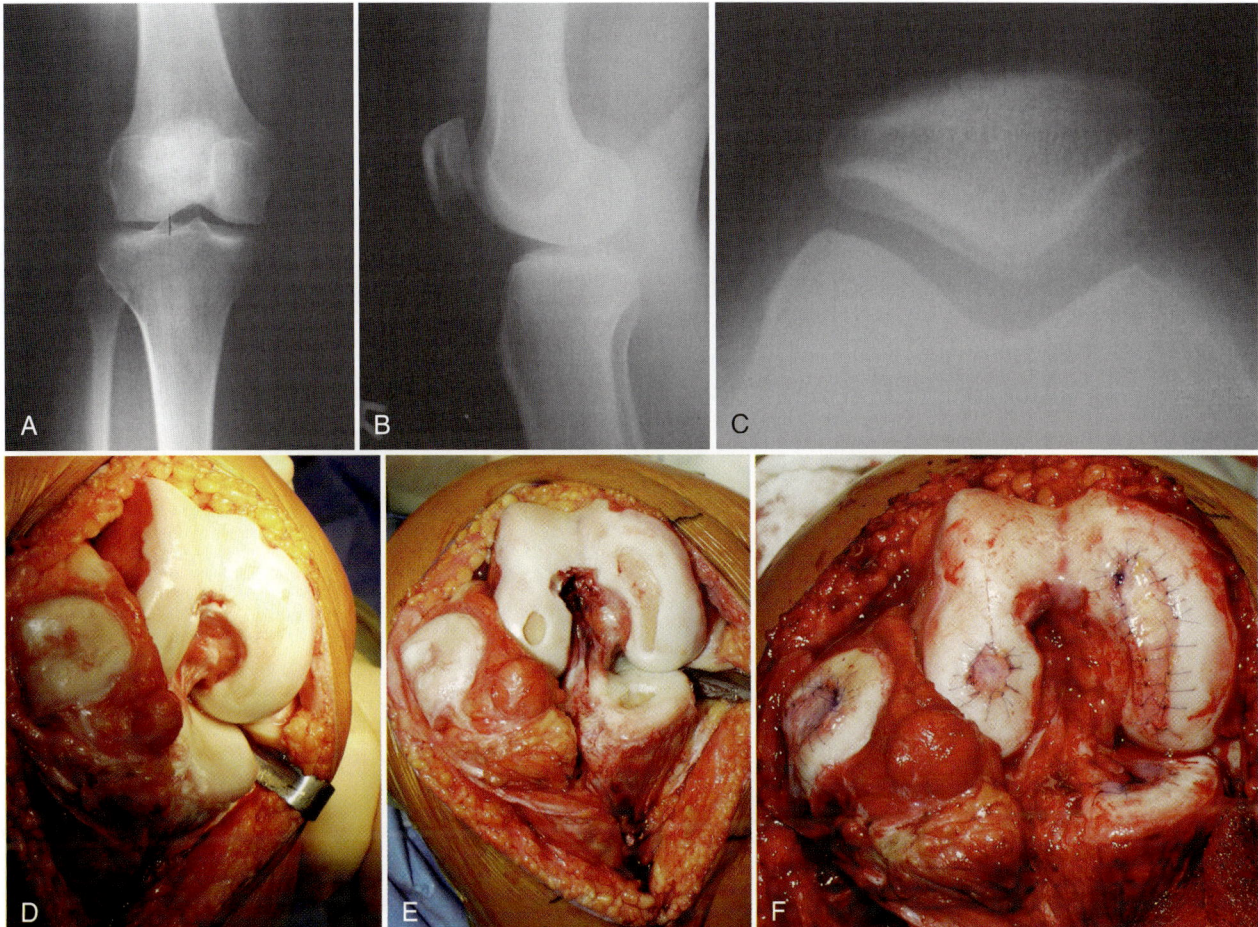

Figure 7-11 Case example demonstrating exposure to posterior weight-bearing condyles and tibial plateau. *A,* Weight-bearing x-ray film of a young woman involved in a motor vehicle accident who had intractable global joint pain. Her joint spaces are normal and her ligamentous exam intact. She has tricompartmental crepitus and joint effusions on clinical examination. *B,* Lateral x-ray film demonstrating intact patellofemoral and tibiofemoral joints. *C,* Intact skyline view of cartilage spaces. *D,* Medial parapatellar arthrotomy is performed with a patellar eversion, and a medial subperiosteal peel maintains the entire medial sleeve intact. This method gives excellent exposure to all the articulations, including the tibial plateau immediately in the posterior medial femoral condyles. *E,* After radical debridement of the articular cartilage injuries back to intact stable cartilage, focal defects are delineated, templated, and measured. *F,* Periosteal harvest from the medial subcutaneous border of the tibia is performed. The defects are microsutured, sealed with fibrin glue, and injected with autologous cultured chondrocytes. Ten years later the patient remains free of pain and discomfort and maintains normal joint spaces radiographically.

attachment of the iliotibial band insertion at Gerdy's tubercle. The patella is subluxed into the medial parapatellar gutter, and the knee is hyperflexed and internally rotated. This will usually deliver the lateral tibial plateau quite well and will expose the posterior lateral femoral condyles. This step may not be possible if the knee is stiff and the tibial tubercle insertion is located very laterally. In this situation, TTO with a subvastus lateral arthrotomy is recommended, which will easily expose the distal lateral femoral condyles and the entire tibial plateau. The meniscus may still need to be taken down and reapproximated after the procedure for tibial plateau injury is completed (Figure 7-12).

ACI plus High Tibial Osteotomy, High Tibial Osteotomy Plus Tibial Tubercle Osteotomy, Distal Femoral Varus Osteotomy

When varus or valgus malalignment is concomitant with a medial or lateral condyle injury, respectively, then a corrective osteotomy is paramount to the success of ACI. This can be done in either a staged or a concomitant fashion. My preference is to perform the procedure all at once. A single longitudinal incision will achieve the exposure for both procedures quite easily. However, it is imperative that if the procedure is done concomitantly, a stable fixation must be obtained at the time of osteotomy surgery so that continuous passive motion (CPM)

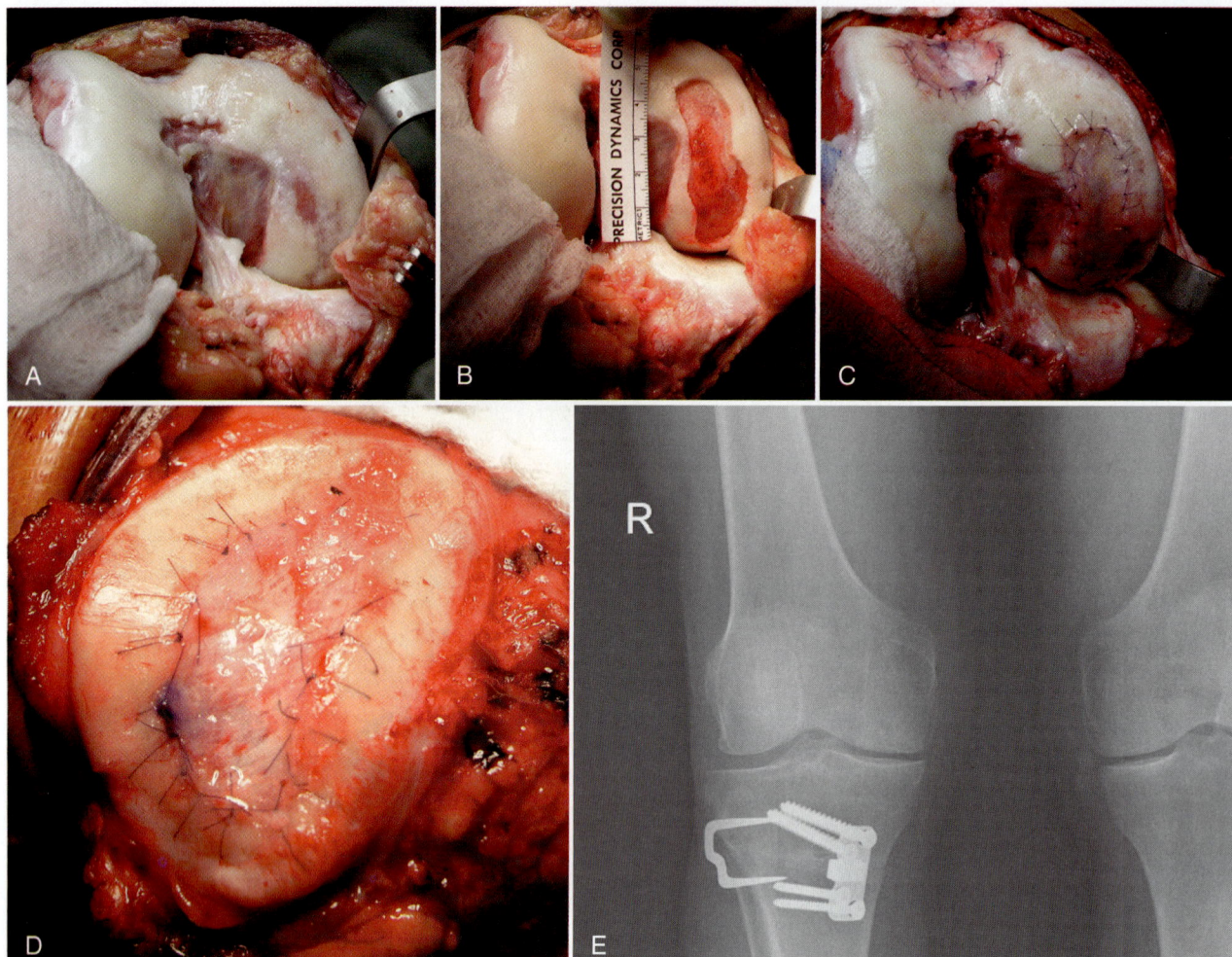

Figure 7–12 Case example of a 19-year-old woman with a twisting work-related injury to the lateral compartment of her right knee. Fat-suppressed images include a coronal magnetic resonance imaging (MRI) scan *(A)* and a sagittal MRI scan *(B)* demonstrating bone marrow edema under the lateral tibial plateau with full-thickness articular cartilage loss to the lateral tibial plateau with an intact femoral surface and meniscus. *C,* Long alignment weight-bearing x-ray films demonstrate valgus malalignment of the right knee with mechanical axis to the lateral tibial spine and 3 degrees of mechanical valgus. *D,* Varus-producing femoral osteotomy and lateral tibial plateau autologous chondrocyte implantation (ACI) are performed. This is performed through a longitudinal incision just to the lateral border of the patella and tibial tubercle. A lateral parapatellar arthrotomy is performed, and the intermeniscal ligament is incised. A lateral subperiosteal peel, which includes the coronary ligament of the lateral meniscus and a portion of the iliotibial band, is performed to the posterior lateral corner of the tibia at the popliteus hiatus of the lateral meniscus. The patella is subluxed into the medial parapatellar gutter, the knee is hyperflexed, and the tibia is internally rotated to deliver the lateral tibial plateau. This technique gives excellent exposure to the entire lateral tibial plateau. Through the same incision proximally the quadriceps is split between the vastus lateralis and the rectus intermedius muscles. The vastus lateralis is dissected laterally to the posterior lateral corner of the femur and the linea aspera. A femoral varus-producing osteotomy is performed through the same dissection, which is an extensile Henry approach to the knee. *E,* Radical debridement of the chondral defect of the lateral tibial plateau exposes its margins circumferentially. Microsuturing of the ACI graft and sealing of its margins with fibrin glue. A single suture is left long laterally to allow injection of the autologous chondrocyte suspension and then is easily closed and sealed over. Final radiographic appearance after femoral varus-producing osteotomy with lateral tibial plateau ACI graft.

and early active range of motion can be pursued immediately postoperatively. Otherwise, a staged reconstruction should be performed.

A common wear pattern is a varus knee with a medial femoral condyle lesion or a varus knee in combination with a trochlea or patellar injury. If the condition is a medial femoral condyle defect with a varus knee, a longitudinal incision is made from the superior medial pole of the patella longitudinally and distally to the inferior aspect of the tibial tubercle (Figure 7–13). A medial parapatellar arthrotomy is performed, the defect is débrided, and a template is made. The template is applied to the periosteum, which has been exposed distal to the pes anserinus tendons, and the periosteum is harvested.

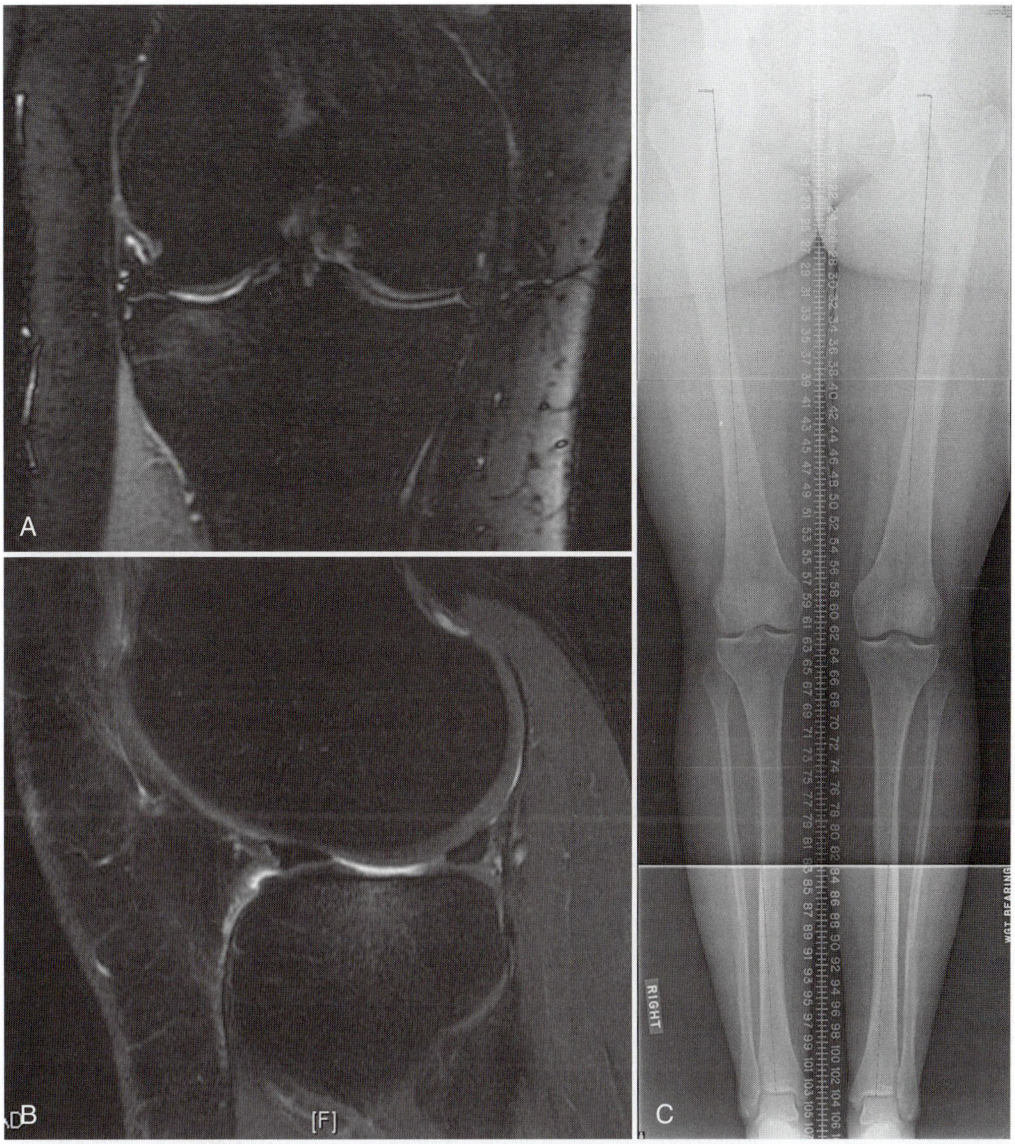

Autologous Chondrocyte Implantation   CHAPTER 7   79

Figure 7-13 Case example demonstrating exposure for osteoarthritic lesions with varus malalignment requiring open wedge tibial valgus-producing osteotomy. *A,* Open appearance of the right knee of a 48-year-old male football coach with intractable medial and anterior joint pain and effusions. A midline incision with a medial parapatellar arthrotomy is performed. The incision is continued distally and subcutaneously to the pes anserinus tendons. *B,* Careful radical debridement of the joint is the most important step in the early arthritic knee undergoing autologous chondrocyte implantation. Note that a lateral intercondylar notchplasty has been performed to prevent impingement of the anterior cruciate ligament when the knee is placed into valgus. Radical debridement of the medial femoral condyle defect preserves the intercondylar osteophytes, which will be used for transosseous suture fixation of periosteum. Intralesional osteophytes are carefully taken down to increase the depth of the chondral defect to maintain a cavity throughout its entire length. *C,* Periosteal microsuturing is performed throughout the length of the medial femoral condyle and the trochlea defects. Note that the final appearance of the joint appears much healthier than the initial appearance. The tibial osteotomy can easily be performed through this single midline incision after the periosteum has been harvested.

Continued

Takedown of the pes tendons and superficial medial collateral ligament is performed in preparation for tibial valgus-producing osteotomy (see Chapter 8). The osteotomy is performed and fixated. The tourniquet is let down, and any bleeders in the soft tissue envelope or the subchondral bone plate in the area to be transplanted are resolved. Careful suturing and transplantation to the medial femoral condyle is performed.

If arthroscopy revealed maltracking of the patella with or without a chondral defect, TTO is performed with a medial subvastus and lateral subvastus arthrotomy elevating the extensor mechanism proximally. The defects are debrided, the periosteum is harvested, and the tibial valgus osteotomy is performed and fixated (see Chapter 8, combined osteotomies). The periosteal covers are microsutured and transplanted. The tibial tubercle is repositioned

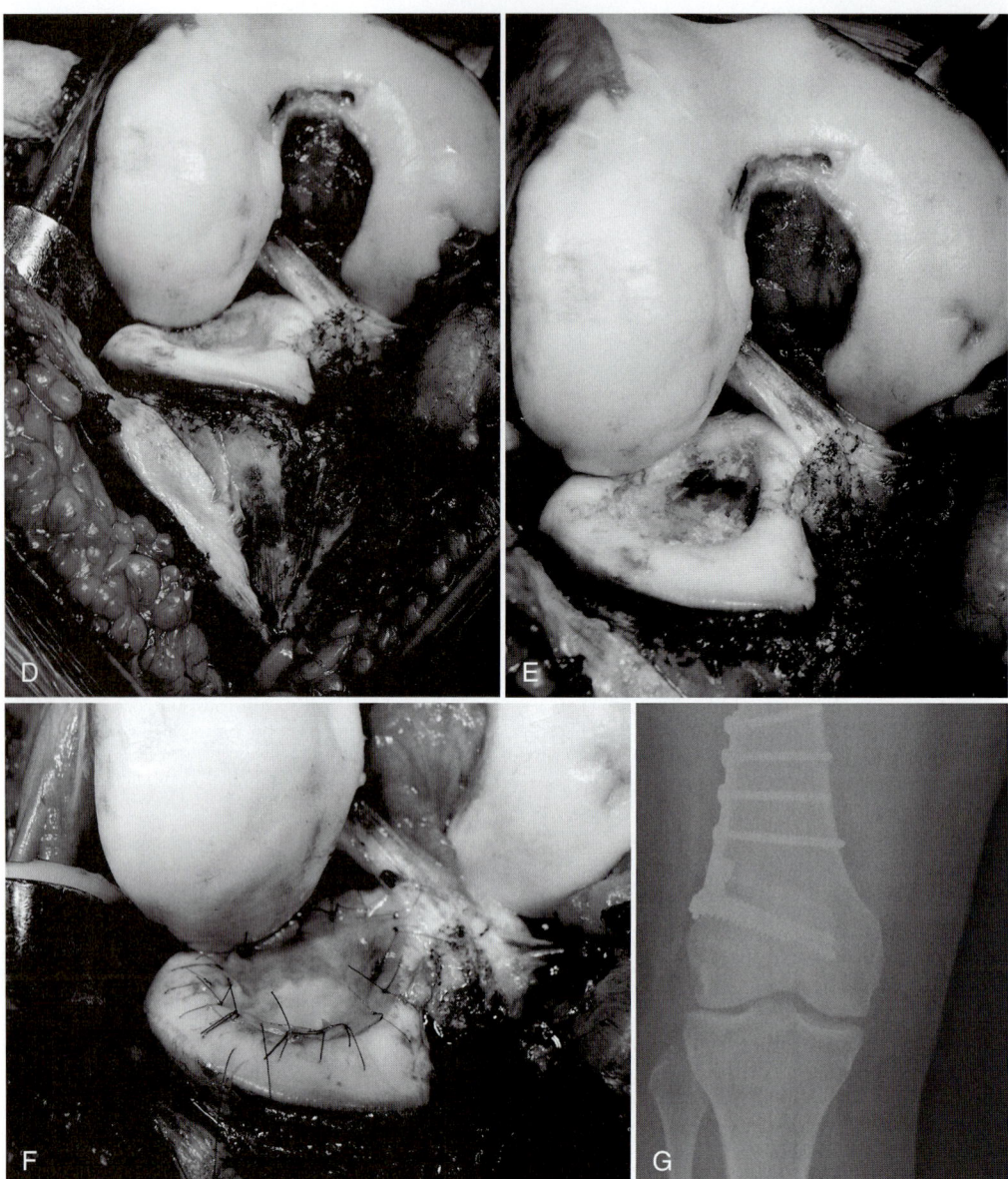

Figure 7–13—cont'd *D,* The periosteum on the patella is sutured to maintain the convex shape of the patella by starting at the midline ridge proximal to distal to maintain the tent-like shape of the periosteum. *E,* Radiographic appearance of the knee 4 years later when the patient returned for treatment of his other knee treated, which now had become equally painful as the right knee originally had been. The right knee has served him without pain and allowed him to return back to coaching and running on the sidelines until the demise of his left knee. The left knee was treated with identical lesions, with excellent clinical outcome.

and centered to normalize the extensor mechanism forces postoperatively.

ACI plus Tibial Tubercle Osteotomy for Posterior Exposure/with Patella/Trochlea ACI

Patellofemoral maltracking combined with a trochlea or patellar chondral injury requires careful preoperative assessment by physical examination and CT or MRI. TTO combined with soft tissue realignment to ensure proper tracking is paramount to successful graft healing. My preference is a longitudinal incision just off the midline laterally. In this way, as the tibial tubercle is anterior medialized a skin incision is placed over the anterior muscle compartment and not over a bony prominence. In the event of wound breakdown, the bone is not exposed and the health of the wound is optimized. A lateral subvastus arthrotomy allows visualization of the posterior femoral condyle, damaged patella, trochlea, or all of these. Assessment of dysplasia of the trochlea can be performed at this time. The laxity of the medial soft tissue envelope also can be assessed. If the medial side of the knee is excessively lax to patellar stability, then a medial arthrotomy is performed, leaving a good cuff of tissue attached to the patellar portion of the extensor mechanism. TTO can then be performed either leaving the distal hinge attached per a classic Fulkerson-type osteotomy or making an oblique distal countercut and elevating the extensor mechanism proximally (Figure 7–14), a posterior lateral osteochondritis dissecans lesion.

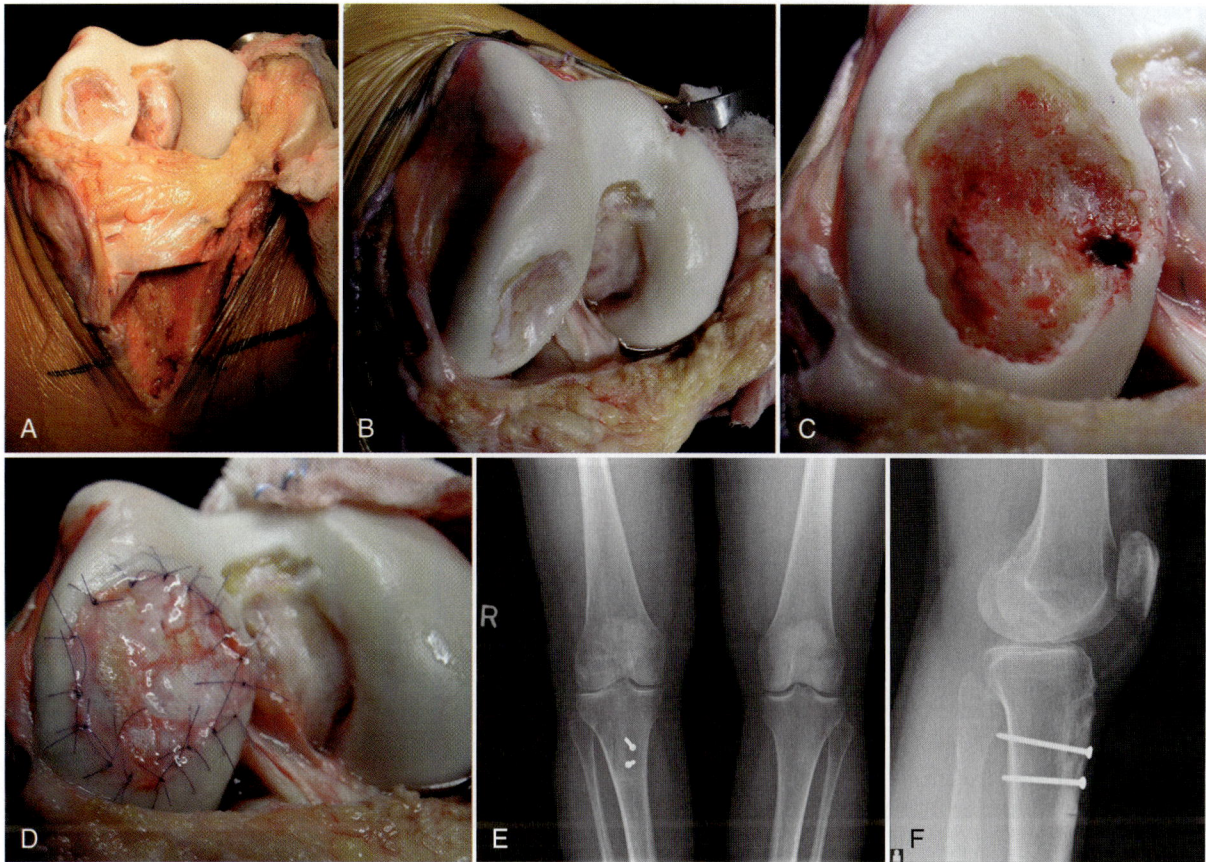

Figure 7-14 Case example of a 39-year-old woman with a large osteochondritis dissecans lesion to the posterior lateral femoral condyle. This case demonstrates the use of tibial tubercle osteotomy to expose a very posterior femoral condyle defect. *A,* Tibial tubercle osteotomy is performed for a length of 6 to 7 cm in cancellous bone as an anterior medialization osteotomy. A lateral subvastus approach is performed, keeping the quadriceps entirely intact. The medial retinaculum is released to the midpatellar pole at the level of the vastus medialis oblique insertion. Hoffa fat pad is released off the anterior tibial interval and anterior to the attachments of the menisci to the tibia. Exposure to the lateral femoral condyles is excellent. The tibial tubercle can be repositioned to a more central location to improve patellar tracking at the conclusion of the case. *B,* View of lateral femoral condyles osteochondritis dissecans from the lateral aspect demonstrates just held posterior the exposure will allow one to go. This is a central lateral femoral condyle osteochondritis dissecans lesion. It is shallow at its margins and no deeper than 6 to 8 mm centrally. This defect will do well with isolated autologous chondrocyte implantation (ACI) without preliminary bone grafting or sandwich technique. *C,* Close-up appearance of the defect after it is radically debrided and the tourniquet is let down to control bleeding. *D,* Final appearance of the ACI graft after microsuturing of the periosteum and sealing with fibrin glue. Anteroposterior *(E)* and lateral *(F)* radiographs demonstrating well-healed tibial tubercle osteotomy and well-preserved tibiofemoral joint space.

Continued

Trochlea debridement and transplantation of the surfaces can then be easily performed. Trochlea articular cartilage is generally 3 to 5 mm thick. In order for postoperative rehabilitation to proceed without patellofemoral catching sensations, the debridement should shape the proximal and distal (or leading and trailing) margins of the defect so that they slope slightly toward the subchondral bone bed, and the medial and lateral margins should be vertical. When a defect is confined to an isolated medial or lateral trochlea facet, then microsuturing a periosteal or collagen membrane flush to the articular surface is easy. However, when the defect crosses the midline sulcus, the order of stitching is important to restore concavity of the trochlea (Figure 7–15). Microsuturing without attention to this step will result in a flat trochlea sulcus and abnormal forces to the membrane with possible early failure.

Similarly, after tibial tubercle proximal ionization with subvastus laterally release, patella debridement and transplantation of the surfaces can be easily performed. The patellar cartilage is generally thicker than the trochlea (5-mm thick), so consideration for restoring the articular surface shape with the microsuturing technique is important (Figure 7–16). The medial and lateral margins of the debrided defect should be vertical to the subchondral bone, and the proximal and distal margins should be slightly sloped to ensure that tracking occurs without mechanical symptoms to the patient. However, circumferential vertical margins are necessary when cartilage is a thin. In this situation, the microsuture technique is even more critical to restoring the normal median ridge of the patella and ensuring that the membrane cover is not bottomed out on the subchondral bone. With this

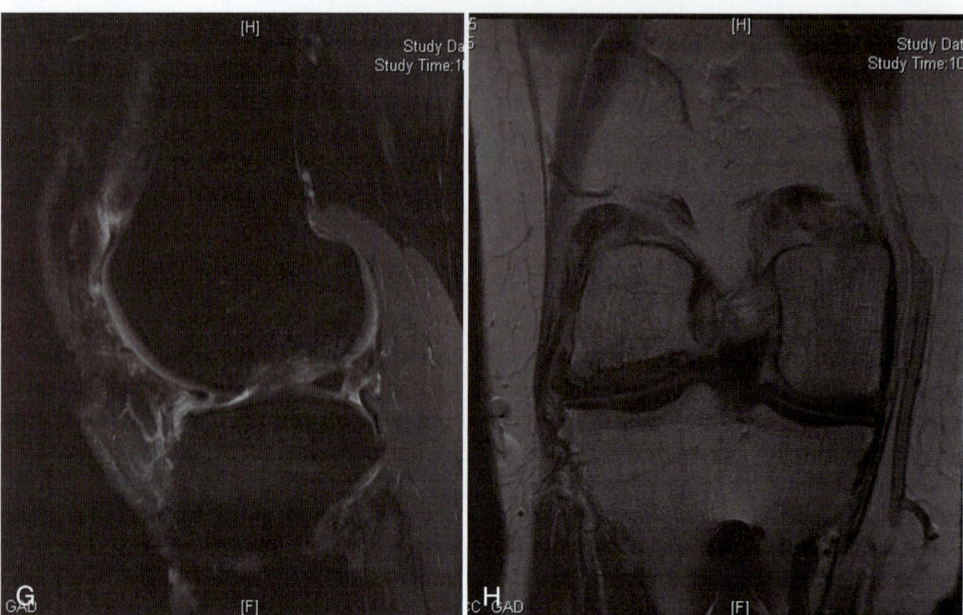

Figure 7-14—cont'd *G*, Two-year postoperative magnetic resonance imaging (MRI) with fat suppression demonstrating excellent cartilage repair fill to the defect. *H*, Coronal MRI scan without fat suppression demonstrating complete fill. The patient remains asymptomatic.

technique, there is always a cavity for the cell suspension to grow to the membrane surface.

At the completion of the transplant, the tibial tubercle is refixated in a central and normalized position for the extensor mechanism. A vastus medialis oblique (VMO) advancement is then performed, bringing the VMO under the medial patellar sleeve to advance the VMO and tension it so that the patella can move 30% of its width medial and lateral in full extension without complete subluxation. The VMO muscle then helps to further elevate the patella away from the trochlea, decompressing it further as a soft tissue sleeve in addition to the TTO elevation. This technique is performed with no. 2 Ethibond sutures using a horizontal mattress stitch (see Chapter 10, Figures 10-25 and 10-27). If trochlea dysplasia is causing continued instability medially and laterally, the medial sleeve repair is taken down and a trochleoplasty is performed as the last step in stabilizing the patellar extensor mechanism. The soft tissue sleeve is readvanced and fixated as before. Congenital trochlear dysplasia is an uncommon factor contributing to patellofemoral maltracking. It is best assessed by preoperative CT scan demonstrating a flattening of the convex superior trochlear capturing entry point. Treatment is surgical by trochleoplasty combined with patellar realignment as necessary (see Chapter 10, Figures 10-33 through 10-35). Results of trochleoplasty for trochlear dysplasia have been excellent.[8]

ACI with Osteochondritis Dissecans, Prior Bone Grafting, or Single-Stage Sandwich Technique ACI

In the case of bony deficiency, as occurs after osteochondral fracture or osteochondritis desiccans, the depth of the bony lesion should be assessed preoperatively by radiography or CT. Osteochondritis desiccans defects on average are 6 to 8 mm deep, including cartilage and bone. However, the margins are gradually sloped to the deepest portion. These defects often do well without bone grafting, using chondrocyte implantation alone (Figure 7-17).[4] However, defects that are more than 1 to 2 cm deep clearly require preliminary bone grafting and healing prior to cartilage resurfacing or a single-stage ACI sandwich technique. In addition, shallow defects with vertical walls, those that have cystic changes deep to the subchondral bone, and those with sclerotic bases from prior marrow stimulation techniques or osteochondral grafting should be considered for bone grafting or sandwich ACI. Autologous bone grafting can be performed either arthroscopically or by open technique (see Chapter 11). An interval of 6 to 9 months is required before second-stage articular resurfacing can be performed. This allows time for the cancellous bone graft to harden as it is loaded with weight bearing after an initial period of 8 weeks of protected weight bearing. In this way, a new "subchondral bone plate" is formed, and minimal, if any bleeding, occurs at the time of preparation of the defect site prior to cell implantation.

The *sandwich technique ACI* was so named because it involves sandwiching autologous cultured chondrocytes between two layers of periosteum (Figure 7-18). When a deep defect requires bone grafting, radical debridement and undermining of the sclerotic or necrotic bone are performed with a high-speed bur with fluid irrigation. The base is drilled to promote vascularization of the defect, and autologous morselized cancellous bone is used to fill the defect up to the level of the subchondral bone plate. A neural patty with thrombin and fibrin

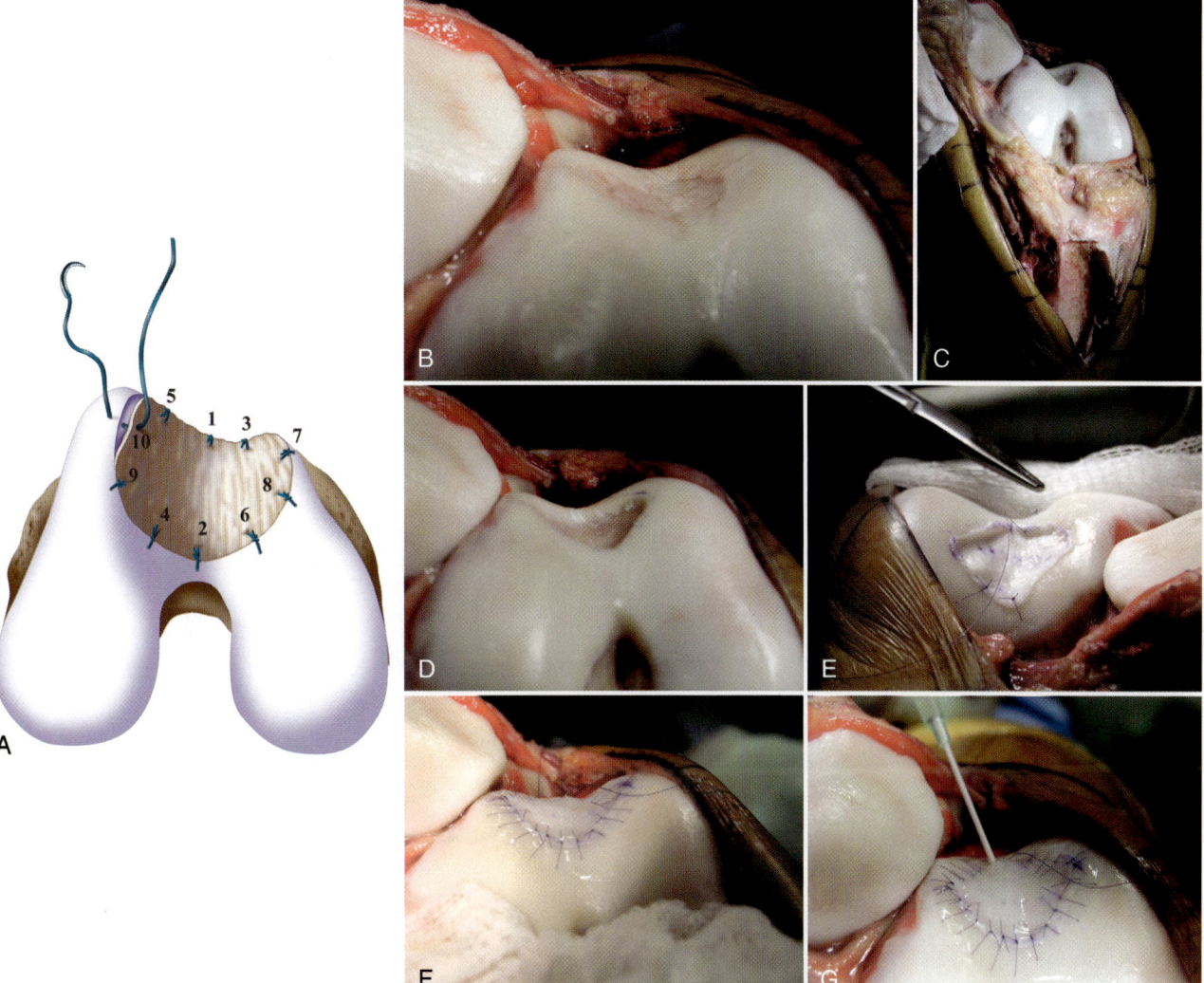

Figure 7–15 Autologous chondrocyte implantation suturing technique to the trochlea, combined with tibial tubercle osteotomy. *A,* When microsuturing a large defect of the trochlea across the midline sulcus, it is important to oversize the membrane in a medial to lateral direction. Suturing in a proximal to distal direction starting at the midline sulcus and working laterally and medially allows restoration of the concavity of the sulcus without undue tension on the membrane and an even depth throughout the entirety of the cartilage defect. *B,* Close-up view of a trochlear defect in the left knee of a 32-year-old man who had undergone an extended tibial tubercle osteotomy as shown in Figure 7–14. *C,* The defect is clearly V shaped and will require a careful suturing technique to the store at the articular topography. *D,* Close-up view after debridement. *E,* Microsuturing should start at the central sulcus proximal and distal (as shown) in an alternating medial and lateral pattern to restore the concavity to the trochlea. *F,* Final appearance of the trochlea membranes sutured in place and sealed with fibrin glue. The superior opening sutures are left long. *G,* Injection of autologous chondrocyte suspension underneath the opening, which was closed after the defect was filled.

glue is applied to the bone graft while the tourniquet is let down. The autologous bone graft is saturated with blood and a surface kept dry. A layer of periosteum or collagen membrane is placed and fixated with fibrin glue or additional transosseous sutures, with the cambium layer facing outward toward the joint. The surface is inspected to ensure that there is no marrow derive bleeding through the membrane and into the defect. A second periosteal layer is sutured flush to the articular cartilage per usual ACI procedure. It is sealed with fibrin glue and checked for water integrity. The saline is aspirated out of the defect, and autologous cultured chondrocytes are injected per ACI. The opening is sutured over and sealed with fibrin glue. The autologous cultured chondrocytes now are located in a bioactive chamber, and the underlying bone deficiency has been restored. The marrow-derived cells are separated from the autologous cultured chondrocytes, which are in a watertight chamber facing the cambium layer of periosteum on both sides.

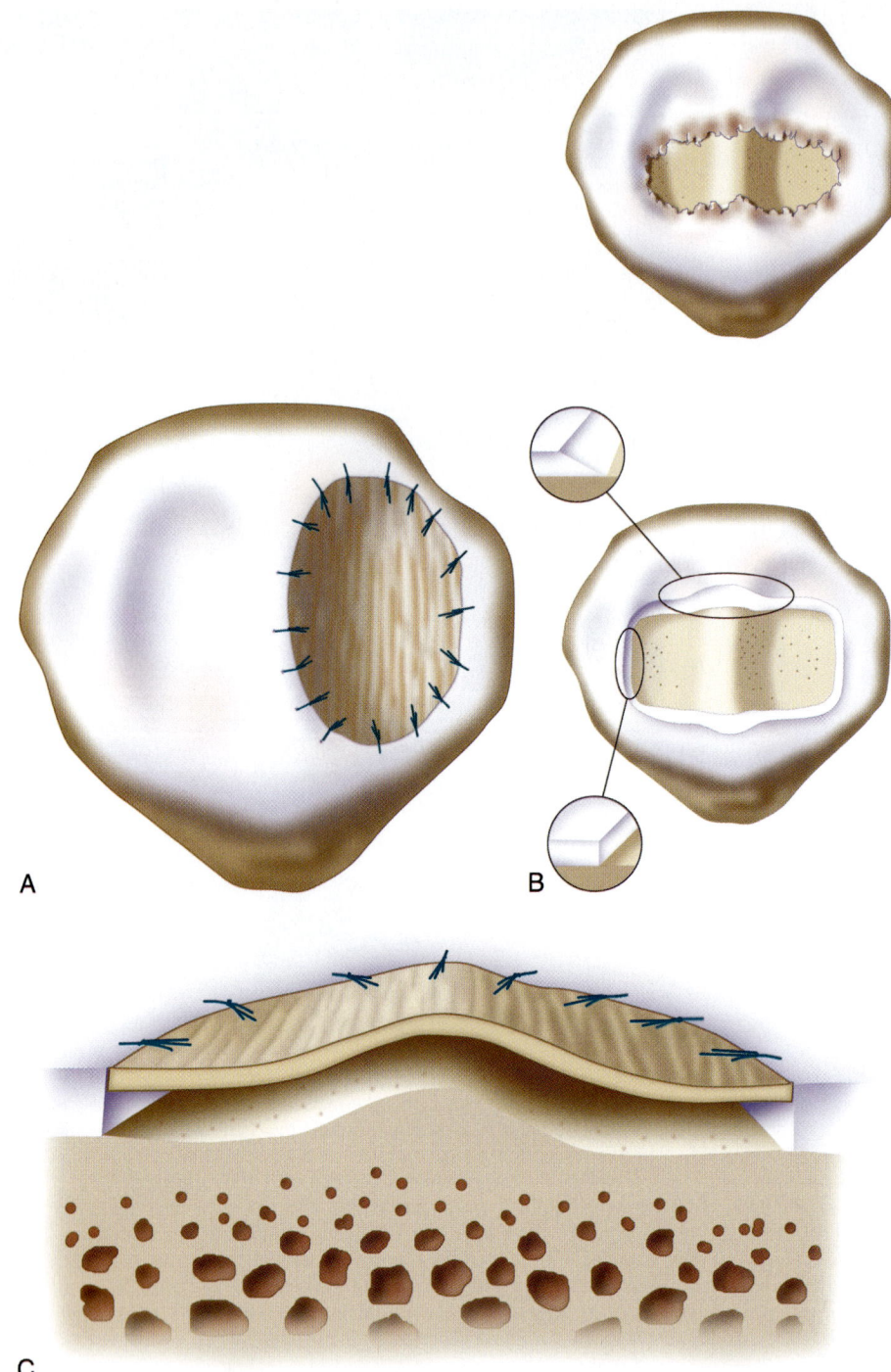

Figure 7–16 Microsuturing techniques for patella defects, combined with tibial tubercle osteotomy. *A,* Isolated medial or lateral patella facet is a flat surface and easy to microsuture flush with the articular surface. *B,* When the defect is large, as in this Fulkerson patella type IV chondral defect (pan-patellar), a good result depends on good debridement technique as well as microsuturing. If the cartilage is thick, bleeding and trailing edge should be slightly beveled to allow easy tracking in the proximal to distal direction and vertically on the medial and lateral margins to allow maximal membrane stability. *C,* As in the trochlea, microsuturing should start at the apex or median ridge of the patella so as to "pitch the tent," then should alternate medially and laterally in a proximal to distal fashion to restore the articular topography of the patella. This technique will maintain a uniform cavity deep to the membrane so that articular cartilage growth develops evenly to the limiting membrane.

Continued

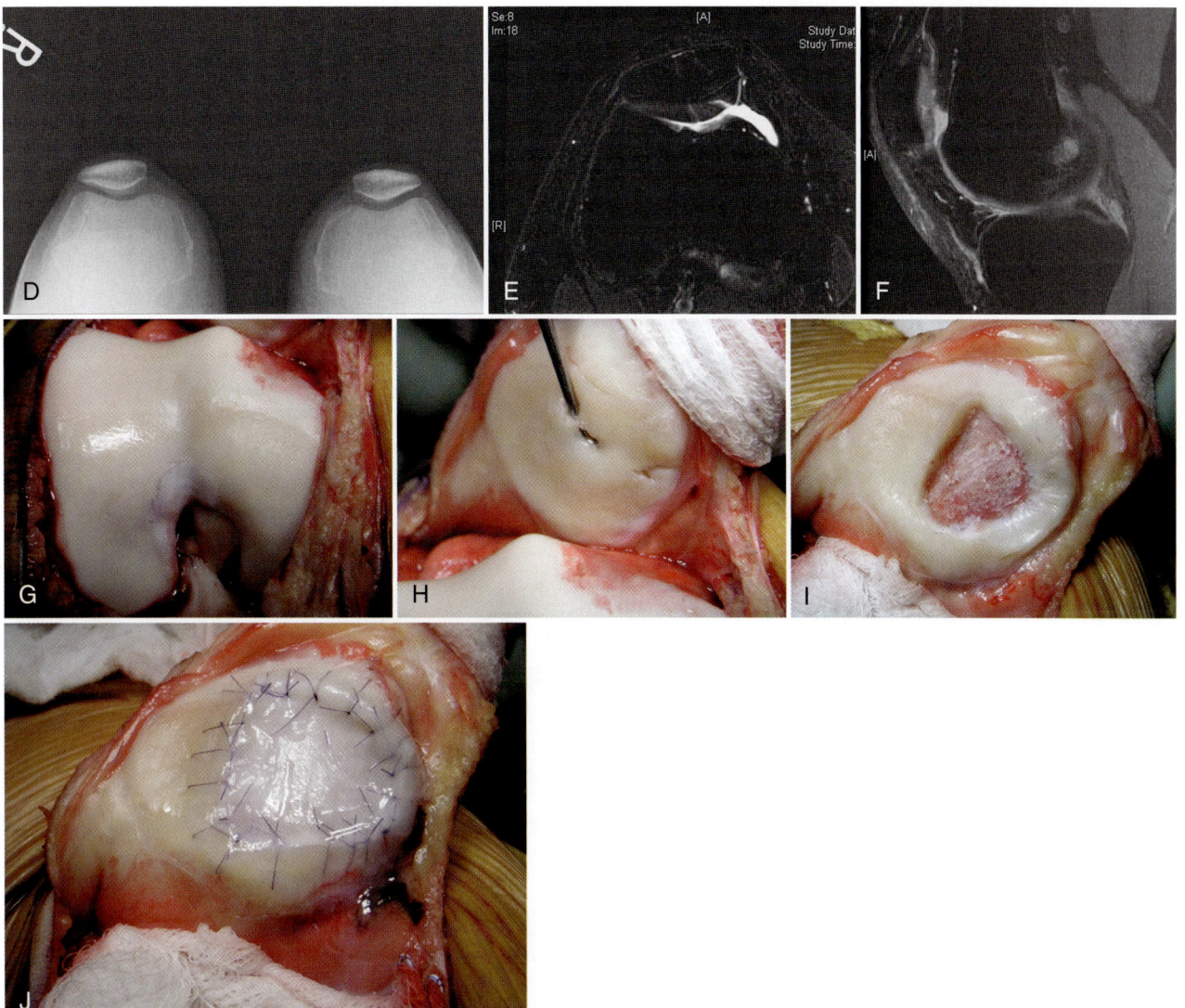

Figure 7–16—cont'd *D*, Case example of a 42-year-old woman with chronic anterior knee pain bilaterally. Skyline x-ray films demonstrate well-preserved joint spaces. *E*, Axial magnetic resonance imaging (MRI) scan with fat suppression demonstrates patellar tilt with fissuring and breakdown of the articular cartilage of the median ridge and medial facet of the patella. *F*, Sagittal MRI scan demonstrates the same patellar damage but intact articular surfaces of the trochlea. *G*, Extensile tibial tubercle exposure reveals an intact trochlea as noted by MRI. A fibrous cover over the biopsy site for autologous chondrocyte implantation is performed at the lateral intercondylar notch. *H*, Metal probe demonstrates delamination and fissuring of the central and medial patellar surfaces. *I*, Radical debridement of the damaged articular cartilage back to native subchondral bone and healthy cartilage margins. *J*, Final appearance of microsuture collagen cover and restoration of articular topography of the patella.

ACI Plus ACL

Cartilage repair in the face of cruciate insufficiency may jeopardize a newly regenerating cartilage graft. Staged or concomitant surgery should be performed with the goal of preventing shear forces and instability episodes from damaging a healing graft.

For any medial femoral condyle defect with ACL insufficiency, my preference is a single open incision from the superior medial pole of the patella to the inferior aspect of the tibial tubercle. A medial parapatellar arthrotomy is performed with the patella then subluxed. An open technique ACL reconstruction is easily performed with only the femoral fixation completed with ACI to the medial femoral condyle (Figure 7–19). Once the autologous cultured chondrocytes are injected into the medial femoral condyle and sealed with fibrin glue, the knee is brought into extension, the tibia is translated posteriorly, and the tibial fixation completes the procedure with wound closure.

For a lateral femoral condyle defect, two choices are available. If the defect is more anterior, I prefer the same approach as that used for a medial femoral condyle, with

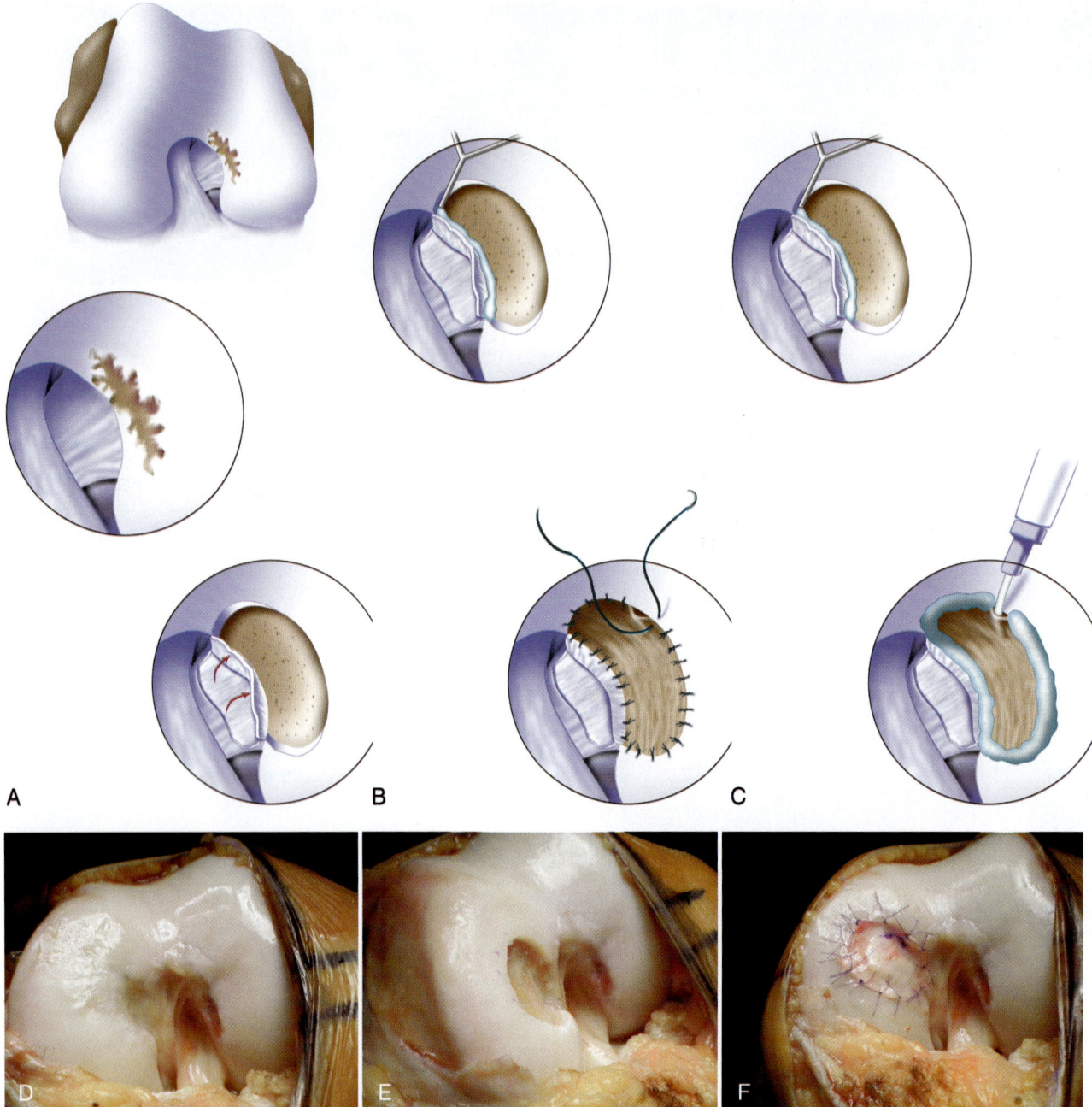

Figure 7–17 Illustrations and examples of the technique for autologous chondrocyte implantation with uncontained osteochondritis dissecans and deep defects requiring a sandwich technique. *A,* Classic location for osteochondritis dissecans is the intercondylar aspect of the medial femoral condyle. After debridement, the defect becomes uncontained. The technique for making this a contained defect involves releasing the synovium off the posterior cruciate ligament and leaving it attached to its intercondylar attachment, as shown in the illustration. *B,* Fibrin glue is placed on the medial aspect of the synovial attachment. The periosteum can then be microsutured to the surrounding articular cartilage and synovial membrane. *C,* It is then sealed with Tisseel fibrin glue, and the autologous cultured chondrocytes are injected. The opening is sutured over and sealed. *D,* Clinical example of a left knee medial femoral condyle osteochondritis dissecans defect. The lesion is uncontained on the synovium of the posterior cruciate ligament (PCL). *E,* After radical debridement, the synovial aspect of the PCL is brought up flush with the articular cartilage off the PCL. *F,* Microsuturing and sealing the defect with Tisseel fibrin glue maintains the defect in a contained fashion.

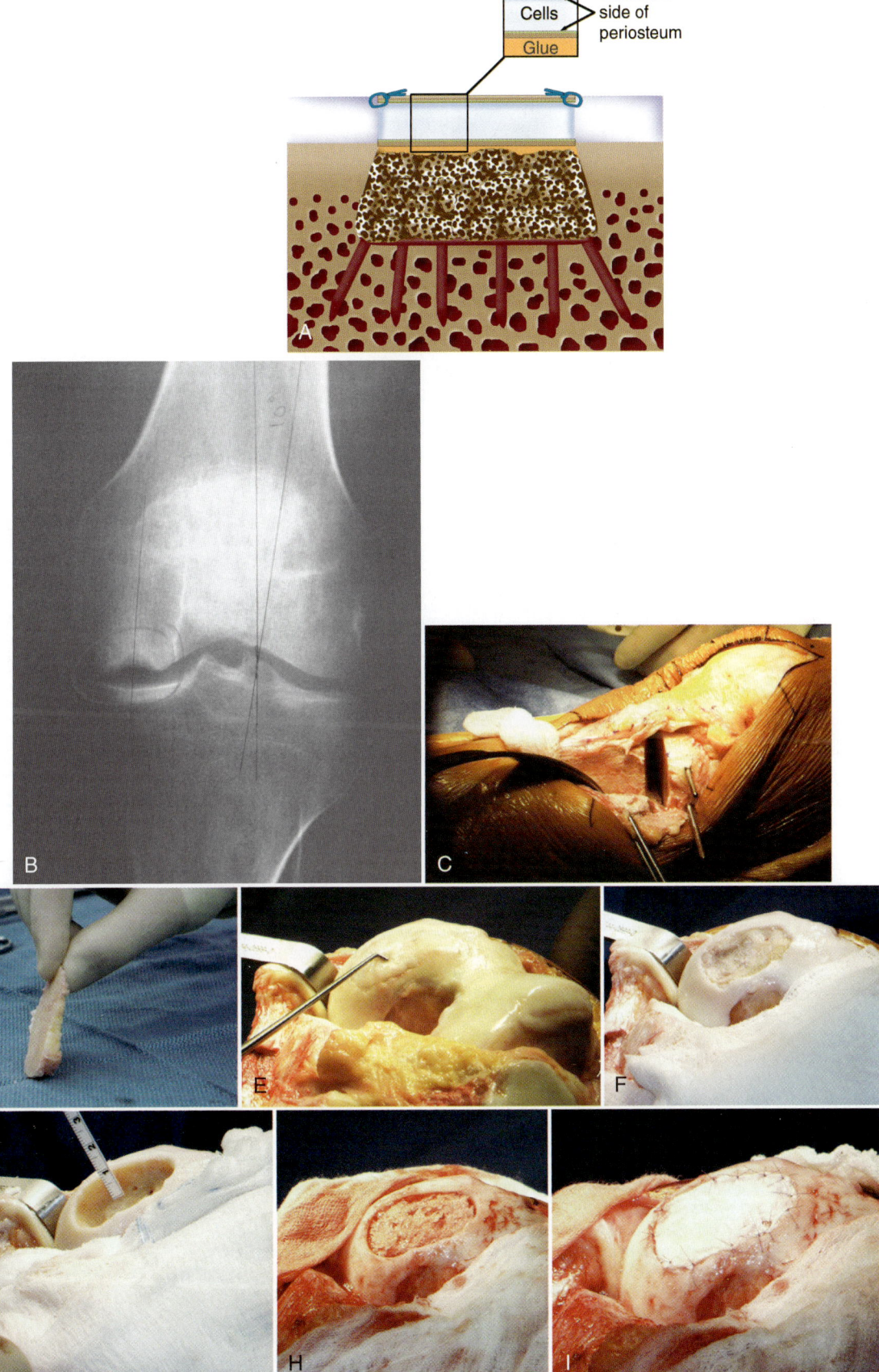

Figure 7-18 Diagrammatic representation and clinical example of a sandwich technique autologous chondrocyte implantation (ACI) for an osteochondral defect. *A,* Diagrammatic representation of the final appearance of an osteochondral defect treated with ACI sandwich technique. As described in Chapter 11, the osseous portion of the defect undergoes radical debridement of the necrotic or sclerotic bone, drilling deep to the osseous defect to promote revascularization, and autologous cancellous bone grafting to the level of the subchondral bone. At the level of the articular surface, a membrane or periosteum is used to contain the marrow-derived cellular response.

Continued

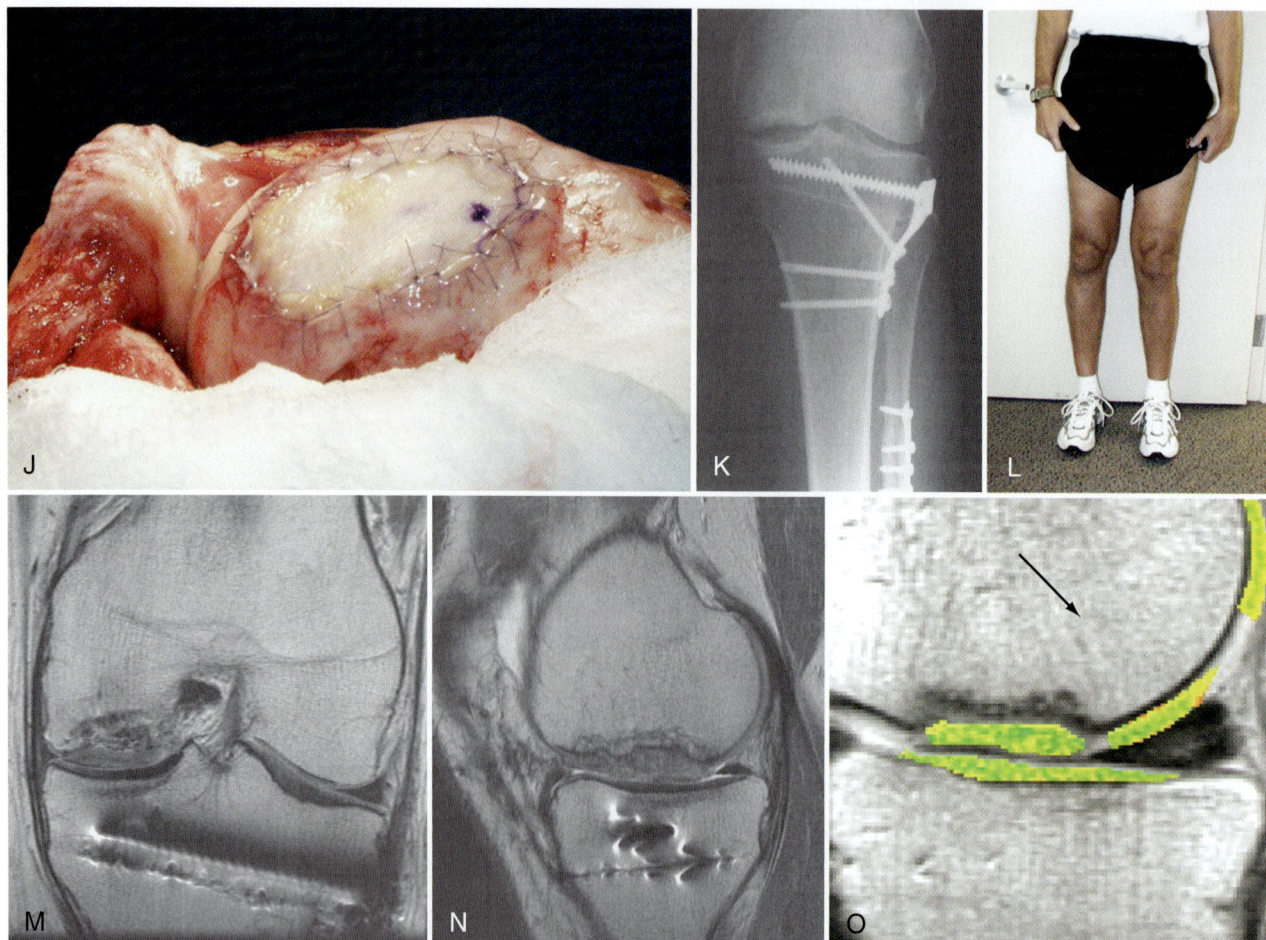

Figure 7-18—cont'd A limiting membrane is sealed to the autologous bone graft with fibrin glue. If periosteum is used, the cambium layer faces the articular surface *(pale green)*. For the second membrane at the level of the articular surface, cambium layer faces deep so that the two layers of cambium tissue are sandwiching the autologous cultured chondrocytes. The underlying marrow response is separated as a watertight separate chamber. *B,* Clinical example of ACI sandwich technique in a middle-aged man with a varus knee and spontaneous osteonecrosis of the medial femoral condyle. The standing anteroposterior (AP) x-ray film demonstrates resorption and collapse of the medial femoral condyle with osteonecrosis *(circled area)*. The mechanical axis falls directly through the center of this lesion (shown). A 10-degree angular correction, to the lateral tibial spine *(intersecting lines)*, is required to unload the lesion by 2 degrees into mechanical valgus. *C,* Lateral view of the proximal tibia bone deficiency demonstrates a 10-degree angular wedge of bone that was removed to allow performance of closing wedge osteotomy. *D,* Autologous bone wedge from the closing wedge osteotomy will be morselized and used as cancellous bone graft to the medial femoral condyle avascular defect after it is radically debrided. *E,* Probe demonstrates the medial femoral condyles avascular necrosis articular surface, which is ballotable and mobile. *F,* Medial femoral condyles and defect after loose articular surface was easily removed. *G,* Defect measured 1 cm deep after radical debridement of necrotic bony bed. *H,* Appearance of medial femoral condyles after cancellous autologous bone grafting and packing to the level of the subchondral bony surface. *I,* Periosteal membrane is sealed to the subchondral bone with Tisseel fibrin glue and tacked peripherally deep to the articular surface. A neural patty is applied with pressure to the periosteal cover while the tourniquet is let down to allow development of a watertight bed to the level that will undergo ACI. *J,* Final appearance after the second periosteal cover, which is microsutured flush to the articular surface. *Blue dot* denotes the superficial fibrous periosteal layer surface of the membrane. The chamber between the two periosteal cambium layers is injected with autologous cultured chondrocytes, and the margins are sealed with fibrin glue. *K,* Standing AP radiograph 1 year after closing wedge valgus-producing osteotomy with ACI sandwich technique to the medial femoral condyle. The joint space is well maintained in the medial compartment. *L,* Frontal view of the clinical appearance of left knee of the patient 1 year after closing wedge valgus osteotomy plus sandwich ACI. Note that the right knee is in slight varus and the left knee is in slight valgus. *M,* Magnetic resonance imaging (MRI) scan proton density, coronal view, demonstrating excellent repair tissue cover of the medial femoral condyles. *N,* Sagittal view demonstrating the same findings as shown in *M. O,* Sagittal delayed gadolinium-enhanced magnetic resonance imaging of cartilage demonstrating proteoglycan content equal to adjacent nontransplanted cartilage. Nine years after surgery, the patient remains pain free and is athletically active.

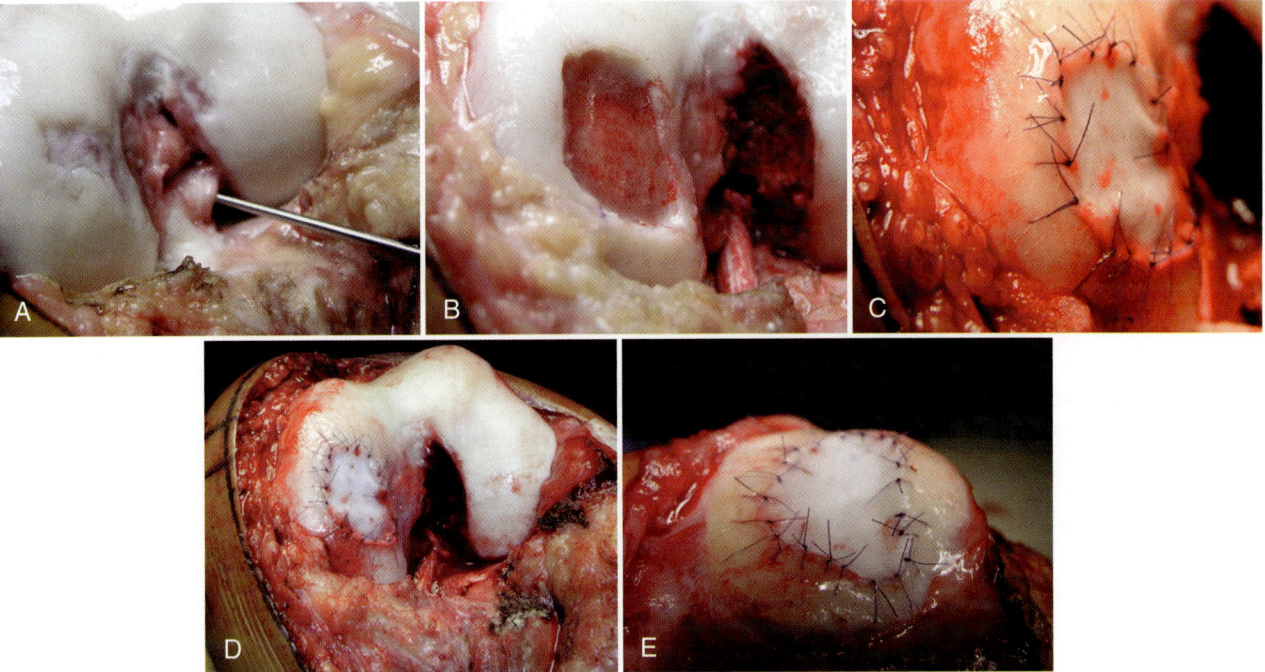

Figure 7–19 Anterior cruciate ligament (ACL) reconstruction with autologous chondrocyte implantation (ACI) to the medial femoral condyle and patella in a 40-year-old man. *A,* Open medial parapatellar arthrotomy, nerve hook demonstrating lax ACL torn off of its femoral attachment. A medial femoral condyle defect with adjacent undermining is evident. *B,* Radical debridement of the damaged articular cartilage to stable margins. When an open medial arthrotomy is performed, my preference is an open ACL reconstruction and open notchplasty. Tunnel placements are easy to acquire and perform. The same landmarks used arthroscopically are used for open technique. I confirm the femoral tunnel placement with the mini C-arm in a lateral position. *C,* Final appearance of ACI grafts microsutured in place on the medial femoral condyle. *D,* ACI appearance on the patella. Two years postoperatively, the patient has returned to pivoting sports and had no limitation.

hyperflexion and eversion of the patella and ACI to the lateral femoral condyle (Figure 7–20). The cells are injected and the patella is reduced, with the knee extended and the tibia posteriorly translated. After femoral fixation for the ACL graft has been accomplished, tibial fixation is performed and the wound closed.

If the defect is more posterior on the lateral femoral condyle, then I prefer an arthroscopically performed ACL, followed by lateral arthrotomy and open ACI to the lateral femoral condyle.

Anterior cruciate rehabilitation is modified to exclude closed-chain resisted strengthening exercises until 3 months after combined surgery to prevent excessive compressive load to the chondral repair site. From 4 to 6 months is required before these exercises can be instituted. Leg presses and squats are avoided for 1 year after surgery. Rehabilitation follows that for ACI, which is the rate-limiting process in recovery.

ACI plus Meniscal Allograft

For meniscal deficiency in combination with articular cartilage injury, I have found that it is much more critical for the lateral than the medial compartment of the knee to transplant the meniscus with the ACI. Medial injuries are frequently accompanied by varus malalignment. I presently have 15 years of results following valgus-producing tibial osteotomy with ACI to the medial femoral condyle in the presence of an absent meniscus. The results show excellent clinical function and no evidence of joint space loss on standing x-ray films.

However, this is not always the case in the lateral compartment. Because of its meniscal dependency, the lateral compartment degenerates rapidly once the meniscus is lost, even in the presence of normal mechanical axial alignment. The progression is much more rapid if valgus malalignment is present.

Meniscal transplantation can be performed arthroscopically using a slot technique, a posterior counterincision for posterior horn fixation followed by open arthrotomy, debridement of the chondral defects, and microsuturing the periosteal membrane and ACI.

I have found it more straightforward to produce a slightly longer midline incision, develop a posterior deep fascial flap, and make the posterior capsular dissection for transcapsular meniscal fixation through a single open incision (see Chapter 12). The defect is debrided and the periosteal suturing performed. A slot technique is easily performed with passage of the meniscus posteriorly and

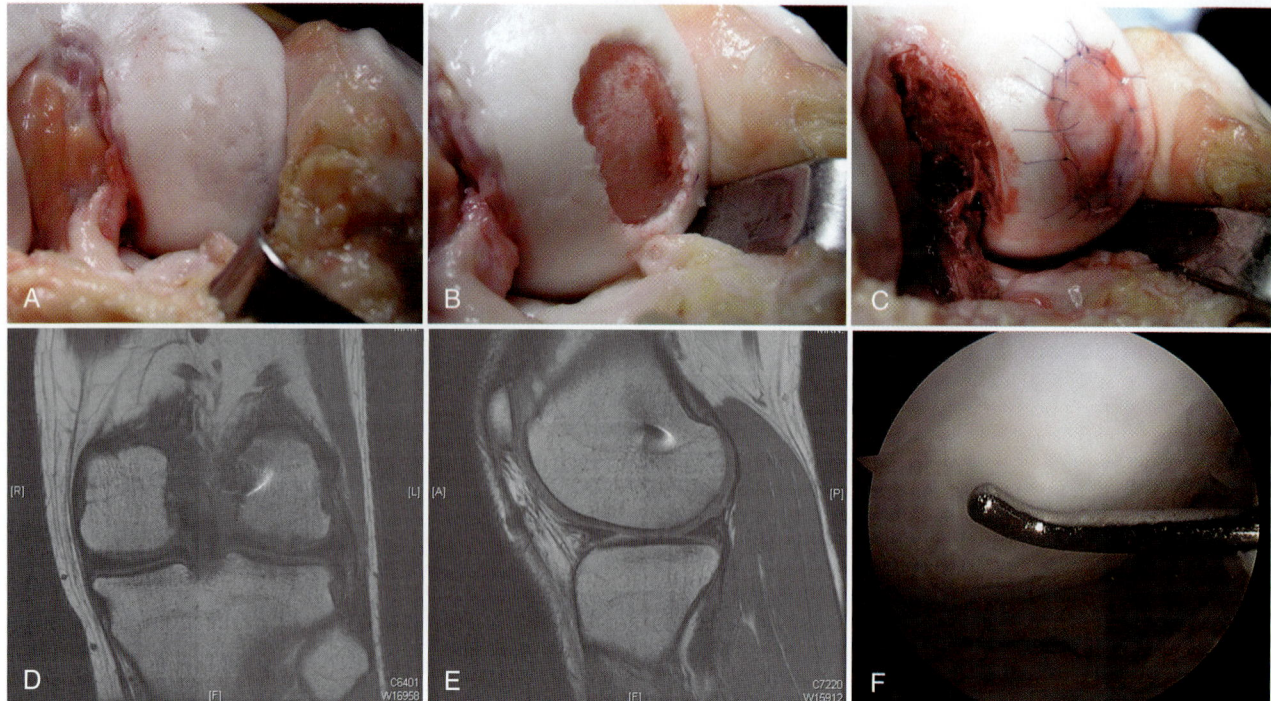

Figure 7-20 Anterior cruciate ligament (ACL) reconstruction with autologous chondrocyte implantation (ACI) to the lateral femoral condyle in an 18-year-old man. *A,* Clinical appearance of the lateral femoral condyles defect as viewed through a medial parapatellar arthrotomy showing a lax ACL, femoral attachment injury. The other option in this case would be an arthroscopic ACL with lateral parapatellar arthrotomy after ACL reconstruction to perform the ACI. *B,* Lateral femoral condyle defect after debridement. *C,* ACL reconstruction with lateral femoral condyle ACI. *D,* Coronal magnetic resonance imaging (MRI) proton density image 1 year after surgery demonstrating excellent ACI repair tissue to the lateral femoral condyle. *E,* Sagittal MRI proton density image 1 year after surgery demonstrating excellent ACI repair tissue. *F,* Confirmation arthroscopy 1 year after surgery. The patient is a high-level athlete and wishes to return to sports. I frequently perform MRI and second-look arthroscopy to confirm that a patient is ready to safely progress to high-level activity.

posterior horn fixation. The body and anterior horn of the menisci are easily repaired to the capsule by open technique. Transosseous fixation sutures can also be placed through the body and anterior horns of the meniscus to the tibial surface, thus preventing postoperative extrusion of the meniscus. ACI is completed when the periosteum is glued and the cells injected. The periosteum is closed and sealed, and the wound is closed. A single setup without arthroscopic equipment makes the procedure quite easy. Excision of any posterior meniscal remnant is usually performed arthroscopically at the time of cartilage biopsy so that it is not necessary at the time of open meniscal transplant with ACI.

ACI after Marrow Stimulation Techniques

We have found that alterations in the subchondral bone are common after drilling, abrasion, and microfracture. The bone may develop large intralesional osteophytes or a thickened sclerotic and near-cortical subchondral bone surface. Occasionally we have encountered subchondral bone cysts at the locations of drill entry or microfracture pick. For these reasons, MRI scan is useful prior to pursuing ACI after marrow stimulation technique to assess the extent of intralesional osteophyte formation and subchondral bone marrow edema and the possibility of cyst formation.

Adequate debridement of the articular defect is the most important aspect of dealing with a previously marrow-stimulated subchondral bone. A radical cartilage debridement back to native cartilage and subchondral bone is the starting point. This identifies the level of native subchondral bone and outlines the size of intralesional osteophyte or sclerotic subchondral bone. Large intralesional osteophytes are removed with a rongeur, and a 5-mm high-speed bur is used to blend in the sclerotic or osteophytic bone to the level of the native subchondral bone. I have found that bleeding in this thickened bone surface is unusual. A template is made of the defect, and the defect is prepared for microsuturing. The tourniquet is let down to assess the vascularity of the subchondral bone and to resolve any excessive bleeding. Neural patties soaked in thrombin and epinephrine, fibrin glue, and electrocautery are used to resolve any bleeding. The periosteal cover is microsutured in usual fashion flush to the articular surface and sealed with fibrin glue. The autologous chondrocyte suspension is injected underneath the membrane, which is sutured over and sealed.

Subchondral cysts, if encountered, are burred out completely. Autologous bone grafting is performed to the area of the cyst, and the surface over the bone graft is sealed with Tisseel fibrin glue and a periosteal membrane. The tourniquet is let down. If all is dry, then a second periosteal cover is sutured over the entire defect, the cells are injected, and the procedure is completed. In this way, a "segmental" ACI sandwich technique is performed in which only the portion of the defect that is bone grafted is sealed watertight with fibrin glue and a periosteal cover to ensure that the entire area to be transplanted is watertight and not contaminated with marrow-derived cells.

ACI in Osteoarthritis, Uncontained Defects, and Sclerotic Subchondral Bone

When treating young patients with more advanced articular injury who have early osteoarthritis, several technically difficult situations may present upon open arthrotomy. Findings in the osteoarthritic knee include large ulcerative focal chondral defects with indistinct borders, chondral defects that become uncontained adjacent peripheral osteophytes, thin peripheral cartilage margins to focal defects, findings similar to those seen with post-marrow stimulation techniques, such as thickened subchondral bone and intralesional osteophyte formation as well as subchondral cysts, and "kissing lesions" (femur on tibia, patella on trochlea, and peripheral osteophytes around the patella that may engage and produce articular injury to the trochlea).

Preoperative assessment of background factors is critical to successful management of these complex reconstructive challenges. One must decide in advance of the surgery whether osteotomy of the tibiofemoral joint or tibial tubercle is required for exposure or unloading of a large defect or kissing defects. Osteotomy will often make the surgical exposure easier when it is planned in advance.

Debridement of articular injuries upon exposure of the knee joint should preserve all peripheral osteophytes because they may be required for management of poorly contained articular cartilage injuries. Transosseous drill holes through peripheral osteophytes on the femur or tibia are commonly required for some of these larger lesions (Figure 7–21). The subchondral bone may be sclerotic and the cartilage margins thin. In this case, I start with a ring curette and remove the sclerotic subchondral bone until the depth of the defect is 2 to 3 mm from the adjacent thinned cartilage. Articular chondrocytes will easily grow to fill these defects with articular cartilage. In this way there is a contained defect and room for growth without undue pressure on the chondrocyte suspension. If the bone is very stiff, a 5-mm high-speed bur is useful provided it is copiously irrigated to ensure no thermal injury is caused to the underlying bone.

Peripheral osteophytes around the patella are usually removed with a small sagittal saw used oblique to the osteophyte so as to not produce a 90-degree surface that will impinge or damage the trochlea. For kissing lesions

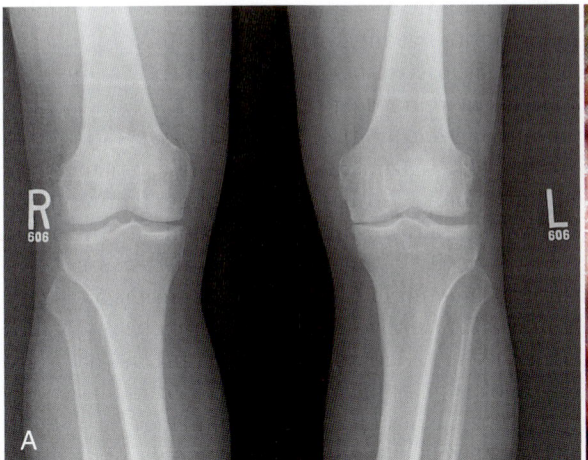
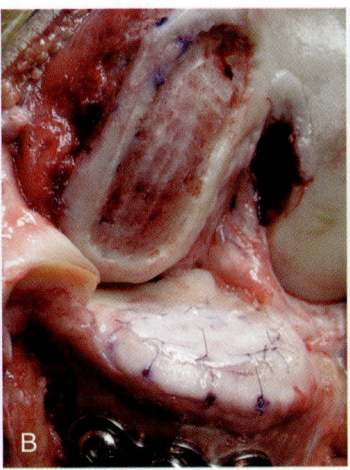
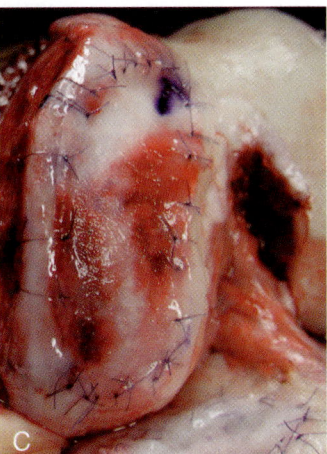

Figure 7–21 Autologous chondrocyte implantation and early osteoarthritis. *A,* Standing anteroposterior x-ray films of a 51-year-old former marathon runner demonstrating near bone-on-bone changes with varus malalignment of the left knee. *B,* Open appearance of the medial compartment of the left knee. Uncontained defects on both the medial femoral condyle and tibial plateau are present. A medial subperiosteal peel was performed, taking down the superficial and deep medial collateral ligaments with a meniscal sleeve. This technique allows exposure of the entire medial joint compartment and concomitant opening wedge tibial valgus osteotomy. The uncontained defects are managed by maintaining the peripheral osteophytes. Transosseous drill holes are performed through the osteophytes using a small C. wire and marking the holes with a blue marking pen as noted. The 6.0 Vicryl sutures are passed through the membrane via the transosseous drill holes and anchored back to the membrane to develop a contained cavity that will accept autologous cultured chondrocytes as noted on the tibial surface. *C,* The membrane on the femoral surface is microsutured using transosseous drill holes through osteophytes to anchor the defect in place.

Continued

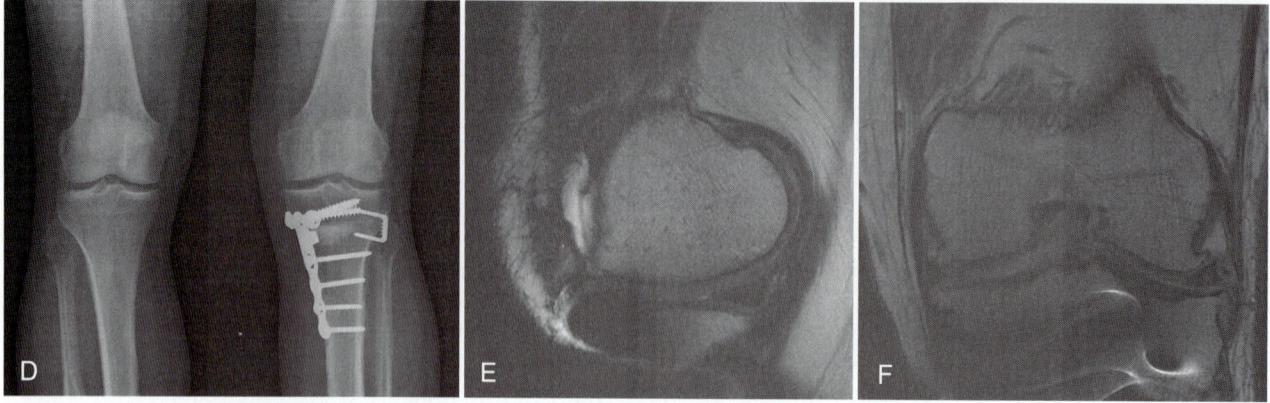

Figure 7-21—cont'd *D*, One-year postoperative weight-bearing x-ray films demonstrating restoration of joint space after transplantation of "kissing" defects. *E*, Sagittal magnetic resonance imaging (MRI) proton density scan demonstrating cartilage repair on the knee or from condyle and tibial plateau. *F*, Coronal MRI scan demonstrating the same findings as in *E*.

in the patellofemoral joint, I routinely perform a decompressive tibial tubercle anteromedialization osteotomy.

If all steps are performed well, then at completion of radical debridement and preparation of the chondral defects for microsuturing of the periosteum or collagen membrane, the knee should look relatively healthy with a few large potholes. Radical debridement and preparation of the arthritic knee are key to successful reconstruction as well as management of background factors. Periosteal suturing to maintain a cavity without the membrane bottoming out on the subchondral bone is essential, and the suture technique is critical.

Early motion of the tibiofemoral joint and patellofemoral mobilizations are critical to the success of these complex reconstructions. Adhesions and arthrofibrosis will jeopardize any good surgical reconstruction. I routinely use antiadhesion membrane (Seprafilm, hyaluronic acid–cellulose, Genzyme Biosurgery; FDA off-label use) on the synovial lining tissues of the joint at the end of the procedure to try to prevent these complications and have found the product to be useful.

AFTER CARE/REHABILITATION

Prophylactic intravenous cephalosporin antibiotics are given for 24 to 48 hours after surgery.

The three main goals in the postoperative period are as follows: (1) range-of-motion exercises to enhance chondrocyte regeneration and decrease the likelihood of intraarticular adhesions, (2) protected graft loading for 6 to 12 weeks after surgery to prevent the likelihood of periosteal overload and central degeneration or delamination of the graft, and (3) isometric muscle exercises to regain muscle tone and prevent atrophy.

CPM is instituted as soon as cell attachment has occurred, generally after 6 hours or the next day. With bearing femoral condyles, CPM is increased to regain a full range of motion as the patient tolerates, with a very slow cycle setting of approximately 2 minutes. This is used for approximately 6 to 8 hours daily for up to 6 weeks postoperatively. This schedule is based on experimental work[9] that demonstrated enhancement of the quality of repair tissue via this modality as well as a clinical work[10] that demonstrated increased repair tissue fill with use of CPM 6 to 8 hours per day for 6 to 8 weeks postoperatively. At this time, the exact quantity and duration of CPM for ACI have not been determined. It is clear, however, that patients are comfortable while they are on CPM machines and that CPM does decrease the likelihood of intraarticular adhesions by motion.

CPM for defects of the trochlea is less aggressive. Initially, CPM is used for a range of 0 to 40 degrees maximum. The remainder of the motion is achieved by the patient dangling the leg over the edge of the bed to regain further motion. CPM from 40 to 70 degrees is not recommended because maximal patellofemoral contact forces occur in this range. However, with collagen membranes this may be increased because these membranes appear to be more resistant to tearing and degeneration. In addition, the surgeon must consider whether the defect is a large pan trochlear lesion or a flat trochlea repair on either the medial or lateral trochlea facet. In these cases, no restriction in range of motion would be required.

Weight bearing for the femoral condyles is protected at weight of leg/"foot-flat" touch weight-bearing status for 6 weeks postoperatively on crutches. Weight bearing is increased to full body weight by 12 weeks postoperatively on the following schedule: weeks 7 and 8⅓ body weight; weeks 9 and 10⅔ body weight; and weeks 11 and 12—full body weight on crutches. Thereafter the patient is instructed to use one crutch in the opposite arm and to switch to a cane when he or she is comfortable. Each patient's progress is individualized and guided by symptoms. If weight-bearing discomfort, catching, locking, or swelling of the knee occurs, then the weight-bearing status and activity level are decreased as tolerated by the patient. These symptoms may indicate that the graft is undergoing overload with stimulation of the subchondral bone, resulting in pain. On average, patients have discarded their canes and are walking relatively comfortably with a small effusion at 4 to 4½ months. Larger lesions take longer for recovery. At this time, nonimpact activities such as long-distance walking, cycling, swimming, and cross-country skiing are encouraged. Running is not permitted until graft hardness is similar to adjacent cartilage, which takes approximately 9 to 12 months on a weight-bearing femoral condyle lesion. Larger lesions make take as long as 18 months. Osteochondritis desiccans may take 18 to 24 months. Deep lesions (e.g., osteochondritis dissecans), large weight-bearing femoral condyles lesions, and those that are bipolar (e.g., tibia femur kissing lesions) usually are protected with an unloader brace to allow earlier weight-bearing and recovery. For osteochondritis dissecans or large femoral condylar lesions, the unloader brace is started approximately 3 months after transplantation. For kissing lesions, the brace is started within the first week after transplant to unload the opposing membrane surfaces initially and progresses as comfort allows. For kissing lesions on the tibia and femur, it is soft in 6 months postoperatively before an unloader brace is discontinued.

Lesions of the trochlea respond slower in the rehabilitation process and healing. Weight-bearing status is allowed at full weight bearing with a knee immobilizer from the onset because the weight-bearing condyles are not affected. Isometric straight-leg lifts are instituted as the patient's comfort allows. Rehabilitation for maintaining decreased patellofemoral contact pressures is encouraged. Active flexion and passive extension are encouraged for the first 6 weeks. At 6 to 8 weeks following surgery, walking backward on the treadmill encouraged. Effusion is more common with trochlea repairs for up to 6 months after surgery. Stationary bicycling with low resistance is allowed as early as 3 weeks postoperatively. Kneeling and squatting are not permitted until 12 to 18 months following surgery, at which time graft hardness is similar to that of adjacent cartilage.

Many patients and their physical therapists are interested in starting weight training in the first year after ACI. I believe much of this mindset has arisen from the accelerated rehabilitation protocols following ACL reconstruction. However, we have taken the stance that the first year after surgery is the time for restoration of functional pain-free mobility for the patient. In this regard, we focus on good tibiofemoral and patellofemoral mobilizations and muscle tone in the first 1 to 3 months postoperatively, attaining muscle tone and function with isometrics as well as stationary bicycling. Gait training ensues between months 3 and 6 postoperatively, and we encourage distance walking as comfort allows, on a treadmill or outdoors, and progress to an elliptical trainer. As long as stationary and outdoor bicycles do not cause pain and effusions within the knee, the resistance on these devices is increased to allow strengthening of the lower extremity without overloading the transplanted knee. Rollerblading is allowed after 6 months if the activity is pain free. Torque-loading activities that involve descending and jumping, such as golfing, racquet sports, and hiking, are not allowed until after 12 months.

After 12 months, inline jogging is permitted if the patient responds favorably without pain or swelling. Pivoting activities such as racquet sports, soccer, and golfing are allowed 14 to 18 months postoperatively. Leg presses and squats are not encouraged at any time unless they are performed at less than the patient's body weight and high repetitions are allowed. We emphasize to patients that they do not have a normal knee but a prepared knee that is improved and better with regard to functionality compared to the preoperative condition. Patients should use symptoms other than those from the knee as a barometer to gauge their activities. We have noted that patients who have excellent muscle tone and strength in their quadriceps and hamstring musculature and maintain them through cycling and elliptical trainer strengthening for life do well many years thereafter. Patients with leg weakness will frequently complain of aching and discomfort in the operated knee.

Strengthening for trochlea lesions should involve short-arc quadriceps strengthening from 0 to 30 degrees of flexion and closed-chain strengthening from the same 0- to 30-degree range of motion. Open-chain resisted quadriceps strengthening should not be permitted for at least 12 months following ACI to the trochlea based on symptoms. I usually recommend that patients never engage in open-chain resisted quadriceps strengthening if they have a patella or trochlea lesion. Closed-chain strengthening is less traumatic and forceful on transplants in these locations and is recommended instead.

COMPLICATIONS

To date, no intraarticular joint infections following ACI have been reported. Complications related to open arthrotomy include intraarticular adhesions, arthrofibrosis of the joint, and occasional superficial wound infections.

Intraarticular adhesions are uncommon except when femoral periosteum from the suprapatellar pouch region is used or the patient has a propensity for keloid formation or arthrofibrosis. These factors may enhance intraarticular fibrosis. If arthrofibrosis with stiffness occurs, a blind manipulation is not recommended. Adhesions are best released with arthroscopic lysis of adhesions after the grafts are visualized (to ensure there are no adhesions to the grafts) (Figure 7–22), followed by a manipulation,

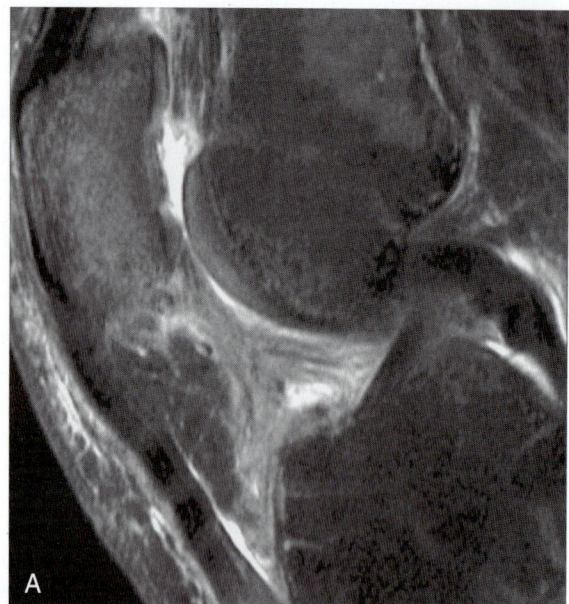
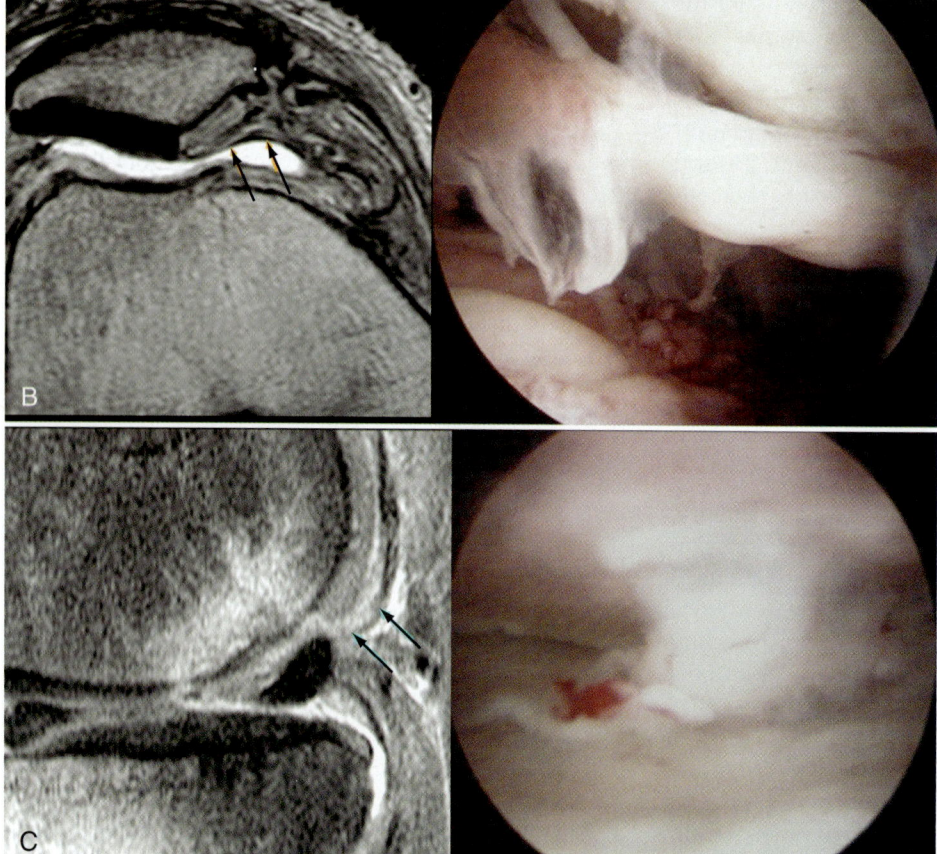

Figure 7-22 Three weeks after autologous chondrocyte implantation (ACI) to the medial femoral condyles patella with tibial tubercle osteotomy, the patients knee becomes very stiff. *A*, Sagittal magnetic resonance imaging (MRI) scan demonstrating dense adhesions from Hoffa fat pad to anterior cruciate ligament. ACI to the patella appears to be intact. *B*, Axial MRI scan of the patella demonstrates adhesions from the medial parapatellar gutter, which is obliterated by scar tissue directly on the transplant surface, noted at the time of arthroscopy *(right)*. *C*, *Arrows* indicate scan adhesions to the medial femoral condyle ACI transplant on sagittal MRI. At the time of arthroscopy, the adhesions are clearly visible attached to the graft *(right)*. A blind manipulation without arthroscopic lysis of adhesions would result in failure of both grafts by intraoperative avulsion from the subchondral bone.

drain placement in a parapatellar gutter for 24 to 48 hours postoperatively, and early CPM.

Periosteal problems may occur in 5% to 40% of cases, and some of them require intervention. In most cases, the catching response settles and the patient remains asymptomatic. This situation likely represents graft remodeling by the patient's activity level alone without delamination.

However, if the catching worsens, then periosteal hypertrophy is likely. The most common problems after ACI are incomplete periosteal graft incorporation to host cartilage and hypertrophic periosteal fibrous layer response. Those not familiar with the varied appearances of periosteal hypertrophy (Figure 7-23) may presume a graft has failed or is soft. However, removing the fibrous

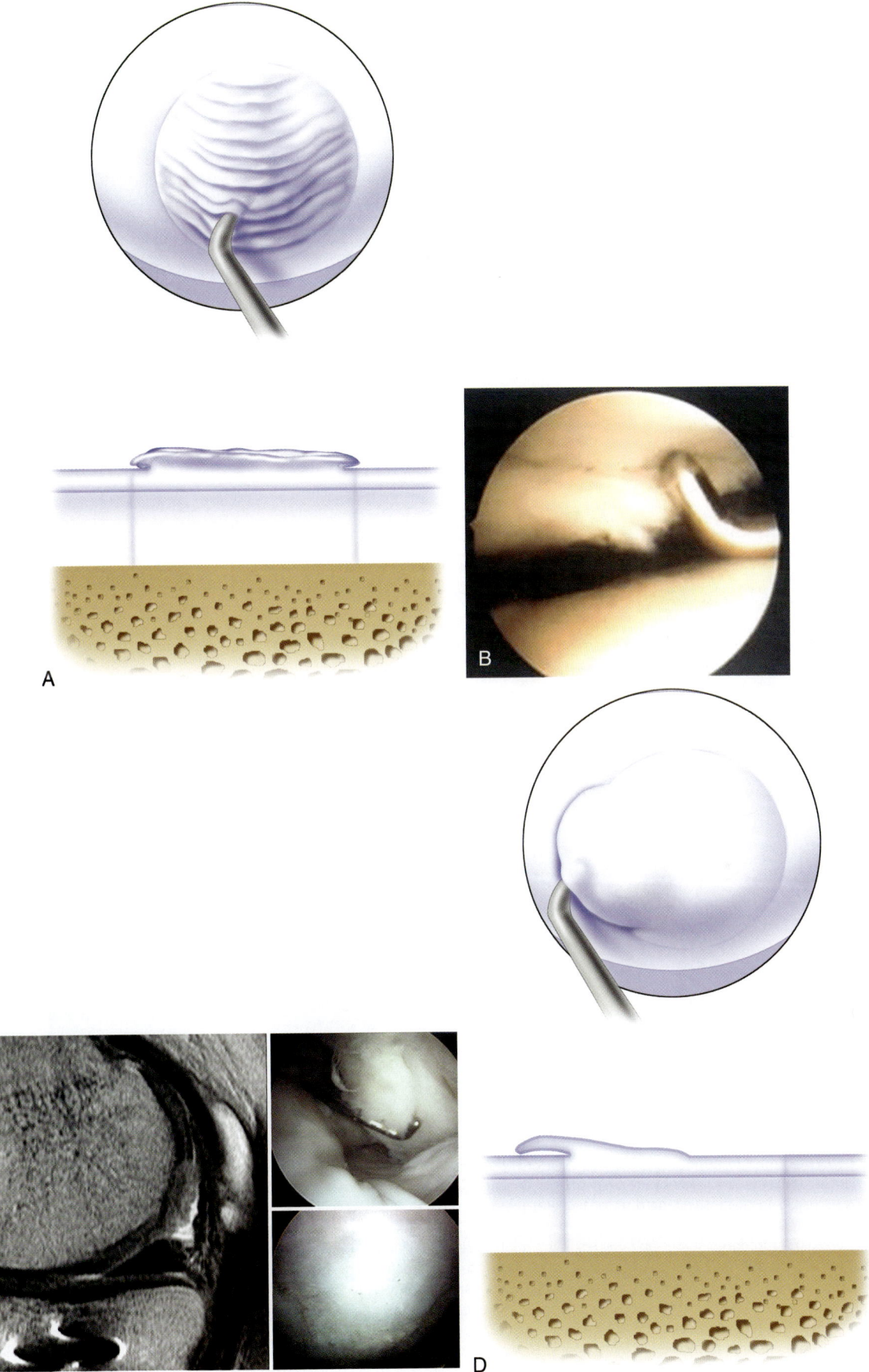

Figure 7-23 For legend see next page

Continued

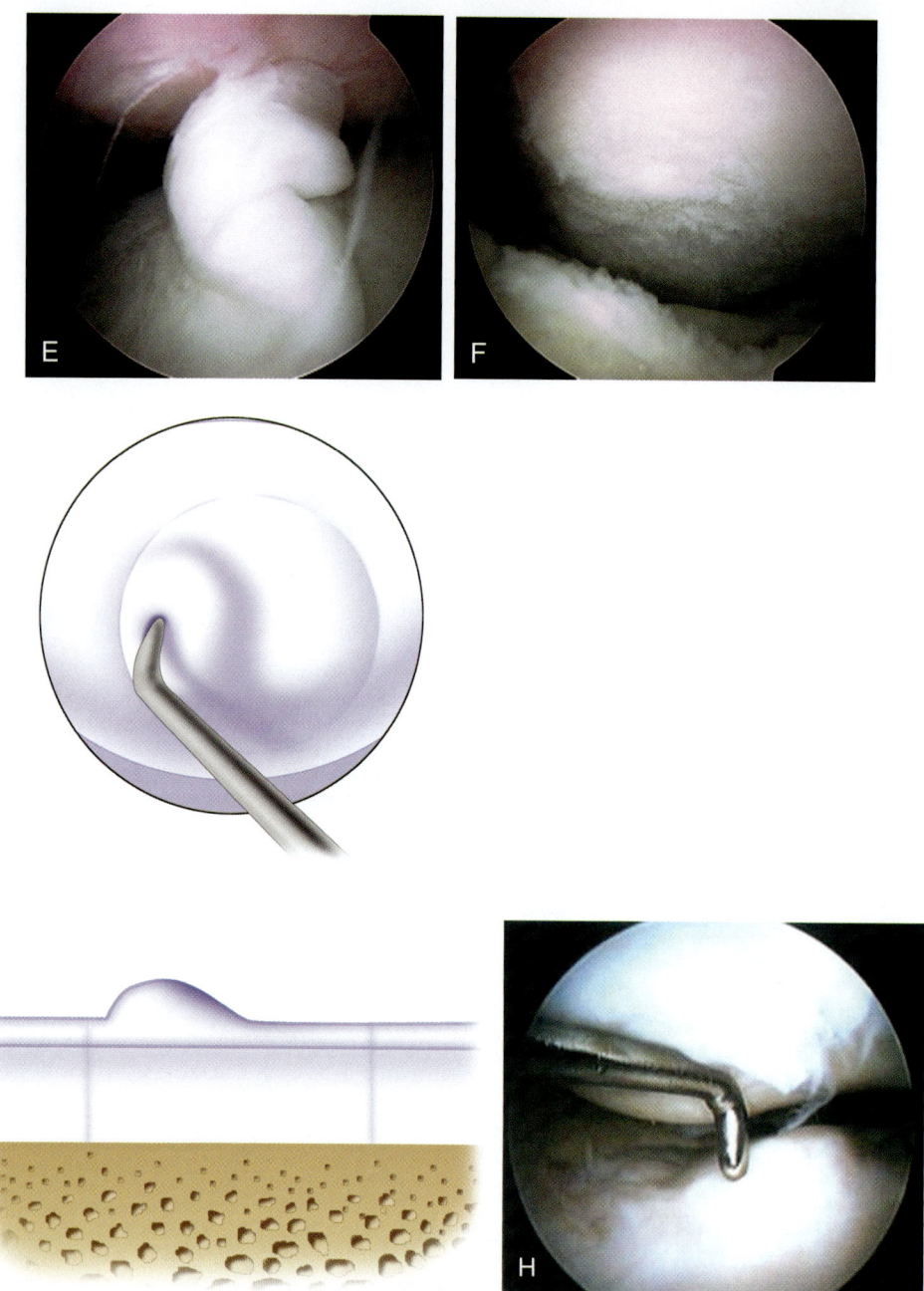

Figure 7-23—cont'd Fibrous layer of the periosteum may undergo overgrowth and have varied appearances, termed onion skinning, overlapping, mounding, or superficial fibrillation. If these appearances are not recognized at the time of arthroscopic evaluation, they may be mistaken for a failed poor-quality autologous chondrocyte implantation (ACI) graft. Takedown of the overgrown fibrous layer with a motorized shaver will result in complete relief of symptoms and will demonstrate healthy repair tissue flush with the native articular surface. Magnetic resonance imaging (MRI) scan is helpful in distinguishing mechanical painful symptoms of overgrowth from a delaminated failed graft. MRI scan is routinely performed prior to arthroscopic management of hypertrophy. In this way, surgical options can be discussed with the patient in advance of treatment if the graft has failed by delamination or degeneration. *A*, Diagrammatic representation of onion skinning. Removing the layered fibrous tissues results in clean, shiny, hard repair tissue at the deep surface. *B*, Arthroscopic appearance of onion skinning. Probe demonstrates the level of native articular cartilage adjacent to overgrown fibrous layer of periosteum. The prominent fibrous layer will be removed flush with the native tissue using a motorized shaver and will result in symptom relief. *C*, Sagittal MRI scanning, proton density, reveals a prominent hypertrophic periosteal surface on the ACI graft. Arthroscopic photos to the *right* demonstrate onion skinning-type hypertrophy, which is removed. *D*, Diagrammatic representation of overlapping hypertrophy. The flap of periosteum on top of native tissue with resulting mechanical catching sensation should be removed. *E*, Arthroscopic appearance of overlapping hypertrophy on the medial femoral condyle ACI graft, which results in a painful snapping sensation in deep flexion. *F*, Medial femoral condyle ACI graft appearance after removal of overlapping hypertrophy. *G*, Diagrammatic representation of mounding hypertrophy. *H*, Arthroscopic appearance of mounding hypertrophy to the lateral tibial plateau ACI graft.

Continued

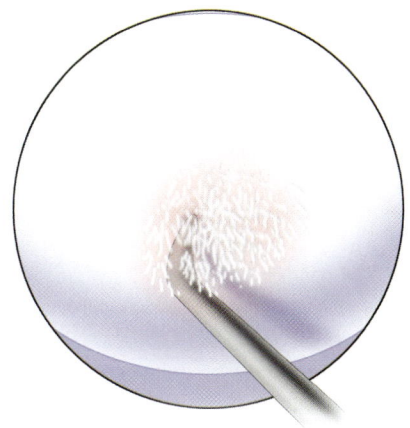

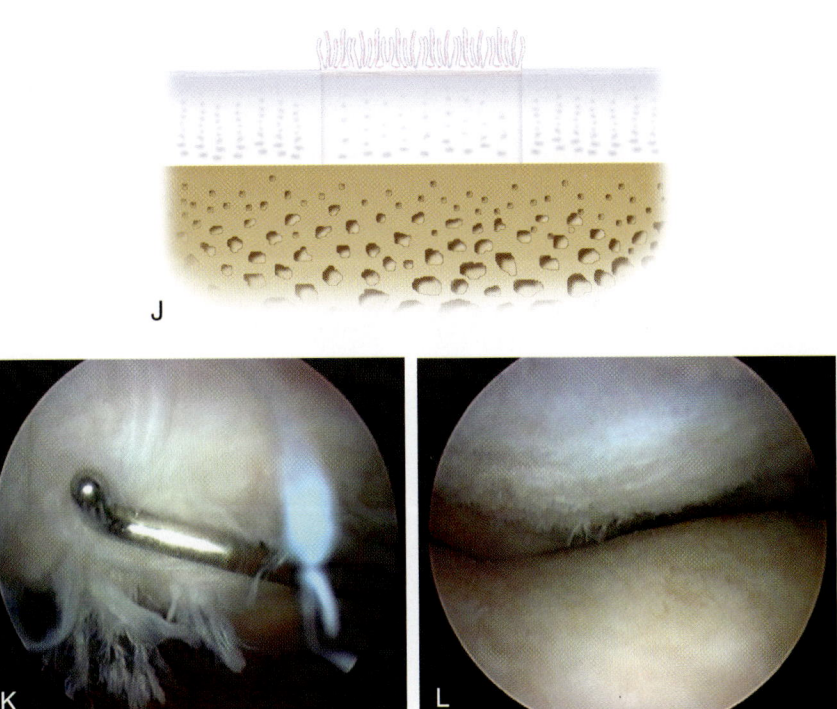

Figure 7-23—cont'd *I,* Mounding hypertrophy to the patella ACI graft viewed arthroscopically *(left)* and by sagittal MRI scan *(right).* *J,* Diagrammatic representation of superficial fibrillation. *K,* Arthroscopic appearance of superficial fibrillation on the patella ACI graft. Superficial fibrillation–type hypertrophy usually results in pronounced crepitus. *L,* Arthroscopic appearance of ACI patellar graft after removal of superficial fibrillation hypertrophy, which results in complete resolution of crepitus, mechanical symptoms, and pain.

overgrowth of the fibrous layer of the periosteum usually will result in complete relief of symptoms and ongoing maturity of the transplanted autologous cultured chondrocytes to firm smooth repair tissue. Clinically, this usually manifests between 3 and 7 months after surgery at the stage of proliferative hypertrophic periosteal healing response. Patients may present with new-onset catching from a previously smooth tracking knee and may have symptoms of pain and effusion. In this case, their activity should be decreased to avoid the symptomatic area. MRI evaluation followed by arthroscopic treatment is recommended.

In the worse-case scenario where a large portion of the graft is delaminated (Figure 7–24) and the remaining portion is intact and adherent to the underlying bone, an open suture repair is not recommended. Instead, arthroscopic sharp incision of the periosteum that is not attached to the subchondral bone should be performed with removal

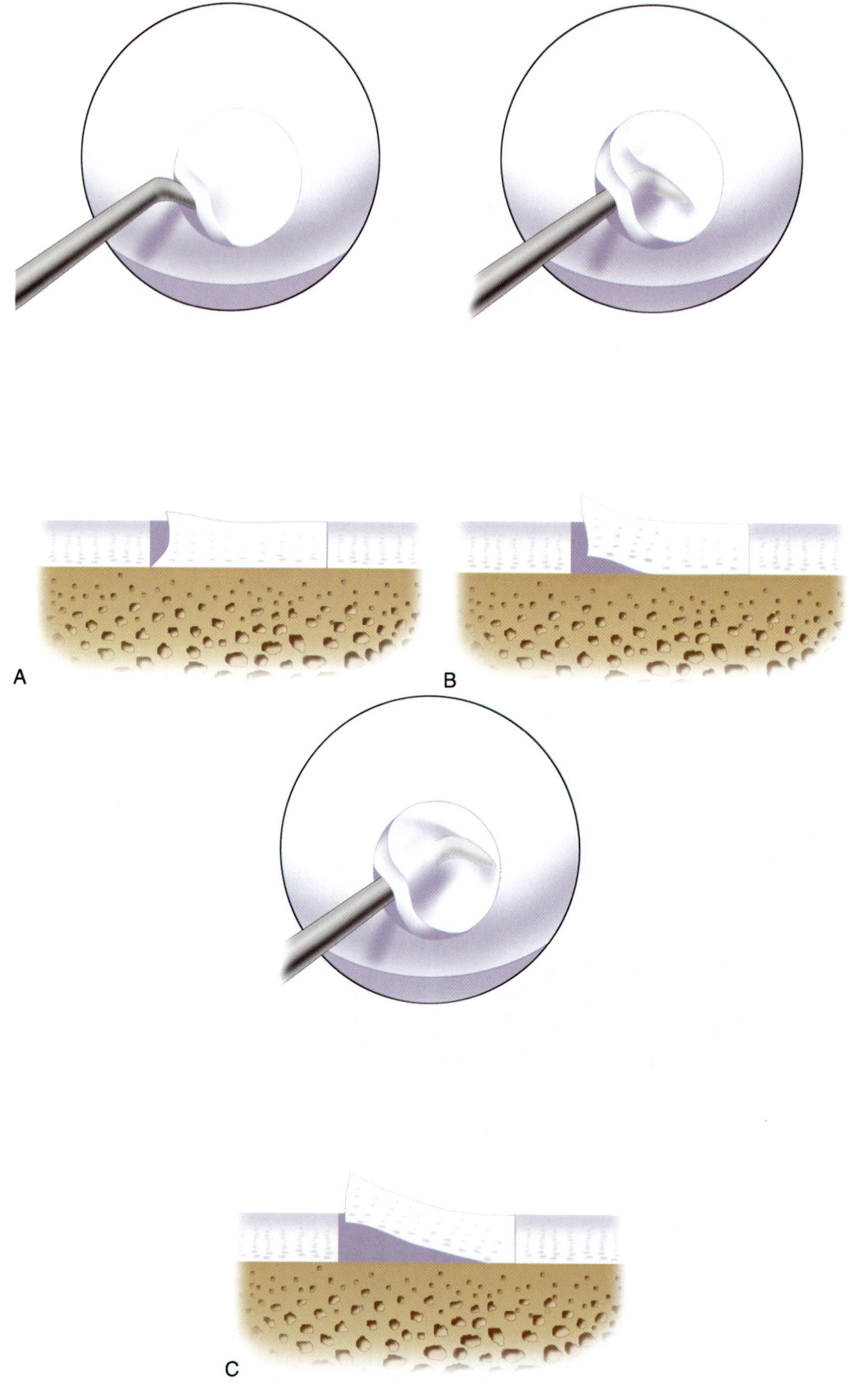

Figure 7-24 Graft delamination usually results in painful symptoms of weight-bearing discomfort and catching. It may be marginal, partial, or complete in severity. Treatment depends on the amount of graft that remains in the size of the defect that ensues. Magnetic resonance imaging (MRI) scan is useful in the diagnosis of graft delamination (see text for details).

Continued

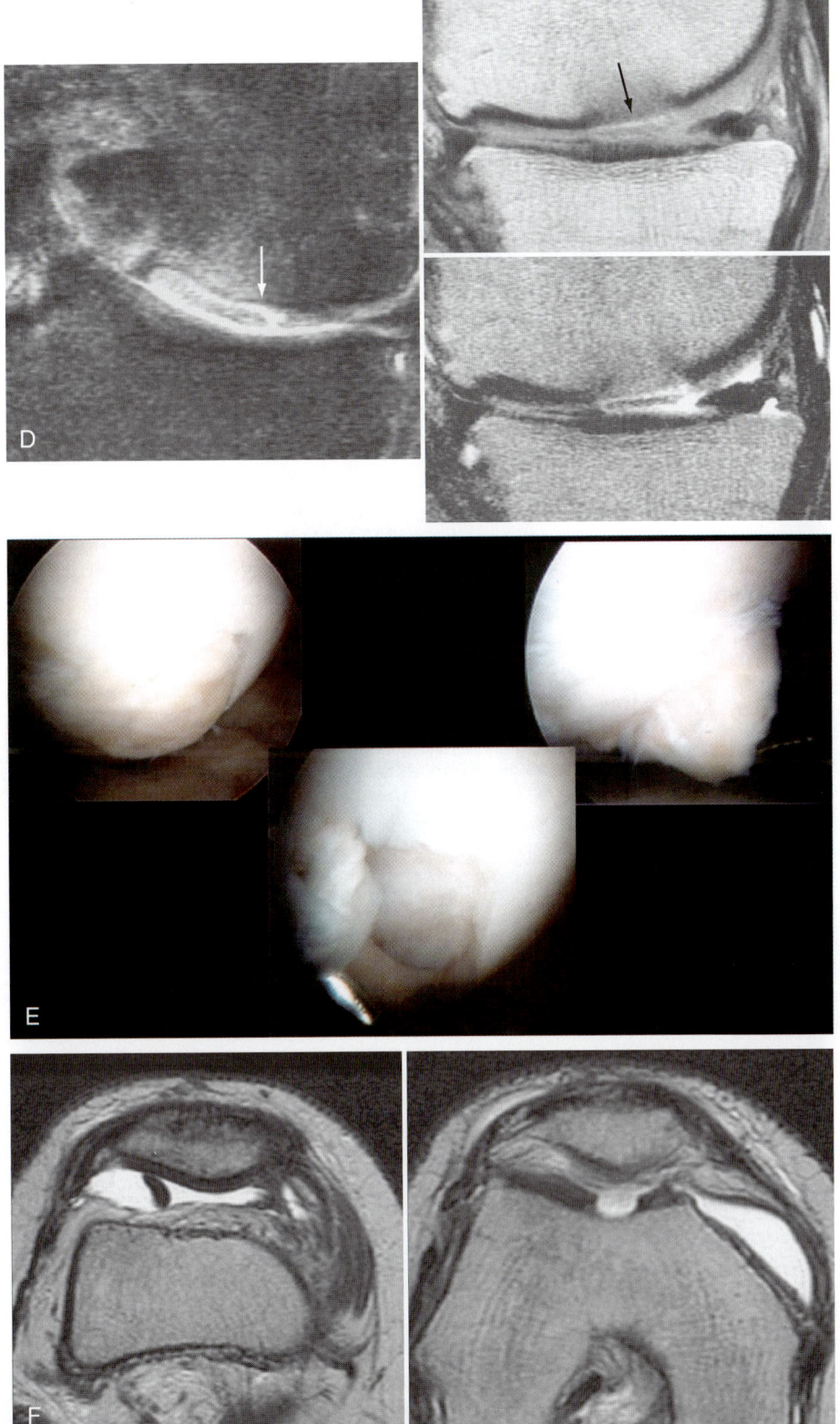

Figure 7-24—cont'd *A,* Diagrammatic representation of a marginal graft delamination. This is usually managed by sharp removal of the graft edge to stabilize the defect and possible marrow stimulation to the defect edge to seal the defect edge with repair tissue. *B,* Diagrammatic representation of a partial graft delamination. *C,* Diagrammatic representation of complete delamination with only edge that remains attached. *D,* Fat-suppressed coronal MRI scan demonstrates a fluid signal *(arrow)* deep to the autologous chondrocyte implantation (ACI) graft. Proton-density MRI scans *(right)* also demonstrate a deep fluid signal indicating poor attachment of the graft to the subchondral bone. *E,* At the time of arthroscopy, the graft appears to be intact *(top left).* However, when a probe is used to assess the stability of the graft, it has become completely delaminated with only and edge attached *(center, right). F,* Axial proton-density MRI scan demonstrates a loose body in the superior patellar pouch *(top).* A clear defect in the trochlea at the site of a small ACI graft and the central sulcus has failed and displaced. These findings indicate complete delamination with loose body.

of the loose flap, leaving behind the integrated chondral graft and any repair tissue underneath the periosteal delamination.

Persistent pain after ACI in a patient who has undergone drilling or microfracture should be investigated by MRI. We have seen late failures from central graft overload and breakdown, delamination, and cyst formation (which is not visible arthroscopically) (Figure 7–25). A slip and fall can result in new articular or meniscal injury and not necessarily be related to the graft despite a history of ACI (Figure 7–26).

CLINICAL OUTCOMES USING ACI

The clinical outcomes that follow include our collaborative results on the use of ACI in adolescents[3] and soccer players[11] as well as personal updated results for the patellofemoral joint,[12] patients older than 45 years,[13] patients treated after marrow stimulation techniques,[14] and the osteoarthritic or salvage group[15] of patients. We have moved on to using a type I–III collagen porcine membrane in an attempt to lessen the incidence of periosteal hypertrophy[16] and report on this topic as well. The cost effectiveness of ACI remains substantiated since its early report in 1998[17,18] based on its durability.[19]

Following institutional review board approval in November 1994, ACI was prospectively evaluated in patients as of March 1995 at our institution. Initially, the expected patient clinical improvement after ACI was not known. Patients with single articular cartilage lesions as well as multiple lesions presented to our clinics. We wished to capture complementary clinical outcomes based on a survey that included overall quality of life, specific knee scores that included sporting activity levels, and well-established outcome scores of arthritis improvement. Patients filled out questionnaires including SF-36,[20] Knee Society Score (KSS),[21] Western Ontario MacMaster (WOMAC) osteoarthritis score,[22] modified Cincinnati rating scale (0–10)[23] activity-based score (Figure 7–27), and patient satisfaction survey (Figure 7–28).

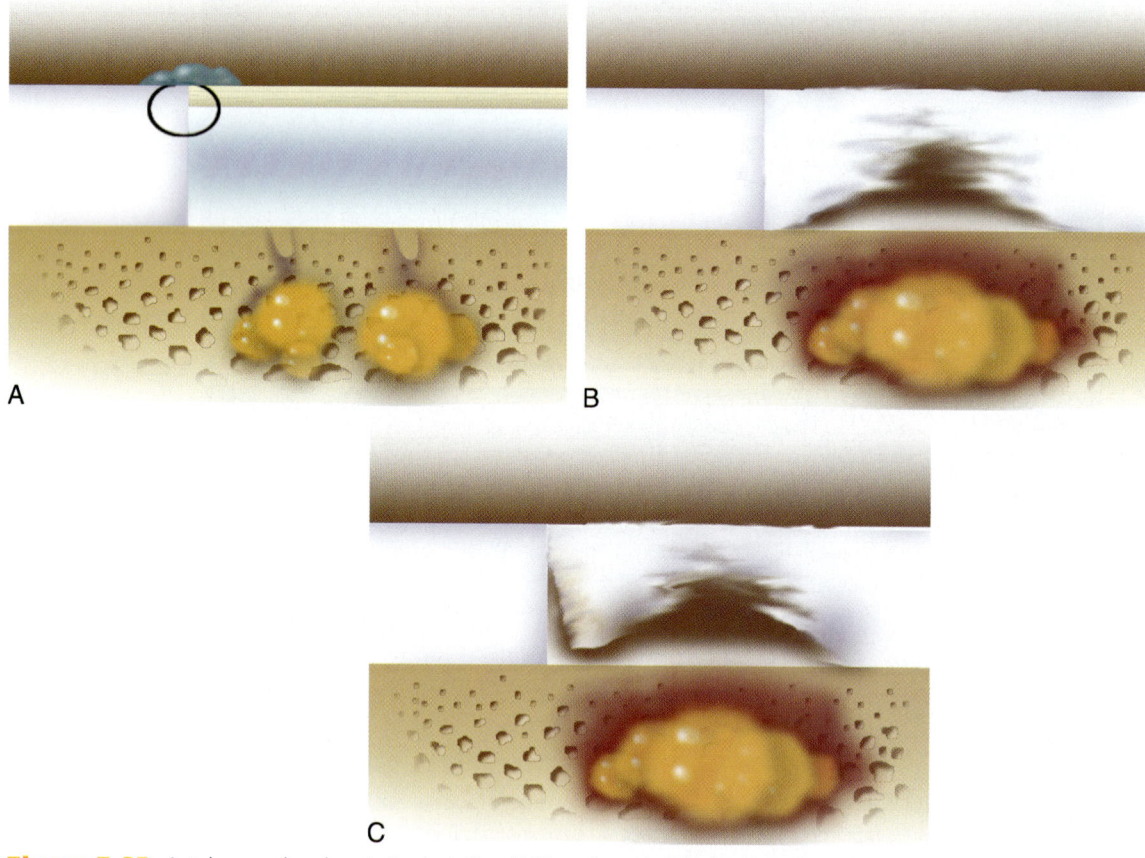

Figure 7–25 Autologous chondrocyte implantation (ACI) grafts may fail after prior microfracture due to cyst formation after microfracture. The cysts may expand after ACI, eventually leading to graft detachment and failure. *A*, Diagrammatic representation of an ACI graft immediately after treatment with prior microfracture. Small subchondral cysts are present at the distal aspect of the pick entry sites. *B*, Cysts expand over time, subchondral bone thickens, and ACI graft attachment debonds. *C*, Eventual detachment of the ACI graft from adjacent cartilage and subchondral bone.

Continued

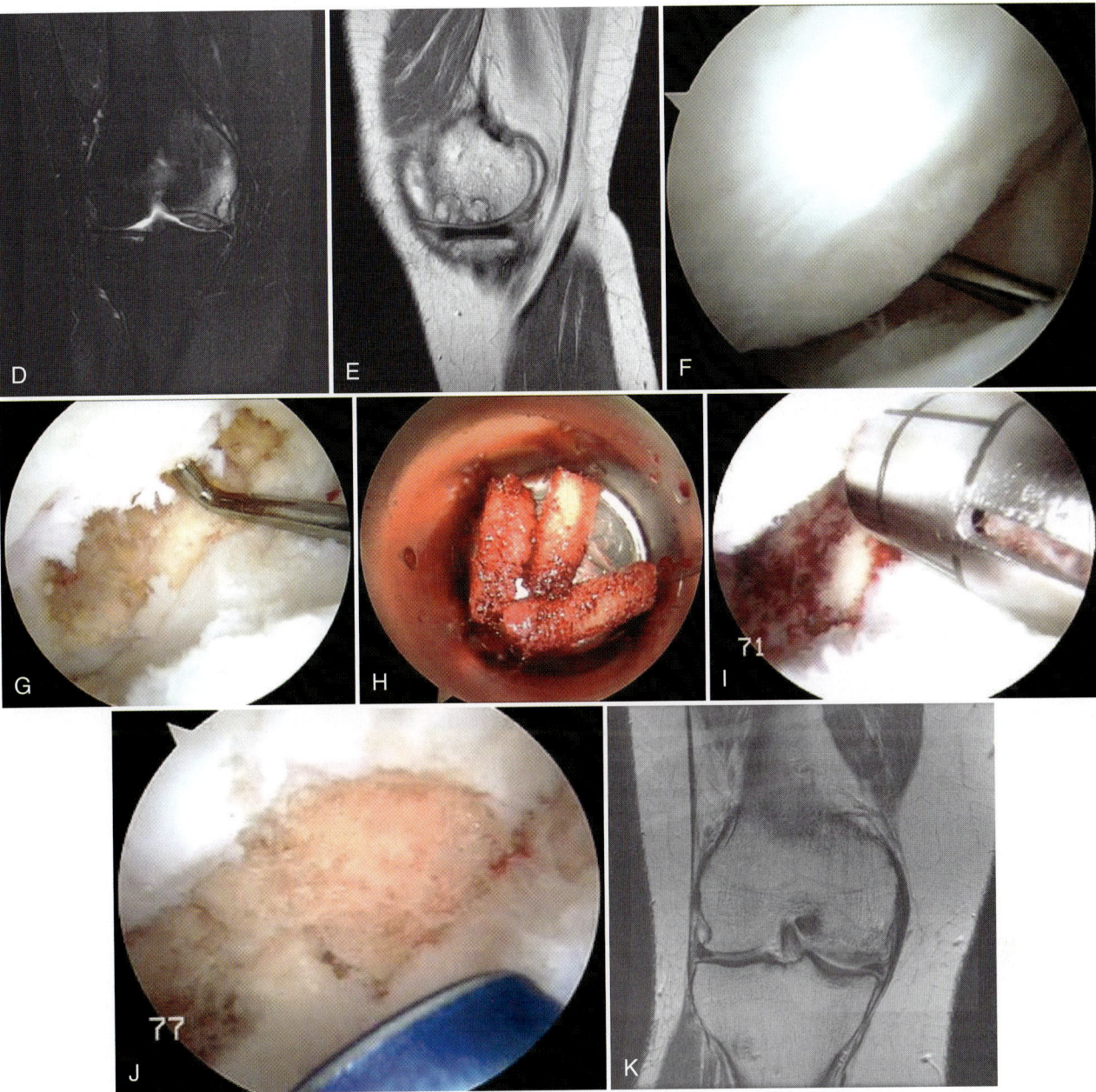

Figure 7–25—cont'd *D,* Magnetic resonance imaging (MRI) scan of a 32-year-old woman 2 years after ACI to the medial femoral condyles that previously had been microfractured. Note intense subchondral edema and developing cyst formation at the margin of the ACI graft to the native articular cartilage. *E,* Sagittal MRI proton-density scan demonstrates large cysts in the medial femoral condyles deep to the ACI graft. *F,* At the time of arthroscopy, the articular surface of the medial femoral condyles anterior cruciate ligament graft appears to be of excellent quality. However, based on the patient's painful symptoms and MRI scan, a problem with ACI graft attachment to native cartilage and subchondral bone on the medial-most aspect of the transplant is known to exist. This is carefully probed and noted to be detached. *G,* Arthroscopic appearance of the defect after the delaminated articular cartilage is removed. The cysts are excavated with a curette. The bony deficiency is apparent after the cyst lining tissue is removed. *H,* Autologous bone graft harvested with a 10-mm-diameter osteochondral autograft transfer system (OATS) harvester from the proximal tibia near Gerdy's tubercle in a specimen cup. *I,* Arthroscopic appearance of the autologous cancellous bone after it has been morselized into small chips, reloaded into the OATS harvester, and packed into the osteochondral defect on the medial femoral condyles. *J,* Arthroscopic appearance of the defect completely filled to the level of the subchondral bone and packed securely with a bone tamp. The tourniquet is then let down, and the patient is rehabilitated as if this were a microfracture technique with 6 weeks of protected weight-bearing and continuous passive motion. *K,* MRI scan, coronal proton-density image, 1 year later demonstrates complete resolution of the subchondral bone cysts and excellent repair tissue fill on the medial femoral condyle. The patient remains symptom free many years later.

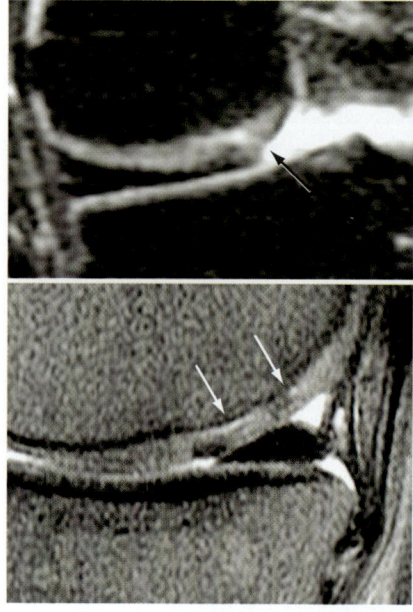
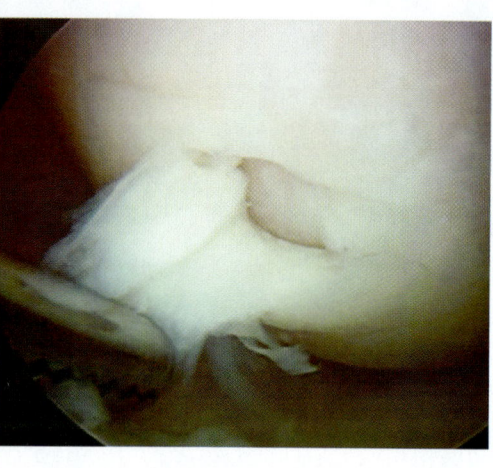

Figure 7-26 Eight months after autologous chondrocyte implantation (ACI) graft to the lateral femoral condyle, the patient has a slip and fall on his driveway. New-onset mechanical catching and pain ensue. The patient feels he has damaged his transplanted knee. Magnetic resonance imaging (MRI) scan demonstrates an intact lateral femoral condyles ACI graft but a new area of subchondral bone detachment of the medial femoral condyles cartilage. MRI fat-suppressed scan shows cartilage detachment from medial femoral condyle *(arrow, upper left)*. Proton-density sagittal image shows cartilage detachment from subchondral bone *(arrows)*. Arthroscopic appearance demonstrates a small chondral flap to the medial femoral condyle, which is debrided and microfractured.

Modified Cincinnati rating scale
Overall condition

Rate overall condition at the present time

2	4	6	8	10
Poor	Fair	Good	Very good	Excellent

2 = Poor — Significant limitations affect activities of daily living
4 = Fair — Moderate limitations affect activities of daily living, no sports
6 = Good — Some limitations with sports but participate; I compensate
8 = Very good — Only a few limitations with sports
10 = Excellent — Able to do whatever I wish (any sport) with no problems

Figure 7-27 Modified Cincinnati rating scale (0–10)[23] activity-based score.

ACI in Adolescents

Twenty patients 18 years or younger with 29 full-thickness articular cartilage lesions in 23 knees were treated with ACI at Boston Children's Hospital and Brigham and Women's Hospital between December 1995 and December 2000.[3] All patients had failed prior conservative and surgical treatment. All patients had undergone at least one surgical procedure before ACI (mean 2.5 procedures, range 1–6 procedures). Patient demographics, defect etiology and characteristics, preoperative duration of symptoms, and surgical history were recorded. Injuries were considered chronic if the preoperative duration of symptoms was greater than 12 months. Preoperative radiographs were obtained for every patient and demonstrated open growth plates at the time of ACI in 60% of the adolescent athletes.

In two patients, the depth of the defect required autologous bone grafting in combination with ACI. Implantation of chondrocytes in these cases was performed using the sandwich technique. Reconstruction of the ACL was performed in one patient at the time of chondrocyte implantation. One other patient had undergone staged ACL reconstruction before autologous chondrocyte transplantation. Meniscal repair was performed in four patients, at the time of chondrocyte implantation in two and as part of the prior surgical procedures in two. TTO was performed concomitantly in one patient. Postoperatively, CPM was initiated within 6 to 12 hours and administered for 2 weeks. Patients were on non–weight-bearing status for 6 to 8 weeks, with gradual progression to full weight bearing by 10 to 12 weeks. Most patients were allowed to return to regular daily activities by 4 months, low-impact activities by 6 months,

Compared to one year ago, how would you rate each operated joint now?			
Much better			
Somewhat better			
About the same			
Somewhat worse			
Much worse			
Compared to before each surgery, how would you rate each operated joint now?			
Much better			
Somewhat better			
About the same			
Somewhat worse			
Much worse			
What is your overall satisfaction level with each joint surgery?			
Very satisfied			
Somewhat satisfied			
Neutral			
Somewhat dissatisfied			
Very dissatisfied			
If you could go back in time and make the decision again, would you choose to have each joint surgery?			
Definitely yes			
Probably yes			
Completely uncertain			
Probably not			
Definitely not			
How would you rate the results of each joint surgery			
Good or excellent			
Fair			
Poor			

Figure 7–28 Patient satisfaction survey for treating osteoarthritis of the knee with autologous chondrocyte implantation.

and running by 9 months. Physically demanding high-impact and pivoting sports were avoided for 12 months.

Patients were evaluated preoperatively and at a mean of 47 ± 4 months postoperatively (range 23–91 months). Functional outcome was determined using established knee scoring systems including the Lysholm score and Tegner activity score. In addition, a questionnaire was used to evaluate the patient's ability for athletic participation and subjective rating of knee function, which was graded as excellent, good, fair, or poor. The level of athletic participation before injury was compared to athletic ability after chondrocyte transplantation.

Twenty adolescent patients with articular cartilage lesions in 23 knees were treated with autologous chondrocyte transplantation. Seventeen patients had unilateral involvement, and three patients presented with bilateral knee articular cartilage lesions. The mean age at chondrocyte transplantation was 15.9 ± 0.3 years (range 12–18 years). There were 15 male and 5 female adolescent athletes. The average duration of symptoms was 21 months (≤ 12 months in 11 [48%] knees, >12 months in 12 [52%] knees). All patients had failed previous conservative and surgical treatment.

Osteochondritis dissecans was the cause of chondral defect in 14 knees. In the remaining nine knees, the cartilage lesions resulted from acute focal trauma associated with pivoting sports such as basketball, football, and soccer. Two (10%) patients had tears of the ACL, and 4 (20%) patients had meniscal injuries. A total of 29 cartilage lesions were observed; the majority presenting as a single lesion, with an average of 1.3 cartilage defects per knee. Average lesion size was 6.4 cm^2.

At latest follow-up, 96% of patients were able to regularly participate in high-impact, pivoting sports at the recreational level or higher. Sixty percent of athletes had returned to the same or higher level of athletic activity than before their injury. Tegner activity scores increased in all patients compared to preoperative values. Lysholm scores were not available before injury but increased significantly from preoperative values of 64 ± 3 points to 87 ± 7 points at latest follow-up ($P < .01$).

Only 33% of adolescents with chronic preoperative symptoms (>12 months) returned to the same level of athletics compared to all adolescents with shorter preoperative intervals ($P < .01$). Postoperative Tegner scores (7.2 ± 0.3 points) and Lysholm scores (85 ± 3 points) in adolescents with chronic symptoms were lower than Tegner scores (8.7 ± 0.2 points, $P < .01$) and Lysholm scores (91 ± 2 points) in adolescents with symptoms ≤ 12 months. The average preoperative duration of symptoms of adolescents who returned to preinjury athletic levels was 15 ± 4 months and lower than in adolescents who failed to return to the same level (31 ± 6 months, $P < .05$). Adolescents with chronic symptoms had undergone an average of 3.2 ± 0.4 prior surgeries compared to 1.6 ± 0.2 in adolescents with acute symptoms ($P < .05$). The number of prior operations also showed significant correlation with the ability to return to preinjury athletics ($r = 0.453$, $P < .05$).

Ninety-six percent of patients rated their results as good or excellent; only one patient reported a fair outcome. This patient presented with moderate genu varum and did not consent to primary realignment. He briefly returned to high-impact athletics after autologous chondrocyte transplantation to the medial femoral condyle and trochlea but developed recurrent symptoms with athletic activities and graft failures. Secondary high tibial osteotomy (HTO) was performed. The patient has not yet returned to high-impact activities at the time of last follow-up and he awaits revision ACI. Other complications included graft hypertrophy, which was observed in 3 (15%) athletes and was successfully treated with arthroscopic chondroplasty in all cases.

ACI in adolescent patients is highly successful when used as a first-line treatment strategy for large chondral defects within the first year of injury. Multiple surgeries in an attempt to be less invasive leads to chronic dysfunction and a poor clinical outcome in those patients.

ACI in Soccer Players

Forty-five soccer players were treated with ACI at participating institutions between March 1988 and August 2000.[11] All athletes complained of acute or chronic symptoms. Baseline evaluation included careful history and physical examination and documentation of type, onset, and duration of symptoms. Demographic data, prior surgical history, and skill level were recorded (Table 7–1). Skill level was divided into recreational and high-level competitive for athletes who participated in high school, collegiate, professional, or national team level soccer.

All patients had full-thickness Outerbridge type IV articular cartilage lesions or osteochondral lesions of the knee demonstrated at arthroscopy. Minimum follow-up duration from the time of implantation was 12 months. At follow-up, the athlete's function was rated using the sports activity-based Tegner scale (Figure 7-29). The ability and time of return to soccer and skill level after articular cartilage repair were recorded. Successful articular cartilage repair was defined as the ability to return to soccer even if not to the previous skill level. Treatment durability was defined as the percentage of players who returned to soccer and maintained this functional status at subsequent follow-up. Adverse events and complications were carefully documented.

Significant improvement of activity scores was observed in greater than 80% of players, confirming the overall functional improvements described after autologous chondrocytes in previous studies. Despite the overall increased function, only one third of the players were able to return to soccer. The return rate was significantly higher in competitive than recreational level players. The return rate among competitive soccer players following autologous chondrocyte transplantation in our study was 83%. Interestingly, the return rate to recreational soccer in our study was significantly lower than at the higher skill level. Significantly prolonged preoperative

Table 7–1 Soccer player demographics undergoing ACI for focal chondral defects after knee surgery.

	All Players	Return	No Return
Gender (%male:%female)	71:29	80:20	63:37
Age (yr)	26 ± 1 (14–43)	22.3 ± 1.6	27.6 ± 1.2
No. of previous surgeries	2.0 ± 0.3 (0–13)	1.5 ± 0.3	2.3 ± 0.5
Skill level (%)			
Recreational	73	16	84
High	27	83$_c$	17
Symptom duration (mo)	26 ± 3.4 (3–96)	16.7 ± 3.8	30.7 ± 4.5
Lesion size (cm^2)	5.7 ± 0.6	5.5 ± 0.8	5.6 ± 0.8
Lesion type (%)			
Single	65	86$_c$	14
Multiple	35	30	70
Lesion location (%)			
Medial femoral condyle	48	37	54
Lateral femoral condyle	23	21	24
Trochlea	13	16	11
Patella	11	16	8
Tibia	5	11	3
Graft failure (%)	13	6	16
Brittberg rating (%)			
Excellent	32	60	18
Good	40	33	43
Fair	23	6	32
Poor	5	0	7

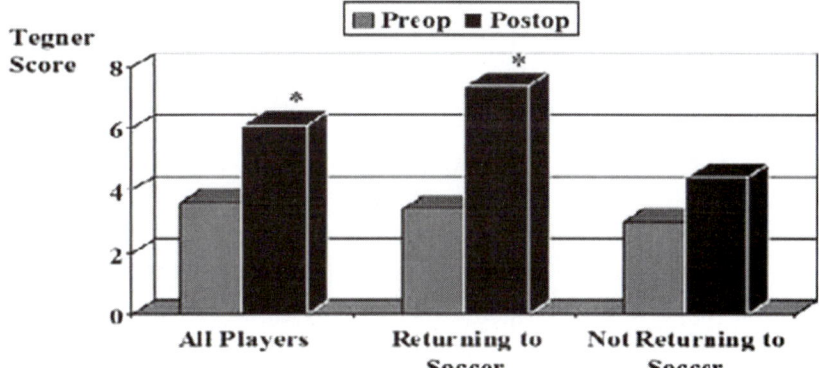

Figure 7-29 Sports activity-based Tegner scale.

morbidity was seen in players who failed to return to soccer after autologous chondrocyte transplantation in our study and could also explain the lower return rate of recreational players in the study. Our data indicate that the longer the time between injury and chondrocyte transplantation, the lower the rate of return to competitive or recreational soccer is. In fact, the success rate effectively doubled if autologous chondrocyte transplantation was performed within 1 year after the onset of articular cartilage injury. This finding confirms previous observations of a significantly better functional outcome if autologous chondrocyte transplantation was performed within 1 year of sustaining the cartilage injury, as in our adolescent patients.

The average time to return to soccer in our study was 18 months, and 87% of returning players were still competing a mean of 48 months postoperatively. Although initial recovery with chondrocyte transplantation may be more prolonged, our data suggest that this cartilage repair technique provides excellent durability even under very high athletic demands. Some world-class athletes who were treated primarily with autologous chondrocyte transplantation within 4 months of injury were able to rapidly return to their preinjury level of play, with excellent long-term durability. These excellent results under maximum demand support the use of autologous chondrocyte transplantation as a primary technique for articular cartilage repair in young active patients. In contrast, when autologous chondrocyte transplantation is used as a salvage procedure in older patients with longstanding preoperative symptoms and multiple prior operations, the results are less predictable. Adjuvant procedures, tibial osteotomy, TTO, and ACL reconstruction all did not affect the return to soccer.

Results of autologous chondrocyte transplantation in soccer athletes are encouraging. An excellent return rate to demanding athletic activity and long-term function, particularly in young, competitive players with short duration of symptoms and fewer prior surgical interventions, is possible. These results are comparable to those reported for microfracture or osteochondral mosaicplasty. Long-term evaluation will help to determine whether restoration of articular cartilage lesions in the knee of soccer players can effectively reduce the high incidence of osteoarthritis in this population.

ACI in the Patellofemoral Joint

Many factors have been implicated as contributing to abnormal pathomechanics leading to pain in the patellofemoral joint. They include patella alta, trochlea dysplasia, increased quadriceps or Q angle with secondary soft tissue problems, weakened or hypoplastic VMO quadriceps muscle with contracted lateral retinaculum, and/or absent redundant medial patellofemoral ligament. These pathomechanics lead to abnormal forces across the patella, resulting in secondary degenerative changes or injury to the articular surfaces of the patellofemoral joint acutely or chronically. Diagnosing and correcting these underlying abnormalities when associated with cartilage injury is crucial to a successful outcome when using ACI for repair of these defects.[12] For these reasons, the early results of resurfacing of the patella with ACI led to good or excellent results in only 2 (29%) of 7 patients treated in the first study introducing autologous chondrocyte transplantation from Sweden in 1994.[1] As patellar tracking was addressed by realignment of the extensor mechanism at the time of transplantation, later reports[19,24] noted that the success rate increased at 2 years to 11 of 17 patients (65% good or excellent results),[24] and at 10 years the results had improved to 13 of 17 patients (76% good or excellent results).[19] Two patients who rated a fair result at 2 years had improved to good results at 3 years, improving the results over time. The importance of correcting the underlying cause of chondral injury cannot be underestimated when attempting surgical correction with cartilage repair techniques.

Anteromedialization of the tibial tubercle has become a useful surgical tool for correcting maltracking and unloading an articular cartilage injury to the patella. Fulkerson and colleagues[25] demonstrated that the anteromedialization TTO successful clinical outcome correlates with the location of the patellar articular lesion (Figure 7–30). In patients with a type I articular cartilage

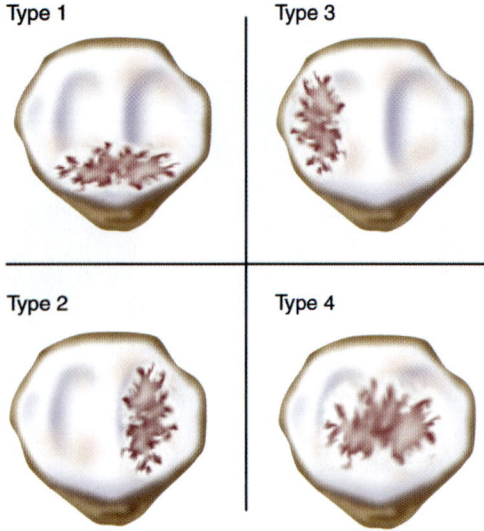

Figure 7-30 Fulkerson classification wear patterns to the patella. Type I and II defects are well managed by anteromedialization tibial tubercle osteotomy (Fulkerson osteotomy). A type I defect involves the inferior patellar pole. A type II defect involves the lateral patellar facet. A type III defect involves the medial patellar facet and is frequently associated with a trochlear defect. A type IV patellar defect is a pan patellar defect. A variant is a proximal pole crush, which occurs in a dashboard impact-related injury. Type III and IV injuries do not do well with isolated Fulkerson osteotomies but are well managed when combined with cartilage repair by autologous chondrocyte implantation.

lesion (inferior patellar pole) or a type II (lateral facet), osteotomy for unloading these two locations had 87% good to excellent subjective results, and 100% of the patients said they would undergo the procedure again. Type III (medial facet) lesions had 55% good to excellent results, and type IV (proximal pole or diffuse) had only 20% good or excellent results. Patients with type I or II lesions were significantly more likely to have good or excellent results than were those with type III or IV lesions. Central trochlea lesions were associated with medial patellar lesions, and all patients with central trochlea lesions had poor results. Workers' Compensation issues diminish the likelihood of this satisfactory outcome by 19%. The authors concluded that the location of the articular patellar cartilage lesion was significantly correlated to the success of anteromedialization TTO.

Localization of the articular cartilage injury at the time of reconstruction is important to determine whether osteotomy surgery alone may predict a successful outcome. Theoretically, cartilage repair to patellar type III and IV lesions as well as the trochlea may improve the clinical outcome for these difficult lesions when associated with patellar maltracking or in the absence of abnormal tracking when no other options exist.

Between March 1995 and July 2002, 248 patients had been treated. One hundred seventy patients had a minimum of 2-year follow-up as of July 2002. Of the 170 patients treated, 45 had treatments involving the patella or trochlea, in isolation or in combination with other lesions, with a minimum of 2 years of follow-up. These group constituted the patients followed up in this study.

Baseline patient demographics were captured, as were outcomes as assessed by several validated outcomes instruments. For all patients, the surgery was photographed in order to assess the appearance of the native chondral injury, the debrided chondral injury, the periosteal patch after completion of suturing, and the injection with autologous cultured chondrocytes. These photographs are maintained in a digital file. The photographs were used to classify the patellar defect location per the Fulkerson classification.[25]

The group consisted of 27 males and 18 females. The average patient age at surgery was 36.9 years (range 15–54 years). The average follow-up was 47.5 months (range 24–86 months). The average number of prior surgeries on the affected knee was 2.5 per patient. Twenty-four percent (11/45) of patients had been treated while receiving Workers' Compensation. There was an average of 2.2 defects per knee, with an average of 2.18 vials containing 12 million cells per vial (26.16 million cells) used to treat each knee. The lesions treated were large, with an average surface area per knee joint of 10.45 cm^2.

Technical issues specific to the surgical procedure of ACI in the patellofemoral joint include a suture technique that restores the surface articular shape of the patella (see Figure 7–16A–C) and the trochlea (Figure 7–15A) as well as soft tissue tensioning at the end of the procedure that allows the normal medial to lateral and proximal to distal patellar glide without overconstricting the patellofemoral joint. An anteromedialization TTO that I prefer is discussed in Chapter 10 (see Figures 7–16 through 7–28). If patellar instability secondary to a dysplastic trochlea remains after anteromedialization TTO and soft tissue stabilization, a trochleoplasty is added to the procedure as described by Peterson et al[8] and illustrated in Chapter 10 (Figures 7–31 and 7–32).

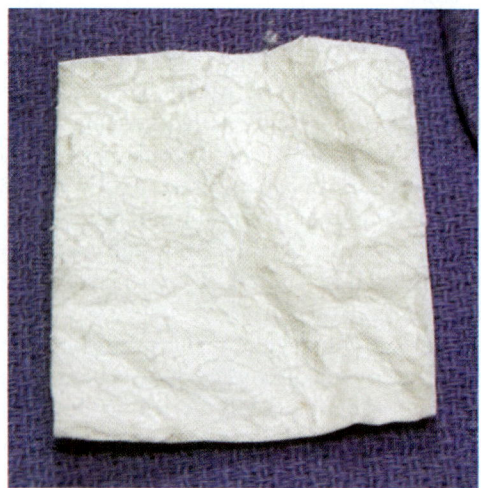

Figure 7-31 Type I–III collagen bilayer membrane (porcine derived; Geistlich Pharma AG, Wolhusen, Switzerland) used as a periosteal substitute for autologous chondrocyte implantation.

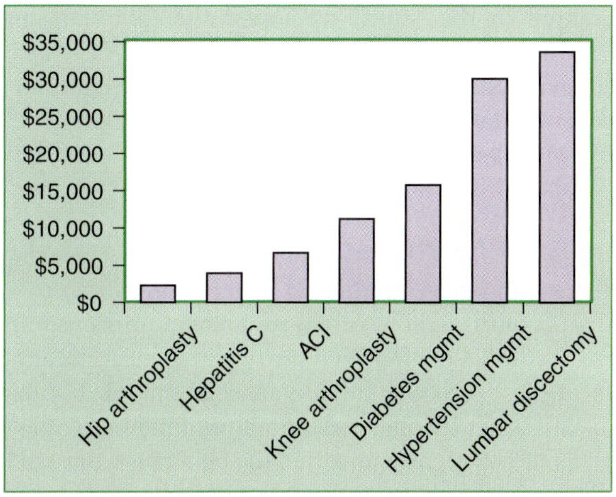

Figure 7-32 Cost-effectiveness chart represented in dollars per quality-adjusted life-years for procedures that are commonly performed and other disease states treated. Despite the cost of autologous chondrocyte implantation (ACI), the clinical improvement and durability of ACI in young patients are pronounced and explain why ACI is so cost effective as a procedure when treating large focal articular cartilage defects compared to other treatment options. (From Minas T: Chondrocyte implantation in the repair of chondral lesions of the knee: economics and quality of life. *Am J Orthop* 1998;27:739–744.)

Osteotomy was performed frequently in this series: 29 (64%) of 45 patients had tibiofemoral malalignment, patellofemoral malalignment, or both. The success of cartilage repair is believed to include normal alignment and tracking. Therefore, if 2 degrees or more of mechanical malalignment from a neutral mechanical axis in the tibiofemoral joint is noted in combination with a large chondral defect, then a varus- or valgus-producing osteotomy is performed with the cartilage repair on the weight-bearing condyles. If evidence of patellar subluxation and tilt with regard to patellar tracking is noted by clinical examination and/or CT scan, then anteromedialization TTO is performed in combination with resurfacing of the patella, trochlea, or both.

Patient failures were defined as poor clinical outcomes accompanied by evidence of graft failure due to delamination from adjacent cartilage and subchondral bone, poor biomechanical properties indicative of fibrous or fibrocartilage repair as evidenced by arthroscopy, or evidence of graft detachment by MRI or arthroscopy despite a good clinical outcome.

When assessing the first 45 patients in whom the patellofemoral joint was treated by ACI with a minimum 2-year follow-up, we found that patient satisfaction was high. Using a patient satisfaction questionnaire, patient overall satisfaction was 71% satisfied, 16% neutral, and 13% dissatisfied. Compared to before surgery, 76% were better, 18% were the same, and 6% were worse. Eighty-seven percent of patients said they would choose the surgery again, and 13% said they would not. Overall, patients rated their results as 71% good or excellent, 22% fair, and 7% poor. Large clinical improvements and statistical significance were seen using the SF-36, KSS, WOMAC score, and modified Cincinnati activity score.

Our series noted that the location of the chondral defect on the patella and trochlea recognize a successful clinical outcome when ACI was used to treat the chondral defect, in addition to realignment when needed, whereas other series did not.[25] In this series, 31 (91%) of 34 patellar lesion locations treated were type III or IV. The other defects were trochlea (n = 11) or kissing patella and trochlea (n = 20). Sixty-four percent of cases involved osteotomy of the tibial tubercle alone or in combination with a valgus-producing tibial osteotomy. The osteotomy effect alone would not account for the high success rate based on Fulkerson's results[25] because of the size and location of the chondral defects.

Three subgroups in our series (patella plus trochlea [n = 4], weight-bearing condyles plus patella [n = 2], and weight-bearing condyles plus trochlea [n = 2]) had a small sample size and the statistics were not very meaningful. However, three other subgroups (patella [n = 8], trochlea [n = 9], and weight-bearing condyles plus patella plus trochlea [n = 20]) demonstrated marked improvement in pain relief and functionality.

The SF-36 physical component summary demonstrated a highly significant improvement in physical well-being after ACI. Emotional well-being as measured by the SF-36 mental component summary was significant for the larger group (n = 20) of weight-bearing condyle plus patella plus trochlea. The WOMAC score, which indicates relief in pain stiffness and swelling, was significant for these three groups, as was the KSS for its knee rating component. Surprisingly, the highest improvement in sports activity rating was seen in the most severely injured knees. This treatment group had the largest surface area of transplantation for knee (15.31 cm^2).

When assessing the overall size of the defects treated, we noted that 35 trochleas with an average surface area of 5.22 cm^2 and 34 patellas with an average surface area of 4.86 cm^2 were treated.

In total, 11 (24%) of 45 patients were defined as having failed, three due to failure of the weight-bearing condyle ACI graft; therefore, 8 (18%) failures were due to a patella or trochlea graft failure. Of the patients treated while receiving Workers' Compensation, 5 (45%) of 11 failed. Three patients underwent prosthetic reconstruction, two patients went on to total knee replacement, and one patient who failed patella transplant underwent an isolated patellofemoral prosthesis. Three patients who had partial graft failures underwent arthroscopic debridement. Five patients with failed grafts underwent revision ACI procedure: two for the trochlea, two for the patella, and one for a medial femoral condyle; they all have undergone successful revision ACI procedures.

In our series of ACI in the patellofemoral joint, 91% of patients with chondral injuries to the patella were type III and IV. Thirty-four patients underwent ACI to the patella with average defect size of 4.86 cm^2. Thirty-five patients underwent ACI to the trochlea with defect size of 5.22 cm^2. Overall, the average surface transplanted per knee was 10.45 cm^2. Patient satisfaction overall was 87% for patients who would choose the surgery again. Seventy-one percent believed their clinical outcome was good or excellent, 22% fair, and, 7% poor.

Three patients failed (two patellar and one medial femoral condyle) and required prosthetic replacement. When failures occurred, they were readily managed by revision ACI when the source of the failure was a robust repair tissue that did not integrate well. If the repair tissue was of poor quality, then we recommend either an osteochondral allograft or a prosthetic reconstruction. Hence, despite initial failure, the final good result was usually obtained by biologic means and preserved the patient's function and joint.

We believe that ACI plays a complementary role, not previously available, for symptomatic pain relief and improved functionality in young patients for whom osteotomy is not successful and prosthetic reconstruction is not desired. Based on the clinical outcomes presented in this study, we found the following algorithm to be useful in the clinical management of patients with patellofemoral disease. A successful treatment is based on identification of (1) patellar tilt, (2) patellar subluxation, and (3) location of chondrosis (see Chapter 10, Table 10–1 for details).

Update on 130 Patients with Patellofemoral ACI

A recent update of the initial 45-patient cohort to 130 patients confirmed our initial results and improved upon them further. One hundred thirty patients had treatment involving the patella or trochlea in isolation or in combination with other lesions, with minimum follow-up of 2 to 9 years. These patients constitute the cohort for this study.

Baseline patient demographics are given in Table 7–2, and outcomes as captured by validated outcomes instruments are given in Table 7–3.

When assessing the overall size of the defects treated, 98 trochleas had an average surface area of 5.8 cm^2, and 63 patellas had an average surface area of 4.72 cm^2. These large areas constituted the majority of the articular surface of those joints.

The procedures failed in 30 (23%) patients, 14 (11%) due to failure of the weight-bearing condyle ACI graft and 16 (12%) by a patella or trochlea graft failure.

Table 7-2 Autologous Chondrocyte Implantation Patellofemoral Subgroup Characteristics

Subgroup	N	Osteotomy	Patellar Defect Location (Type I–IV)	Surface Area Transplanted (cm^2)	Average Age (yr)
Patella	14	TTO-7	1 Type II 8 Type III 5 Type IV	5.10	38
Trochlea	15	TTO-7	N/A	4.74	34
Patella + trochlea	5	TTO-3	3 Type III 2 Type IV	12.69	48
Weight-bearing condyle + patella	19	TTO-6 HTO-1 HTO+TTO-5	1 Type II 7 Type III 11 Type IV	10.23	39
Weight-bearing condyle + trochlea	52	TTO-10 HTO-6 HTO+TTO-4	N/A	13.05	38
Weight-bearing condyle + patella + trochlea	25	TTO-7 HTO-1 HTO+TTO-6	4 Type II 10 Type III 11 Type IV	15.84	39
Total	130	63/130 (48%)	57/63 Type III + IV (90%)	11.03 cm^2 (average per knee)	37.5

All trochlea (n = 98), average surface area = 5.8 cm^2.
All patella (n = 63), average surface area = 4.72 cm^2.
Osteotomy was performed in this series (63/130 [48%]) of patients who had tibiofemoral malalignment (high tibial osteotomy [HTO]), patellofemoral malalignment (tibial tubercle osteotomy [TTO]), or both (HTO-TTO). Based on the patient satisfaction survey, overall satisfaction was 82%, with 11% neutral and 7% dissatisfied; 86% thought they were better, 8% the same, and 6% worse; 88% of patients said they would choose the surgery again, 4% were uncertain, and 8% said they would not. Overall, the patients rated their results as 80% good or excellent, 18% fair, and 2% poor.
N/A, trochlea is not applicable to patellar defect location classification.

Table 7-3 Overall Outcome Scores for Autologous Chondrocyte Implantation in the Patellofemoral Joint

Outcome Measures	Preoperative	Postoperative	P Value
SF-36 PCS	33.88	41.01	<.0001
SF-36 MCS	48.92	53.13	<.0001
WOMAC	38.06	21.27	<.0001
KSS–knee	51.83	79.72	<.0001
KSS–function	62.35	82.08	<.0001
Modified Cincinnati	3.58 (range 1–8)	6.03 (range 1–10)	<.0001

Large average clinical improvement was found using the Medical Outcomes Study 36-Item Short-Form Health Survey (SF-36) Physical Component Summary (PCS) and Mental Component Summary (MCS); Knee Society Score (KSS); Western Ontario MacMaster (WOMAC) osteoarthritis score; and modified Cincinnati activity score. Of these four rating measurements, only the WOMAC score is designed to decrease with patient improvement; the others increase. All of these results were statistically significant.

Twelve (9%) patients had prosthetic reconstruction. Eight (6%) patients underwent revision ACI for graft failure, 5 (4%) patients had no further treatment for partial graft failure, and 5 (4%) patients went on to develop new chondral defects. Of these five patients with new defects, two had ACI, one an allograft, one an arthroscopic abrasion, and the last patient awaits ACI.

The failure rate of ACI in the patellofemoral joint appears to be no different than in the tibiofemoral joint in our series. However, the clinical outcomes, good as they are—80% good or excellent, 18% fair, and only 2% poor—are less than in the tibiofemoral joint. This is common among different series and treatments. My preferred treatment in the patellofemoral joint remains ACI because of the high patient satisfaction and clinical outcomes.

ACI in Patients Older than 45 Years

Background: ACI has become an accepted option for treatment of full-thickness chondral defects of the knee in carefully selected patients. Current recommendations limit this procedure to younger patients, yet many patients older than 45 years wish to remain active and preserve their joint. The purpose of this study was to determine whether increasing patient age adversely affected clinical outcome in this patient group.[26]

Methods: Patients 45 years and older were treated with ACI involving the weight-bearing femoral condyles, patella, and trochlea, in isolation or in combination.

Results: Fifty-six patients 45 years and older were treated with ACI between February 1995 and February 2005. The average patient age at index surgery was 48.6 years (range 45–60 years). The minimum follow-up was 2 years (mean 4.7 years, range 2–11 years). The cohort consisted of 36 males and 20 females. The mean transplant size was 4.7 cm^2 per defect (range 1–15.0 cm^2) and 9.8 cm^2 per knee (range 2.5–31.6 cm^2). There were 8 (14%) failures and a need for additional surgical procedures in 24 (42%) patients. At the latest available follow-up, 72% of patients rated themselves as good or excellent, 78% felt improved, and 81% would again choose ACI as a treatment option.

Conclusion: Our results suggest that ACI can provide good clinical results even in older patients but is associated with a significant rate of reoperation for arthroscopic treatment of adhesions and graft hypertrophy.

This review of prospectively collected data details the clinical and functional outcomes of ACI in 56 patients older than 45 years with a minimum follow-up of 2 years. The overall failure rate of 14% is comparable to prior reports on the results of ACI in younger patients.

Overall, patients rated their outcomes at the latest available follow-up as 72% good or excellent, 15% fair, and 13% poor. Seventy-eight percent felt improved by the surgery, and 81% would choose to undergo ACI again. Only 8% felt their knee was worse than before the surgery, and another 8% would not choose to have ACI again if they were in a similar situation. When subcategorized into simple, complex, and salvage groups, clinical improvement was seen in all three categories across all scores. Despite having the highest absolute changes in each of the functional scores, none of the improvements seen in the simple subcategory reached statistical significance due to the small number of patients (n = 3) in this group. For the complex and salvage subcategories, all scores showed significant improvements at the time of latest follow-up; no significant relationship was found between complexity of defect and clinical outcome. The greatest improvement in sports activity rating was found in the most severely involved knees. Failure of treatment occurred in 8 (14.3%) of the 56 patients. Surprisingly, only one failure occurred in the 16 patients treated for kissing lesions, resulting in a failure rate (6.25%) lower than the average failure rate across all patients. Of the patients treated under Workers' Compensation, 6 (40%) of 15 had failed procedures, reflecting a significantly higher failure rate compared to patients with a non–work-related history. In the non-Workers' Compensation patients, two of 41 failed for a failure rate of 5%, which is similar to that of the group younger than 45 years. Of note, 5 of the 6 patients treated in the Workers' Compensation group who had failed had a prior marrow stimulation technique, which may have been the most significant aspect of the treatment failure in this group. Our data demonstrated that a higher failure rate with ACI will occur after prior marrow stimulation technique.[14]

With an average transplant size of 4.7 cm^2 per defect and 9.8 cm^2 per knee, the lesions treated were substantial and generally larger than those reported in other studies of patients who, on average, were more than a decade younger. Our finding of an overall failure rate of 14% is similar to existing data from younger patient populations. We previously published our experiences with ACI in a younger patient cohort with an average age of 36 years, average transplant size of 4.3 cm^2 per defect, and overall failure rate of 13%.

Most patients in this age group present to our office specifically to avoid, or postpone, prosthetic replacement, so a randomized controlled study comparing cartilage repair with joint replacement was not feasible. A younger patient group treated at our institution by the same surgeon with identical technique and outcomes instruments showed similar results.[7] The strengths lie in the very complete and long follow-up with multiple validated outcome instruments; all patients were operated by a single surgeon with extensive experience in cartilage repair. To our knowledge, this is the first detailed report on the clinical outcome of ACI in an older age group.

Conclusion

In older patients, metabolic cell activity is assumed to be lower and defects are often large and chronic in nature, adding to concerns about the efficacy of cartilage repair procedures in these patients. Treatment of older patients with cartilage defects has traditionally consisted of palliation, osteotomy, or joint replacement. With an aging population now comes an increasing number of patients who wish to remain active and are less willing to accept the limitations associated with joint replacement or who dislike the comparatively large angular corrections of isolated osteotomy. The study focuses on this group of patients who are beyond the current recommendations for cartilage repair but either are unwilling or are biologically too young to undergo joint replacement. We chose 45 years as our threshold because this age has developed as a common insurance limit for ACI, even though it is not strongly supported by data.

Our results indicate that ACI is a reliable technique for treatment of patients 45 years and older with symptomatic, large full-thickness chondral defects of the knee. Careful indication and correction of associated malalignment are essential for a successful outcome. Patients require careful counseling with regard to the long and complex rehabilitation, the likelihood of additional surgery, and the functional gains that can be reasonably expected in order to avoid disappointment.

Prior marrow stimulation in this age group, especially in Workers' Compensation patients who may have undergone prolonged and problematic treatment and have prolonged symptoms, should be of concern. In our series, the failure rate in non–Workers' Compensation patients was only 8% versus 40% in Workers' Compensation patients, 5 of 6 of whom had prolonged symptoms and prior marrow stimulation.

ACI for Joint Preservation in Patients with Early Osteoarthritis: 2- to 11-Year Follow-up

Perhaps the most gratifying use of ACI is in the management of injured young athletes with early osteoarthritis, young arthritics, and young people with old knees. This group of patients is outside the realm of sports medicine and is too young to undergo prosthetic arthroplasty. These patients may still obtain successful pain relief, functional improvement, and quality of life after undergoing ACI.

Young patients with early osteoarthritis who wish to remain functionally active have limited treatment options. Existing studies examining the use of ACI have included patients with early degenerative changes, for which encouraging results have been reported.[7,27] However, no study has specifically investigated the outcome of ACI in this challenging population. We hypothesize that ACI reduces pain and improves function in young, early-stage osteoarthritic patients while delaying the need for joint replacement surgery.[15]

For patient selection, we first chose all ACI patients who had completed a minimum follow-up of 2 years; however, patients who had failed within the first 2 years after their procedure were also included in the study. From this group, we selected those who had been categorized radiographically or clinically as having early osteoarthritic disease at the time of ACI. Radiographically, patients were eligible if they had peripheral intraarticular osteophyte formation and/or 0% to 50% joint space narrowing as defined by Ahlback stage 0 or 1 classification.[28] Patients were also included if they had normal radiographs but evidence of bipolar (kissing) lesions or generalized chondromalacia noted at the time of surgery. From the database of the 328 patients treated with ACI within the study period, 153 patients (155 knees) fulfilled the criteria and were enrolled in study. There were no exclusion criteria, and all eligible patients were analyzed.

Autologous Chondrocyte Implantation

Patients with 2 degrees or more of malalignment were treated by realignment osteotomy and overcorrected by 2 degrees to unload and optimize the mechanical environment of the compromised compartment. We intentionally avoided more significant overcorrection by 3 to 5 degrees as recommended for isolated osteotomy due to the risk of overload and accelerated failure of the contralateral compartment. Patients with patellofemoral defects had a concurrent anteromedialization TTO, lateral release, and VMO advancement if there was evidence of patellar subluxation and tilt as noted by physical examination, radiography, and/or CT scan assessment.

Outcome Measures

Our standard outcome measures were prospectively collected. In addition, we analyzed clinically important patient-perceived improvements. *Minimal clinically important difference* was defined as the smallest difference in score that patients perceive as beneficial.[29,30] According to previously published studies, the minimal clinically important difference of improvement in patients with osteoarthritis of the knee was defined as a 17% to 22% change from baseline WOMAC subscale scores.[29,31]

Results

Patient and Defect Characteristics

A total of 153 patients with 155 treated knees were included in the study. Patients in this cohort were, on average, 38.3 years of age at the time of implantation; there were 70 females and 83 males. Mean patient age was 38.3 years. On average, 2.1 defects were treated per knee. The mean defect size was 4.9 cm^2, and the total area per knee was 10.4 cm^2. Fourteen percent (22/153) of patients were receiving Workers' Compensation. An average of 2.1 defects per knee with an average defect size of 4.9 cm^2 and a total treated surface area of 10.4 cm^2 per knee joint was treated. When considering only the size of the primary, or largest, lesion in each joint, average size increased to 6.7 cm^2. Lesions were most commonly located in the following location, by order of incidence: medial femoral condyle, trochlea, patella, and lateral femoral condyle. Bipolar (kissing) lesions were present in 27% (42/155) of knee joints. In addition to ACI, many concurrent procedures were performed, most commonly to correct tibiofemoral malalignment in 31% (48/155) and patellar maltracking in 28% (44/155) of implanted knees.

Treatment Failures and Revision Surgery

For the purposes of this study, treatment failure was conversion to a prosthesis because this was the primary reason patients in this group sought treatment—to avoid prosthetic arthroplasty. Twelve (8%) knees were considered treatment failures and were revised to partial (2) or total (10) joint replacements at an average of 38 months (range 9–118 months) after ACI. The reasons for revision included complete graft failure in three patients, inadequate pain relief in one patient, and progression of osteoarthritic disease beyond the originally transplanted defect area in eight patients.

Eight percent (12/155) of knees treated in ACI patients met the criteria for treatment failure due to revision with partial or total knee arthroplasty; six of these patients received payments through Workers' Compensation, resulting in a failure rate of 27.3% (6/22) in that subgroup. ACI in non–Workers' Compensation patients failed at a rate of 4.5% (6/133). Kaplan-Meier survivorship for the group is shown in Figure 7–33.

Outcome Measures

The 92% of knees that were not considered treatment failures experienced statistically significant changes in WOMAC pain and function scores from baseline to follow-up that exceeded the definition of minimal clinically important difference (Table 7–4).

Excluding patients whose treatments failed, the mean improvement in the 20-point WOMAC pain score and the 68-point WOMAC function score was 4.9 points (51% improvement) and 15.7 points (53% improvement), respectively. More specifically, the proportion of patients who experienced severe or extreme pain while walking on a flat surface decreased by 73% whereas the percentage of patients with similar pain walking up and down stairs decreased by 76%. Similar reductions were seen in the proportion of patients who had severe or extreme difficulty descending stairs, ascending stairs, bending to the floor, and walking on a flat surface, decreasing by 78%, 75%, 73%, and 74%, respectively.

Statistically significant improvements in mean score change also were observed for the modified Cincinnati knee rating system, KSS function scale, KSS pain scale, and all eight SF-36 domain scales (see Table 7–4 and Figure 7–34). Furthermore, 91.6% of patients were satisfied with their outcome after treatment with ACI, 90.2% rated their knees better than before the surgery, and 91.3% would have the same procedure again.

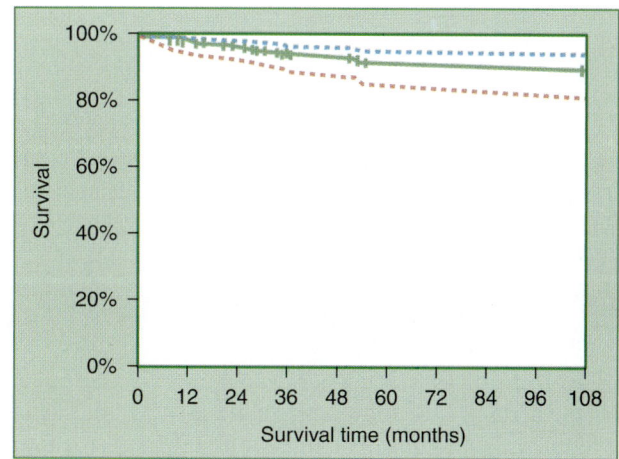

Figure 7-33 Kaplan-Meier survival curve and 95% confidence interval for survival of autologous chondrocyte implantation over time.

Table 7-4 Functional Scores Preoperatively, at 24 Months, and at Latest Follow-up

	Preoperative (n = 143)	24-Month Follow-up (n = 143)	Latest Follow-up (>2 yr) (n = 132)	P value
Modified Cincinnati	3.6 (1–8)	6.1 (2–10)	6.7 (2–10)	<.001
KSS–knee	59.0 (24–100)	82.6 (45–100)	88.0 (50–100)	<.001
KSS–function	60.6 (15–100)	74.2 (40–100)	79.4 (40–100)	<.001
WOMAC–pain	9.6 (0–20)	5.8 (0–16)	4.7 (0–17)	<.001
WOMAC–stiffness	3.9 (0–8)	2.7 (0–7)	2.4 (0–8)	<.001
WOMAC–function	29.4 (2–62)	17.3 (0–51)	13.7 (0–49)	<.001
SF-36 PCS	37.2 (23–60)	44.0 (25–60)	45.4 (9–60)	<.001
SF-36 MCS	38.4 (9–55)	41.3 (9–53)	43.8 (9–56)	<.001

Data are given as mean (range).
KSS, Knee Society Score; modified Cincinnati, modified Cincinnati activity score; n, number of patients at the respective time point; SF-36, Medical Outcomes Study 36-Item Short-Form Health Survey, Physical Component Summary (PCS) and Mental Component Summary (MCS); WOMAC, Western Ontario MacMaster osteoarthritis score.

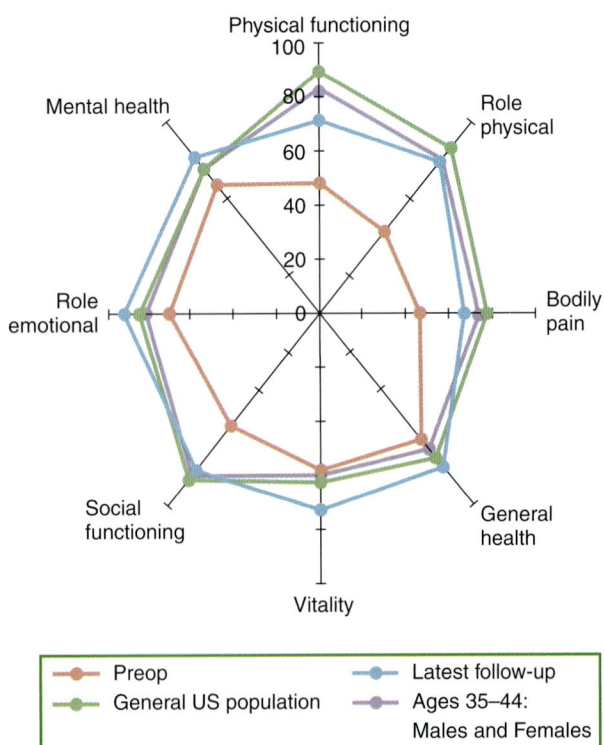

Figure 7-34 Medical Outcomes Study 36-Item Short-Form Health Survey domain scores for autologous chondrocyte implantation patients preoperatively and at the time of latest follow-up. Reference values for the general U.S. population and patients aged 35–44 years.

Additional Analyses

Additional analyses were performed to test the effect of concurrent osteotomy procedures on the functional outcome of ACI. Both patients with and those without concurrent osteotomies experienced significant improvement in all functional scores (P < .001). There were no significant differences between patients without osteotomies and individual subgroups of patients with isolated HTO, isolated TTO, or a combination of both. Comparing patients with HTO and patients who had undergone TTO demonstrated significantly better outcomes for the HTO group at final follow-up (Table 7–5) when considering absolute levels; however, TTO patients started with worse scores.

The results from this study demonstrate that ACI results in statistically significant and clinically relevant reductions in pain and improvement in function while delaying the need for knee arthroplasty for more than 5 years in 92% of patients. Careful and thorough discussion of the invasive surgical procedure, the complex rehabilitation and long recovery, and the high likelihood of repeat surgery is paramount to ensure a reasonable level of patient expectations and satisfaction with the outcome. Given the limited treatment options for this subset of patients, ACI may be a plausible treatment for young osteoarthritic patients to delay the need for joint replacement surgery in the hope of obviating subsequent revision surgery, which is associated with much less satisfactory outcomes than primary procedures.

Our data suggest that ACI in patients with early osteoarthritis results in clinically relevant and statistically significant reductions in pain and improvement in function. Ninety-two percent of patients were functioning well 5 years postoperatively and were able to delay the need for joint replacement. Given the limited number of treatment options for this subset of patients, ACI may offer improved quality of life for young osteoarthritic patients.

In this prospective cohort study with 2- to 11-year follow-up, we hypothesize that ACI reduces pain in young patients with early osteoarthritic changes. Our hope is to use ACI to delay the need for primary knee

Table 7-5 Functional Scores for Osteotomy Groups Preoperatively and at Latest Follow-up

	Preoperative			Latest Follow-up (>2 yr)		
	HTO (n = 29)	TTO (n = 23)	P value	HTO (n = 27)	TTO (n = 23)	P value
Modified Cincinnati	3.4	3.3	0.9	7.3	6.1	0.002
KSS–knee	61.7	52.9	0.03	92.0	84.1	0.02
KSS–function	64.5	59.1	0.2	82.6	74.3	0.04
WOMAC–pain	9.5	11.5	0.08	3.3	6.2	0.01
WOMAC–stiffness	4.1	4.9	0.1	1.9	3.2	0.01
WOMAC–function	30.0	34.9	0.2	10.8	19.7	0.007
SF-36 PCS	36.7	35.6	0.6	48.6	43.3	0.03
SF-36 MCS	39.1	38.4	0.7	43.7	43.7	0.99

Data are given as mean.
P values compare the two groups at each time point.
HTO, high tibial osteotomy; KSS, Knee Society Score; modified Cincinnati, modified Cincinnati activity score; n, number of patients at the respective time point; SF-36, Medical Outcomes Study 36-Item Short-Form Health Survey, Physical Component Summary (PCS) and Mental Component Summary (MCS); TTO, tibial tubercle osteotomy; WOMAC, Western Ontario MacMaster osteoarthritis score.

replacement until the patient is older, when the replacement might outlast the patient's lifetime, thus avoiding the need for revision surgery.

ACI in Patients after Marrow Stimulation Techniques

When I first started to perform ACI in 1995, patients who were typically sent to me had failed multiple previous treatment options and were considered to have failed the standard of care at the time, which included drilling, abrasion, and the recently introduced microfracture technique as a marrow stimulation to promote fibrocartilaginous repair in an articular defect. I noted thickened and sclerotic subchondral bone plates after debridement of the fibrocartilage repair tissue, remaining fibrous tracts within drill holes, and occasionally intralesional osteophyte formation that was very prominent and sometimes above the adjacent articular surface. My concern with taking down these intralesional osteophytes was the possibility of creating bleeding and mixing marrow-derived cells with end-differentiated chondrocytes, thus contaminating the cell suspension and resulting in recurrent fibrocartilage repair instead of hyaline repair tissue. I initially used a bone tamp to impact the prominent bone flush with the adjacent subchondral bone to create a cavity for the recipient cells. However, I noted that several of the transplants filled the defect and then delaminated, leaving behind a very visible sclerotic subchondral bone that had been impacted. I then removed the intralesional osteophyte with a rongeur and used a high-speed bur to thin out the subchondral bone to the adjacent level of subchondral bone. I was surprised to see that bleeding was minimal given that the bone is very cortical. Despite this finding, failures from delamination, central breakdown of the graft over the area of stiffening, and occasional deep cystic formation occurred, with failure of the transplant. These failures did not seem to occur with articular defects that had not previously been marrow stimulated.

I hypothesized that the osteochondral unit had been affected by the marrow stimulation technique, which lessened the success rate of integration to the subchondral bone of ACI and caused a change in the subchondral bone such that its load-absorbing capacity was altered, and that the overlying repair tissue was subject to central overload and breakdown.

We reviewed my series of ACI in systematic fashion to compare patients who had undergone prior microfracture, abrasion, or drilling and compared them a control group of patients who had not. A summary of our findings is presented.

Increased Failure Rate of ACI after Previous Treatment with Marrow Stimulation Techniques

Background: Marrow stimulation techniques, such as drilling and microfracture, are first-line treatment options for symptomatic cartilage defects. Common knowledge holds that these treatments do not compromise subsequent cartilage repair procedures with ACI. We present our experience with ACI after prior marrow stimulation.[14]

Hypothesis: Cartilage defects pretreated with marrow stimulation techniques will demonstrate an increased failure rate.

Study Design: Case control, level 2 study.

Methods: This study reviewed prospectively collected data for the first 321 consecutive patients treated at our institution with ACI for full-thickness cartilage defects who have reached more than 2 years of follow-up. Patients were grouped based on whether or not they had undergone prior treatment with a marrow stimulation technique. Outcomes were classified as complete failure if more than 25% of a grafted defect area had to be removed in later procedures due to persistent symptoms. This includes treatment with revision ACI, allograft transplantation, and partial or total knee replacement.

Results: A total of 522 defects in 321 patients (325 joints) were treated with ACI. Average patient age was 35 years (range 13–60 years). There were 185 men and 136 women, with an average follow-up of 55 months (range 24–144 months). On average, there were 1.7 lesions (range 1–5) per patient with a transplant area of 4.9 cm^2 (range 0.5–21 cm^2) per lesion and 8.2 cm^2 (range 1–30.5 cm^2) per knee. One hundred eleven of these joints had previously undergone surgery that penetrated the subchondral bone: microfracture (n = 25), abrasion chondroplasty (n = 33), and drilling (n = 53). Two hundred fourteen joints had undergone no prior treatment that affected the subchondral bone and served as control. Within the marrow stimulation group, there were 29 (26%) failures compared with 17 (8%) failures in the control group ($P < .001$).

Conclusion: In our review of 321 patients, defects that had undergone prior treatment affecting the subchondral bone failed at a rate three times that of nontreated defects. The failure rates for drilling (28%), abrasion arthroplasty (27%), and microfracture (20%) were not significantly different ($P > .5$), possibly due to the lower number of microfracture patients in this cohort (25/110 marrow stimulation procedures). Our data demonstrate that marrow stimulation techniques have a strong negative effect on subsequent cartilage repair with ACI and therefore should be used judiciously in larger cartilage defects that could require treatment with ACI in the future.

The marrow stimulation group of patients were very similar to the control group in all ways, as noted in Table 7–6. The failure rates in the two treatment groups as well as the failure rates among different categories of patients being treated are noted in Table 7–7.

Interestingly, even within the group of 29 knees that had failed ACI after prior treatment with MST, 14 were implanted for isolated defects and 15 for multiple defects. Among these 15 knees, there were a total of 35 implanted defects, some of which had been marrow stimulated and some of which had not. Specifically, 17 had previously been marrow stimulated (13 knees with one defect each and 2 knees with two defects each), and 18 lesions had not been treated prior to ACI. Because all knees had at least one marrow-stimulated defect and one untreated defect, we used the untreated defect as an internal control. Sixteen of the 17 marrow-stimulated defects failed compared with 2 of the 18 previously untreated lesions.

We have noted that marrow stimulation techniques do "burn bridges." We have noted that prior marrow stimulation techniques do alter the osteochondral unit. The subchondral bone is either hypertrophic with an internal osteophyte, thickened and sclerotic, or the pick holes or drill holes develop into subchondral cysts with eventual failure of the grafts (Figure 7–35). Accordingly, these techniques should be used when they have the highest chance of success and will not compromise a future reconstruction if they fail.

Table 7-6 Patient Demographics for Control Group (No MST) and Previously Marrow-Stimulated Group (Prior MST)

	No MST	Prior MST	P value
No. of knees/no. of patients	214/211	111/110	
Average age (yr)	35.0 (9.2, 13–60)	35.4 (10.1, 14–55)	.7
Gender (male/female)	124/87	61/49	.6
Average follow-up time (mo)	54 (27, 24–132)	56 (30, 24–144)	.4
Average no. of defects per knee	1.7 (0.9, 1–5)	1.7 (0.8, 1–4)	.9
Average defect size (cm^2)	4.6 (2.7, 0.5–21)	5.2 (3.1, 0.7–16.8)	.2
Average transplant area per knee (cm^2)	7.9 (5.0, 1.0–28.3)	8.6 (5.9, 1.5–30.5)	.3
Workers' Compensation patients	28 (13%)	24 (22%)	.1
Patients lost to follow-up after 2 years by defect category			
Simple	3 (1%)	2 (2%)	>.5
Complex	16 (8%)	12 (11%)	
Salvage	6 (3%)	4 (4%)	

Data are given as (SD, range) or number (%).

Table 7-7 Failure Rates for Control (No MST) and Marrow-Stimulated (MST) Groups

	No MST	Prior MST	*P* value
Overall	214 (17, 8%)	111 (29, 26%)	<.001
Simple defects	18 (2, 11%)	9 (1, 11%)	N/A
Complex defects	97 (9, 9%)	56 (17, 30%)	<.01
Salvage defects	99 (6, 6%)	46 (11, 24%)	<.01
Subanalyses			
Osteochondritis dissecans lesions	23 (2, 9%)	20 (6, 30%)	N/A
Workers' Compensation patients	28 (4, 14%)	24 (9, 38%)	N/A
Previous microfracture		25 (5, 20%)	
Previous abrasion arthroplasty		33 (9, 27%)	>.5
Previous drilling		53 (15, 28%)	

All values are given as no. overall (no. of failures, % failure).
N/A, insufficient power to calculate.

Modes of Failure

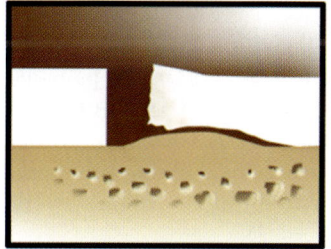 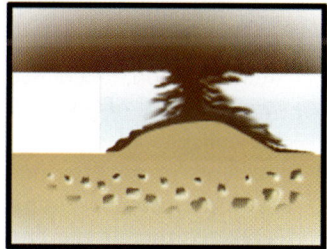 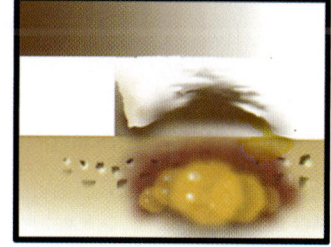

Figure 7-35 Modes of failure after marrow stimulation: delamination *(left)*, intralesional osteophyte *(center)*, subchondral cyst *(right)*.

Microfracture yields the best results in patients who have defects smaller than 2 to 3 cm², on the weight-bearing femoral condyle, in patients younger than 40 years, in relatively acute defects less than 1 year from injury. Chronic degenerative large lesions and locations on the patella, trochlea, and tibia do not do well. A simple debridement as a first-step treatment option may be adequate for these types of lesions prior to recommending ACI or fresh osteoarticular allograft for these locations.

Use of a Type I–III Collagen Membrane for ACI Compared to Periosteum

At present, the most frequently encountered postoperative adverse event associated with ACI is periosteal hypertrophy, followed by adhesions and arthrofibrosis. A randomized prospective British study comparing collagen-covered ACI (ACI-C) versus periosteal-covered ACI (ACI-P) noted a dramatic decrease in periosteal hypertrophy.[32] In this group of 68 patients with a mean age of 30 years old, 33 patients were randomized to ACI-P and 35 patients to ACI-C. Mean defect size was 4.5 cm². All patients were followed up at 24 months. Clinical and functional assessment showed 74% of patients had good or excellent results after ACI-C compared with 67% after ACI-P at 2 years. Arthroscopy at 1 year also demonstrated similar results for both techniques. However, 34.6% of the ACI-P grafts had periosteal graft hypertrophy that required shaving for hypertrophy compared with none of ACI-C grafts at 1 year.

With a hypertrophy rate greater than 40% in our series of multiple defects per knee, we sought to assess the use of an off-label, type I–III collagen membrane cover similar to that used in the British study.

After obtaining informed consent from the patient and IRB approval for data collection, we proceeded with the use of a type I–III collagen membrane for ACI in our patients and compared the results to the incidence of hypertrophy using periosteum in the prior 100 patients.

Our early results at 1 year were presented at the Eighth International Cartilage Repair Society Meeting, Miami, Florida, May 2009.[33] A prospective comparative study using a type I–III collagen membrane (ACI-C) to traditional periosteal-covered ACI (ACI-P) was performed. The last 100 ACI performed prior to June 2007 were compared with all ACI performed after June 2007 with a minimum one-year follow-up (54 knees). The endpoints were reoperation within the first year for symptomatic cover-related issues and the failure rate in the first year. A comparison of clinical outcomes will be assessed at 2-year follow-up and are not presented at this time.

The membrane used was produced by Geistlich Pharma AG (Wolhusen, Switzerland). It is of porcine origin (peritoneum), is semipermeable, has a type I/III collagen bilayer structure, and is bioabsorbable (Figure 7–30 and Tables 7–8 through 7–10).

There is no appreciable difference in the failure rate between techniques, confirming prior reports from Britain demonstrating a drastic lowering of the reoperation rate for cover-related problems (6% vs 52%), with no difference in the failure rate in the first year (1% vs 1.9%).

Table 7–8 Patient demographics undergoing ACI-P, ACI-C.

	ACI-P	ACI-C	P value
No.	100	54	
Age (yr)	34.5	37.6	.06
Defect number	1.9	2.1	.25
Defect size (cm^2)	4.6	4.8	.5
Defect total surface area (cm^2)	8.8	10.2	.16

Defect size characteristics and demographics of patients treated are not appreciably different.
ACI-C, autologous chondrocyte implantation collagen-covered; ACI-P, autologous chondrocyte implantation periosteal-covered.

Table 7–9 ACI membrane hypertrophy after ACI-P, ACI-C.

	ACI-P	ACI-C	P value
Intervention for hypertrophy	52%	5.6%	1.6E-09

Dramatic decrease in incidence of periosteal hypertrophy using autologous chondrocyte implantation collagen-covered (ACI-C) is seen.
ACI-P, autologous chondrocyte implantation periosteal-covered.

Table 7–10 Failure rate after ACI-P, ACI-C.

	ACI-P	ACI-C	P value
Failure rate in first year	1 (1%)	1 (1.9%)	.66

ACI-C, autologous chondrocyte implantation collagen-covered; ACI-P, autologous chondrocyte implantation periosteal-covered.

Further follow-up of this cohort of patients and review will determine whether the clinical outcomes differ at 2 years. A collaborative multicenter study is presently underway to determine 2-year outcome data differences if they exist.

We combined our results from a three-center study[16] in order to review the combined results with different practice patterns for a "threshold" to intervene for periosteal hypertrophy versus membrane-related problems and found a similar marked decrease in periosteal-related problems with no difference in failure rates. These demographics are summarized in Table 7–11.

Both groups were comparable with regard to age at time of implantation with ACI and average defect size (see Table 7–11). Patients treated with collagen membrane ACI had significantly more defects than those treated with periosteal ACI, resulting in a larger total area per knee implanted. The specific reoperation rate for cover-related issues, such as hypertrophy and periosteal delamination, decreased from 25.7% (77/300 patients) with the use of periosteum to 4.9% (5/103) with the use of collagen membrane ($P < .0001$). A total of 7 (2.3%) patients were considered treatment failure after ACI with periosteum compared with 4 (3.9%) patients in the collagen membrane group ($P = .2$).

ACI-C appears to be a reasonable substitute for periosteum. Our 2-year multicenter outcomes data will verify whether there is any decreased outcome as a result of this substitution. However, European studies do not demonstrate any differences, and we do not anticipate any either.

CLINICAL COST EFFECTIVENESS OF ACI

ACI has proven clinically effective in restoring hyaline-like cartilage to isolated chondral defects of the knee; however, no studies have quantified the quality of life or economic outcomes of this procedure. This study prospectively examined efficacy and quality of life in 44 patients undergoing ACI for full-thickness cartilage lesions and calculated the average cost per additional quality adjusted life year.[17] The 12-month results of ACI treatment demonstrated improvement in patient function as measured by both the KSS (23% mean improvement [114.02–140.67], $P < .001$) and the WOMAC osteoarthritis score (33% mean improvement [35.30–23.82], $P < .05$). Quality of life as measured by the SF-36 Physical Component Summary was dramatically enhanced from 33.32 prior to

Table 7–11 Demographic Data of Study Groups

	ACI-P (n = 300)			ACI-C (n = 103)			P value
	Mean	Min	Max	Mean	Min	Max	
Age at ACI (yr)	31.9	13.5	56.0	32.4	14.2	54.0	.762
Gender (male/female)	162/138			51/50			
No. of defects	1.5	1.0	5.0	1.8	1.0	5.0	.001
Defect size (cm^2)	4.6	0.7	36.0	4.7	0.5	19.2	.645
Total defect area (cm^2)	6.7	1.4	36.0	8.5	0.5	29.9	.004

ACI-C, autologous chondrocyte implantation collagen-covered; ACI-P, autologous chondrocyte implantation periosteal-covered.

biopsy to 41.48 12 months postimplant ($P < .05$). Improvement on all three scales was maintained from 12 to 24 months. Estimated cost per additional quality-adjusted life-year (QALY) was $6,791. This cost-effectiveness ratio was minimally sensitive to reasonable changes in effectiveness, patient age, and procedural cost and remained very cost effective even when assumptions were less favorable than in the base case. Cost effectiveness of ACI compares favorably with other interventions for chronic diseases, such as intensive therapy for diabetes ($16,000/QALY) and interferon-α for hepatitis C ($4,000/QALY), and is more cost effective than many commonly reimbursed interventions, such as therapy for mild hypertension ($30,200/QALY) and lumbar discectomy for treatment of herniated intervertebral disc ($33,900/QALY). ACI improves patient quality of life and is an appropriate, cost-effective treatment for cartilage lesions of the knee.

At the time this study was performed, only 1-year follow-up data of clinical outcome measures (including SF-36 standardized outcome, which was used to calculate the utility value for QALY) were available. To date, ACI grafting has been very durable,[19] with clinical outcomes improving to a maximal medical endpoint in the tibiofemoral joint after 2 years and in the patellofemoral joint at 3 years. As the clinical outcomes continue to improve up to 3 years, the utility calculated would also be more favorable and the procedure more cost effective. Despite the increased costs for the procedure and the cell culture process, after sensitivity analysis the conclusion does not change: ACI is very cost effective because it dramatically improves the quality of life for patients and is a durable procedure. It is very cost effective compared to other standard surgical and medical treatments that are considered the "standard of care" for patients (Figure 7–31).

SUMMARY

Articular cartilage once injured does not heal, a finding that has been known for more 200 years.[34] ACI provides a durable hyaline repair tissue when patients are carefully chosen, background factors responsible for the chondral injury are addressed surgically at the time of ACI, and a careful surgical technique and rehabilitation are performed.

ACI clearly has outstanding clinical results in juvenile athletes and high-level soccer players when the injury is treated by ACI within the first year of injury. Delays in treatment or multiple treatments result in lesser clinical outcomes for reasons that are not yet clear.

ACI in the patellofemoral joint has been successful for a difficult treatment management problem when careful attention is given to patellar tracking. ACI has been successful for pan-patellar injuries (Fulkerson type IV patella) and medial patellar facet injuries (Fulkerson type III patella). It is effective in managing defects of the trochlea, which was a problem area until the advent of ACI. ACI has a complementary role in managing patellofemoral chondral defects in maltracking knees for which realignment osteotomy alone is not successful.

Patients older than 45 years continue to do favorably. We have found that for the patient who is physiologically young and active with a localized chondral defect, the success rate after treatment remains 95%. However, for the patient who was previously microfractured and is on Workers' Compensation, the success rate drops to 60%. This finding more likely is secondary to microfracture performed in the Workers' Compensation group, but separating the two factors is difficult.

Young arthritics pose a particular management dilemma because these patients frequently are too young to be considered for prosthetic arthroplasty, and traditional sports medicine techniques are not effective in alleviating pain by repairing articular cartilage. This group of patients is generally older (39 years) and requires large areas of surface repair (average 11 cm^2). The clinical outcomes in this group have been very positive, with a patient satisfaction rate of 87% overall. Seven percent of this group went on to prosthetic replacement over the course of this study.

Marrow stimulation techniques appear to alter the osteochondral unit. If a surface treatment such as ACI is subsequently performed, the success rate drops from 92% for a native chondral defect to 74% for a chondral defect previously treated by a marrow stimulation technique that has failed. When all other factors are controlled, it appears that marrow stimulation techniques, irrespective of the type (abrasion, drilling, or microfracture), jeopardize the success with ACI. Therefore, it is recommended that microfracture be used for lesions that are smaller than 2 to 3 cm^2 and are confined to the femoral condyles in patients younger than 40 years with acute lesions that are known to do the best with this technique. Failed marrow stimulation technique remains a treatment dilemma. Alterations in the management of the subchondral bone, such as thinning of the bone prior to ACI or replacing the osteochondral unit with a sandwich technique ACI or osteoarticular allograft, may be more suitable. Further research is required.

A bioabsorbable type I–III collagen membrane that is replacing periosteum in ACI appears not to diminish the clinical outcomes but improves upon the problem of periosteal hypertrophy. This was demonstrated in a randomized controlled trial comparing the two membrane covers.[32] We confirmed in a prospective matched comparison that our hypertrophy rate is dramatically diminished and nearly abolished.

At this time, ACI remains an open procedure requiring careful surgical preparation and microsuturing of the membranes. Background factors must be addressed and managed. Careful rehabilitation will then result in a good clinical outcome. Next-generation ACI techniques will involve cell-seeded membranes that are arthroscopically delivered. They will improve upon the ease of recovery for patients, the universal application of the techniques by surgeons, and hopefully the clinical outcomes. These new techniques represent exciting advancements and are addressed in Chapter 14.

REFERENCES

1. Brittberg M, Lindahl A, Nilsson A, et al. Treatment of deep cartilage defects in the knee with autologous chondrocyte transplantation. *N Engl J Med.* 1994;331:889–895.
2. Minas T, Marchie A, et al. *SF-36 as a predictor of clinical outcome after autologous chondrocyte implantation in the knee.* Toronto Ontario Canada: International Cartilage Repair Society; (poster) 2001.
3. Mithofer K, Minas T, Yeon H, et al. Functional outcome of knee articular cartilage repair in adolescent athletes. *Am J Sports Med.* 2005;33:1147–1153.
4. Peterson L, Minas T, Brittberg M, et al. Treatment of osteochondritis dissecans of the knee with autologous chondrocyte transplantation: results at two to ten years. *J Bone Joint Surg Am.* 2003;85-A (suppl 2):17–24.
5. Curl WW, Krome J, Gordon ES, et al. Cartilage injuries: a review of 31,516 knee arthroscopies. *Arthroscopy.* 1997;13:456–460.
6. Minas T, Nehrer S. Current concepts in the treatment of articular cartilage defects. *Orthopedics.* 1997;20:525–538.
7. Minas T. Autologous chondrocyte implantation for focal chondral defects of the knee. *Clin Orthop Relat Res.* 2001;(suppl 391):S349–S361.
8. Peterson L, Karrlson J, Brittberg M, et al. Patellar instability with recurrent dislocation due to patellofemoral dysplasia results after surgical treatment. *Bull Hosp Joint Dis Orthop Inst.* 1988;48:130–139.
9. O'Driscoll SW, Salter RB. The induction of neochondrogenesis in free intra-articular periosteal autografts under the influence of continuous passive motion. An experimental investigation in the rabbit. *J Bone Joint Surg Am.* 1984;66:1248–1257.
10. Rodrigo J, Steadman R, Fulstone H. Improvement of full-thickness chondral defect healing in the human knee after debridement and microfracture using continuous passive motion. *Am J Knee Surg.* 1994;7:109–116.
11. Mithofer K, Peterson L, Mandelbaum BR, et al. Articular cartilage repair in soccer players with autologous chondrocyte transplantation: functional outcome and return to competition. *Am J Sports Med.* 2005;33:1639–1646.
12. Minas T, Bryant T. The role of autologous chondrocyte implantation in the patellofemoral joint. *Clin Orthop Relat Res.* 2005;436:30–39.
13. Rosenberger RE, Gomoll AH, Bryant T, et al. Repair of large chondral defects of the knee with autologous chondrocyte implantation in patients 45 years or older. *Am J Sports Med.* 2008;36:2336–2344.
14. Minas T, Gomoll AH, Rosenberger R, et al. Increased failure rate of autologous chondrocyte implantation after previous treatment with marrow stimulation techniques. *Am J Sports Med.* 2009;37:902–908.
15. Minas T, Gomoll AH, Solhpour S, et al. Autologous chondrocyte implantation for joint preservation in patients with early osteoarthritis. *Clin Orthop Relat Res.* 2010;468:147–157.
16. Gomoll AH, Probst C, Farr J, et al. Use of a type I/III bilayer collagen membrane decreases reoperation rates for symptomatic hypertrophy after autologous chondrocyte implantation. *Am J Sports Med.* 2009;37(suppl 1):20S–23S.
17. Minas T. Chondrocyte implantation in the repair of chondral lesions of the knee: economics and quality of life. *Am J Orthop.* 1998;27:739–744.
18. Lindahl A, Brittberg M, Peterson L. Health economics benefits following autologous chondrocyte transplantation for patients with focal chondral lesions of the knee. *Knee Surg Sports Traumatol Arthrosc.* 2001;9:358–363.
19. Peterson L, Brittberg M, Kiviranta I, et al. Autologous chondrocyte transplantation. Biomechanics and long-term durability. *Am J Sports Med.* 2002;30:2–12.
20. Ware Jr JE, Sherbourne CD. The MOS 36-item short-form health survey (SF-36). I. Conceptual framework and item selection. *Med Care.* 1992;30:473–483.
21. Insall JN, Dorr LD, Scott RD, et al. Rationale of the knee society clinical rating system. *Clin Orthop Relat Res.* 1989;248:13–14.
22. Bellamy N, Buchanan WW, Goldsmith CH, et al. Validation study of WOMAC: a health status instrument for measuring clinically important patient relevant outcomes to antirheumatic drug therapy in patients with osteoarthritis of the hip or knee. *J Rheumatol.* 1988;15:1833–1840.
23. Noyes FR, Barber SD, Mooar LA. A rationale for assessing sports activity levels and limitations in knee disorders. *Clin Orthop Relat Res.* 1989;246:238–249.
24. Peterson L, Minas T, Brittberg M, et al. Two- to 9-year outcome after autologous chondrocyte transplantation of the knee. *Clin Orthop Relat Res.* 2000;374:212–234.
25. Pidoriano AJ, Weinstein RN, Buuck DA, et al. Correlation of patellar articular lesions with results from anteromedial tibial tubercle transfer. *Am J Sports Med.* 1997;25:533–537.
26. Rosenberger RE, Gomoll AH, Bryant T, et al. Repair of large chondral defects of the knee with autologous chondrocyte implantation in patients 45 years or older. *Am J Sports Med.* 2008;36:2336–2344.
27. Minas T. Autologous chondrocyte implantation in the arthritic knee. *Orthopedics.* 2003;26:945–947.
28. Ahlback S. Osteoarthrosis of the knee: a radiographic investigation. *Acta Radiol.* 1968;(suppl 277):7–72.
29. Angst F, Aeschlimann A, Michel BA, et al. Minimal clinically important rehabilitation effects in patients with osteoarthritis of the lower extremities. *J Rheumatol.* 2002;19:131–138.
30. Jaeschke J, Singer J, Guyatt G. Measurement of health status. Ascertaining the minimal clinically important difference. *Control Clin Trials.* 1989;10:407–415.

31. Goldsmith CH, Boers M, Bombardier C, et al. Criteria for clinically important changes in outcomes: development, scoring and evaluation of rheumatoid arthritis patient and trial profiles. OMERACT committee. *J Rheumatol*. 1993;20:561–565.
32. Gooding CR, Bartlett W, Bentley G, et al. A prospective, randomized study comparing two techniques of autologous chondrocyte implantation for osteochondral defects in the knee: Periosteum covered versus type I/III collagen covered. *Knee*. 2006;13: 203–210.
33. Gomoll A, Probst C, Bryant T, et al. *Decreased surgical re-intervention rate for hypertrophy after ACI with use of the BioGide collagen membrane*. Paper #15.3.3. Presented at the 8th World Congress of the International Cartilage Repair Society. May 23–26, Miami, Florida: 2009.
34. Hunter W. On the structure and diseases of articulating cartilage. *Phil Trans R Soc Lond B Biol Sci*. 1743;9:267.

PART 3

SURGICAL MANAGEMENT OF BACKGROUND FACTORS

Chapter 8

Tibial Osteotomy

Tom Minas, MD, MS

ARTHRITIS AND MALALIGNMENT

WHY OSTEOTOMY?

TECHNIQUE-RELATED ISSUES AGAINST HIGH TIBIAL OSTEOTOMY

PATIENT-RELATED ISSUES

PROCEDURAL PLANNING

    Preoperative Planning for Angular Correction of Tibial Osteotomy

    Cartilage Repair, Osteoarthritis, Instability

TECHNIQUE SELECTION FOR HIGH TIBIAL OSTEOTOMY

SURGICAL SETUP AND HOSPITAL COURSE

ANATOMIC CONSIDERATIONS

CLOSING WEDGE OSTEOTOMY

OPENING WEDGE OSTEOTOMY

OPENING WEDGE HIGH TIBIAL VALGUS OSTEOTOMY ACCOMPANIED BY

ANTEROMEDIALIZATION TIBIAL TUBERCLE OSTEOTOMY

REVERSE DOME TIBIAL VALGUS OSTEOTOMY

    Postoperative Care

OSTEOTOMY FOR INSTABILITY: THE SAGITTAL CORRECTION

ACL LAXITY WITH VARUS

CONCLUSION

ARTHRITIS AND MALALIGNMENT

The premise of knee osteotomy surgery is to correct malalignment at the site of the deformity and relieve pressure on the overloaded or arthritic compartment. In general, medial compartment osteoarthritis of the knee coexists with a varus knee secondary to deformity in the metaphysis of the tibia. The joint line is generally horizontal to the floor. Femoral varus is unusual but may occur secondary to metabolic bone disease (e.g., rickets) or trauma; it usually is excluded by long alignment x-ray films. Therefore, tibial osteotomy is usually performed for varus leg alignment with medial compartment overload or osteoarthritis.

Similarity, valgus malalignment of the knee with lateral compartment osteoarthritis usually coexists with deformity in the distal femur, which consists of dysplasia or hypoplasia of the lateral column of the distal femur. Usually the joint line is directed superiorly and laterally. Osteotomy through the distal femur corrects the deformity at its location and produces a horizontal joint line. If a varus proximal tibial osteotomy were to occur in this situation, further superior lateral joint line obliquity usually results, with risk of subluxation of the tibia on the femur. Although Coventry reported on the use of proximal tibial varus osteotomy for valgus osteoarthritis of the knee, he recommended that this procedure be performed for deformity less than 10 degrees and noted the risk of subluxation.

WHY OSTEOTOMY?

In 1994, the Centers for Disease Control and Prevention[1] reported that by the year 2020, osteoarthritis will have the largest increase in numbers of new patients of any disease in the United States. Approximately 60 million persons aged 45 to 64 years (referred to as *baby boomers*) constituting 20% of the U.S. population are at risk. Total knee arthroplasty has become one of the most commonly performed procedures with reproducibly good results in the United States. This is largely due to generically designed anatomic implants with universal knee instrumentation. Prior to the development of total knee replacement, high tibial osteotomy was commonly performed. However, in 2008, 220,000 total knee replacements were performed in patients younger than 55 years, and a total of 450,000 total knee replacements were performed overall. As good as total knee replacement is, patient satisfaction remains only approximately

80%. With the inherent problems of prosthetic arthroplasty failure due to polyethylene osteolysis, mechanical loosening, joint infection, and problematic revision surgery secondary to ligamentous laxity or bone deficiency, reevaluation of joint preservation techniques led to the resurgence of osteotomy and cartilage repair surgeries as well as more bone-sparing partial prosthetic arthroplasties.

Tibial osteotomy had been a procedure routinely performed in patients older than 50 years with tibial varus malalignment and medial unicompartmental disease. In the series by Coventry et al,[2] the average age of patients undergoing tibial osteotomy was 63 years. However, today it would be difficult for surgeons to perform tibial osteotomy in patients of a similar age given the reproducible long-term results with total knee arthroplasty in that age category.

However, unicompartmental arthrosis is becoming prevalent among patients in their 20s, 30s, and 40s. As baby boomers age and activity levels remain high because of their interest in sports, injuries to the anterior cruciate ligament (ACL), meniscus, and articular cartilage predispose to unicompartmental disease in patients much younger than those treated in the past. The average age of patients undergoing high tibial osteotomy for bone-on-bone medial compartment disease in my practice was 44 years.[3] Unicompartmental and total knee arthroplasty cannot offer these patients long-term, high-level functional activity.

Sharma et al[4] demonstrated that the risk of progression of unicompartmental osteoarthritis with malalignment is four times more common in a varus than a neutrally aligned knee and five times more common in a valgus than a neutrally aligned knee over a 18-month time course, with evidence of progression on standing radiographs. Osteoarthritis in the malaligned limb with unicompartmental disease remains a problem in the young athlete and adult. Tibial osteotomy remains the procedure of choice in the limb with unicompartmental osteoarthritis with malalignment.

A long-term Swedish study evaluating the natural course of arthrosis of the knee over 20 years noted that 61% of patients with Ahlback stage 1 osteoarthrosis (50% joint space narrowing) would have progression of disease; the remaining 39% would remain stable without further reduction in joint space.[5] Fifty-seven percent of patients with Ahlback stage 0 arthrosis, defined as osteophytes or subchondral bone sclerosis with normal joint space, would not progress over time. Patients with more advanced cases, Ahlback stages 2, 3, 4, and 5, would progress over time.

If tibial osteotomy is to be used in treatment algorithms designed to help these young patients, then the technique-related problems and patient-related issues that led to disfavor with tibial osteotomy in the past must be avoided.

TECHNIQUE-RELATED ISSUES AGAINST HIGH TIBIAL OSTEOTOMY

Arthroplasty surgeons have conceptual difficulty with osteotomies because of the potential for making the arthroplasty more challenging and for compromising the results of primary arthroplasty. Issues that have led to problems include placement of skin incisions, patella baja (infera)–infrapatellar tendon contracture, contracture of the lateral ligament and posterolateral corner with release of the proximal tibial fibular joint, obliquity of the joint line, and distortion of the upper anatomy of the tibia (Figure 8–1). Excessive valgus correction also has resulted in difficulty with arthroplasty balancing of the flexion–extension gap and obtaining adequate alignment and increases the risk of perineal nerve palsy. The total joint literature is abundant with reports of inferior outcomes following tibial osteotomy to primary total joint replacement. However, other investigators have reported that results are equivalent but that experienced surgeons using modified surgical techniques are needed in order to obtain results equal to those of total knee replacement as a primary procedure. If osteotomy surgery is to be pursued for cartilage repair or for treatment of instability or unicompartmental arthritis in young patients, then the eventuality of total knee replacement must not be compromised or made more difficult.

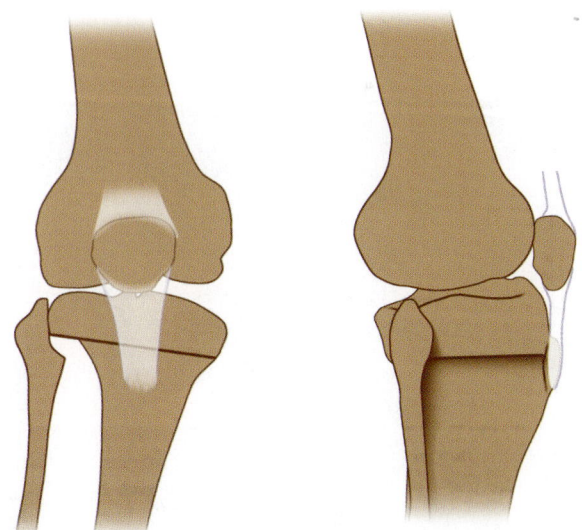

Figure 8–1 Common sequela of the classic closing wedge Coventry osteotomy with cast immobilization postoperatively. Metaphyseal–diaphyseal mismatch, proximalization of the fibula with lateral collateral laxity, patella infera, and marked overcorrection into valgus are present. These aspects of the osteotomy are unfavorable to patients because of cosmetic issues and functional issues and are deterrents to surgeons because of difficulties with performing total knee replacement in the future.

PATIENT-RELATED ISSUES

Closing wedge osteotomy with staple fixation and postoperative casting in full extension often leads to patient dissatisfaction that arises predominantly from overcorrection in valgus with cosmetic disfigurement (Figure 8–2). Release of the proximal tibiofibular joint leads to lateral laxity, which results in the sensation of a sloppy knee secondary to posterolateral ligament instability. Cast immobilization leads to difficult ambulation and return to work as well as the technique-related problems previously discussed: patella baja (infera) and lateral contracture with decreased motion. These problems can be avoided or eliminated by appropriate procedural osteotomy technique selection, patient selection, and careful preoperative and postoperative planning and care. Renewed interest in joint preservation and cartilage repair have led to innovative new osteotomy techniques that are more precise, have improved technical ease, and provide reproducible results.

PROCEDURAL PLANNING

In a multivariate analysis of predictors of good outcome, Coventry et al[2] found that long-term outcome was determined by mechanical correction to 8 degrees or more of tibiofemoral valgus and patient weight less than 1.32 of ideal body weight.[2] Rinonapoli et al[6] noted that longevity was proportional to the stage of disease at the time of osteotomy. Updated reports with experimental cadaveric loading have demonstrated similar findings.[7] The authors found that when tibiofemoral alignment was shifted from varus to valgus alignment, decreases in medial contact pressure and medial contact area occurred. For defect chondral sizes 10 to 20 mm, all contact pressures within the medial compartment were shifted to the lateral compartment at between 6 and 10 degrees of tibiofemoral valgus. Contact pressures were found to concentrate around the defect rims for all defect sizes. From 6 to 10 degrees of tibiofemoral valgus was recommended as the optimal axial alignment favoring cartilage repair.

My experience has been similar. If the patient is relatively slim (i.e., ideal body weight less than 1.32 times normal), is a nonsmoker, is highly motivated, and has unicompartmental medial disease with varus deformity, then he or she is a good candidate for osteotomy surgery. An arc of range of motion of 90 degrees or more is desired. Patellofemoral symptoms are acceptable if they can be resolved with concomitant tibial tubercle osteotomy. Attention to clinical varus thrust and baseline leg length discrepancy is important.

Preoperative x-rays films (Figure 8–3) include long axial alignment x-ray films on 54-inch cassettes to include the hip, knee, and talus as a standing film in extension. Rosenberg 45-degree bent posteroanterior, standing AP, lateral, and skyline films and radiograph measurements of leg length are important.

The mechanical axis is measured from the center of the femoral head to the center of the talus. If this axis falls through the medial joint compartment with evidence of peripheral osteophyte formation, flattening of the articulation, subchondral bone sclerosis, and/or joint space narrowing, then the patient is a candidate for osteotomy surgery if he or she does not have subluxation of the tibiofemoral joint or lateral symptoms. Lateral symptoms must be assessed to disprove lateral compartment degenerative changes or meniscal tear. If in doubt, high-resolution magnetic resonance imaging (MRI) scan is the most sensitive method for assessing the lateral and patellofemoral compartments.

Preoperative Planning for Angular Correction of Tibial Osteotomy

Consider the normal tibiofemoral alignment of the knee. A neutral mechanical access requires that a line pass from the center of the femoral head through the center of the knee into the center of the ankle (Figure 8–4). This assumes that the neck shaft angle at the hip joint is within normal limits, 130 to 135 degrees, and that the tibiofemoral axis at the knee is 5 to 7 degrees of valgus.

My desired angular correction for medial osteoarthritis (Figure 8–5) is to place the mechanical axis through the center of the lateral intercondylar spine or just to the downslope of this area. This is 2 degrees overcorrected

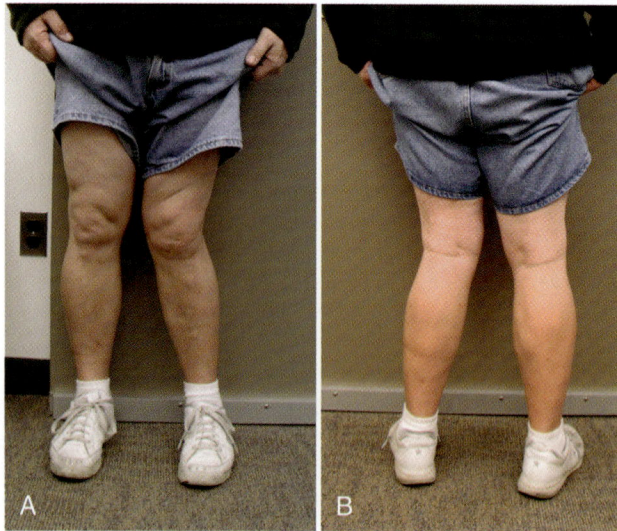

Figure 8-2 Frontal and rear views of patient standing after tibial osteotomy. This patient had left knee medially based pain with a neutrally aligned lower extremity. He underwent a closing wedge valgus tibial osteotomy and was very dissatisfied with the procedure due to his altered gait pattern as a result of overcorrection into too much valgus. His medially based pain did not resolve.

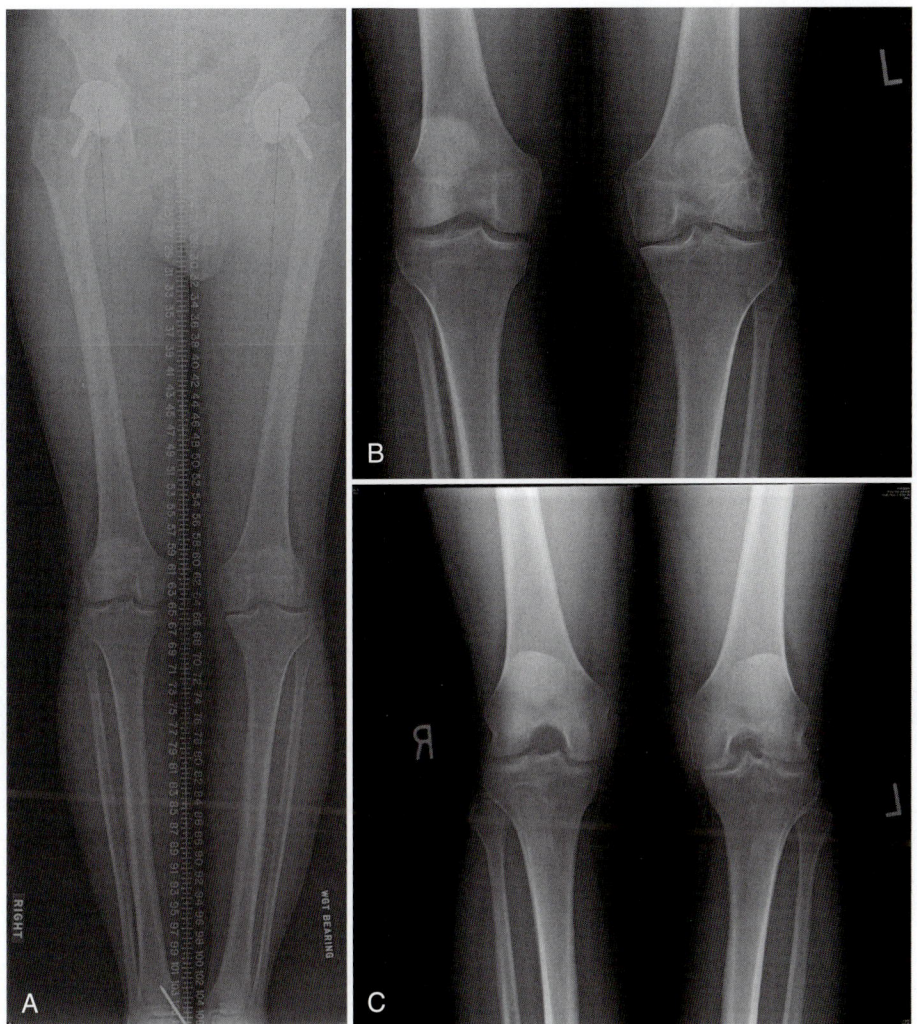

Figure 8-3 Standard series of x-ray films used to evaluate a patient for tibial valgus osteotomy. This 54-year-old police officer, who had undergone hip resurfacing procedures, wishes to remain physically very active and avoid total knee replacement. *A,* Long axial alignment x-ray films demonstrate that the left knee is in mechanical varus with the mechanical axis falling into the medial compartment with medial compartment joint space narrowing. *B,* Standing anteroposterior (AP) view. Evidence of previous anterior cruciate ligament reconstruction is noted with tibial and femoral tunnels present. *C,* Standing posteroanterior Rosenberg views demonstrate loss of posterior cartilage space on the medial joint compartment typical for a chronic anterior cruciate ligament (ACL)-deficient knee as normal where pattern for the medial compartment is anterior and medial noted on the standing AP x-ray film.

Continued

from a neutral mechanical axis. It is different than the classic teaching, which recommends that the mechanical axis pass through the Kurosaka point at 62% across the width of the tibia. I believe this is overcorrected to a level that is cosmetically unacceptable to patients and alters the kinematics of the patient's athletic endeavors so that they are difficult to perform. If the osteotomy is performed for a cartilage repair procedure with an intact joint space, the mechanical axis should pass through the center of the knee joint and should not overcorrected. In addition to the mechanical axis, consider the tibiofemoral axis. From previous basic science research, a 6- to 10-degree tibiofemoral valgus angle is sufficient to unload a medial compartment.[7] If there is varus in the proximal femur, the knee alignment can be markedly overcorrected by looking only at the mechanical varus of the overall leg alignment.

Assuming that the proximal femur has a normal neck shaft angle, my preferred technique for calculating the angular correction is as follows (Figure 8–6). A simple angular correction as measured on the long axial standing films is performed by passing a line from the center of the femoral head to the desired axis at the knee joint (e.g., lateral intercondylar spine). A second line from the center of the talus then intersects this same point. The acute angle between the two is the angular correction desired. Ligamentous instability of the medial complex and ACL should be assessed so

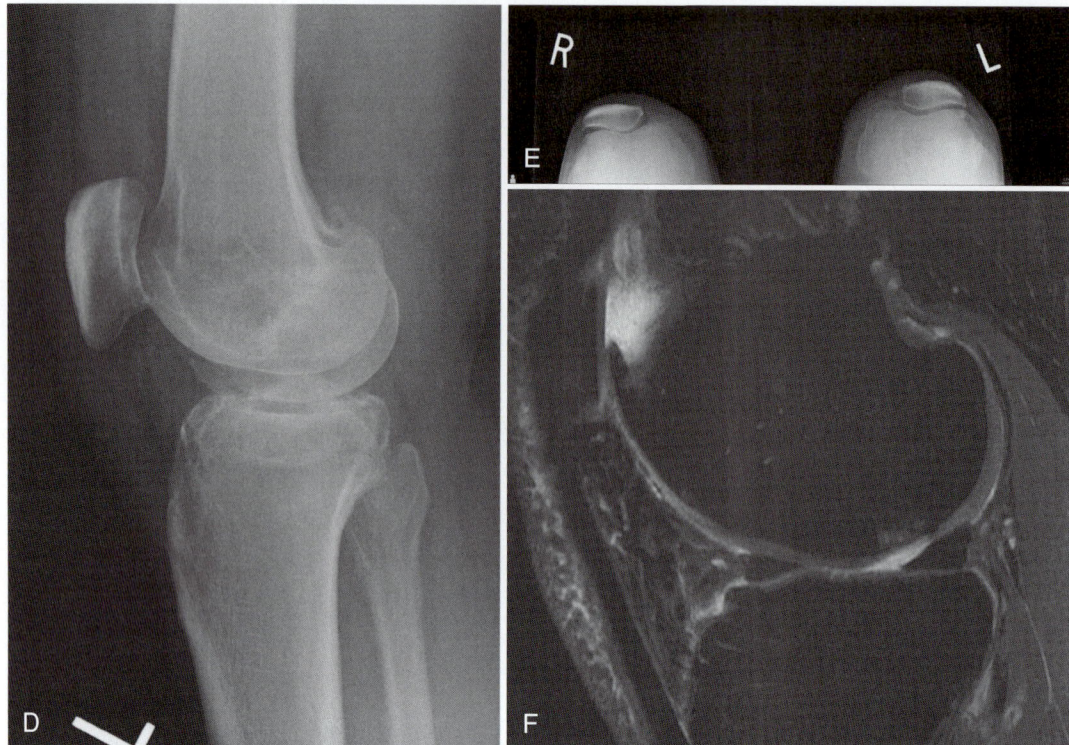

Figure 8–3—cont'd *D,* Lateral x-ray film further demonstrates central posterior erosion of the tibiofemoral joint on the medial compartment and the formation of a "cupula" (cupping of the joint). Loss of the intercondylar notch is also noted with chronic ACL-deficient knees. *E,* High-resolution magnetic resonance imaging (MRI) scan performed with a 1.5-T magnet demonstrates full-thickness articular cartilage loss in the center of the lateral femoral condyles with underlying bone marrow edema. The cartilage defect measures approximately 2 cm long by 1 cm wide. This defect is associated with laterally based discomfort in the patient. *F,* As tibial valgus-producing osteotomy loads the lateral tibiofemoral compartment, the MRI scan here is useful because it demonstrates that the osteotomy is contraindicated in this patient.

that laxity, if present, can be accounted for at the time of osteotomy to ensure that marked overcorrection does not ensue.

Cartilage Repair, Osteoarthritis, Instability

Interest in the use of tibial osteotomy has been renewed. Patients are maintaining higher levels of fitness and aerobic activity as they age and generally wish to preserve their joints as long as possible. Newer techniques of both opening and closing wedge tibial osteotomy give predictable angular corrections with reliability. This increased technical accuracy lessens the risk of complications, make the pursuit of joint preservation more appealing for both surgeon and patient. Three broad categories of indications for osteotomy surgery presently exist. It is generally agreed that cartilage repair in the presence of malalignment usually results in failure because the source of cartilage breakdown in the first place is generally malalignment in addition to other traumatic factors such as meniscal deficiency, ACL injury, or articular cartilage injury. Therefore, osteotomy has become an adjuvant procedure that has been deemed necessary when the articular cartilage injury undergoing repair is greater than 2 degrees of malalignment if the lesion is greater than 2 cm^2 with a cell-based treatment such as microfracture or autologous chondrocyte implantation. The goal of realignment osteotomy with cartilage repair without evidence of joint space narrowing is restoration of normal mechanical alignment and mechanics to the knee joint prior to bringing the mechanical axis to the midline or restoring at least 6 degrees of tibiofemoral valgus.[7] When bone-on-bone changes are present on x-ray film and joint preservation with cartilage repair is not indicated, osteotomy remains effective as a pain-relieving procedure that still allows improved levels of activity. However, overcorrection is recommended in this situation, with 2 degrees of overcorrection to the lateral tibial spine being my preferred amount. Anteroposterior instability may be improved upon by altering the tibial slope when performing osteotomy surgery for recurvatum or hyperextension deformity secondary to neuromuscular disorder or anatomic joint line deformity by performing flexion osteotomies. ACL-deficient knees or knees with fixed flexion deformities may be improved upon by extension osteotomies either in isolation or in combination with tibial valgus osteotomies.

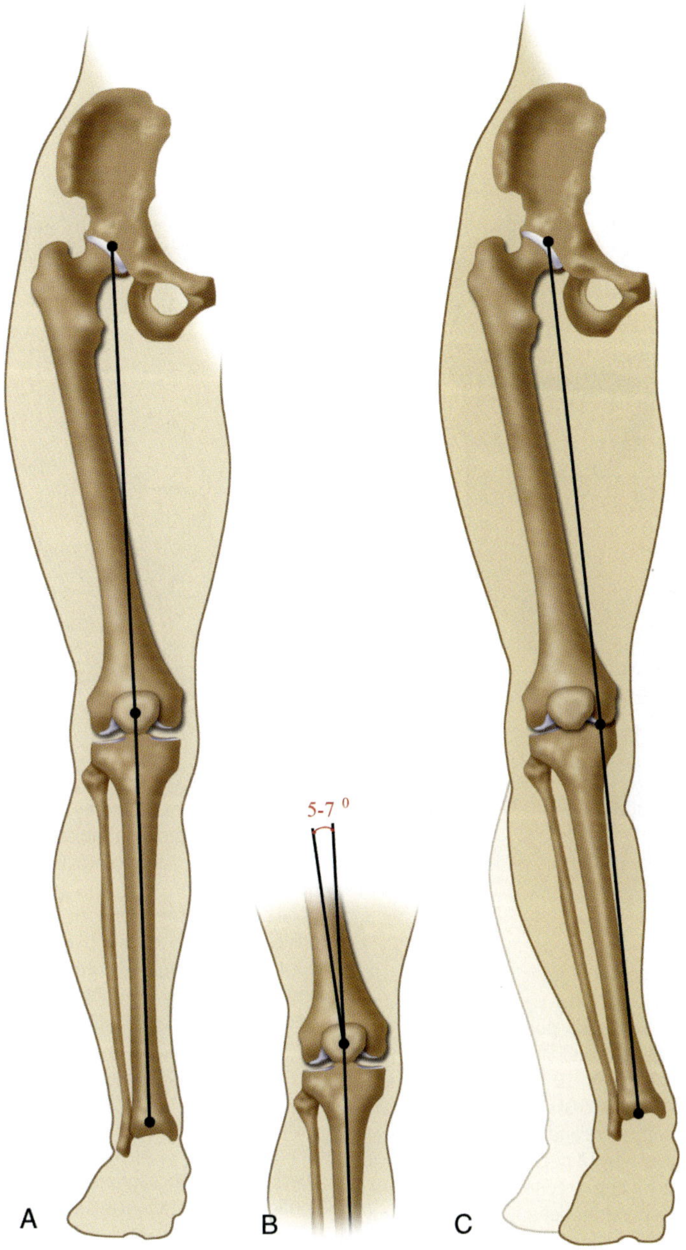

Figure 8-4 *A*, Normal mechanical axis. A line drawn through the center of the femoral head to the center of the talus should fall to the center of the knee. This assumes a normal hip neck shaft angle of 130 degrees and a tibiofemoral valgus anatomic axis angle of 5 to 7 degrees *(B)*. *C*, Varus mechanical axis.

TECHNIQUE SELECTION FOR HIGH TIBIAL OSTEOTOMY

Factors to consider when performing proximal tibial valgus osteotomy include leg length discrepancy, medial joint laxity, ACL laxity, presence or absence of an osteochondral defect on the medial femoral condyle, joint line obliquity, a patient who is a prior smoker or presently is smoking, opiate requirements at baseline, and a cooperative and compliant patient. Recent basic science work evaluating the effect of open versus closing wedge osteotomy on changes in load distribution across the knee have demonstrated that with less than 5-degree osteotomy correction, the closing wedge provided superior results in load transfer from medial to lateral compartments than that seen with an opening osteotomy. However, at 10-degree osteotomy correction, no significant difference in load transfer in the knee compartments was seen between opening versus closing wedge osteotomy.[8]

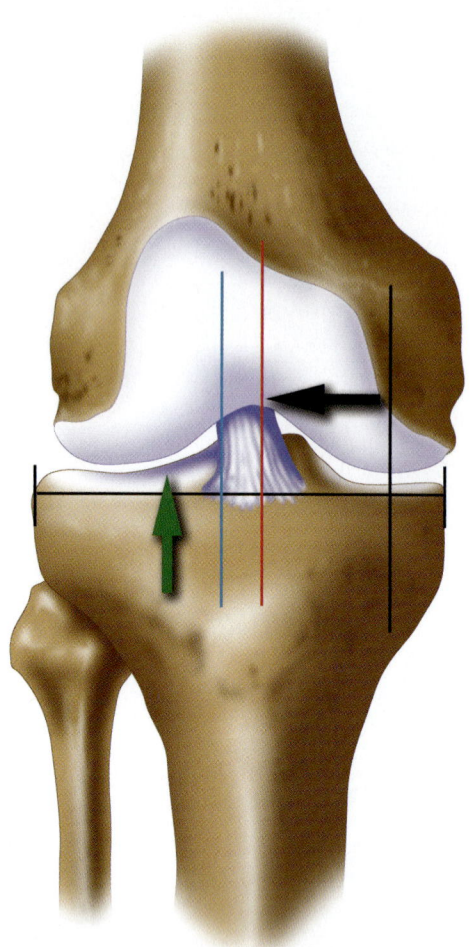

Figure 8–5 Mechanical axis correction. Classic mechanical axis correction for tibial valgus-producing osteotomy is recommended by several authors to pass through the Kurosaka point at 62% across the width of the tibia *(broad green arrow)*.[12] This results in a tibiofemoral valgus angle of approximately 10 to 12 degrees. My preference is to correct the mechanical access to the midline *(red line)* when correcting the varus with cartilage repair for a focal medial defect and to only overcorrect by 2 degrees to the lateral tibial spine if the patient has a very large medial femoral condyle chondral defect, "kissing" medial chondral defect, or established osteoarthritis with greater than 50% loss of the joint space on weight-bearing-x-ray films.

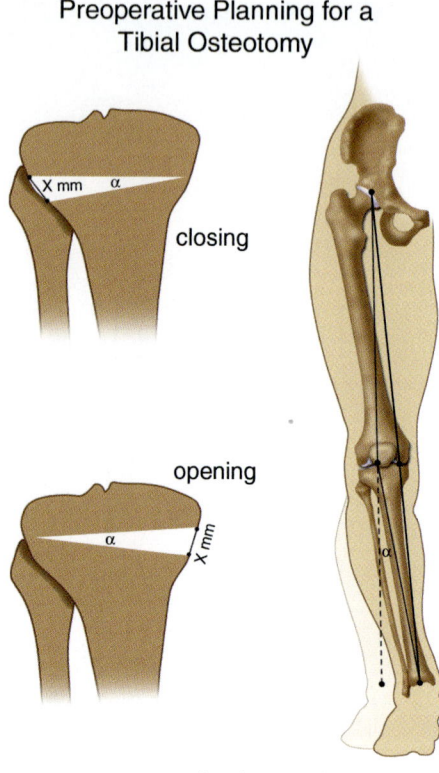

α = angle of correction

Figure 8–6 Osteotomy is a straightforward procedure when the varus is in the proximal tibial metaphysis, which is the most common situation. A line is drawn from the center of the femoral head to the desired point of correction (see Figure 8–5), in this case, the lateral tibial spine, to the proposed position of the foot, at the center of the ankle. The angle between the center of the talus and the proposed position is the angle of correction, α. Using calibrated digital x-ray films and commercially available web-based software (Centricity, General Electric, Waukesha, WI), the actual opening in the millimeters, *x*, can be calculated for a opening wedge osteotomy. Similarly, the exact number of millimeters for angle α for a closing wedge osteotomy can be calculated or the angle taken directly off the osteotomy closing wedge calibrated angular system, which is typical. Intraoperative check with clinical appearance of the limb after osteotomy as well as intraoperative checks with long alignment wires or rods under fluoroscopic control confirm accurate angular corrections.

With regard to the patient-related factors, I presently exclude patients who are smoking or are taking baseline opiates from osteotomy surgery because of the difficulty in postoperative pain management for both surgeon and patient due to the possibility of delayed or nonunion of the tibia with persistent pain. Patient who have unrealistic expectations about recovery after surgery, return to work, or inability to use crutches also should not be considered for osteotomy surgery.

The technique of open wedge tibial valgus osteotomy has become my preferred technique. It addresses the deformity where it occurs on the medial aspect of the metaphyseal–diaphyseal junction of the proximal tibia. It does not distort the anatomy of the upper tibia so that total knee replacement is more easily performed than after traditional closing wedge Coventry osteotomy. When performed for early osteoarthritis, medial joint laxity can be corrected easily, and secondary laxity of the ACL can be lessened by decreasing the sagittal slope of the tibia by placing the osteotomy fixation device more posteriorly. However, it requires special care to ensure that the hamstring insertions are not overly tightened by lengthening the medial column of the tibia or by increasing the patellofemoral contact forces with large opening corrections. In addition, it requires the use of bone graft at the osteotomy site, which increases the time to union of the osteotomy. Opening wedge osteotomy can increase leg length, which is advantageous if the leg is short at the baseline but can be problematic otherwise. The average time to union of a tibial opening wedge osteotomy is 10 to 12 weeks and that of a closing wedge osteotomy is 6 to 8 weeks. This may be a factor in procedure selection for a patient who must return to work in a physical capacity at an earlier time. These technical details will be discussed further.

Closing wedge osteotomies are presently performed for corrections less than 10 degrees, specifically for conditions of osteochondritis dissecans, large osseous bone cysts, or avascular necrosis of the medial femoral condyle. The autologous bone graft that is harvested with the osteotomy is used as the restorative bone graft for the osteochondral defect on the medial femoral condyle. In this way, malalignment is corrected and the osseous defect is repaired in a single setting (see Chapter 6). Other indications for a closing wedge osteotomy include patients who previously were smokers and laborers who require a quick return to work (i.e., cancellous bone to cancellous bone healing usually occurs within 6–8 weeks).

A reverse dome osteotomy, as popularized by Paley,[9] is very powerful for large corrections of 15 to 30 degrees. It has the advantage of maintaining the anatomy of the upper tibia and correcting large deformities. It is technically demanding and requires a freehand technique with a concomitant fibular osteotomy and a fixed-angle device for fixation or an external fixator. It usually is longer to heal (3–4 months).

SURGICAL SETUP AND HOSPITAL COURSE

Osteotomies are performed on a radiolucent table, which allows visualization of the hip, knee, and ankle, accompanied by image intensification. Epidural anesthesia is used during and for 24 hours after surgery. Drains are left under the muscle compartments only until less than 30 cc of serous drainage over 8 hours (sometimes 2–3 days), then the drains are removed to prevent muscle compartment syndrome. Patients are placed on deep vein thrombosis (DVT) prophylaxis during the surgery with Venodyne foot pump compression (to avoid calf muscle compression), given light graduated compression stockings with a light gauze dressing only, and started on oral warfarin (Coumadin) for 3 weeks postoperatively starting the day of surgery. Upon discontinuation of epidural anesthesia the first morning postoperatively, transitioning of the patient for good pain management is critical. We use intravenous ketorolac (Toradol) 30 mg every 8 hours for six doses and 5–10 mg oral oxycodone every 3 hours for the first week postoperatively. Patients are generally discharged home on postoperative day 3 in a removable hinge knee brace, a continuous passage motion machine, and two crutches for touch weight-bearing with foot flat to the ground and weight of the leg supported. Ice cryotherapy is generally very helpful for swelling and discomfort. Narcotics use lessens after the first week only at bedtime and before physical therapy but are generally used for up to 6 weeks postoperatively. Acetaminophen is generally adequate otherwise. It is recommended that patients take a multivitamin supplement with vitamin D, 1,000 mg of calcium daily, and avoid nonsteroidal antiinflammatory drugs, which may delay osteotomy healing. As noted earlier, we do not perform osteotomies on patients who are cigarette smokers because of the known risk of nonunion.

ANATOMIC CONSIDERATIONS

When performing high tibial osteotomy, avoidance of neurovascular injuries and compartment syndrome is critical. Understanding the course of the femoral artery and its normal and abnormal anatomy as well as the course of the peroneal nerve is important to prevent damage from an oscillating saw blade during performance of the procedure. Upon performing a closing wedge osteotomy, I inadvertently cut through a small artery located directly on the back of the tibia. A vascular consult was obtained, the tourniquet was let down, and Doppler pulses of the foot revealed a good distal circulation. The small vessels were tied off, and no further sequela occurred. Further investigation revealed that the vessel was an aberrant anterior tibial artery (Figure 8–7). Review of the malpractice cases against osteotomies in the Boston area revealed two cases of arterial injury resulting in (1) a compartment syndrome of the anterior musculature requiring excision of the anterior muscle compartment and tendon transfer to the foot and (2) avascularity to the foot resulting in amputation. I then collaborated with my radiology colleagues to investigate the incidence and significance of the aberrant anterior tibial artery.[10] The angiographic literature has reported a prevalence of high division of the popliteal artery from 3% to 8%. Our MRI surveillance of 1,116 knees revealed a 2.1% incidence (23/1116) of an aberrant anterior tibial artery lying directly on the posterior cortex of the tibia deep to the popliteus muscle. The vessel is an embryologic remnant of the deep popliteal artery that had undergone developmental arrest.

Another recent study using Duplex ultrasonography on 100 knees in 50 patients visualized the popliteal artery at the level of total knee arthroplasty, 1 to 1.5 cm distal to the articular surface, which moved only 1.4 mm further posterior at 90 degrees of flexion in 76% of knees but was closer to the posterior cortex in 24% with flexion.[11] At the level of the tibial osteotomy, 1.5 to 2 cm distal to the articular surface, 85% of the arteries moved further away posterior at 90 degrees of flexion by only 1.7 mm; however, 15% moved closer to the tibia at 90 degrees of flexion. Hence, because it is technically more difficult to perform an osteotomy at 90 degrees of flexion and there is no guarantee the vessels will not be brought closer to the tibia and placed at greater risk for injury, I prefer to perform the osteotomy in full extension after dissecting out the back on the knee, protecting the neurovascular structures with sponges and retractors. I then perform an accurate and safe osteotomy, fixing the osteotomy in full extension to ensure that a fixed flexion deformity does not arise, which may occur if fixation is performed with the knee flexed and constitutes a large mistake when performing osteotomy surgery.

CLOSING WEDGE OSTEOTOMY

Several companies presently use calibrated osteotomy jigs in 1- and 2-degree increments, thus allowing very accurate reproducible Coventry wedge, closing osteotomy corrections. A closing wedge osteotomy can generally be performed without elevation of the tibial tubercle for up to a 10 degrees of angular correction. Removal of the medial portion of the fibular articular surface, leaving the proximal tibiofibular joint capsule intact, is preferred with corrections of 8 degrees or less (Figure 8–8). It is difficult to accept corrections

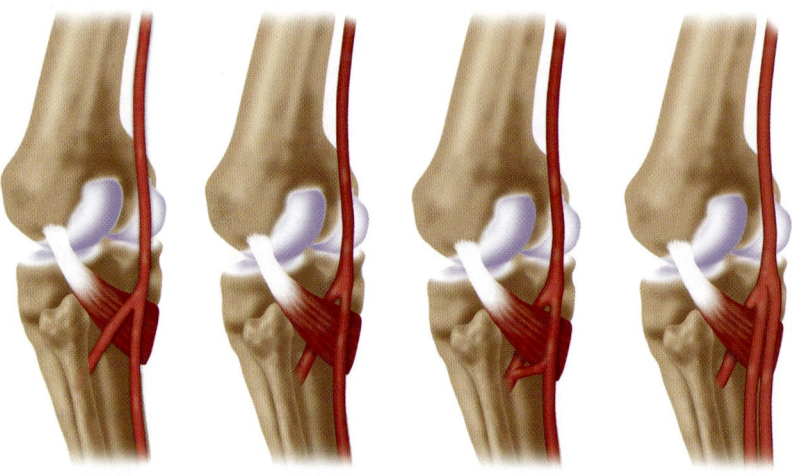

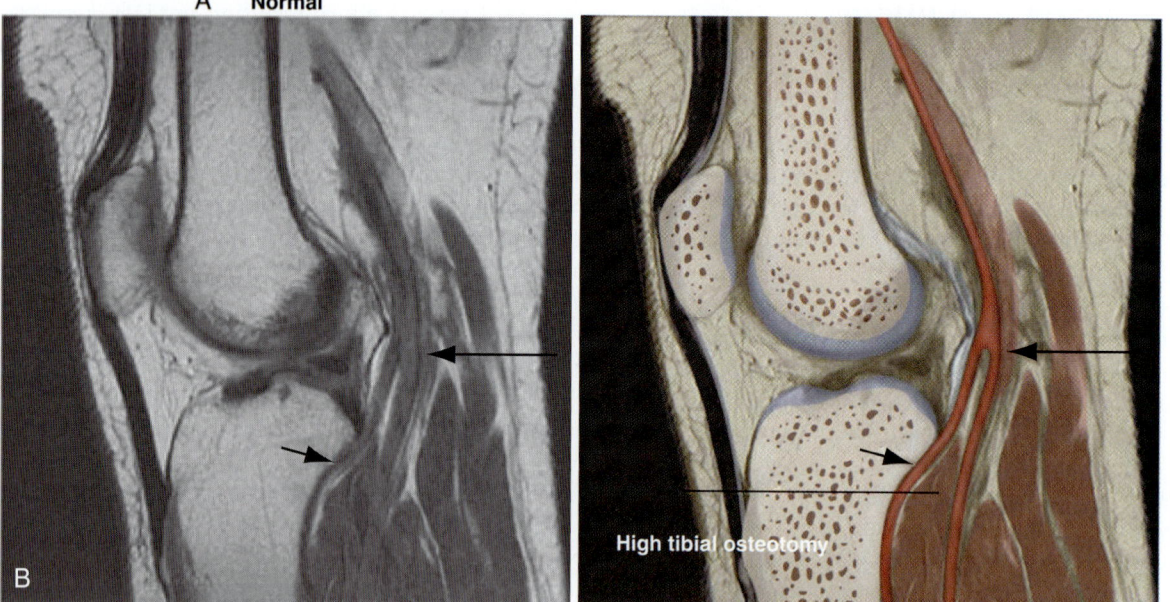

Figure 8-7 *A*, Variations of an aberrant tibialis anterior artery. A division of the popliteal artery into the tibialis anterior artery and the peroneal artery trunk may be aberrant, with the tibialis anterior artery going deep to the popliteus muscle and lying directly on the posterior tibial cortex as noted. This vessel may then be inadvertently transected during procedures on the upper and of the tibial metaphysis. It is especially at risk during tibial osteotomy. An aberrant tibialis anterior artery occurs in approximately 2.1% of knees.[10] *B*, Magnetic resonance imaging (MRI) scan and corresponding diagram illustrate the aberrant anterior tibial artery deep to the popliteus muscle lying directly on the posterior cortex of the tibia is at risk with the usual position of high tibial osteotomy.

Continued

Aberrant Anterior Tibial Artery

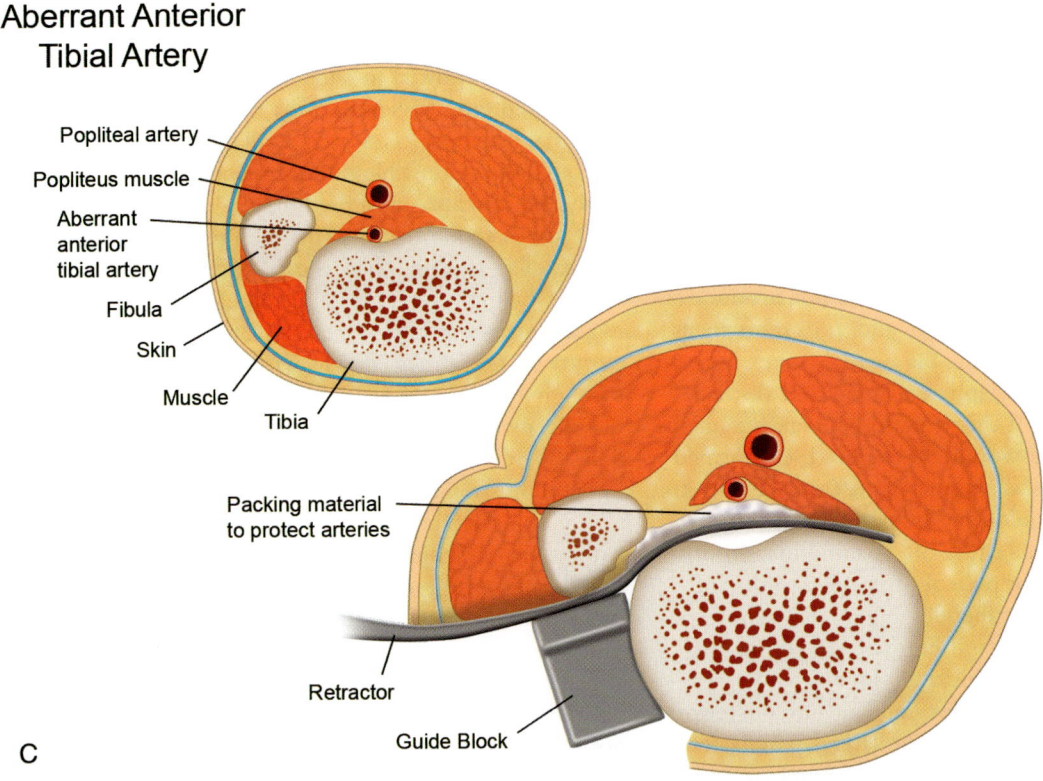

Figure 8-7—cont'd *C*, Careful posterior subperiosteal dissection of the tibia protects an aberrant anterior tibial artery from injury. The incidence of this variation is 2.1%[10] and can be visualized on preoperative MRI scan.

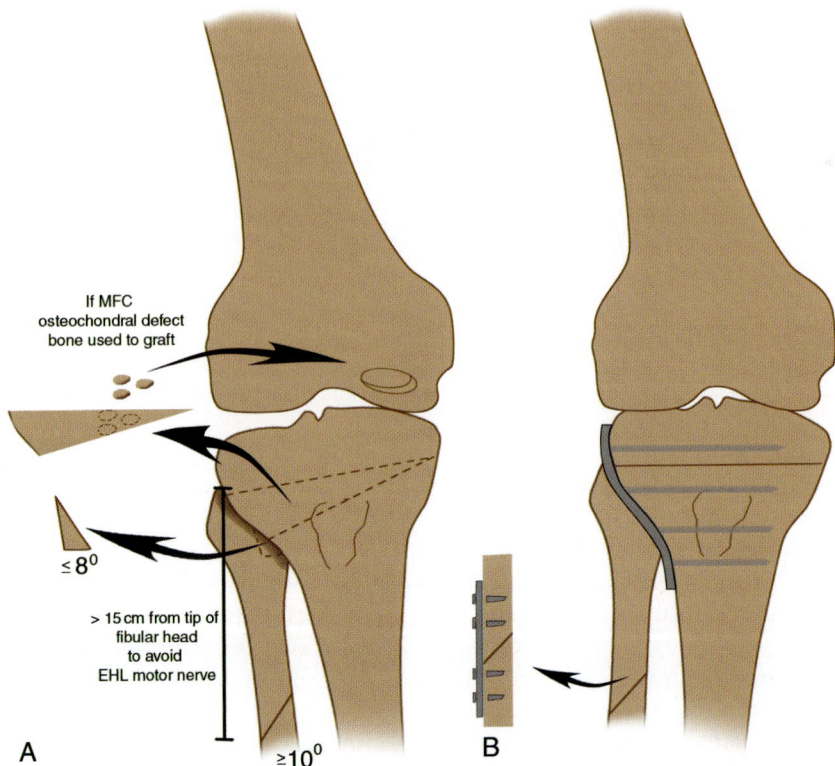

Figure 8-8 *A*, The current primary indication for a closing wedge tibial valgus osteotomy is to provide bone or a medial femoral condyle bone grafting of an osteochondral defect and restore the alignment of the leg to neutral mechanical alignment. If the angular correction it is 8 degrees or less, then the medial aspect of the fibular articular surface is removed. If the correction is greater than 10 degrees, a midshaft fibular osteotomy is performed and then fixated *(B)*.

of 10 degrees or greater without performing a midshaft fibular osteotomy so as to allow an easy closing osteotomy. Otherwise the surgeon would completely release the proximal tibiofibular joint, rendering the lateral ligamentous complex lax and the fibula migrating proximally above the lateral tibiofemoral joint line. For osteotomies between 10 and 14 degrees, the tubercle is generally elevated and a retrotubercular osteotomy is performed. This allows the osteotomy to be performed lower down on the tibial surface so as to not produce a metaphyseal–diaphyseal mismatch and not remove as much bone. However, this puts the medial cortex at risk for fracturing as it is in diaphyseal bone and displacement of the osteotomy. If this were to happen, a medial plate or fixation staple would be required, performed with concomitant midshaft fibular osteotomy. Fixation of both osteotomies would then be performed.

A skin incision is made just off the midline slightly laterally from the superior pole of the patella to the inferior aspect of the tibial tubercle. Figure 8–9 shows a stepwise surgical approach, and Figure 8–10 shows postoperative x-ray films. Full-thickness medial and lateral flaps are made to the posterior medial and posterior lateral corner of the knee joint. The lateral patella tendon margin is dissected sharply to the anterior tibial crest and along the anterior compartment muscle fascia. A second deep incision is made transversely from the anterior aspect of the proximal tibiofibular joint, transversely to the patella tendon below Gerdy's tubercle. The anterior lateral muscle compartment is subperiosteally dissected from distal to proximal, with an elevator used distally and sharp knife dissection on the metaphysis. The anterior and inferior aspects of the fibular head are subperiosteally dissected, leaving the joint capsule of the proximal tibiofibular joint intact. The posterior aspect of the tibia is subperiosteally dissected and extracapsularly dissected to the back of the knee joint is packed full of saline-soaked sponges to protect the neurovascular structures. The patella tendon is skeletonized to its insertion on the tubercle. The iliotibial band is reflected proximally off of Gerdy's tubercle to the coronary ligament of the lateral meniscus. Stay sutures are used to hold the soft tissues (iliotibial band) proximally.

If the angular correction is 8 degrees or less, the calibrated jig is applied to the proximal tibial joint margins and a transverse cut is made to but not through the medial cortex. The angled cut is then made to the medial cortex in extension as the posterior structures are packed off with sponges.

If the correction is 10 degrees or greater, a separate 3- to 5-cm incision is made between the superficial posterior muscle compartment and the lateral compartment at the level of the midshaft fibula, through the skin and the fascia only. Blunt finger dissection is made to the posterior lateral corner of the fibula where the periosteum is sharply incised with a knife and a circumferential subperiosteal dissection is performed. Retractors are applied to the fibula. An oblique osteotomy is made with a sagittal saw, and the osteotomy is allowed to slide on itself once the proximal tibial osteotomy is closed. This is then fixated, after the proximal osteotomy is fixated, with a one-third semitubular four-hole plate. This allows ease of comfort postoperatively and rapid union of the fibula.

If the osteotomy of 10 degrees or greater intersects the patellar tendon, then the tibial tubercle is osteotomized, leaving it intact distally and elevating it. The closing wedge osteotomy is then performed. The osteotomy closure is performed slowly with a compression device through an L-plate so as not to fracture and make unstable the medial cortex (the cortex is usually predrilled). The tubercle is refixated with 1- or 2- to 3.5-mm screws in a compression mode through the posterior cortex. Usually, if some lateral patella facet disease is present along with this, a full-thickness lateral release is performed and the closing wedge bone graft is placed under the tibial tubercle in order to elevate it.

The sponges are removed, the tourniquet is let down, and electrocautery is used for any bleeders. Hemovac drains (two arms) are placed in the wounds. One is placed posterior to the tibia, loosely reapproximating the iliotibial band to the superior aspect of the anterior lateral muscle compartment. The anterior aspect of the muscle fascia is left completely opened. Closure of the subcutaneous tissues and the skin follows. A second drain is placed in the wound flap outside of the muscle compartment. The drains are left in place for 3 days postoperatively. During the first 48 hours, a continuous epidural pain management program is monitored by a 24-hour pain service. The muscle compartments are clinically inspected every 4 to 8 hours and as needed. Venodyne foot pumps are used immediately after surgery to diminish swelling and DVT risk. They are the preferred mechanical compression device because they improve venous return without applying pressure on the muscle compartments.

OPENING WEDGE OSTEOTOMY

Opening wedge osteotomy is presently the preferred osteotomy because of its technical ease, highly accurate dial-in correction, and lack of deformity to the proximal tibia, which presumably will result in an easier conversion to total knee replacement in the future. It is especially useful if there is leg length shortening on the affected side and joint line obliquity inferomedially with a varus thrust because it restores leg length and produces a horizontal joint line. It is performed proximal to the pes anserinus insertion in an oblique fashion directed toward the proximal tibiofibular joint but not through the lateral cortex and above the tibial tubercle (Figure 8–11). Opening wedge osteotomies can be performed up to approximately 20 degrees; however, at

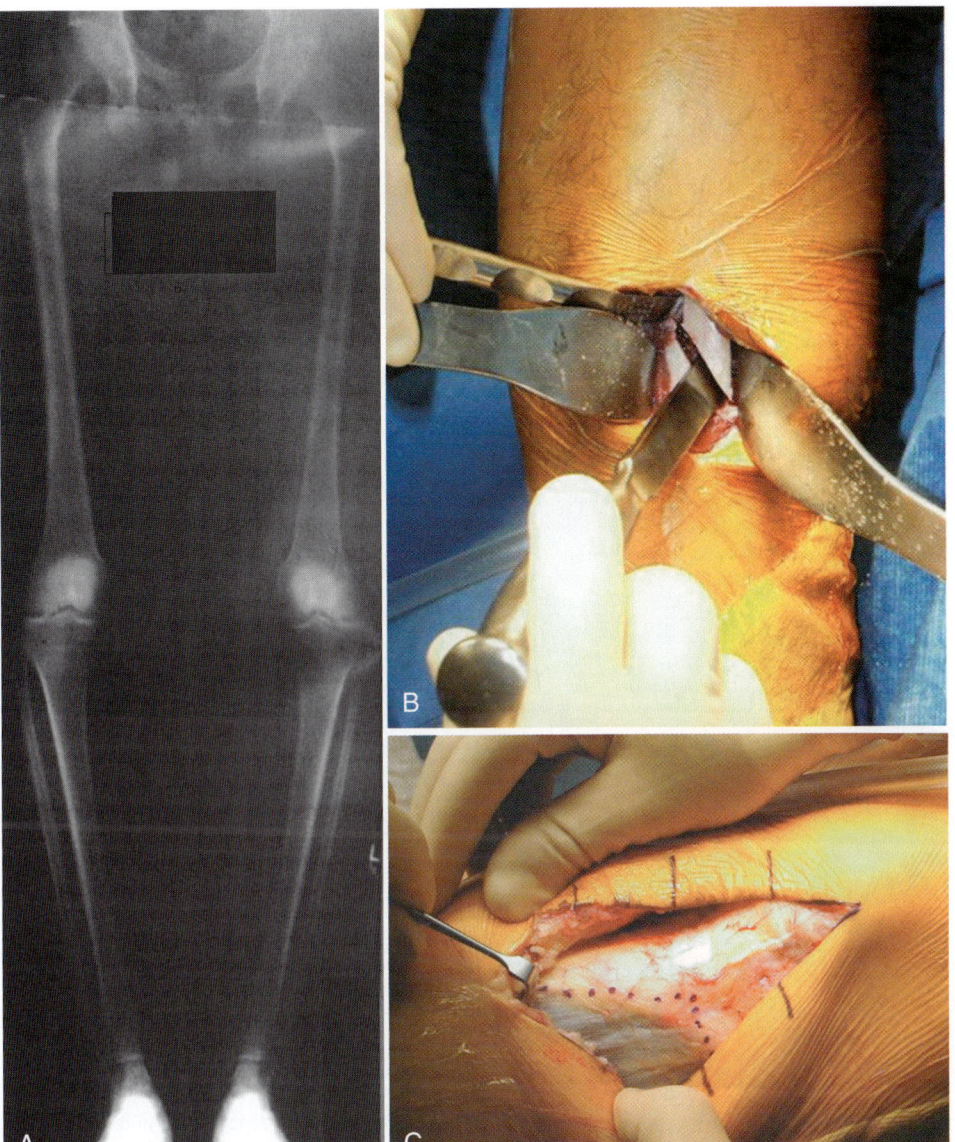

Figure 8-9 *A,* Long alignment 54-inch x-ray films demonstrating marked varus malalignment of both knees in a 30-year-old man. The left knee has medially based pain. A 10-degree angular correction places the mechanical axis to the lateral tibial spine, thus unloading the medial compartment, which has early joint space narrowing. *B,* A 3-cm skin incision is made at the level of the midshaft of the fibula at least 15 cm distal to the fibular head to avoid injury to the motor nerve of the extensor hallucis longus muscle. This is made at the junction of the lateral and posterior muscle compartments. A blunt finger dissection is all that is required to reach the posterior lateral corner of the fibula, which contains the fascial attachments. These are sharply incised longitudinally, and a subperiosteal dissection to the deep and superficial aspect of the fibula reveals the bone (clearly noted in the figure). A small sagittal saw creates an oblique osteotomy to the deep cortex, which is opened with an osteotome, and allows easy motion of one segment relative to the other. *C,* A longitudinal incision is made at the level of the superior lateral pole of the patella to the inferior aspect of the tibial tubercle. Full-thickness flaps at the level of the fascia are performed around the tibia to the posterior medial aspect of the upper tibia and to the posterolateral aspect. The proposed takedown of the anterolateral muscle compartment is identified as noted by the sterile marking pen dots on the photograph. *D,* The anterolateral muscle compartment is sharply taken down subperiosteally to the posterior lateral corner of the tibia and the proximal tibiofibular joint. The iliotibial band attachment to Gerdy's tubercle is also subperiosteally dissected sharply with a knife as a single flap to the level of the coronary ligament of the lateral meniscus and then sutured onto the capsule to keep it out of the way. The infrapatellar fat pad is released off the anterior tibia to identify the pretibial bursa and protect the patellar tendon. *E,* A small elevator is placed along the posterior proximal tibiofibular joint capsule. The anterior aspect of the fibular head is carefully subperiosteally dissected. The inferior half of the joint capsule of the proximal tibiofibular joint is released anteriorly and posteriorly through the anterior approach. This allows the proximal portion of the fibula to mobilize minimally when the fibular osteotomy is later fixated with a one-third semitubular plate. If this correction was 8 degrees or less, a fibular osteotomy would not be required, and the osteotomy correction would be achieved entirely through excision of the medial third of the proximal fibular articular surface, leaving only the proximal capsule attached to the tibia. This allows the osteotomy of the tibia to close without proximal migration of the fibula and resultant laxity of the fibular collateral ligament and popliteus tendon attachments. In addition, the posterior muscle compartment is sharply subperiosteally dissected off the back of the tibia to protect the neurovascular structures. A small wet sponge is placed in a distal to proximal direction directly on the bone and extracapsularly on the posterior joint line.

Continued

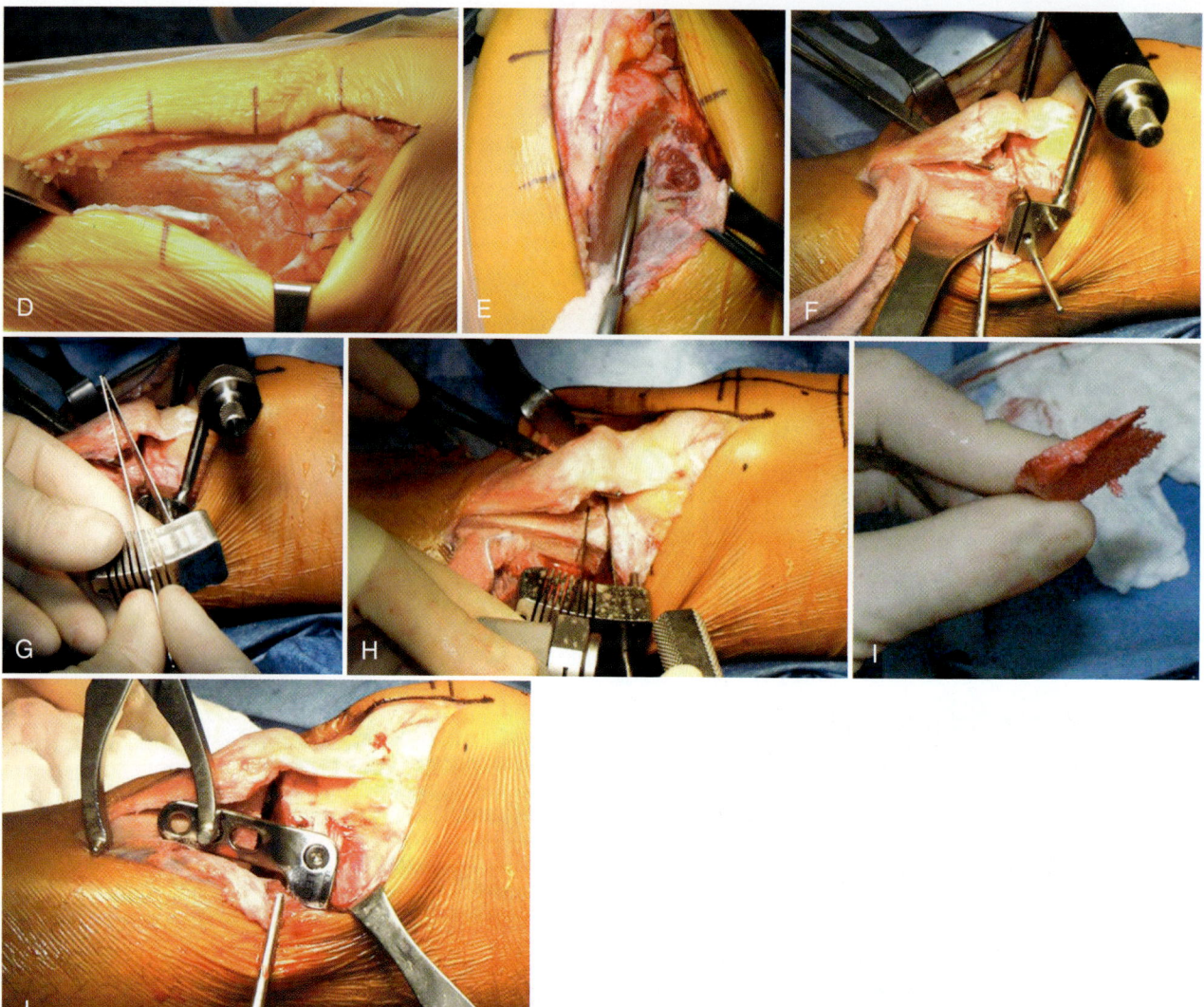

Figure 8-9—cont'd *F*, A transverse tibial tubercle osteotomy is first performed 1 cm posterior to the anterior cortex with the distal hinge remaining intact. This allows the transverse component of the osteotomy to be performed further distally on the metaphysis, thereby removing less bone with the same angular correction. In addition, the tibial tubercle may be either elevated using the bone that has been extracted from the tibial closing wedge osteotomy or just medialized to improve patellar tracking. A radiolucent calibrated jig is placed across the medial and lateral aspects of the tibia parallel to the joint line and confirmed on image intensification. The transverse osteotomy is performed to the medial cortex through both the anterior and posterior cortices, protecting the posterior neurovascular structures with sponges that had been packed on the posterior cortex after it had been carefully subperiosteally dissected. In this way, any aberrant tibialis anterior vessel on the posterior cortex is avoided. *G*, Most closing wedge osteotomy jigs are calibrated in varying increments. This jig is calibrated from 6 to 20 degrees in 2-degree increments. The saw blade as shown, when placed through the jig, will need to the opposite tip at which the transverse osteotomy rests, in this case the medial proximal cortex of the tibia. *H*, With the second calibrated jig now applied to the proximal cut, a second bony cut is made 10 degrees to the first to the opposite medial cortex through both anterior and posterior cortices. This is checked under image intensification as the procedure is being performed to ensure that the medial cortex is not being violated. *I*, Using a 0.25-inch osteotome at the level of the proximal and distal closing wedge osteotomy cuts, the bony fragment is easily removed. Note that this 10-degree fragment, which has been removed from the metaphysis at a more distal location, is quite small. Therefore, the metaphyseal–diaphyseal mismatch is very small and the distortion of the upper end of the tibia is minimized. If a total knee replacement were required in the future and offset tibial stem likely would not be required, then the procedure would be facilitated by the utilitarian midline incision that is used for the osteotomy instead of a classic hockey stick–type incision. *J*, The osteotomy is slowly closed after the medial cortex has been multiply drilled with a 3.2-mm drill bit to ensure that a controlled closure occurs. After the proximal two 6.5-mm screws have been placed in the plate, a compression clamp is attached to the offset L-plate used with the system. The midshaft fibular osteotomy is carefully palpated and through its separate incision to ensure that it moves easily and allows closure of the tibial osteotomy. When the osteotomy is completely closed, the distal two screw holes are placed. If the medial cortex is cracked, a staple can be placed at that site to prevent translation of the tibial shaft laterally or opening up of the medial cortex. The other option is to use an oblique lag screw through the oblong hole within the plate, which was performed in this case for added stability and to prevent breakage of the medial side.

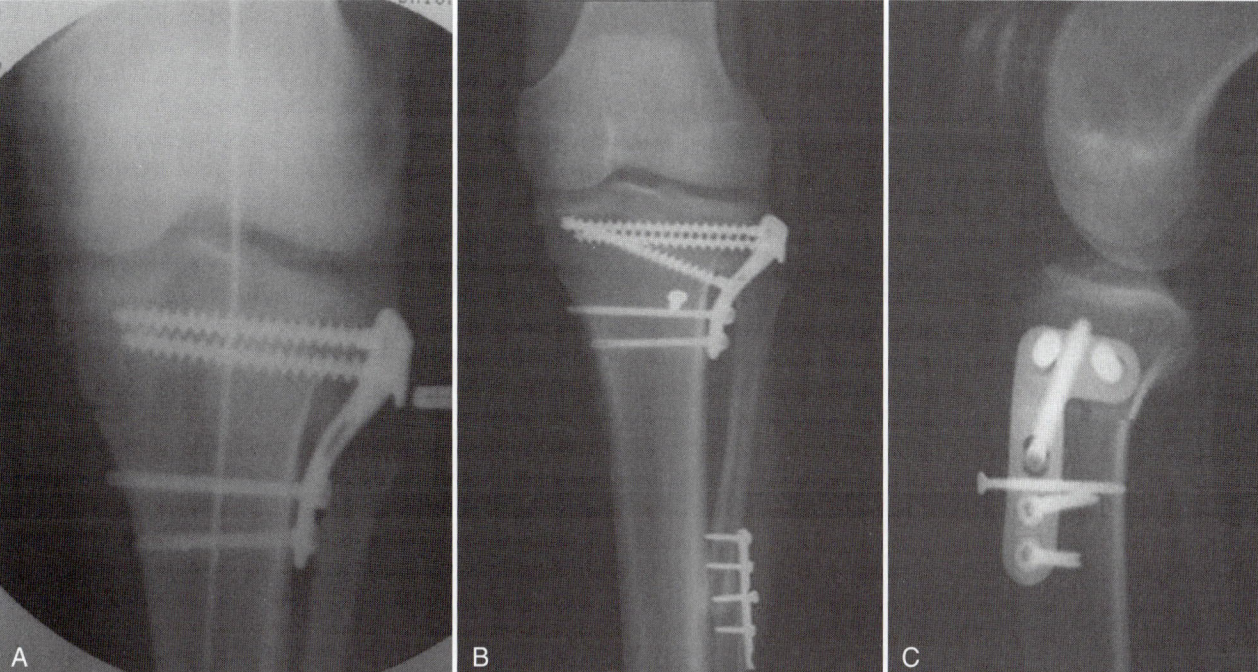

Figure 8-10 *A,* Intraoperative check is performed using a Bovie cord on the radiolucent table from the center of the femoral head to the center of the talus at the ankle joint to ensure that the proposed angular correction is made to the lateral tibial spine, as planned preoperatively. *B,* Tibial tubercle is slightly medialized to ensure central patellar tracking and fixated with a single anterior to posterior lag screw to the posterior cortex of the tibia. The fibula is separately plated with a small one-third semitubular plate. X-ray film shows the final radiographic appearance. Note the minimal deformity of the upper end of the tibia and the location of the proximal fibula at its native position, ensuring that the posterior lateral ligamentous complex has not been made lax. *C,* Final radiographic appearance on lateral x-ray film. Note that the tibial tubercle osteotomy in this case was performed to facilitate a lower osteotomy position and not to specifically unload the patellofemoral joint. For corrections less than 10 degrees, a tibial tubercle osteotomy is generally not used unless the position of the patellar tendon attachment is very proximal and near the joint line. In that situation, a tibial tubercle osteotomy would be useful to protect the patellar tendon from injury.

greater than 10 degrees the pes anserinus tendons must be released off the medial subcutaneous border of the tibia in order to allow the medial column to lengthen and not develop a flexion deformity due to soft tissue tightness. Similarly, the extensor mechanism also undergoes tightening with increasing opening wedge osteotomy. This can be resolved by performing a tibial tubercle osteotomy and replacing it at its proximal-most native position or a modified retrotubercular osteotomy. In this way, the extensor mechanism tension is not increased and thus does not cause excessive force on the patellofemoral joint and loss of flexion (Figure 8–12).

A longitudinal incision is made from the superior medial pole of the patella to the inferior aspect of the tibial tubercle. Figure 8–13 shows a stepwise surgical technique for opening wedge tibial valgus osteotomy. A full-thickness medial subcutaneous flap is made, then pes anserinus tendons are identified on the subcutaneous border of the tibia medially. The superior aspect of these tendons is incised and the tendons retracted. A transverse incision is made through the periosteum in the deep portion of the medial collateral ligament from the posterior aspect of the tibia to the anterior aspect of the tibia, proximal to the pes insertion. The medial collateral ligament (MCL) is subperiosteally dissected to within 1 cm of the joint line, leaving the deep and superficial aspects of the medial collateral ligament intact. The patella tendon is skeletonized on its insertion, distally. With the knee flexed in a figure-of-four position, the posterior aspect of the tibia is dissected and extracapsularly dissected. The past tendons are reflected in the posterior or medial direction and left only at tear posterior attachment to the tibia. The gastrosoleus muscle origin on the exposed posterior aspect of the knee is sharply released off the back of the tibia, allowing a careful subperiosteal dissection across the tibia from medial to lateral to the proximal tibiofibular joint. Small wet sponges are packed behind the knee to the level of the lateral tibiofibular joint and proximally to the level of the joint. This is easily palpated.

Under image intensification, a guidewire is placed obliquely at the level of the metaphyseal–diaphyseal junction, proximal to the patella tendon insertion, to the level of the proximal tibiofibular joint. If the patellar tendon insertion is very proximal, then a retrotubercular osteotomy is performed. This is done by making an axial saw cut at the level of the patellar tendon insertion, followed by a medial to lateral saw cut 1 to 2 cm distal to this at a level 1 cm posterior to the anterior tibial

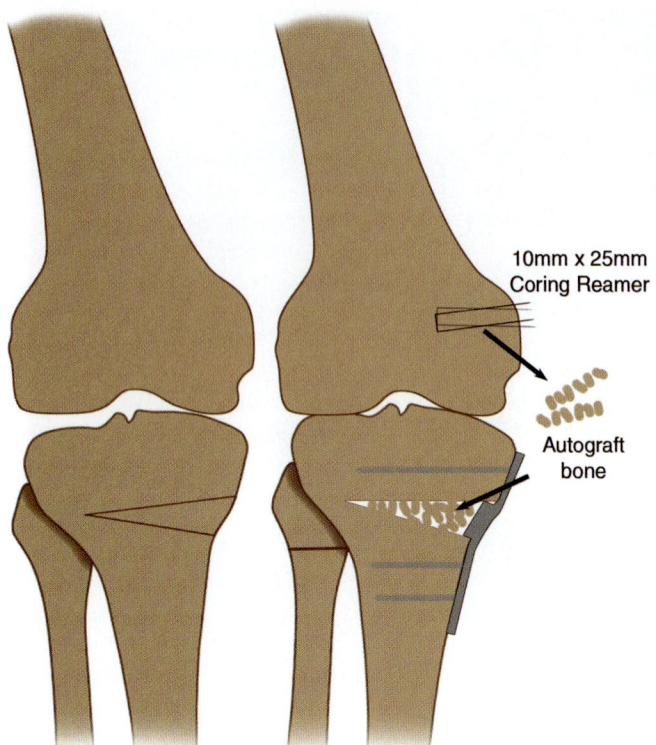

Figure 8-11 Step 1: Oblique cut is made to proximal fibular head at least 2 cm distal to lateral tibial plateau. Step 2: After osteotomy is opened and plated, autograft bone harvested with a core reamer or osteochondral autograft transfer system (OATS, Arthrex Corp., Naples, FL) can be used to take bone from the distal femoral metaphysis to graft the proximal tibia. The donor femur is backfilled with a combination of allograft cancellous chips and demineralized bone matrix.

tubercle cortex. In this way, the tibial tubercle is still attached to the distal fragment. A saw cut is then made on top of the guidewire with the knee in full extension, visualized under image intensification guidance, to but through the lateral cortex of the tibia. Opening wedge tines are used to open the medial aspect of the tibia. The correct amount of angular correction is documented with an intraoperative guidewire assessment placing a Bovie cord wire from the center of the femoral head to the center of the talus falling through the lateral intercondylar spine. This will coincide with the desired degree of angular correction. Puddu plates are then placed, and 6.5-mm cancellous screws are used proximally through the plate and 4.5-mm screws are placed distally. I have found that the to do plate used for the femur is more robust because it has three proximal screws and four distal screws about the osteotomy site. I have used it for several years on the tibia without failure of the plate or loss of correction. It is a low-profile implant and usually is not felt by the patient. Cancellous autograft dowels are placed at the osteotomy sites at the anterior and posterior cortices taken from the distal femoral metaphyses above the MCL origin, and allograft cancellous bone is packed deep within the osteotomy surfaces. The tourniquet is then let down, and an excellent marrow "blush" of marrow elements permeates the allograft bone; no irrigation is used as to not lose any of these bone-forming cells and elements. I have found that healing is similar to that with autograft bone, and I have not used iliac crest bone since 2001.

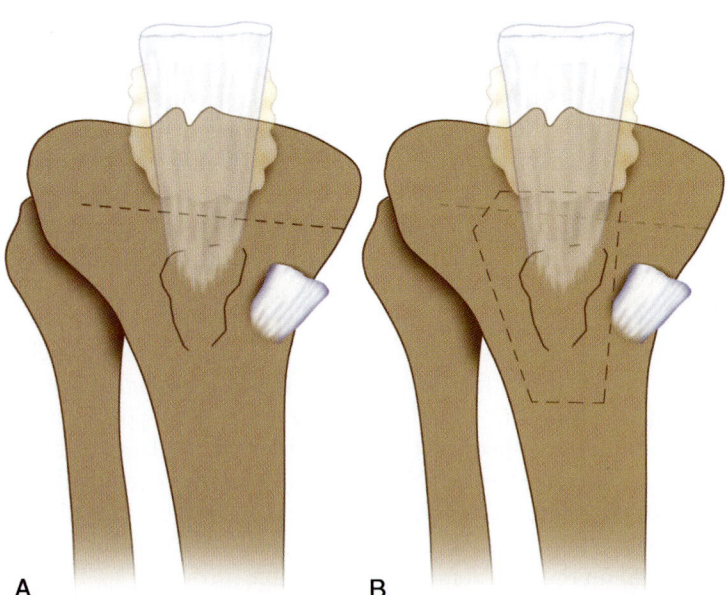

Figure 8-12 *A*, Step 1: *Dotted line* represents the proposed level of the tibial opening wedge valgus-producing osteotomy from the metaphyseal–diaphyseal junction of the proximal tibia to the proximal tibiofibular joint. *B*, Step 2: Outline of the proposed level of the tibial tubercle anteromedialization osteotomy (Fulkerson osteotomy) with a transverse proximal countercut and a oblique distal countercut, followed by the medial to posterolateral osteotomy typical of the Fulkerson osteotomy. The steepness will vary depending on the amount of anteriorization versus medialization required for extensor mechanism unloading and proper tracking. The posterior lateral cortex of the tibia must always remain intact.

Continued

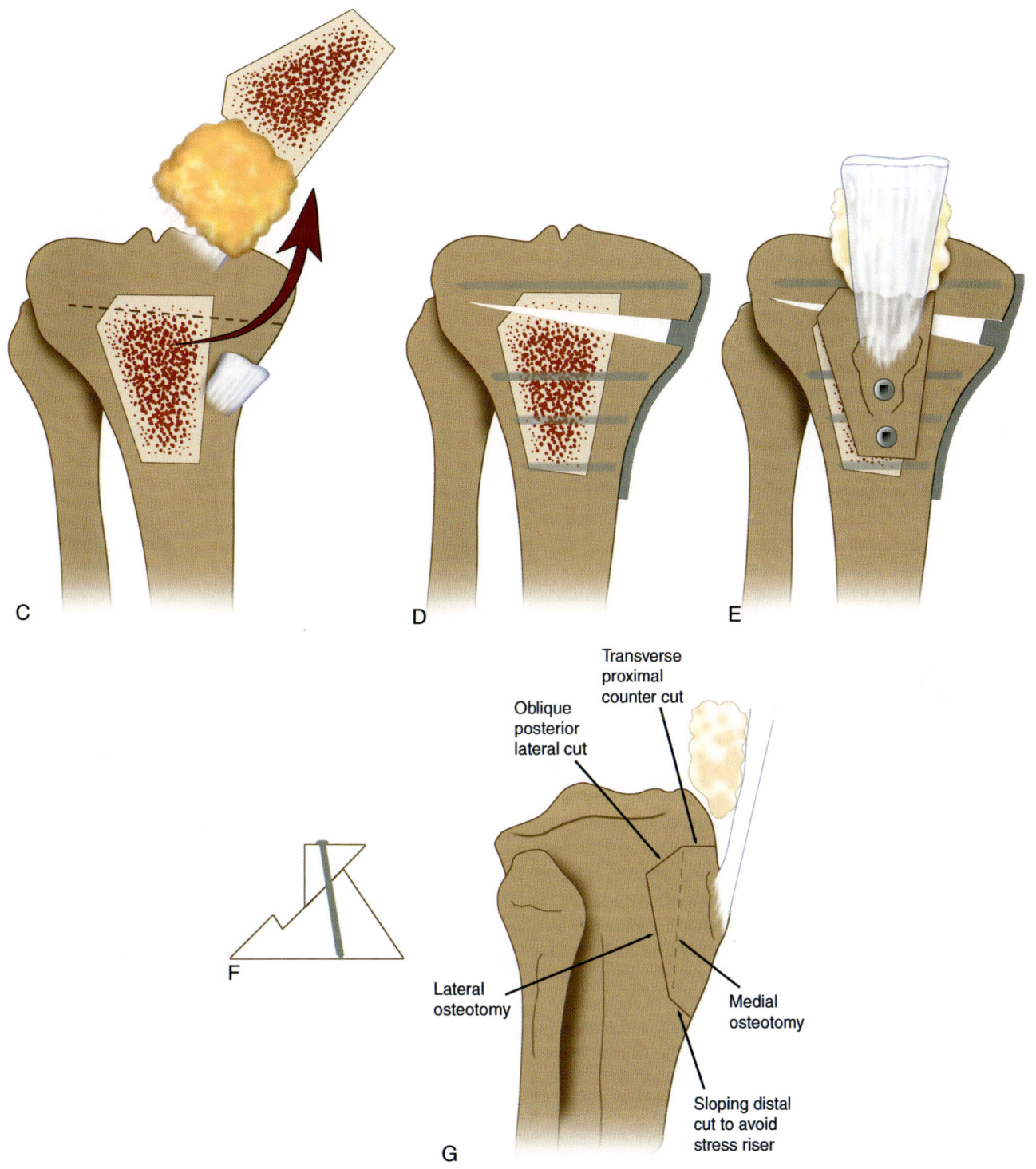

Figure 8–12—cont'd *C,* Step 3: Tibial tubercle osteotomy is performed, and the Hoffa fat pad is released off the anterior tibial interval anterior to the intrameniscal ligament and the origins of the anterior horns of the medial and lateral menisci. A lateral subvastus arthrotomy is performed in order to visualize the joint and unload the patella. A medial subvastus arthrotomy is performed to the level of the insertion of the vastus medialis obliquus on the joint capsule. *D,* Step 4: Opening wedge tibial valgus-producing osteotomy is performed and fixated. *E,* Step 5: Tibial tubercle is replaced to the level of its original proximal transverse countercut and positioned in the anterior and medial directions necessary to centralize and unload the tibial tubercle. Pointed reduction forceps or a K-wire holds the tubercle in position while two anterior to posterior lag screws are used to fixate the tibial tubercle. Note that the distal cut of the tibial tubercle is not a straight anterior to posterior transverse cut but slopes distally and anteriorly to avoid a stress riser and potential postoperative stress fracture at this position. Usually a gap is present at this position and is bone grafted with a combination of demineralized bone matrix and cancellous allogeneic bone chips. *F,* Cross-sectional appearance of the tibia at the level of the tibial tubercle after it is mobilized and fixated. The deficient lateral bone stock is replaced with demineralized bone matrix as is the overhanging medial tibial tubercle supplemented underneath its overhang. The medial periosteal sleeve, which includes the past anserinus tendons, is cold over the bone graft substitute and reattached to the patellar tendon on the tibial tubercle so as to provide a smooth medial subcutaneous border with no bony prominences (see technique of tibial tubercle osteotomy in Chapter 10). *G,* View of the tibial tubercle osteotomy from the lateral side. The distal aspect of the tibial tubercle osteotomy is sloped anteriorly so as to lessen the stress riser and possibility of postoperative fracture. The proximal countercut is transverse to allow the osteotomy to "lock in" when finally positioned and lessen the chance of proximal migration postoperatively, thus aiding in the stability of the osteotomy.

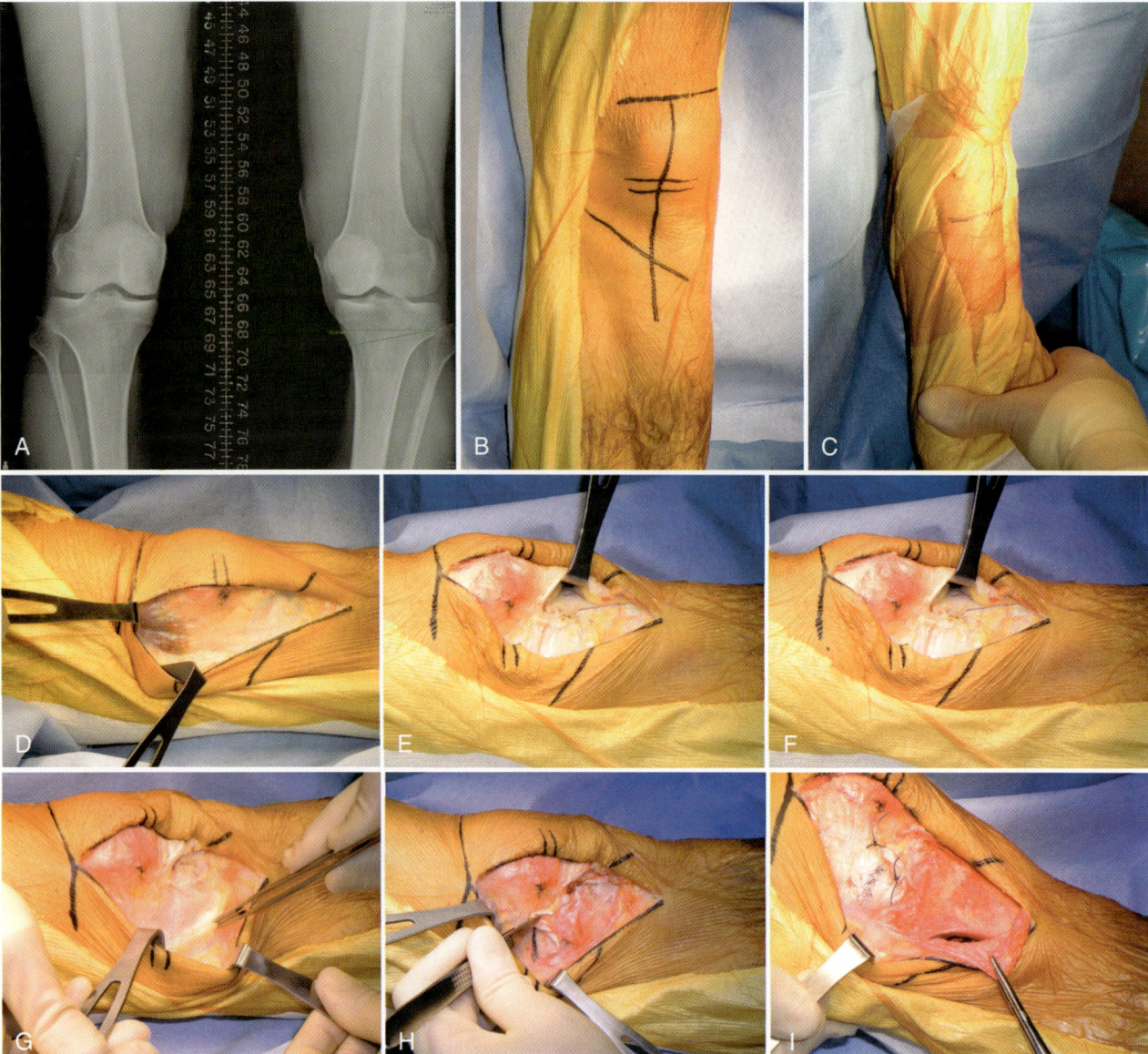

Figure 8–13 *A,* Digital long x-ray films demonstrating varus alignment used to calculate the opening wedge correction that will place the mechanical axis through the lateral tibial spine of the knee. Digital templating of this standing anteroposterior (AP) x-ray film demonstrates that an 11-degree angular correction places the mechanical axis through the center of the knee, corresponding to a 12.5-mm opening wedge tibial valgus-producing osteotomy. *B,* Intraoperative skin incision demonstrates the extent of the incision. Oblique marking indicates the pes anserinus tendon insertions on the subcutaneous border of the tibia. *C,* The center of the ankle is separately marked and confirmed by fluoroscopy. *D,* Medial subvastus exposure to the distal femur is prepared for harvesting of autologous bone graft for tibial valgus osteotomy. The soft tissue flaps are directly down to fascia and remaining full-thickness fasciocutaneous flaps that are well vascularized. *E,* A periosteal dissection is made just above the femoral origin of the medial collateral ligament (MCL) in preparation for cancellous bone graft harvesting with a dowel harvester. *F,* In preparation for the tibial osteotomy, the medial border of the patellar tendon is dissected into the infrapatellar bursa to the tendinous insertion on the tibial tubercle. *G,* The proximal border of the pes anserinus tendons is localized. *H,* A sharp subperiosteal dissection release is made to the pes anserinus tendons off their insertion distally and posteriorly to the tibia. The superficial medial collateral ligament is transected and subperiosteally dissected in a proximal direction to within 1 cm of the joint line, which is marked with a sterile marking pen. They are then held out of the way of the osteotomy with stay sutures. The knee is placed in a figure-of-four position so that the posterior soft tissue envelope can be sharply subperiosteally dissected off the posterior tibial cortex in a lateral direction to the proximal tibiofibular joint. *I,* The tendons are held with Kocher forceps while the origin of the soleus muscle is sharply incised off the back of the tibia and the posterior structures are dissected sharply off the back of the tibia.

Continued

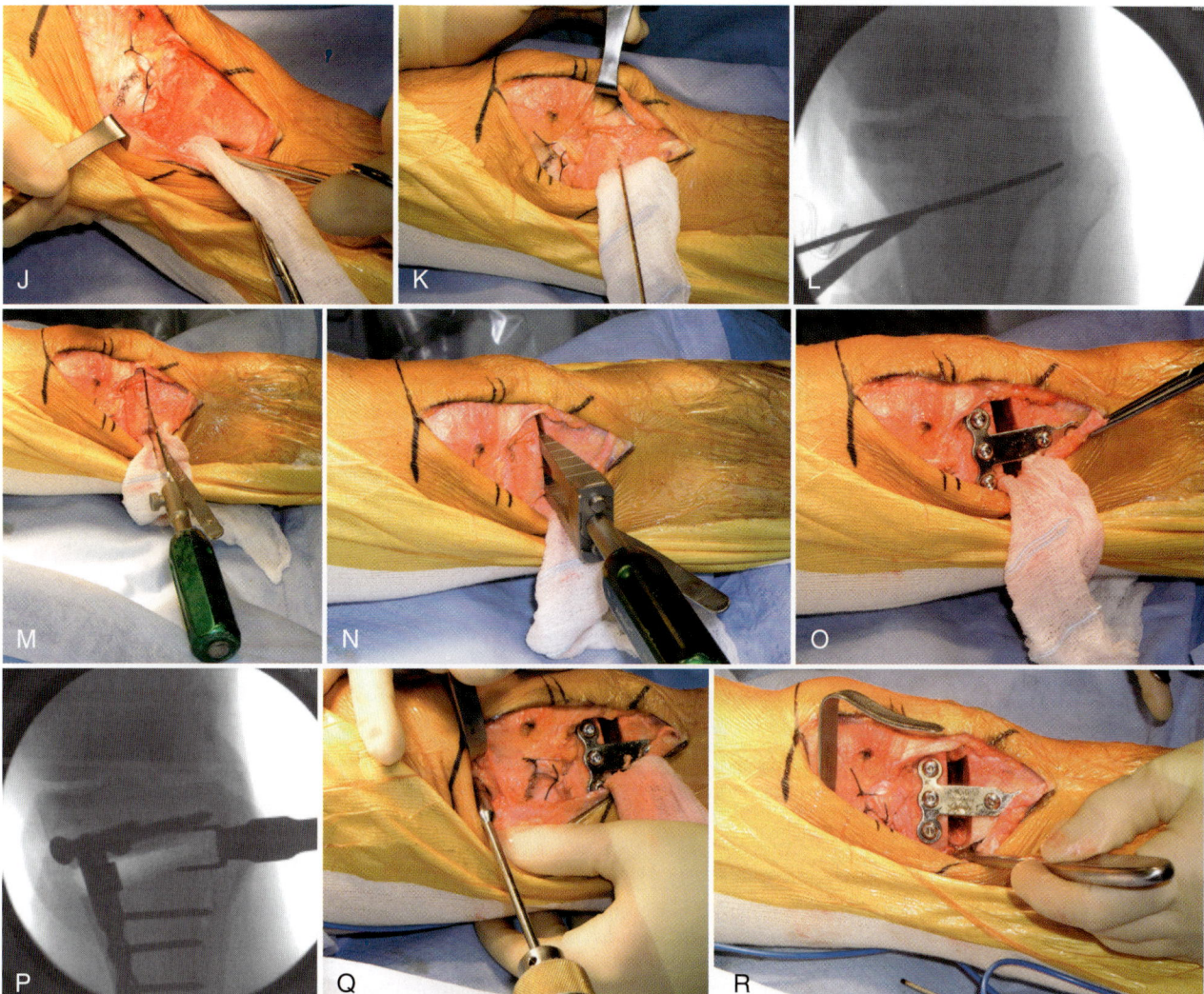

Figure 8-13—cont'd *J,* A small saline-soaked sponge is packed directly against the posterior aspect of the tibia, protecting the neurovascular structures before osteotomy. *K,* In preparation for the tibial osteotomy, a guidewire is directed to the midportion of the proximal tibiofibular joint and confirmed under image intensification while the knee is in full extension to allow good oscillating saw control. The pin is then broken away short of the cortex, the leg is stabilized, the guidewire is used to stabilize the saw blade at first the anterior cortex, and then the posterior cortex is cut two thirds of the way to the opposite cortex. A large osteotome is used for the final one third as to not broach the lateral cortex but to leave it intact so that the osteotomy can hinge on the intact cortex and proximal tibiofibular joint capsular tissues. *L,* The breakaway pin is well positioned in the metaphyseal bone of the proximal tibia at the level of the tibiofibular joint. There is at least a 2.5-cm space to the lateral tibial joint line to ensure that there is not an insufficiency fracture into the articular surface. The proposed osteotomy goes to the soft spongy lateral cortex of the metaphysis and not the diaphysis, where it is more likely to crack and displace. *M,* A broad osteotome is used to complete the osteotomy to but not through the lateral cortex. This is confirmed on image intensification. Note that the medial cortical osteotomy opens up symmetrically anteriorly and posteriorly. If not, then concern would be raised that the osteotomy was not completed either anteriorly or posteriorly, which would make for a difficult angular correction. *N,* With counterpressure at the level of the proposed osteotomy and a slight valgus force at the level of the ankle, the opening wedge tines are gently impacted in the direction of the lateral cortex, ensuring that full extension of the knee is always obtained. A bolster under the ankle is used to confirm this fully extended knee position. *O,* I prefer a femoral T Puddu plate on the tibia because of its improved fixation and low profile when the desired correction is obtained. *P,* When large opening corrections are required, a prophylactic lateral staple is applied through the same midline anterior incision. This is also used in the event of a lateral cortical fracture or displacement. If this were to occur, the osteotomy position would be closed laterally and the staple applied. *Q,* An 11-mm diameter harvester is used through a single cortical entry to harvest several 20-mm autologous cancellous bone dowels from the distal metaphysis of the femur. *R,* The autologous bone graft dowels are positioned both anteriorly and posteriorly at the cortical margins to enhance cortical bony union and prevent any movement of allograft cancellous bone chips into the soft tissue envelope.

Continued

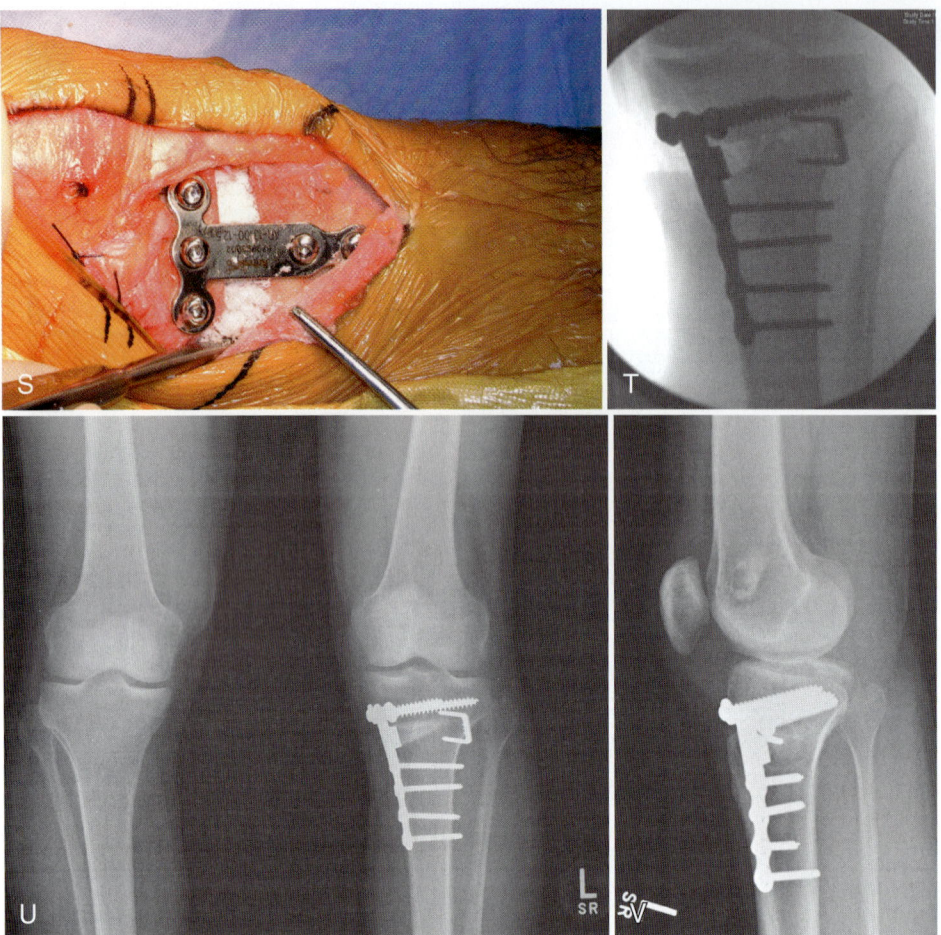

Figure 8-13—cont'd S, Final appearance after cancellous allogeneic bone chips are used to fill the central void of the osteotomy and the donor bone graft site. Drains are now positioned posterior to the tibia and one in the subcutaneous envelope. The pes tendons are loosely reattached to the superficial MCL and medial retinacular sleeve with interrupted suture. The tourniquet is then let down, and the marrow elements permeate the entire bone graft site with marrow stem cells, which enhance the union of the construct. No irrigation is used on this area. Small bleeders are cauterized, and a light dressing with a compression sock is supplied from toes to groin. A cryotherapy sleeve is applied over the knee and then a knee immobilizer accompanied by a Venodyne pump is applied for deep vein thrombosis prophylaxis. Continuous passage motion is started the following day. T, Immediate postoperative appearance of the osteotomy. U, V, Radiographic appearance of osteotomy 1 year after surgery, in the anteroposterior (U) and lateral (V) views.

OPENING WEDGE HIGH TIBIAL VALGUS OSTEOTOMY ACCOMPANIED BY ANTEROMEDIALIZATION TIBIAL TUBERCLE OSTEOTOMY

Combined osteotomies are performed when either large corrections are required (i.e., 10–20 mm opening wedge) or specific patellofemoral maltracking or lateral facet cartilage wear is present. If the tibial tubercle is left attached to the tibia and a large opening wedge osteotomy is being performed above the patellar tendon insertion, the patella will be effectively distalized, increasing contact forces across the patellofemoral joint and resulting in pain and articular cartilage wear. In this situation, a retrotubercular osteotomy can be performed, leaving the tubercle attached to the proximal fragment, or the entire tubercle can be removed and placed back at its proximal-most insertion to correct for patellar alignment. This is diagrammatically demonstrated in Figure 8–12.

REVERSE DOME TIBIAL VALGUS OSTEOTOMY

For corrections of 15 degrees or greater, I prefer a reversed dome osteotomy below the tibial tubercle with a midshaft fibular osteotomy. This is a very powerful osteotomy because it does not distort the upper anatomy of the proximal tibia and thus does not compromise future reconstruction.[8] It is technically the most difficult to perform of the three types of tibial osteotomies described here and has a longer time to osseous union (3–4 months). It usually requires a fixed-angle device, such as blade plate fixation, to allow for a stable correction (Figure 8–14).

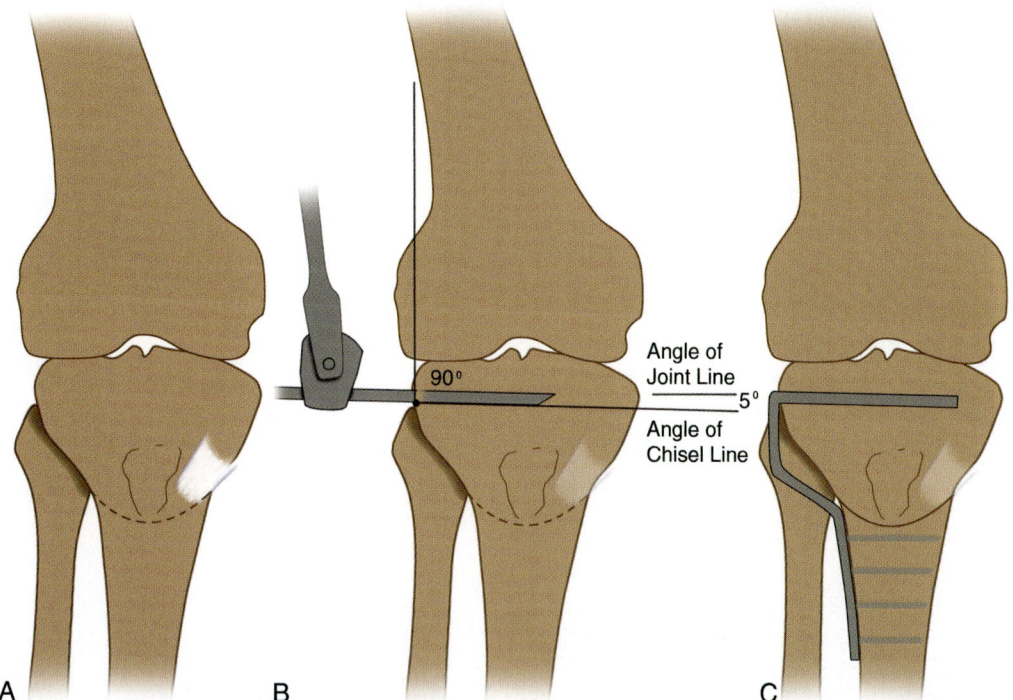

Figure 8-14 *A–C,* Reverse dome osteotomy. When a corrective osteotomy requires 15 degrees or greater, a reverse dome osteotomy[8] performed below the level of the tibial tubercle has allowed a very large angular correction of up to 30 degrees without distorting the proximal tibial geometry for eventual total knee arthroplasty. A midshaft fibular osteotomy is also required, and a fixed-angle device such as a 90-degree offset blade plate is used for fixation. *A,* Step 1: Upper end of the tibia is exposed. The arc of rotation to the metaphysis of the medial and lateral tibial plateau below the tibial tubercle is outlined and marked on the tibia with a marking pen. *B,* Step 2: Under image intensification guidance, a guidewire is placed parallel to the tibial articular surface and up to 5 degrees divergent from the surface to produce a tibiofemoral angle of 0 to 5 degrees of valgus. A seating chisel for blade plate placement is seated to the depth desired. *C,* Step 3: A 90-degree offset blade plate is placed and fixated, a reticulated compression device is used to compress the osteotomy, and the desired angular correction is obtained. The fibula is fixated with a one-third semitubular plate.

The exposure is similar to closing wedge valgus osteotomy. Figure 8–15 shows stepwise surgery for a reverse dome tibial valgus osteotomy. However, depending on the location of the proposed arc of the osteotomy on the proximal medial tibia, the pes anserinus tendons may have to be subperiosteally released in a posterior medial direction per an opening wedge tibial valgus osteotomy in order for the tendons to slide proximally and not be injured during the reverse dome osteotomy portion of the procedure. Prior to osteotomy, however, the chisel for the 90-degree blade is placed at the desired obliquity to the tibiofemoral joint, usually with a 15- to 20-mm offset to the tibia. The correction is determined by the angle of entry into the tibia relative to the tibial plateau surface. Usually a 5- to 7-degree tibiofemoral axis is desired, which requires entry 5 to 7 degrees parallel to the tibial plateau surface. The shaft of the tibia is then brought to the proximal fragment after the osteotomy, and the desired correction is obtained. After chisel placement, the reverse dome osteotomy is made, usually with a series of drill holes through a premade drill guide from anterior to posterior. The drill holes are connected with small ⅛-inch osteotomes, first the anterior cortex followed by the posterior cortex and then the midshaft fibular osteotomy. The blade plate is then placed, and the angular correction is made under manual valgus force, distracting and reapproximating the tibial osteotomy. An articulated compression device is used through the blade plate to provide compression to the osteotomy in order to obtain the angle of correction desired. Postoperative wound care and analgesics are the same as for the other tibial osteotomies described.

Postoperative Care

Patients generally stay in the hospital 3 to 4 days after high tibial osteotomy. Deep muscle compartment drains are left in place for 3 days postoperatively with 48 hours of epidural. If the drains fall out, then the epidural is immediately discontinued so that compartment status can be carefully monitored and clinical examination performed. Continuous passive motion begins the second day after surgery to help restore motion. The patient is generally sent home with a continuous passive motion machine for 3 weeks postoperatively unless intraarticular work is added. Continuous passage motion is used for 6 weeks to prevent adhesions and enhance cartilage repair or health. Nonsteroidal antiinflammatory medications

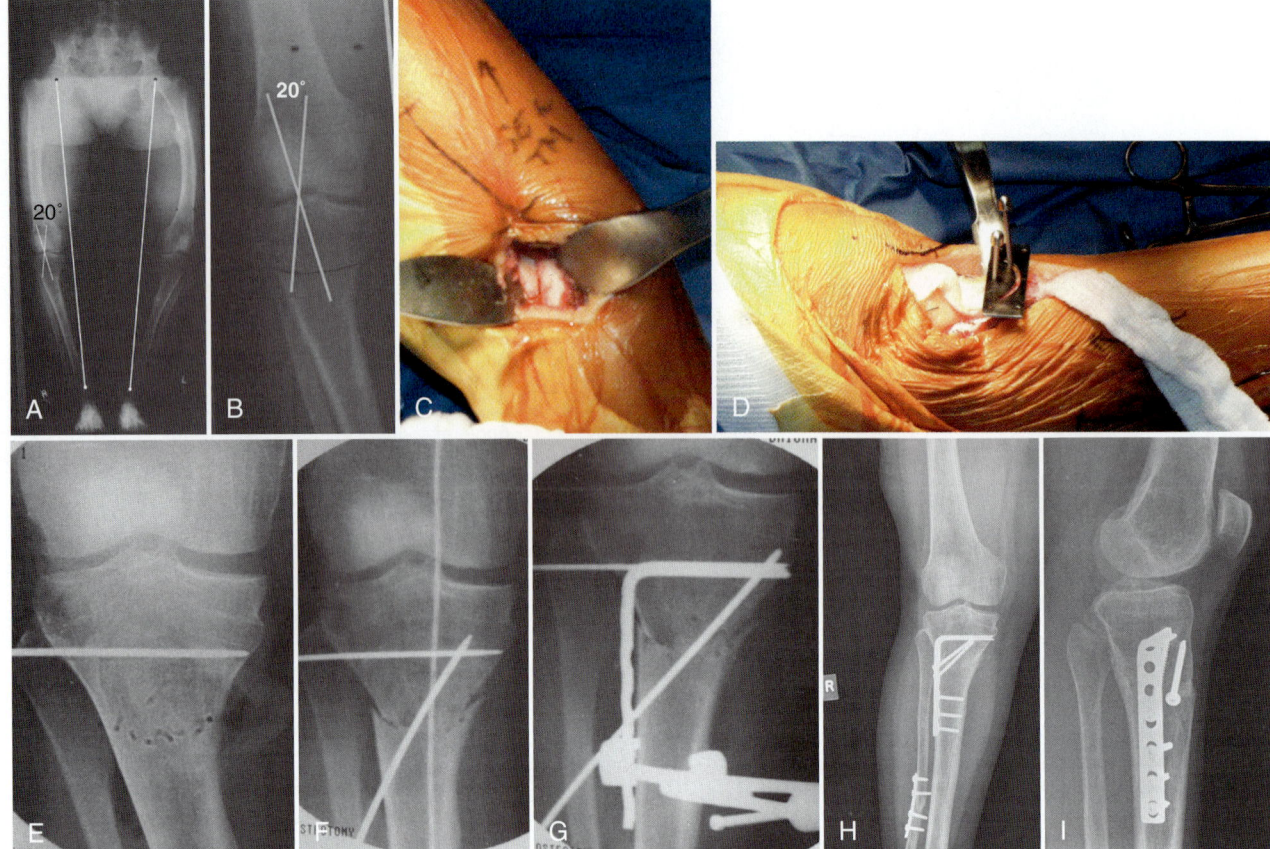

Figure 8–15 *A*, Long alignment films in a 31-year-old woman with familial vitamin D-resistant rickets. X-ray films demonstrate severe varus malalignment with mechanical axis falling outside of the medial aspect of the knee joints. Presently the right knee is very symptomatic with medially based pain. There is mild deformity in the femur with varus bow malalignment but more so in the proximal tibia. *B*, A 20-degree angular correction is required to place the mechanical axis through the lateral tibial spine unloading the medial compartment. This can be performed partly through the femur and the tibia. In this case, the decision was made that because the femoral contribution to the deformity was not severe (unlike the left knee), the correction would be performed entirely through the tibia with a reverse dome tibial valgus osteotomy. The outline of the proposed dome osteotomy is demonstrated in the metaphysis of the proximal tibia. This will be performed below the level of the tibial tubercle around a center of arc of rotation that is at the center of the knee. *C*, A midshaft fibular osteotomy is first performed at the junction between the superficial posterior muscle compartment and the lateral muscle compartment in an oblique fashion. *D*, Several different crescentic jigs are available that match the width of the proximal metaphyseal curve. An appropriate jig is chosen, and several small drill holes are made centrally through the tibia from anterior to posterior to be used to connect the dots with a thin sharp 0.25-inch osteotome. *E*, Fluoroscopic radiograph taken after the dome drill holes were made through the tibia. Because the patient is of very small stature, a pediatric blade plate guidewire is placed parallel to the joint line to produce a 90-degree cannulated blade plate. Sponges are placed behind the tibia after a dissection is made to take down the anterolateral muscle compartment and to release the superficial medial collateral ligament and the pes anserinus tendon attachments to the medial aspect of the tibia. The osteotomy is performed from anterior to posterior with a osteotome. The distal fragment is gently distracted hinged around the dome osteotome and placed on the lateral side to produce the desired correction. *F*, Fluoroscopic radiograph after the fragment was fixated with a temporary K-wire at the proposed level of correction. A Bovie cord has been placed from the center of the femoral head to the center of the talus at the ankle, demonstrating that the mechanical axis falls to the medial tibial spine. This is believed to be an adequate correction for this severe deformity. *G*, A 90-degree cannulated pediatric blade plate (no offset available) is applied to the proximal fragment, and an articulated compression device is placed distally to compress the two fragments together before screws are placed. *H*, Final appearance of the tibia 1 year after osteotomy surgery. Note minimal deformity in the upper tibia despite such a large angular correction. This formation does not jeopardize any potential future reconstructive needs for the patient. *I*, Lateral radiography after reverse dome tibial valgus producing osteotomy.

are not used following surgery because they may interfere with bone healing. Patients remain on touch weight-bearing until radiographic evidence of bony healing is seen, then a graduated weight-bearing program is allowed.

OSTEOTOMY FOR INSTABILITY: THE SAGITTAL CORRECTION

Tibial osteotomy is also very powerful in the sagittal plane. Opening and closing wedge osteotomies may be performed to correct hyperextension of the knee and lessen posterior cruciate ligament (PCL) insufficiency with a flexion osteotomy (Figure 8–16) or decrease a flexion deformity of the knee and lessen ACL insufficiency with extension osteotomy (Figure 8–17). If ACL insufficiency is present, then the more posterior the slope, the more likely the tibia will translate forward. Lessening this tibial slope with an extension osteotomy lessens the tendency for anterior translation of the tibia. Similarly, the tibia tends to slide posteriorly with minimal posterior slope in a PCL-insufficient knee with femoral rollback. Increasing tibial slope with a flexion osteotomy lessens the likelihood of posterior tibial translation. These principles can be used for hyperextension deformities of the knee as well as fixed flexion deformities around the knee. They can be combined with valgus-producing tibial osteotomies but will increase the complexity of the osteotomy.

ACL LAXITY WITH VARUS

The ACL-injured knee frequently has varus alignment and often an increased tibial sagittal slope. This puts ACL reconstruction at increased risk for failure.

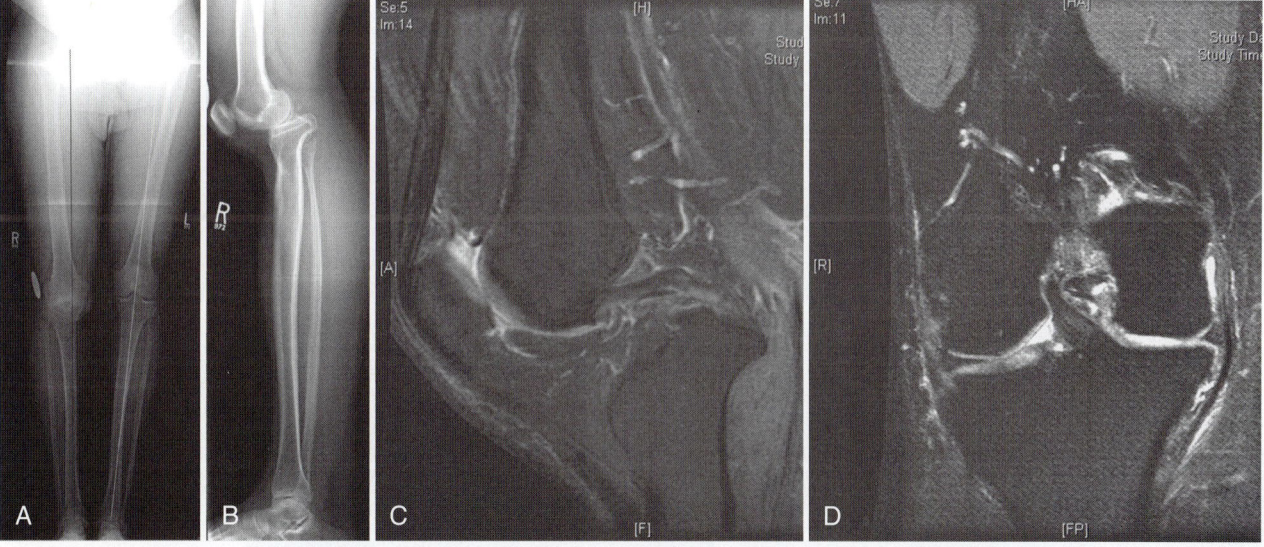

Figure 8–16 *A*, Recurvatum/posterior cruciate ligament (PCL) insufficiency. Long axial alignment x-ray films in a 50-year-old man who has experienced difficulty with weight bearing over the last 6 months. He has experienced hyperextension instability of his knee. A femoral fracture sustained when he was a boy had been treated by skeletal traction with a tibial traction pin. The tibial traction pin was applied through the proximal tibia, presumably injuring his anterior epiphyseal plate and resulting in growth arrest anteriorly and a deviated sagittal tibial slope. His joint line is not visible on standing anteroposterior (AP) or long alignment AP x-ray films. *B*, Weight-bearing x-ray films in the lateral plane demonstrate posterior translation of the tibia with a tibial upslope in the sagittal plane secondary to anterior tibial growth plate arrest after pediatric use of a tibial skeletal traction pin. *C*, Magnetic resonance imaging (MRI) in the sagittal plane demonstrates that the posterior cruciate ligament and the articular surfaces of the patellofemoral joint are intact. *D*, Coronal MRI demonstrating intact collateral ligaments and anterior cruciate ligament with loss of articular cartilage on the medial femoral condyle. *E*, This case demonstrates the need for corrective osteotomy by increasing the posterior sagittal slope. This patient had a reversed sagittal slope with an upslope in the posterior direction secondary to an anterior tibial epiphyseal arrest from a traction bow. The principles for correction require restoration of a posterior sagittal slope with an anterior to posterior osteotomy leaving the posterior hinge intact until the recurvatum disappears, which is noted immediately intraoperatively (see panel *G*). The same technique can be performed to prevent posterior translation of a tibia in a patient with symptomatic posterior cruciate instability accompanied by medial compartment osteoarthritis. A tibial valgus-producing osteotomy is performed with the osteotomy opened more anteriorly than posteriorly. In this manner, the tibial slope is increased, and PCL instability is lessened in addition to unloading the damaged medial compartment.

Continued

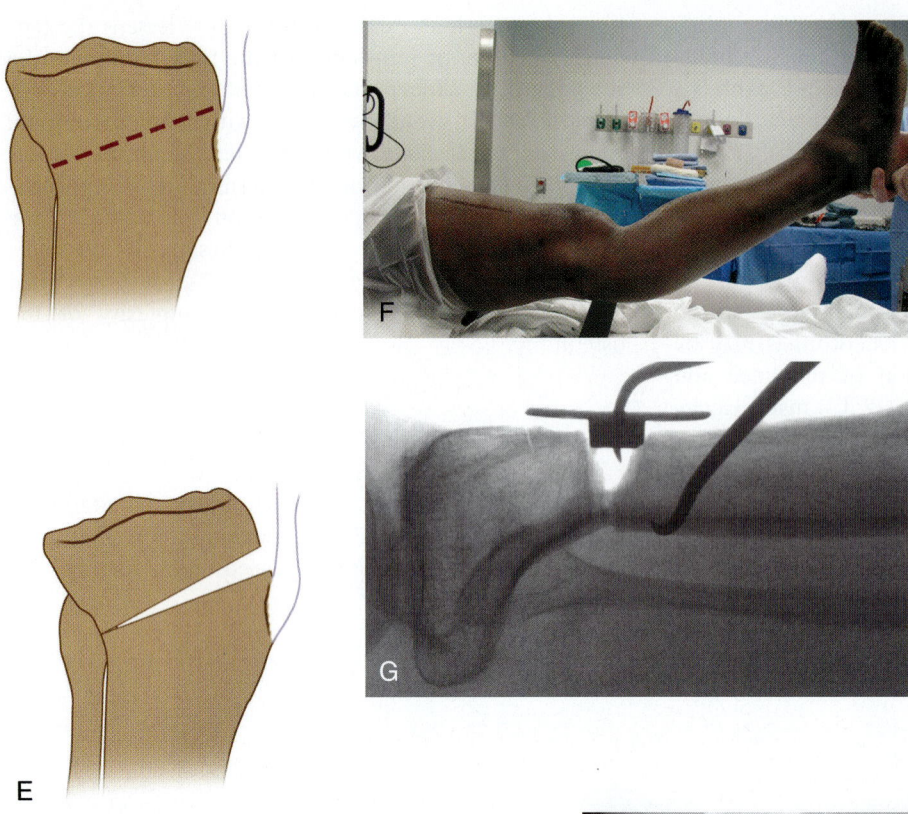
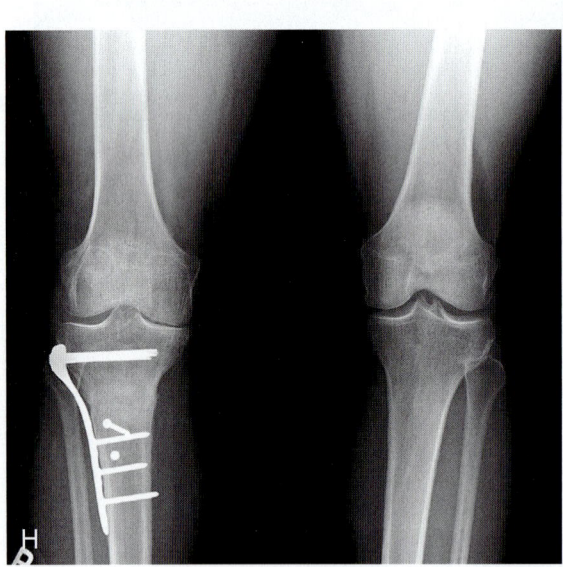
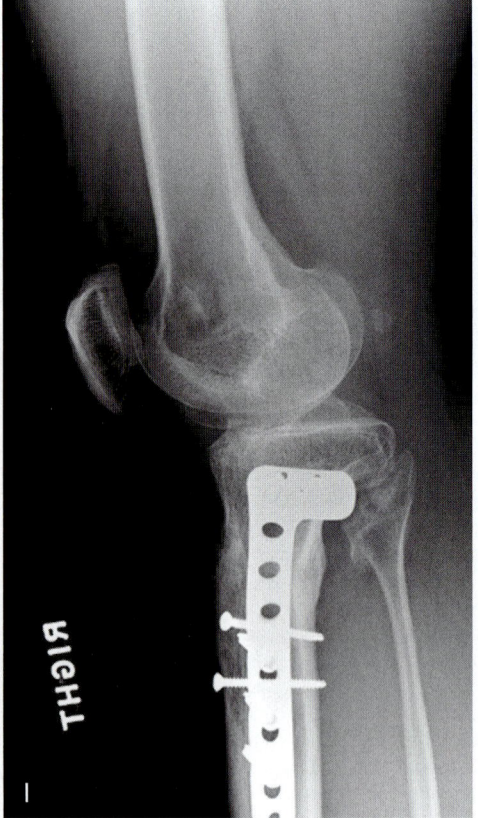

Figure 8-16—cont'd *F,* Clinical evaluation of the knee during operative correction with approximately 30 degrees of hyperextension deformity. *G,* Anterior flexion osteotomy is performed after taking off the tibial tubercle to gain exposure at the level of the deformity at the metaphyseal–diaphyseal junction. The osteotomy is opened anteriorly until full extension without hyperextension is obtained. A spacer plate of the appropriate anterior opening is applied to temporarily confirm the osteotomy position as noted. *H,* Postoperative (AP views) appearance 1 year after surgery. Osteotomy is solidly united demonstrating tangential articular joint views. A locking plate was used for the fixation. *I,* Lateral x-ray film demonstrates a 0-degree tibial slope without hyperextension deformity and a fever that is centrally located on the tibia and is not subluxed anteriorly. The patient remains asymptomatic many years later.

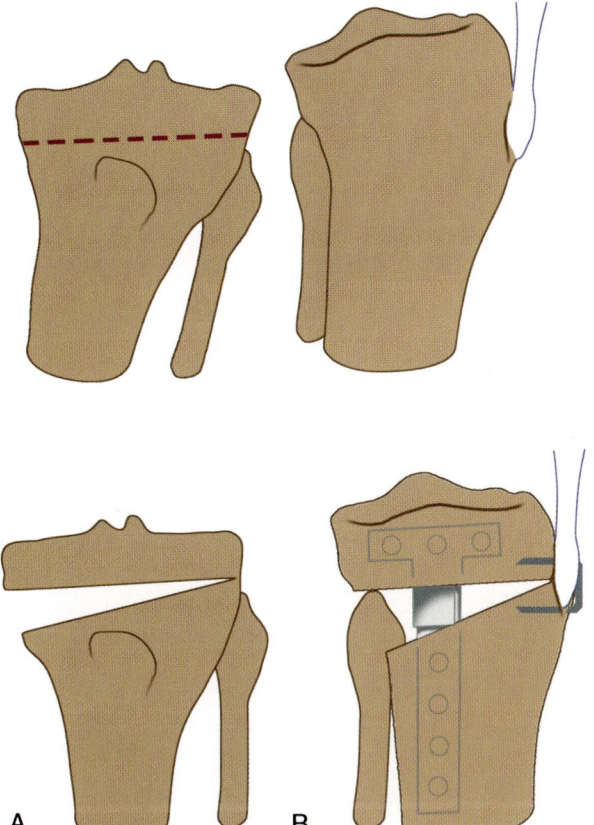

Figure 8–17 Anterior cruciate ligament (ACL) insufficiency is frequently associated with increased posterior tibial sagittal slope. *A*, Frontal view. A valgus-producing osteotomy in an ACL-deficient knee decreases the posterior sagittal slope. *B*, Lateral view. A tibial valgus-extension osteotomy will assist in stabilizing the tendency toward anterior translation of the tibia by preferentially opening the osteotomy posteriorly as shown.

Articular injury at the time of ACL disruption is often on the medial compartment of the joint; therefore, reconstruction will require attention to all background factors for successful clinical outcome. Restoring neutral alignment in the frontal plane will optimize the chance of success of cartilage repair in the medial compartment or osteoarthritic degenerative change in the medial compartment. Improving and restoring to normal amounts (3–5 degrees), the sagittal slope, by decreasing the sagittal slope will decrease the tendency toward anterior translation of the tibia. In this situation, an opening wedge valgus-producing tibial osteotomy in combination with an extension osteotomy may be performed by placing the opening wedge plate more posteriorly, thereby decreasing the sagittal slope of the tibia. An anterior staple may help prevent anterior opening. Using a small sagittal saw to make a rectangular space for a rectangular spacer block plate posteriorly by taking some extra bone away from the distal fragment ensures that the slope is lessened. Intraoperative radiography or fluoroscopy to assess the lateral view of the tibia and the sagittal slope is necessary for confirmation (see diagrammatic representation in Figure 8–17).

CONCLUSION

Using the techniques described, I have found high tibial osteotomy to be safe and reproducible, and does not jeopardize future prosthetic reconstruction of the knee joint. It was originally indicated for unloading medial compartment osteoarthritis with varus deformity. This indication still applies; however, improved osteotomy techniques provide accurate corrections with minimal cosmetic disfigurement or change in the shape of the proximal tibia. In addition, the indications now include optimizing the success of cartilage repair for medial lesions in the varus knee with mechanical correction to normalize the mechanical environment of the joint and place the mechanical axis to neutral alignment. Exciting improvements in osteotomy include an understanding of the effect of altering the sagittal slope of the tibia to improve stability in the anteroposterior plane of the knee joint.

When performed accurately, high tibial osteotomy is a reproducible and satisfying procedure that may optimize the outcome of cartilage repair and joint instability, alleviate the pain of osteoarthritis, and allow improved levels of activity with joint preservation.

REFERENCES

1. Centers for Disease Control and Prevention. Arthritis prevalence and activity limitations—United States, 1990. *JAMA*. 1994;272:346–347.
2. Coventry MB, Ilstrup DM, Wallrichs SL. Proximal tibial osteotomy. A critical long-term study of eighty-seven cases. *J Bone Joint Surg Am*. 1993;75:196–201.
3. Korbyl R, Minas T. Clinical Outcomes after high tibial osteotomy in young active patients. Presentation at the Harvard Hip and Knee Course, Boston, MA, September 2003.
4. Sharma L, Song J, Felson DT, et al. The role of knee alignment in disease progression and functional decline in knee osteoarthritis. *JAMA*. 2001;286:188–195.
5. Sahlstrom A, Johnell O, Redlund-Johnell I. The natural course of arthrosis of the knee. *Clin Orthop Relat Res*. 1997;152–157.
6. Rinonapoli E, Mancini GB, Corvaglia A, et al. Tibial osteotomy for varus gonarthrosis. A 10- to 21-year followup study. *Clin Orthop Relat Res*. 1998;353:185–193.
7. Mina C, Garrett Jr WE, Ricardo P, et al. High tibial osteotomy for unloading osteochondral defects in the medial compartment of the knee. *Am J Sports Med*. 2008;36:949–955.
8. Ogden S, Mukherjee DS, Keating MM, et al. Changes in load distribution in the knee after opening wedge or closing wedge high tibial osteotomy. *J Arthroplasty*. 2009;24:101–109.
9. Paley D. *Principles of deformity correction*. Berlin: Springer-Verlag; 2002.
10. Klecker RJ, Winalski CS, Aliabadi P, et al. The aberrant anterior tibial artery, Magnetic resonance appearance, prevalence, and surgical implications. *Am J Sports Med*. 2008;36:720–727.
11. Shetty AA, Tindall AJ, Qureshi F, et al. The effect of knee flexion on the popliteal artery and its surgical significance. *J Bone Joint Surg Br*. 2003;85-B:218–222.
12. Dugdale TW, Noyes FR, Styer D. Preoperative planning for high tibial osteotomy: Effect of lateral tibiofemoral separation and tibiofemoral length. *Clin Orthop*. 1992;271:105–121.

# Chapter 9

Femoral Varus Osteotomy

Tom Minas, MD, MS

INTRODUCTION
INDICATIONS
PLANNING
OPENING WEDGE VARUS FEMORAL OSTEOTOMY

Technique and Aftercare
REVERSE DOME FEMORAL VARUS OSTEOTOMY
CLOSING WEDGE VARUS FEMORAL OSTEOTOMY: CLASSIC TECHNIQUE

DISTAL FEMORAL VARUS CLOSING WEDGE OSTEOTOMY FOR VALGUS MALALIGNMENT WITH OSTEOCHONDRAL REPAIR
SUMMARY

INTRODUCTION

The valgus knee (Figure 9–1) is usually secondary to hypoplasia of the lateral femoral condyle resulting in a superior lateral directed joint line. Corrective osteotomy is most appropriately performed at the level of the deformity to restore a joint line that will be parallel to the floor. For this reason, correction of valgus malalignment is performed through the femur. As in tibial corrective osteotomies, osteotomies may be closing wedge, opening wedge, or reverse dome. Each has advantages and disadvantages. The clinical outcomes following femoral osteotomies parallel those of tibial osteotomies; however, femoral osteotomies are much less common, as is the literature on them.[1,2] One possible reason is that the disease pattern frequently involves the patellofemoral joint when the knee is in valgus, and correction of both arthritic conditions is technically more demanding and less predictable.

INDICATIONS

Femoral varus-producing osteotomy is indicated for unloading a laterally based articular cartilage defect, pain secondary to lateral compartment overload, or lateral compartment osteoarthritis with intact medial and patellofemoral articulations. Unlike tibial osteotomy, which is very effective for addressing instability such as anterior cruciate ligament or posterior cruciate ligament secondary to sagittal slope correction, changing the flexion or extension of the distal femur has no influence on instability. Overall, femoral osteotomies are technically more challenging to perform because of the larger soft tissue envelope, the longer lever arm, which can displace the osteotomy as it is being performed, and its proximity to the articular surface of the trochlea and the femoral artery. My choice of which type of femoral osteotomy to use is dependent on the degree of correction, the leg length discrepancy, and the need for bone grafting of an osteochondral defect. Like opening wedge tibial osteotomies, an opening wedge femoral osteotomy is technically easier to perform than closing wedge or reverse dome osteotomies because it allows a "dial-in" accurate correction. It has the disadvantage of requiring the use of bone graft; however, I have found that allograft materials (specifically a combination of cancellous allograft bone chips with demineralized bone matrix) heal in the same amount of time as autograft bone.

I use opening wedge femoral osteotomies for corrections up to 15 degrees because I have found that for greater corrections, the distal fragment has a tendency to flex as it remains hinged on the medial side at the level of the adductor tubercle, which is in a relatively posterior axis. In addition, the iliotibial band starts to become very tight as corrections greater than 15 degrees are attempted. A shortened leg length on the affected side is another relative indication for use of an opening wedge varus-producing osteotomy, which tends to equalize leg lengths.

Femoral Varus Osteotomy CHAPTER 9 147

The supracondylar reverse dome osteotomy remains a powerful osteotomy for large angular corrections and is my choice for corrections greater than 15 degrees.[3] It requires the use of an angled blade plate to obtain stable fixation or use of another fixed-angle device.

Closing wedge varus-producing femoral osteotomies heal more rapidly than the other two types of osteotomies and provide a source of autogenous bone graft if an osteochondral defect of the lateral femoral condyle requires osseous bone grafting. If the affected leg is long, a closing wedge osteotomy is preferred to equalize leg lengths.

PLANNING

The goal of femoral osteotomy correction is similar to that of tibial valgus-producing osteotomy. If weight-bearing x-ray films demonstrate intact joint spaces and valgus malalignment is present with mechanical axis forces through the lateral compartment, then correction of the mechanical axis is made to the midline if an articular cartilage defect is being unloaded (Figure 9–2). This normalizes the forces across the joint. If joint space narrowing is present or a large articular cartilage defect is undergoing repair, then the aim is to unload the lateral compartment by only 2 degrees, which corresponds to the medial tibial spine. In this way, premature wear of the medial compartment is less likely.

Long alignment x-ray films in a double-stance anteroposterior phase are required for calculating angular correction (Figures 9–3 and 9–4). A line from the center

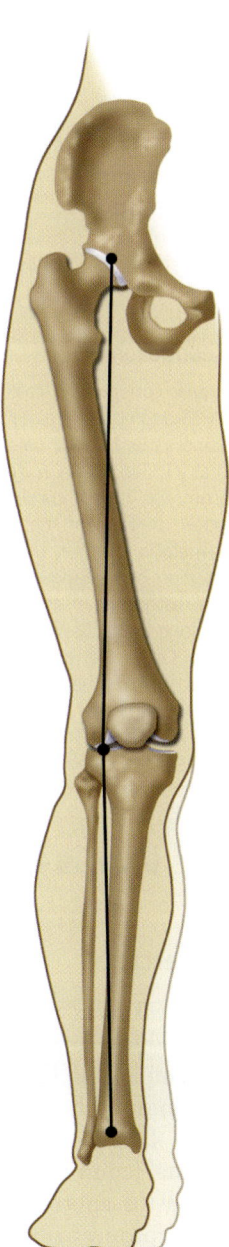

Figure 9–1 Valgus mechanical alignment is associated with hypoplasia of the lateral femoral condyle and a superior lateral directed joint line.

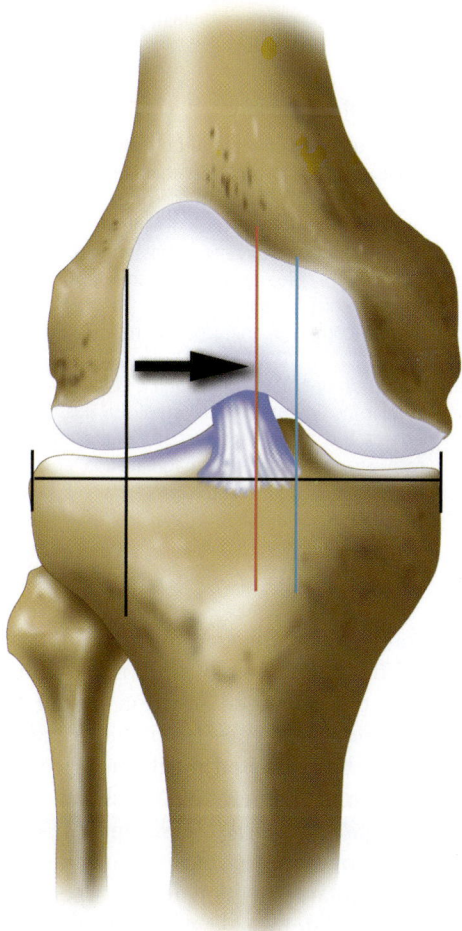

Figure 9–2 The desired mechanical axis correction is to the midline of the knee (*red line*) in a situation of cartilage repair with no joint space narrowing of the lateral compartment or a 2-degree overcorrection to the medial tibial spine (*blue line*) when osteoarthritis or joint space narrowing is present.

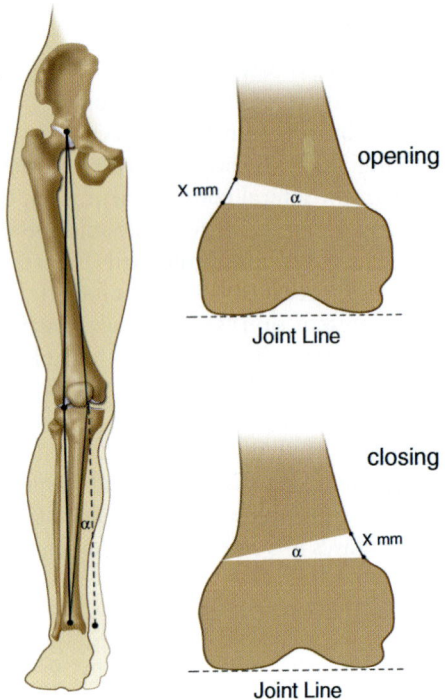

α = angle of correction

Figure 9–3 The angle of correction for a varus-producing femoral osteotomy is measured on a long alignment x-ray film. The angle from the existing center of the ankle to the proposed mechanical axis at the knee (see Figure 9–2) and back to the new position of the ankle represents the angular correction. This angle is applied to the level of the opening or closing wedge osteotomy on the distal femoral metaphyseal–diaphyseal junction. The measurements in millimeters, x, is the correct opening or closing osteotomy. Opening wedge systems generally have spacer plates in millimeters that correspond to the preoperative planning. Closing wedge systems usually have angular increments on the osteotomy jigs that accurately measure in degrees the angular correction. Digitized x-ray systems with built-in software, calibrated for magnification error, make the planning very straightforward (General Electric web-based Centricity software [GE Healthcare, Waukesha, WI]).

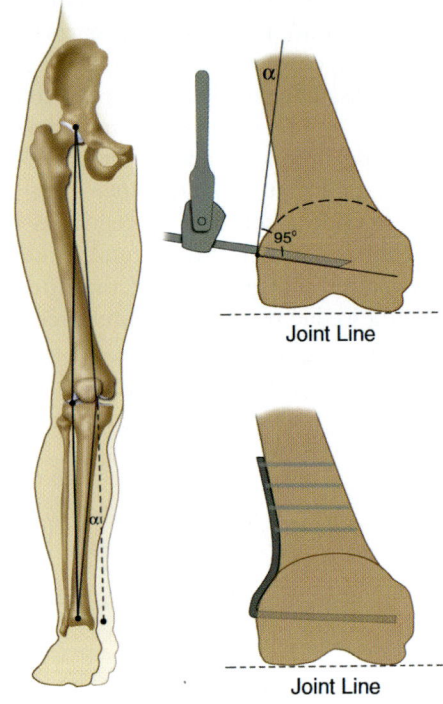

α = angle of correction

Figure 9–4 The angular correction is calculated and identical to obtained in Figure 9–3. A 95-degree blade plate is used for fixation of a supracondylar reverse dome varus femoral osteotomy, although other fixed-angle devices, such as a locking plate, may be used. The corrective angle α is measured from the lateral cortex of the femur to the intersection of the proposed position of the 95-degree angled blade plate. Generally, angled metallic triangles that have the angle α are placed along the plate portion of the angled blade plate. This allows placement of a guidewire along the plane of the entry blade. The seating chisel then passes along the guidewire prior to the supracondylar femoral dome osteotomy. Once the osteotomy is completed, the 95-degree blade plate is placed along the tract of the seating chisel, and the alignment of the leg is corrected with a varus force until the plate portion fits flush to the lateral femoral cortex. An articulated compression device is applied, the osteotomy site is compressed, and screw fixation completes the stabilization of the osteotomy.

of the femoral head is projected to the desired mechanical axis of either the center of the knee or the medial tibial spine to the proposed position of the foot. An angular correction then goes from the existing center of the ankle to the proposed mechanical axis point at the knee and then to the new ankle position. This acute angle is the *angular correction*. This angular correction is converted to opening or closing millimeters using digital x-ray templates to plan for an opening wedge osteotomy on the lateral side of the distal femur or a closing wedge osteotomy on the medial side of the femur above the adductor tubercle and trochlea. This angle also allows planning for placement of a chisel for use of an angled blade plate relative to the tibial femoral joint line (see Figure 9–4).

OPENING WEDGE VARUS FEMORAL OSTEOTOMY

Technique and Aftercare

An opening wedge femoral varus-producing osteotomy is performed through a midline incision. Figure 9–5 shows an appropriate case example, and Figure 9–6 outlines the surgery in stepwise fashion. The deep exposure can be performed through a lateral subvastus approach to approach the lateral distal femur for an extraarticular surgery. The lateral subvastus approach can be combined with a tibial tubercle osteotomy to expose the entire distal femur and joint without a muscle split. I usually use a lateral parapatellar arthrotomy to expose the distal lateral femur as well as the patellofemoral articulation.

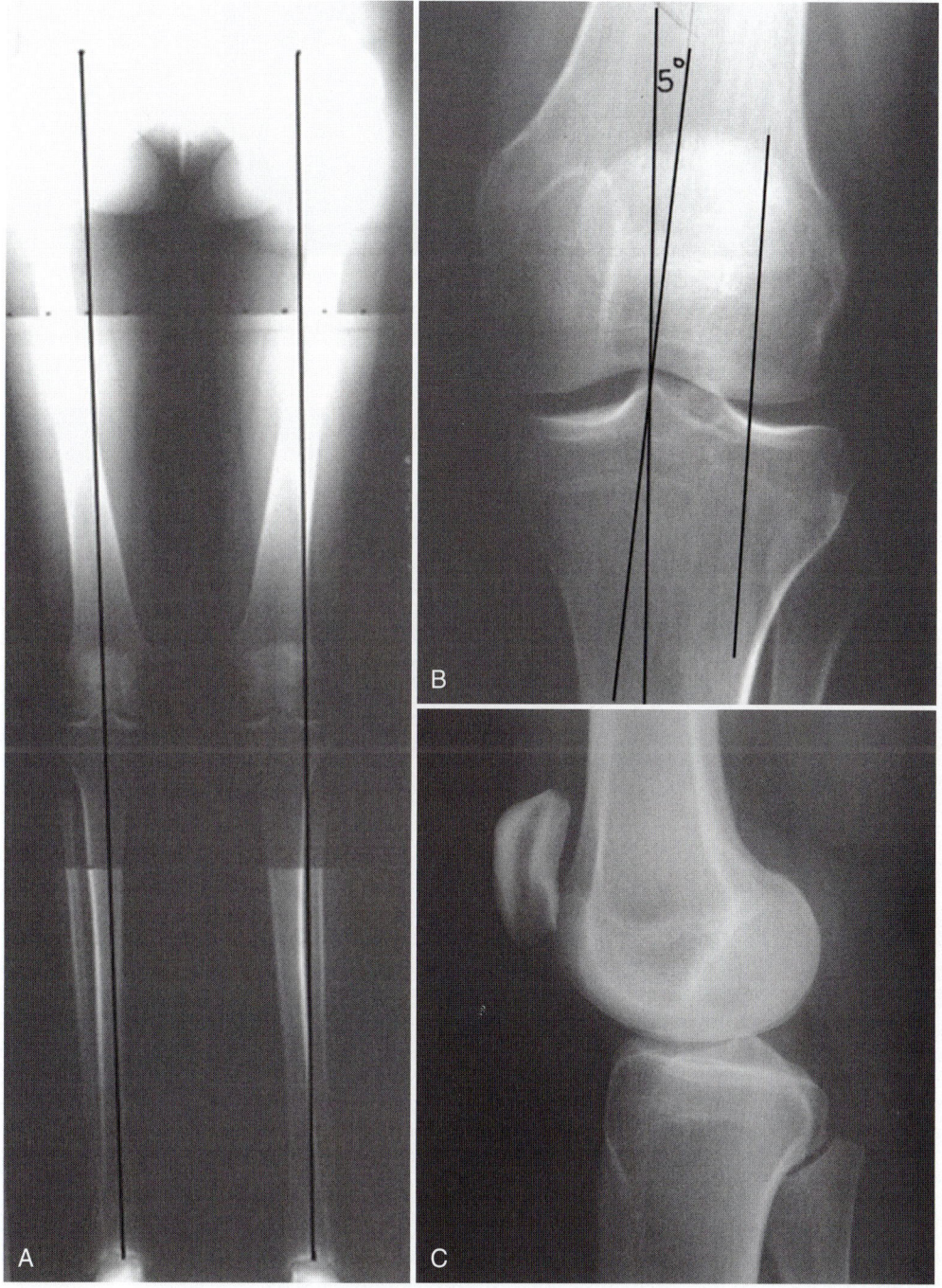

Figure 9-5 *A,* Long alignment x-ray films of a 6-foot 1-inch, 23-year-old woman who has experienced disabling anterior and lateral knee pain for 9 months. Her clinical appearance shows that she has valgus malalignment to her left leg with equal leg lengths, patellofemoral lateral maltracking with subluxation and tilt of the patella, and a positive J-sign as she flexes her knee from a fully extended position. She has a positive patellar compression test, mild crepitus, lateral joint line tenderness, and a stable knee to collateral and anteroposterior testing. *B,* Mechanical axis to the left knee falls through the center of the lateral tibiofemoral compartment. A 5-degree angular correction is required to place her mechanical axis to the medial tibial spine. *C, D,* Lateral and skyline x-ray films demonstrate mild patella alta with a well-centered patella on a 45-degree tangential skyline x-ray film with intact joint spaces.

Continued

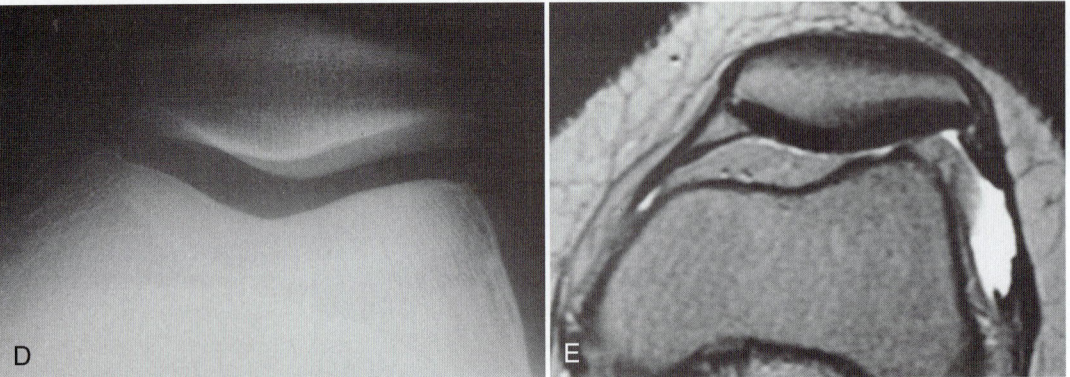

Figure 9-5—cont'd *E,* Corresponding axial magnetic resonance scan demonstrates intact articular surfaces to the patella and trochlea with lateral patella subluxation. A combined varus femoral osteotomy in addition to anteromedialization of the tibial tubercle (see Figure 9-6) is planned to unload and normalize the joint forces and thereby alleviate the patient's symptoms.

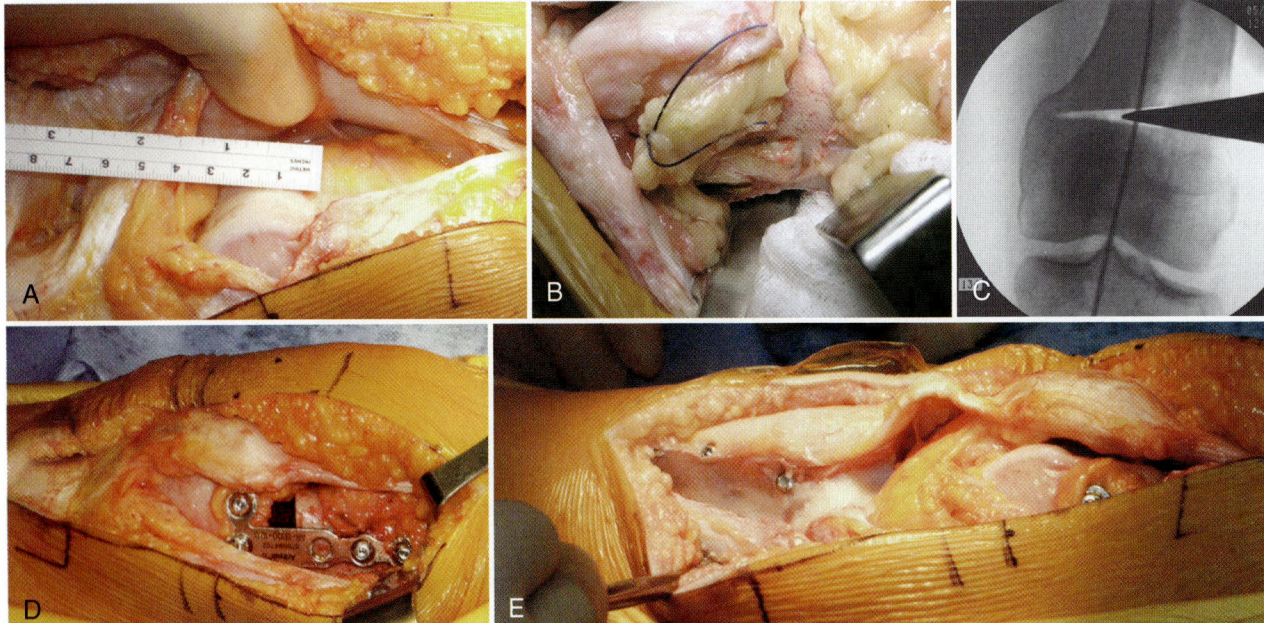

Figure 9-6 *A,* Midline surgical approach was performed to the knee. (The foot is to the *left* of the image and the head on the *right*.) A lateral parapatellar arthrotomy demonstrates lateral wear of the trochlea and exposes the distal lateral femur. *B,* In preparation for a distal femoral varus osteotomy, the intermuscular septum is dissected sharply off the linea aspera on the lateral side for an opening wedge osteotomy (and the distal medial femur to the adductor tubercle on the medial side when performing a closing wedge osteotomy). With the knee flexed and the intermuscular septum released off the sharp posterior lateral distal corner of the femur, it is very easy to digitally sweep off the fatty area and any tissue and neurovascular structures off the back of the femur all the way to the adductor tubercle on the opposite side. Small wet sponges and a retractor are easily placed directly on the back of the femur to protect the neurovascular structures prior to use of an oscillating saw for the distal femoral osteotomy. The osteotomy is performed with the knee in full extension, easily stabilized by an assistant, with minimal risk to the neurovascular structures posteriorly and with good saw control anteriorly to avoid the trochlea. *C,* Opening wedge tines are gently impacted to the desired level of opening that is preoperatively planned. The assistant provides counterpressure on the medial side of the knee so as to not break through the metaphyseal medial hinge. An intraoperative check using a Bovie guidewire from the center of the femoral head to the center of the ankle passes to the desired level at the medial tibial spine. In addition, the clinical appearance of the leg appears to be neutral to minimal varus. At this time, the osteotomy can be fixated in its desired position and bone grafted. *D,* Once the femoral osteotomy is stabilized with internal fixation, the tracking of the patella is assessed after valgus alignment is corrected with a full-thickness lateral release being left open. In this case, the patella continues to track laterally, there is thinning of the articular surface of the trochlea laterally, and it is believed that an unloading tibial tubercle osteotomy is necessary to centralize and unload the lateral patellofemoral facet. Autologous bone graft from the left iliac crest was used to bone graft the femoral osteotomy in this patient, who was treated in 2003. Since then, combined allograft cancellous bone chips and demineralized bone matrix have been used as an allograft mixture. The allograft mixture is placed in the defect at the completion of the osteotomy and prior to release of the tourniquet. When the tourniquet is released, marrow-derived elements permeate the allograft mixture completely with bone-forming cells and growth factors. I have found the allograft mixture heals as quickly as autologous bone graft. I have used this mixture in place of autologous bone graft and have noted it lessens the morbidity of the procedure. *E,* Fulkerson (anteromedial tibial tubercle osteotomy, see Chapter 10) osteotomy with the distal hinge intact is performed. Three 3.5-mm cortical screws are used to lag the osteotomy in place. Stable fixation is obtained, and continuous passive motion starts the next day.

A key part of the exposure is to protect the posterior neurovascular structures. This can be performed by releasing the vastus lateralis attachment to the lateral intermuscular septum and the linea aspera distally for 3 cm off the back of the femur sharply. With the knee flexed, the posterior structures on the back of the femur are easily dissected with a finger bluntly. Small wet sponges are packed behind the femur along with a Hohmann retractor to protect the femoral artery and the other neurovascular structures. A breakaway notched guidewire is placed across the femur from the supracondylar lateral position of the proposed osteotomy just proximal to the trochlea across to the adductor tubercle on the medial side. The supracondylar synovium is split and subperiosteally dissected, leaving a cuff attached distally to the trochlea. Methylene blue is used in a longitudinal fashion at the level of the osteotomy to mark the correct rotation. The guidewire is then broken at one of its notches near to lateral femoral cortex, and the leg is kept in full extension with the posterior neurovascular structures protected with a Hohmann retractor and sponges. An oscillating saw is used to cut obliquely across the femur along the path of the guidewire under direct visualization and image intensification on a radiolucent operating room table. The last 1 cm is cut using an osteotome to the medial cortex but not through it at the level of the metaphyseal bone so as to allow "a greenstick-type" opening without fracture and displacement of the two fragments. Opening wedge tines or laminar spreaders are used to gently open the lateral cortex to the desired amount per the preoperative plan. When the desired opening is attained, a secondary check is made with intraoperative assessment by clinical appearance and image intensification assessment using a solid rod or Bovie cord that extends from the femoral head to the talus at the ankle to assess the desired mechanical axis. (An opening of 15 mm is generally the maximum that can be performed based on tightness of the lateral structures of the knee, especially the iliotibial band. More than this a reverse dome osteotomy should be considered.) A femoral Puddu plate with the desired opening spacer block is applied to the distal femur and fixated with distal cancellous screws and proximal cortical screws or a locking plate. Bone graft supplement is used to fill the defect. My preference is a combination of cancellous allogenic bone chips and demineralized bone matrix. I stopped using autograft bone in 2003 and have found that union is predictable and as fast as with autograft, without the associated morbidity to the patient. The supracondylar synovium is sutured overtop of the bone graft such that it remains outside of joint space. The tourniquet is then let down, and the bone marrow elements permeate the bone graft, enhancing its biologic capacity to heal. Antiadhesion membrane is placed directly on top of the synovium to prevent postoperative adhesions. Suction drains are placed in the soft tissue envelope subcutaneously. I generally do not close the lateral retinaculum adjacent to the patella so as not to cause increased mechanical pressures across the patellofemoral joint. A tight subcutaneous closure is performed. A light dressing and a hinged knee brace, combined with cryotherapy, are used postoperatively. Deep vein thrombosis prophylaxis in the form of oral warfarin (Coumadin) is used for 3 weeks postoperatively, maintaining the international normalized ratio at a prophylactic level of 1.5 to 2.0. Continuous passive motion and touch weight-bearing are used for 6 weeks postoperatively. A check x-ray film is taken postoperatively at baseline and at 6-week and 10-week x-ray opening (Figure 9–7). Wedge femoral osteotomies generally heal solidly between 10 and 14 weeks. Partial weight bearing is allowed starting at 6 weeks based on the appearance of radiographic union. Full weight bearing is not permitted until solid healing has occurred as seen by x-ray film.

REVERSE DOME FEMORAL VARUS OSTEOTOMY

The reverse dome distal femoral varus-producing osteotomy as described by Paley[3] is my preferred osteotomy for correction greater than 15 degrees. The osteotomy is based on the "center of rotation arc" around a central point at the center of the knee. By creating a

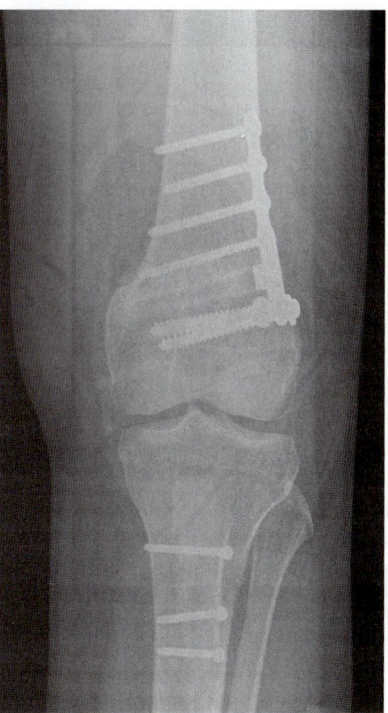

Figure 9–7 Final radiographic appearance 6 months after femoral varus osteotomy and tibial tubercle osteotomy. The patient has become pain free and continues to function well at latest follow-up 6 years later.

circular osteotomy about this center that captures the width of the medial and lateral distal femoral metaphyseal flares, the lower leg can be rotated about this pivot point without appreciable distortion of the femoral anatomy. The soft tissue structures remain balanced and are not overly tightened. Future reconstruction with total knee arthroplasty is not compromised. Figure 9–8 shows diagrammatic representations of the surgical technique. Figure 9–9 show a clinical example.

CLOSING WEDGE VARUS FEMORAL OSTEOTOMY: CLASSIC TECHNIQUE

A diagrammatic representation of a classic femoral closing wedge osteotomy is illustrated in Figure 9–10. The surgical stepwise technique used in a patient is shown in Figure 9–11 and performed as shown in Figure 9–12. An anterior incision is made to the knee and a medial subvastus arthrotomy performed. This allows exposure to the distal femur and to the joint. The distal aspect of the medial intermuscular septum at its insertion on the adductor tubercle and supracondylar femur is released off the posterior aspect of the femur. With the knee flexed, a blunt finger dissection sweeps away the neurovascular structures off the back of the femoral cortex, where they can be protected with small wet sponges and a retractor, as well as one to retract the anterior quadriceps so that good circumferential visualization is adequate. A guidewire is placed parallel to the tibial femoral joint for the placement of a 90-degree offset blade plate chisel. The entry site is started with three 4.5-mm drill bits. This should be located at least 2.5 cm above the joint line and above the intercondylar notch so as not to penetrate the intercondylar anterior and posterior cruciate ligaments. The chisel tract is then made at least 50 to 60 mm deep.

The femoral osteotomy is performed at least 2.5 cm above the proposed blade plate chisel entry site to allow adequate bone bridge during compression of the

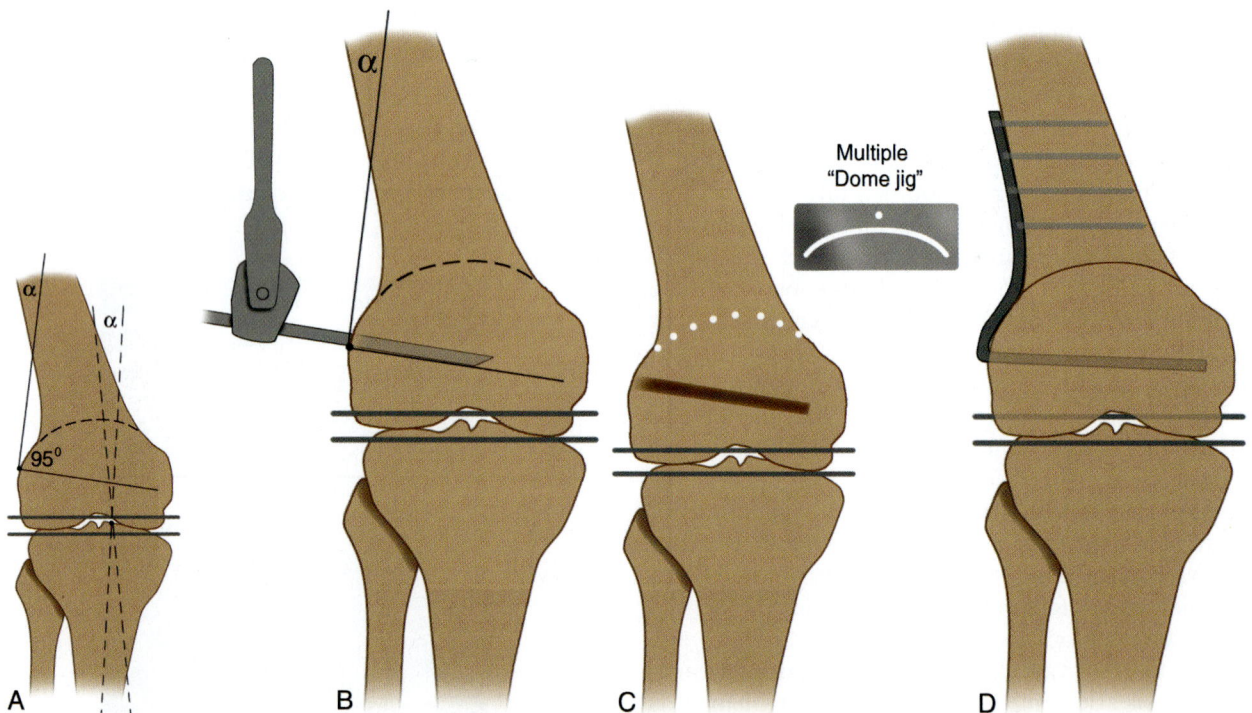

Figure 9–8 *A,* Step 1: Desired angular correction for the femoral osteotomy angle α is calculated per Figure 9–3. I prefer to use a 95-degree angled blade plate for accurate fixation for a reverse dome osteotomy. The seating chisel entry to the distal femoral metaphysis is key for correction of the osteotomy. Using a 95-degree angled blade plate, a guidewire can be placed along the path of the blade entry, noting the correction angle α between the plate and the lateral femoral cortex, which usually can be referenced with a metallic angled triangle used for osteotomies. *B,* Step 2: The seating chisel for the blade plate is introduced along the path of the guidewire in the usual fashion of drilling the outer cortices and seating the chisel inward and outward under fluoroscopic guidance to ensure the path is along the guidewire. *C,* Step 3: Several crescentic domes are applied to the distal femoral metaphysis until an appropriate arc that matches the metaphyseal width is chosen. This is pinned to the anterior femur. Multiple 2-mm drill holes are made, penetrating from anterior to posterior cortex in semicircular fashion. The posterior aspect of the knee neurovascular structures are protected using radiolucent retractors and small wet sponges. The dots are connected with 0.25-inch narrow osteotomes, and the distal fragment is mobilized through the osteotomy. *D,* Step 4: With the osteotomy now mobilized with osteotomes, the leg is gently manipulated with traction and a varus force until the leg is straight. The blade plate is applied through the previous chisel tract, the plate portion is applied against the lateral femoral cortex, an articulated compression device can be used to apply further compression if necessary, and the screw fixation stabilizes the osteotomy.

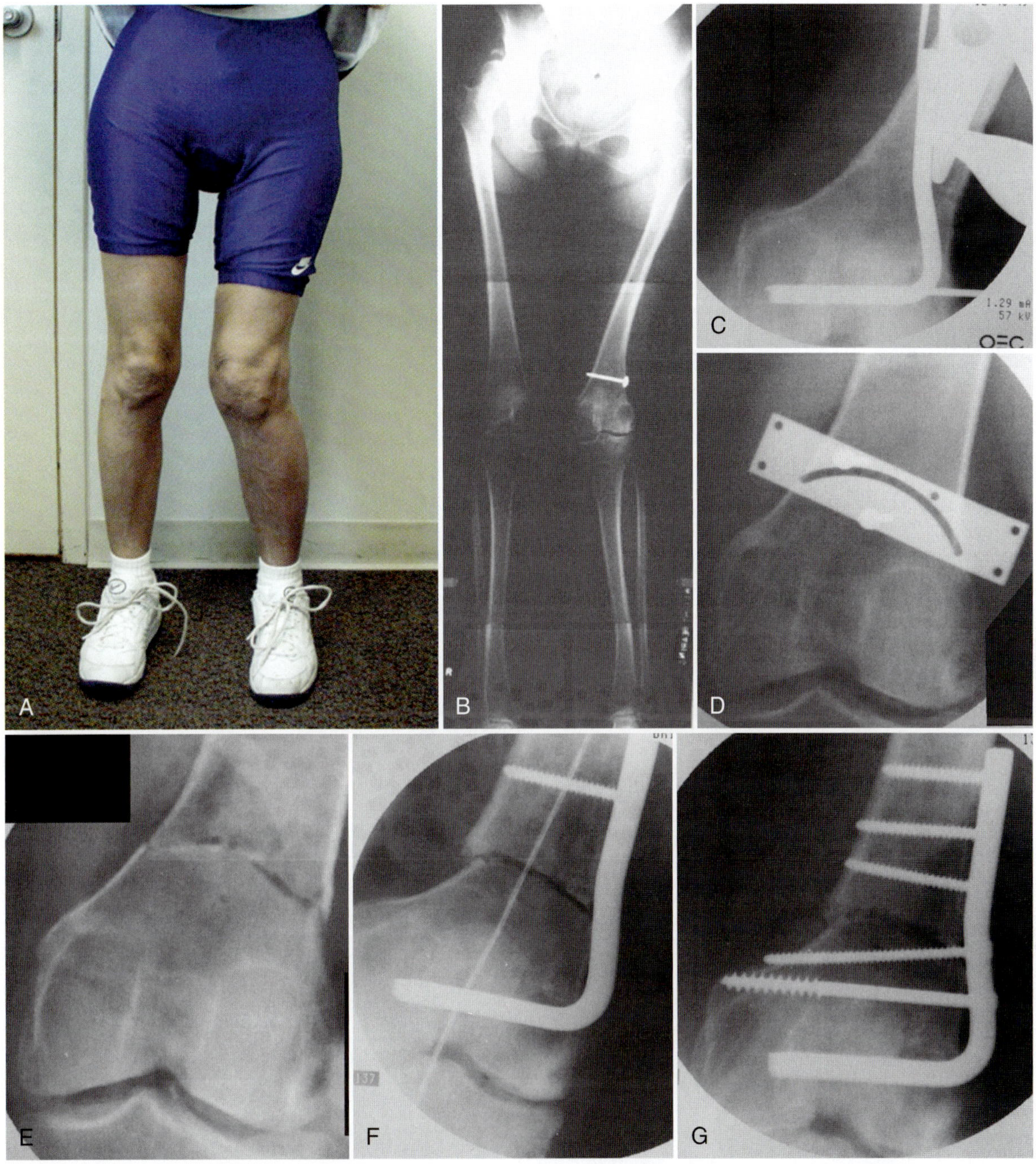

Femoral Varus Osteotomy   CHAPTER 9   153

Figure 9-9 *A,* A 36-year-old woman who had undergone left knee anterior cruciate ligament reconstruction for instability. She has a mild form of congenital insensitivity to pain with arthritis of her right hip as well as her left knee with valgus malalignment. The knee experiences mild discomfort and persistent instability. A varus femoral osteotomy will be performed for a 20-degree angular correction with a supracondylar reverse dome femoral osteotomy and blade plate fixation. *B,* Long alignment x-ray films of the patient shown in panel A. *C,* A guidewire is placed in the proposed path of the blade portion of the 95-degree angled blade plate with a 20-degree angled triangle parallel to the lateral cortex, which delineates the angle of correction for this osteotomy. A blade plate seating chisel is used to enter the distal femur along the plane of the guidewire to provide an appropriate angle correction for the osteotomy. *D,* Intraoperatively, a jig with an appropriate arc of radius is applied to the distal femur with two pins for fixation in preparation for the osteotomy. The supracondylar osteotomy is performed with 2-mm drill bit perforations from anterior to posterior. The back of the knee is protected with retractors and small wet sponges. *E,* A ¼-inch osteotome is used to connect the dots from anterior to posterior until the distal femoral fragment is mobilized. The distal fragment is mobilized with osteotomes through the osteotomy site with gentle traction on the foot and a varus force on the distal fragment until the limb is almost straight. The blade plate is applied to the distal fragment from the previous chisel tract until the plate portion lies flush to the femoral cortex. The osteotomy site is compressed and reduced accurately to ensure that there is no flexion or extension of the distal fragment, and screw fixation is performed for stabilization.

Continued

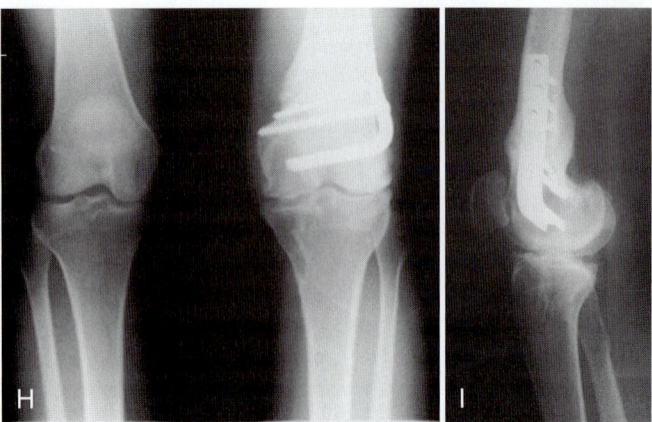

Figure 9-9—cont'd *F*, Intraoperative confirmation of correction of the mechanical axis using a Bovie cord from the center of the femoral head to the center of the talus falls through the center of the knee. *G*, Final intraoperative appearance of the osteotomy when the fixation is complete. *H*, *I*, Radiographic appearance of the healed osteotomy 1 year after surgery in frontal and lateral x-ray projections. One year after surgery, robust callus formation is noted around the osteotomy site. The anatomy of the distal femur is not distorted, so it will not jeopardize future reconstruction with total knee arthroplasty if necessary. This is a key advantage to reverse dome osteotomy about the knee.

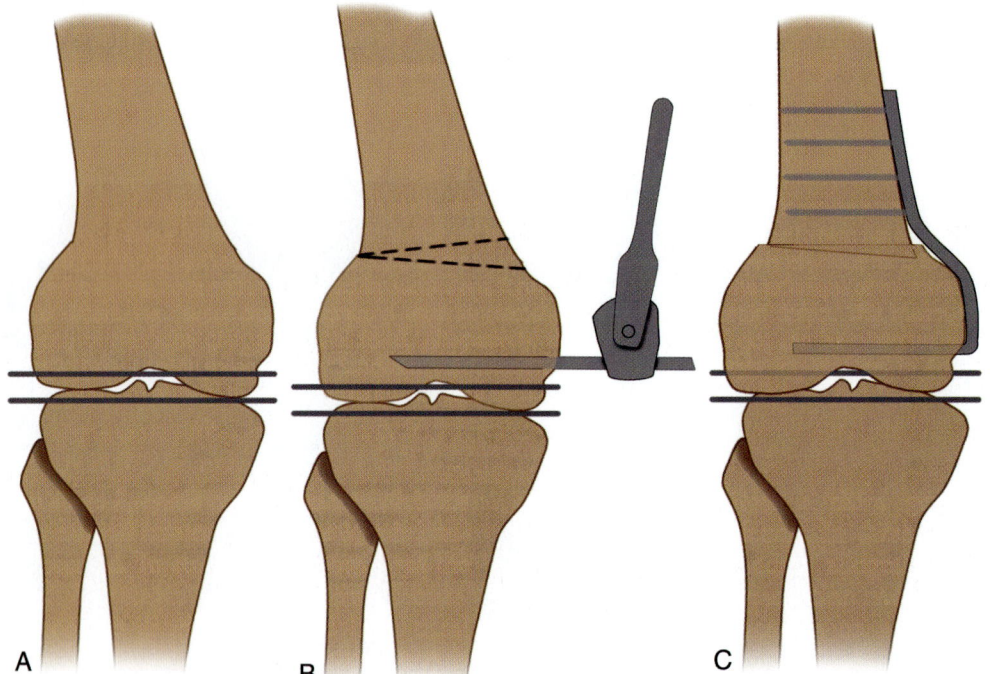

Figure 9-10 *A*, Step 1: With a medial subvastus arthrotomy performed to expose the joint line and the proximal distal medial aspect of the femur, a guidewire is placed along the joint line and one parallel to this into the bone above the intercondylar notch as a guide for the direction of the blade plate chisel. *B*, Because of the trapezoidal shape of the distal femur with the anterior aspect being narrow and the posterior aspect being broad, it is important to ensure that the seating chisel is placed parallel to the shaft of the femur (anterior third of the distal condyles). As the seating chisel is inserted parallel to the guidewire (panel *A*), it should not pass more than two thirds across the width as confirmed on image intensification so that it does not break through the opposite lateral cortex on the more narrow anterior aspect of the femur. Once the seating chisel has exited the distal femur, a transverse osteotomy above the trochlea to the lateral cortex is performed. A 5-mm wedge medially based is removed after a proximal cut is performed to the opposite apex, leaving the lateral cortex intact. *C*, The 90-degree offset blade plate is seated completely to the distal fragment. Axial compression on the lower leg will allow the proximal shaft of the femur to impale itself within the softer cancellous bone of the distal fragment until the plate portion of the fixed angle device rests against the medial cortex of the proximal fragment of the distal femur. An articulated compression device is not used on the medial aspect of the femur because it would put the femoral artery at risk as it exits Hunter's canal at the distal third of the femur. Screws are placed to complete the fixation of the osteotomy. It is not uncommon for the lateral cortex to break during the compression and stabilization of the blade plate device. With newer medially based precontoured locking plates available, the classic technique is generally not recommended because the mechanical access correction is less precise. The osteotomy can be closed and fixated with a precontoured medially based locking plate for a precise and accurate correction.

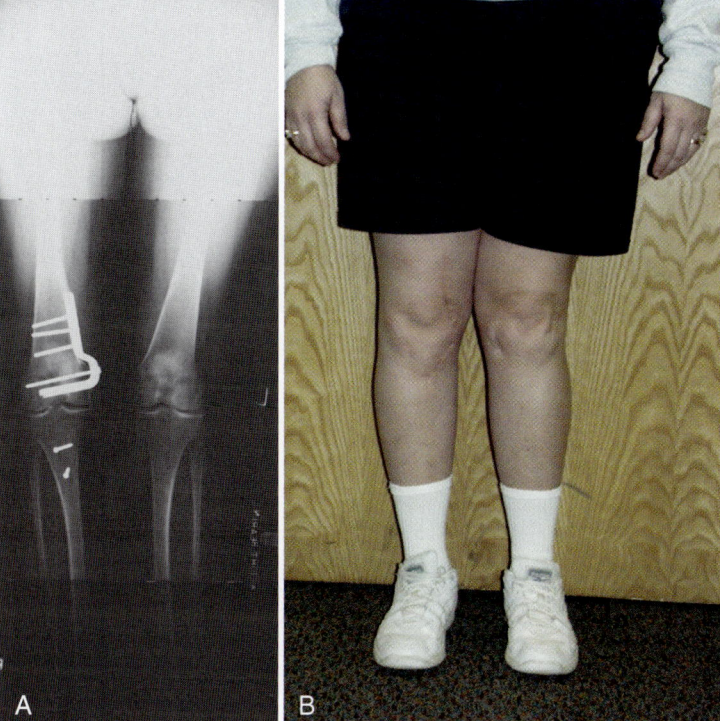

Figure 9-11 *A,* Long alignment frontal x-ray films of a 44-year-old woman who had undergone a closing wedge femoral osteotomy with tibial tubercle osteotomy on the right knee for lateral tibiofemoral osteoarthritis and lateral patellar facet osteoarthritis. She now presents with valgus alignment and lateral and anterior pain in the left knee. *B,* Clinical appearance of the lower extremities 4 years later. The patient now is symptomatic on the left side. She was pleased with the pain relief and clinical appearance provided by the osteotomy and wished to pursue osteotomy for the same problem in the opposite left knee at the age of 48 years. A classic closing wedge femoral osteotomy with 90-degree angled offset blade plate is performed as described by Gross and Hutchinson.[2,4]

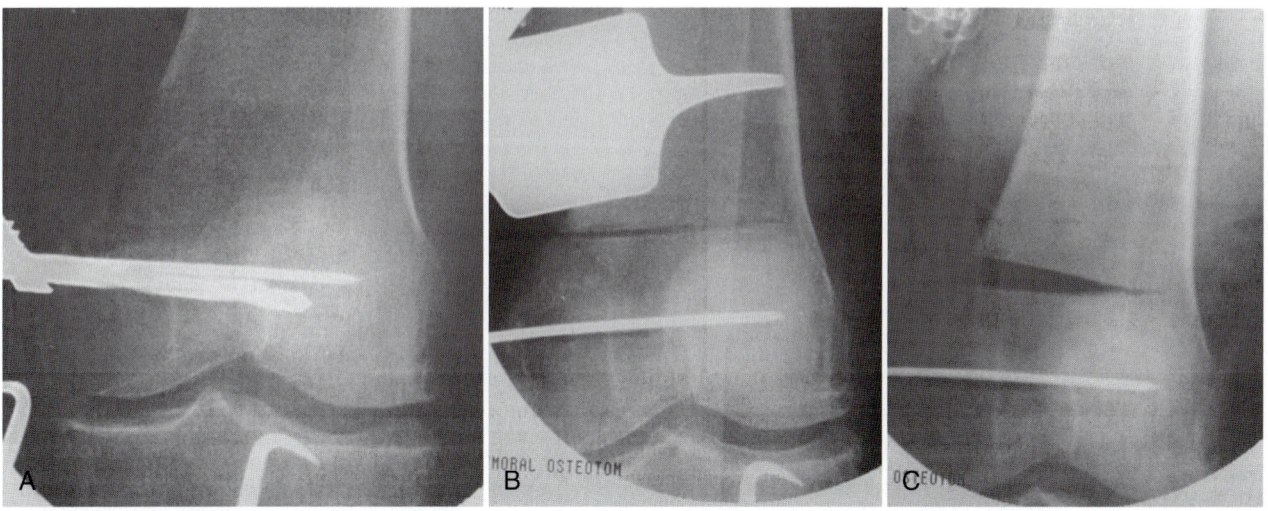

Figure 9-12 *A,* A triple drill guide is used collinear with the guidewire, which is parallel to the joint line, from a medial subvastus approach to the distal femur. This prepares a cortical pathway for the seating chisel to enter the distal femur and be led by the guidewire. *B,* The seating chisel is introduced with a slap hammer back and forth along the distal femur to prevent it from becoming jammed within the dense cancellous bone. It is then removed, and the proximal closing wedge osteotomy is performed. A transverse osteotomy is performed under direct visualization of the anterior cortex to the lateral cortex, leaving this intact. The anterior dissection involves a transverse incision from medial to lateral across the supracondylar synovium, then subperiosteally dissecting it distally toward the trochlea and proximally for 1 cm to allow reapproximation of the synovium over the osteotomy once it is closed and completed. The posterior neurovascular structures are protected with small wet sponges. *C,* A 5-mm medially based osteotomy is performed by freehand technique to meet the opposite lateral osteotomy site. The bone wedge is then removed.

Continued

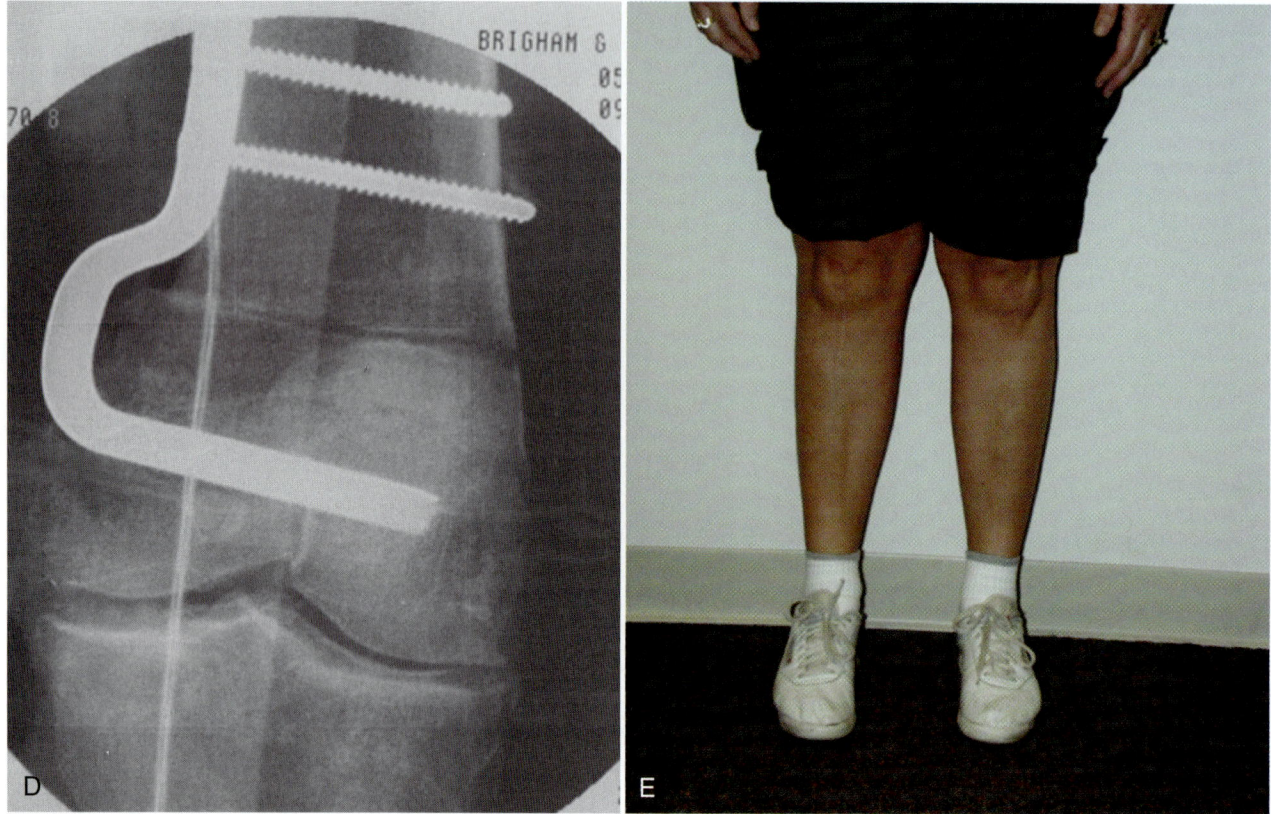

Figure 9-12—cont'd *D*, The 90-degree offset blade plate is chosen by the offset, which is measured from the medial aspect of the femur to the cortical shaft when a trial closing reduction is performed. The blade plate is seated and axial compression applied once more until the plate portion rests upon the medial cortex of the proximal fragment. Bone-holding clamps may be required, and cortical fixation is performed with 4.5-mm screws. In this case, the lateral cortex fractures, which is common because of the compression required to close the osteotomy and implode the proximal shaft into the distal fragment. This is of no consequence because the fixation is stable and the device is rigid and not a tension band device. The mechanical axis is checked intraoperatively on the radiolucent table using a Bovie cord from the center of the femoral head to the center of the ankle, which in this case falls into the center of the medial joint compartment. This is more than is usually recommended with this technique but is common using the classic closing wedge technique with a 90-degree blade plate. *E*, Final clinical appearance after correction with osteotomy on both knees. The patient has only slight varus, equal leg lengths, and good pain relief.

osteotomy so that the blade chisel does not break through into the osteotomy site. The lateral cortex is left intact. A small wedge of bone approximately 5 mm wide is taken from the proximal fragment.

The 90-degree offset blade plate is inserted and compressed axially such that the proximal fragment impales the distal fragment until the plate portion fits to the proximal cortical fragment. Screws are used to fix the plate to the proximal fragment. This produces a tibiofemoral axis of 0 degrees, with the femur collinear to the tibia. Mechanical access will depend on the varus at the hip and its offset. It may actually be through the center of the medial compartment or outside of the medial compartment, depending on the proximal femoral anatomy. A closing wedge osteotomy with the technique as described by Gross and Hutchinson[4] will produce a tibiofemoral angle of 0 degrees. This is the result because the 90-degree blade plate is positioned parallel to the articular surfaces and the fragment is closed down until the plate portion fits to the femoral cortex, always producing a tibiofemoral axis of 0 degrees. It is a simple and reproducible technique that provides excellent fixation stability. However, it does not take into account the neck shaft angle of the hip joint and deformity in the proximal femur and therefore may result in overcorrection into varus, which may lead to premature wear of the medial compartment. This may present a larger problem for a younger patient undergoing cartilage repair surgery in whom a more accurate angular correction to neutral or at the medial tibial spine may be required. This technique does not allow for such precise correction. A calibrated osteotomy correction device may be required for a closing wedge osteotomy fixed with a tension band plate for precise corrections, as will be described in the next section.

DISTAL FEMORAL VARUS CLOSING WEDGE OSTEOTOMY FOR VALGUS MALALIGNMENT WITH OSTEOCHONDRAL REPAIR

At this time, I rarely use a 90-degree blade plate fixation with closing wedge osteotomy. Although a blade plate offers excellent fixation stability, in case of malplacement of the chisel portion of the device, the plate may not sit flush on the femoral cortex medially, or the angular correction of the osteotomy may change and the lateral cortex may break in so doing. In addition, impaling the proximal cortex into the distal metaphysis is not as simple as it sounds.

For these reasons, I presently use a calibrated jig that allows precise angular correction as planned preoperatively. This is performed from the medial side of the distal femur as described through a medial subvastus arthrotomy or a medial parapatellar arthrotomy. The fixation device can be either a contoured locking plate (Synthes TomoFix medial locking plate [Synthes, Solothurn, Switzerland]) or a tension band L-plate (Figure 9–13).

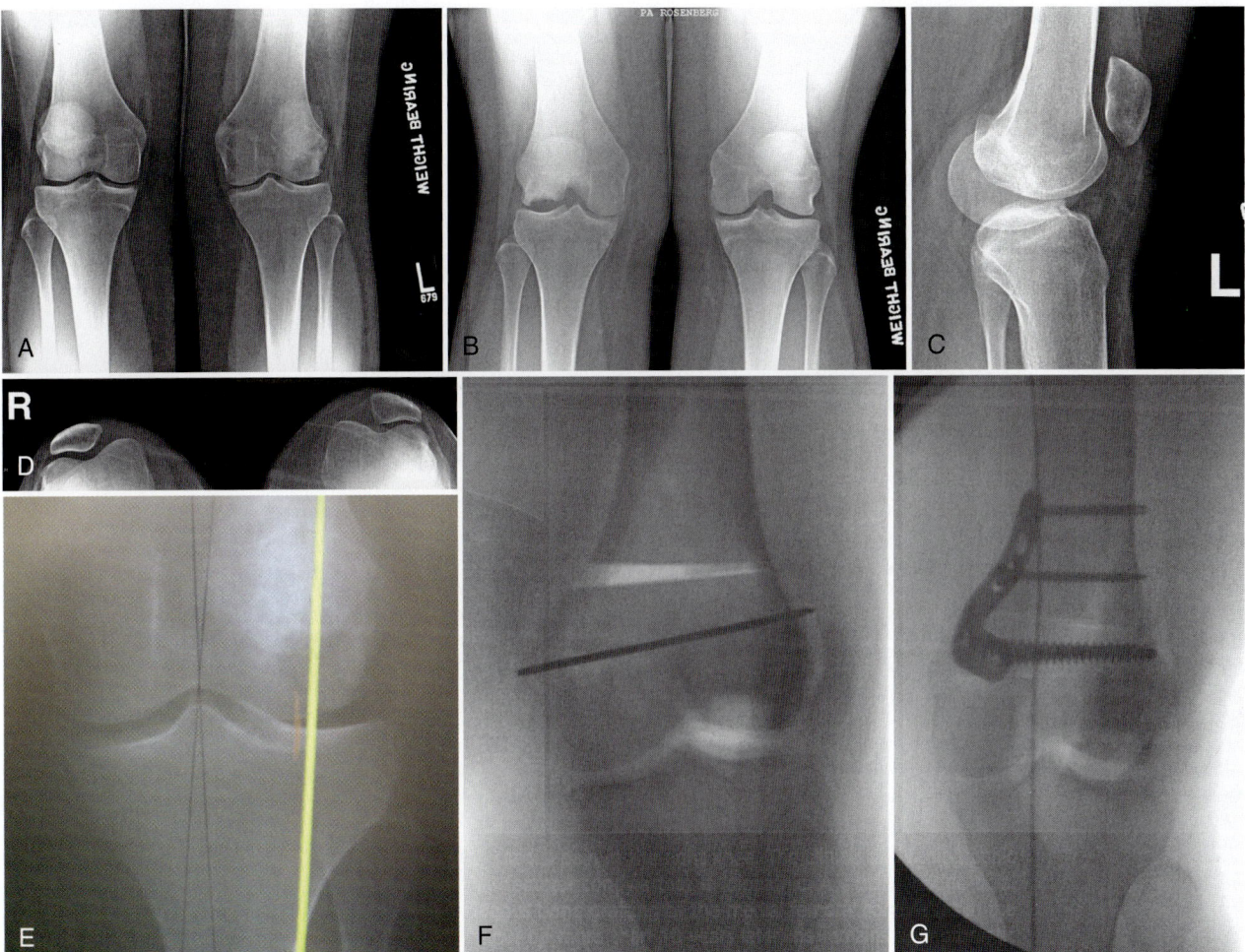

Figure 9–13 *A, B,* Standing anteroposterior *(A)* and posteroanterior *(B)* x-ray films of a 17-year-old girl with osteochondritis dissecans of the posterior lateral femoral condyle. Fragmentation of the osteochondritis dissecans has been removed arthroscopically and leaves an osseous and cartilaginous defect to the lateral femoral condyle. *C, D,* Lateral *(C)* and skyline *(D)* x-ray films of the left knee demonstrate the posteriorly located osteochondritis dissecans lesion on the lateral femoral condyle and the evidence of patellar tilt of the left knee. *E,* Close-up view taken from a long-leg alignment x-ray film of the left knee demonstrates the mechanical axis *(yellow line)* falls through the center of the lateral femoral condyle. Any type of cartilage repair to the osteochondritis dissecans lesion would be at risk of premature failure without mechanical axis correction to the medial tibial spine (the defect is large with early joint space narrowing noted on Rosenberg posteroanterior views), and an 8-degree angular correction is necessary. *F,* Supracondylar 8-degree closing wedge varus-producing osteotomy has been performed. The lateral cortex remains intact. *G,* The osteotomy is closed with a tension band L-plate used for proximal tibial osteotomies contoured to the proximal femur. Note that the intraoperative mechanical axis is successful in placing the axis to the medial tibial spine as preoperatively planned. (I would use a medially based locking contoured plate, now available, because it fits more precisely and is more rigid.) The bone taken from the osteotomy is used as an osseous repair for the lateral femoral condyles osteochondritis dissecans lesion.

Continued

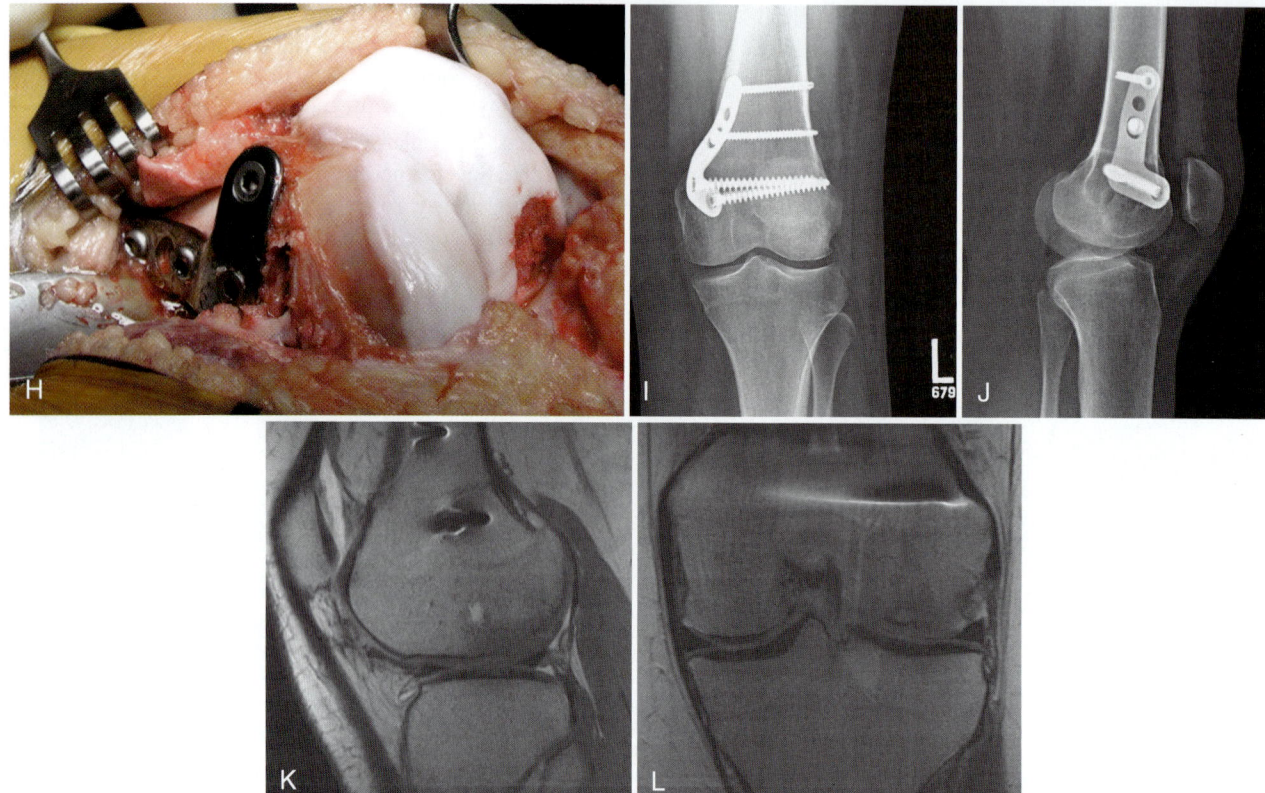

Figure 9-13—cont'd *H,* Intraoperative appearance through a medial peripatellar arthrotomy of the L-plate used as a tension band plate placed on the medial side of the joint in combination with autologous bone grafting to the lateral femoral condyle osteochondritis dissecans. *I, J,* Final anteroposterior and lateral radiographs after osseous union of the osteotomy site and lateral femoral condyle osteochondritis dissecans lesion. *K, L,* No further cartilage repair was required for the osteochondritis dissecans lesion in this patient. The patient's own bone marrow cells under the influence of cartilage rehabilitation with continuous passive motion and protected weight bearing gave the patient a fibrocartilaginous surface, and the patient became asymptomatic. High-resolution magnetic resonance imaging (MRI) scanning ensured the existence of a repair surface and not an empty bony defect (sagittal and coronal proton-density fast-spin echo images). The patient remains asymptomatic and has returned to sporting activities. A biopsy for cultured articular chondrocytes was taken at the time of the open reconstruction for the possibility of failure of the fibrocartilaginous surface repair and the need for second-stage autologous chondrocyte implantation (ACI). However, 4 years later, the patient remains asymptomatic. She is followed with annual clinical examinations to assess for crepitus, swelling, and other symptoms and by annual x-ray films with standing anteroposterior and flexed posteroanterior views to assess for the potential of joint space narrowing. If symptoms or clinical findings were to develop, high-resolution MRI scan would be repeated after the first 2 years with the possibility of arthroscopy for confirmation and cartilage repair with ACI or fresh osteoarticular allograft as deemed necessary.

At this time, my indication for a closing wedge distal femoral varus-producing osteotomy is usually for a leg aligned in valgus with a lateral osteochondral defect. This is performed to obtain the desired varus correction to unload the defect and autologous bone graft for the osseous defect through the same incision without the need for supplemental autologous bone graft source. The distal femoral metaphyseal bone is of excellent quality and is a good source of autologous bone graft. The example in Figure 9-13 illustrates such a case.

SUMMARY

Distal femoral varus osteotomy can be performed for either valgus deformity with lateral osteoarthritis or valgus deformity with cartilage or osteochondral repair to the lateral joint compartment. Long alignment x-ray films confirm that the deformity is in the distal femoral metaphysis with a superior and lateral directed joint line.

Deformity correction of the mechanical axis is to the midline for cartilage repair with an intact lateral joint line or to the medial tibial spine when there is joint space loss or a large chondral defect in the lateral tibiofemoral compartment. Marked overcorrection is not desired.

Opening wedge femoral osteotomy is generally used for corrections up to 15 degrees for cartilage or arthritic lateral disease with valgus malalignment. Closing wedge femoral osteotomy is generally used when there is a need for autologous bone grafting to the lateral tibiofemoral compartment or there is a long leg on the affected side. Presently this is performed only occasionally. A supracondylar reverse dome osteotomy is generally used for corrections of 15 to 30 degrees with a lateral 95-degree blade plate fixation. This is a very powerful osteotomy that does not distort the anatomy of the distal femur. This procedure should always be considered so that future reconstruction (e.g., total knee arthroplasty) is not jeopardized. Femoral osteotomy is technically more difficult to perform than tibial osteotomy but is very reproducible.

REFERENCES

1. Healy WL, Anglen J, Wasilewski S. Distal femoral varus osteotomy. *J Bone Joint Surg Am*. 1988;70:102–109.
2. McDermott A, Finkelstein JA, Farine I, et al. Distal femoral varus osteotomy for valgus deformity of the knee. *J Bone Joint Surg Am*. 1988;70:110–116.
3. Paley D. *Principles of deformity correction*. Berlin: Springer-Verlag; 2002.
4. Gross AE, Hutchinson CE. Realignment osteotomy of the knee-part one: distal femoral varus osteotomy for osteoarthritis of the valgus knee. *Oper Tech Sports Med*. 2000;8:122–126.

Chapter 10

Patellofemoral Malalignment, Tibial Tubercle Osteotomy, and Trochleoplasty

Tom Minas, MD, MS

INTRODUCTION

HISTORY

PHYSICAL EXAMINATION

PHYSICAL THERAPY

IMAGING STUDIES

IDENTIFY THE PATHOMECHANICS: SUCCESSFUL SURGERY

ISOLATED PATELLAR TILT: LATERAL RELEASE

PATELLAR TILT AND SUBLUXATION WITH OR WITHOUT CHONDROSIS

   Fulkerson Type I and II Chondrosis: Anteromedialization TTO

   Type III and IV Chondrosis: Anteromedialization TTO plus Autologous Chondrocyte Implantation

   Modified Surgical Technique of Anteromedialization TTO–Fulkerson

SURGICAL TECHNIQUE

TROCHLEA DYSPLASIA

PATELLAR TILT AND SUBLUXATION: RADIOGRAPHIC LOSS OF JOINT SPACE, PATELLOFEMORAL REPLACEMENT WITH OR WITHOUT TTO, AND PATELLOFEMORAL PROSTHETIC ARTHROPLASTY

SUMMARY

INTRODUCTION

This chapter is designed to offer the practicing orthopedist a practical management approach to dealing with patellofemoral disease. The key to successful treatment relies on an accurate diagnosis of the underlying pathomechanics responsible for the pain.

Chronic patellofemoral pain is a common and problematic management issue. The term *chondromalacia* has often been applied to individuals suffering from anterior knee pain. However, chondromalacia, meaning "soft cartilage," as a pathologic entity may not even be present. Pain is a multifactorial perception. It is important to ensure that the pain is local and not referred, that it is not due to a local soft tissue inflammatory or neurogenic process, and that it arises from the patellofemoral joint. This is usually determined by a careful history and physical examination. The emotional well-being of the patient may modify the subjective response of pain. Even with obvious patellofemoral pathomechanics, if physical therapy has not been performed adequately to address these problems, then a repeat course of carefully directed physical therapy is worthwhile.

Many factors have been implicated as a source of abnormal forces across the patellofemoral joint. They include patella alta, trochlea dysplasia, an abnormally increased quadriceps (Q) angle with secondary soft tissue problems, and weakened or hypoplastic vastus medialis oblique quadriceps muscle with contracted lateral retinaculum. These pathomechanics lead to abnormal forces across the patella, resulting in secondary degenerative changes or injury to the articular surfaces with cartilage defects of the patellofemoral joint acutely or chronically.

The prevalence of patellofemoral cartilage defects is controversial because the percentage of lesions that become sufficiently symptomatic to prompt evaluation is unknown. Several studies have reported the presence of high-grade focal chondral defects in 11% to 20% of knee arthroscopies. Among these defects, 11% to 23% were located in the patella and 6% to 15% in the trochlea.[1–3] A group investigating asymptomatic National Basketball Association players with knee magnetic resonance imaging (MRI) found articular cartilage lesions in 47%, with patellar lesions in 35% and trochlear lesions in 25% of players; however, only approximately half of these defects were characterized as high-grade lesions.[4]

These reports emphasize the importance of a thorough history and physical evaluation of the entire kinetic chain from pelvis to foot, a gait analysis, and assessment of all knee structures (tendons, ligaments, and soft tissues) before attributing a patient's symptoms solely to the presence of a chondral defect.

HISTORY

Patellofemoral articular defects frequently present as anterior knee pain. Patients often report the pain is located retropatellar, peripatellar, occasionally radiating "down the shin bone," or, in the case of trochlear defects, posteriorly in the popliteal area. Secondary pain may derive from synovial or capsular irritation from joint distension secondary to an effusion or exposed subchondral bone overload from a chondral defect. Thus, in light of the secondary nature of pain, other factors may also contribute so that assigning a percentage of pain to the cartilage pathology can be difficult. Large defects can cause clicking or popping, giving way, and activity-related swelling. Distension of the joint often causes an aching sensation, with loss of motion and function but not necessarily complaints of pain. Standard patellofemoral symptoms are often reported, such as increased pain with prolonged flexed knee position and stair climbing, as maximal patellofemoral forces occur in the flexed knee position when patellar engagement in the trochlea is greater than 30 degrees (Figure 10–1). Patients are approximately evenly split in reporting a traumatic versus a more gradual onset of symptoms. Participation in sports was the most common inciting event associated with the diagnosis of chondral lesions. Patellar dislocation is associated with damage to the articular surface, with chondral defects of the patella seen in up to 95% of patients (Figure 10–2).[5] It is my opinion that patellar dislocations usually occur due to baseline mechanical abnormalities with increased Q angles and/or dysplasia of the trochlea. Despite the history of trauma, usually a minor twist occurs during participation in sports. Patients often report extended courses of physical therapy, bracing and taping, or prior knee surgery.

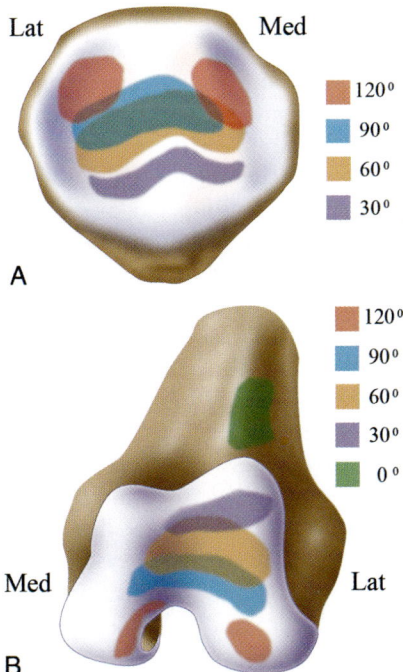

Figure 10-1 *A*, Portions of the patella that are engaging at different angular degrees of flexion. *B*, Corresponding portions of the trochlea that are engaging with the patella at different angular degrees of flexion. (Modified from Aglietti P, Insall JN, Walker PS, et al: A new patella prosthesis. Clin Othop 1975;107:175).

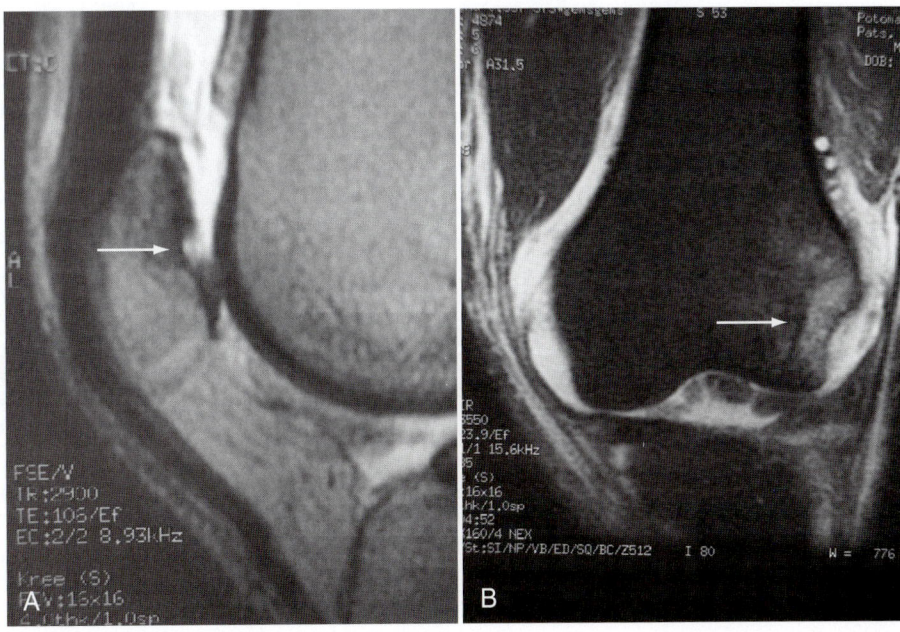

Figure 10-2 *A*, Sagittal MRI scan demonstrating central full-thickness articular cartilage loss *(arrow)*, following patellar dislocation. *B*, Coronal MRI scan with fat suppression, demonstrating intense bone marrow edema at the location of the patellar dislocation at the distal lateral trochlea *(arrow)*. This is a classic MRI appearance of the articular injury patterns following patellar dislocation.

PHYSICAL EXAMINATION

Gait abnormalities, such as intoeing and hip abductor weakness, are frequently seen in this patient population, especially adolescents, as is an increase in femoral anteversion and valgus malalignment of the lower extremity. Adaptations in gait, such as hip and knee external rotation and contractures of the hip abductors and iliotibial band, are also seen. Traditionally, the Q angle (Figure 10–3) has been used in the evaluation of patellofemoral symptoms. Many different methods of measuring this angle have been reported, and the high interobserver variability makes it of questionable usefulness.[6,7] As described, the Q angle should be evaluated in both full extension and approximately 30 degrees of flexion because, in some cases, a laterally subluxated patella in full extension can falsely decrease the Q angle (the patella should be repositioned in the central sulcus before measuring the Q angle). My preference is to examine and measure the Q angle is full extension with the patella manually reduced in the trochlea with medially directed force on the patella; I call this the "thumb reduction test." Ask the patient to contract the quadriceps, and you can see and feel the patella sublux laterally. Q angles in asymptomatic patients are 14 degrees in males and 17 degrees in females.[8] Quadriceps wasting, especially of the vastus medialis, is common in longstanding patellofemoral symptoms. Recently, more emphasis has been placed on core muscle weakness, especially of the hip abductors, hip extensors, and pelvic stabilizers. Weakness in this group can be demonstrated by asking the patient to single-leg stand on the affected limb, which results in a pelvic drop on the contralateral side. In addition to poor pelvic support, dynamic internal rotation of the femur and dynamic valgus positioning of the limb can be observed. Activity-related swelling and, in particular, a joint effusion indicate more advanced disease. Palpation of the medial and lateral retinaculum can elicit pain. The lateral structures often are contracted (tested by attempting to reverse patellar tilt), whereas the medial soft tissues can be attenuated (e.g., chronic patholaxity of the medial patellofemoral ligament). Patellar mobility, tilt, and subluxation should be assessed and quantified medially and laterally. Normally the patella should be able to "glide" 30% of its width medially and laterally without the patient experiencing apprehension of a subluxation or dislocation. Catching with mobilization of the patella against the trochlea is suggestive of larger defects. Knee range of motion usually is preserved but may be inhibited by pain or large effusions in acute cases. The J-sign (the patient slowly extends the knee from full flexion, and the patella subluxes laterally once it leaves the constraints of the trochlear groove near full extension) may occur in normal patients but is exaggerated in patients with patellar maltracking. It often implies incompetence of the medial restraining structures, including the medial patellofemoral ligament.

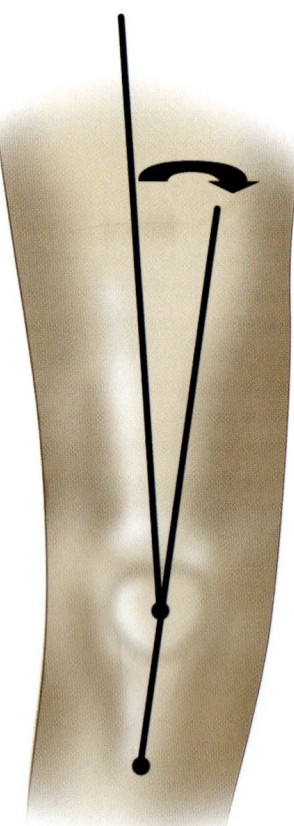

Figure 10–3 Diagrammatic representation of the quadriceps or Q-angle. A line drawn from the anterior-superior iliac spine to the central pole of the patella, (with the patella reduced in the trochlea in full extension), following an angle from the central patella pole to the patellar tendon insertion at the tibial tubercle. This angle averages 14 degrees in men and 17 degrees in women. (Aglietti P, Insall JN, G. C: Patellar pain and incongruence; measurements of incongruence. Clin Orthop. 1983;176:217-224.)

PHYSICAL THERAPY

The goal of physical therapy is to restore soft tissue balance in the patellofemoral joint, including muscular and capsuloligamentous balance often remote from the joint. Rehabilitative exercises should include a stretching regimen to restore flexibility of the quadriceps, hamstrings, and iliotibial band, as well as patellar mobilizations as needed to optimize capsular structure balance (e.g., reverse tilt) of the quadriceps and patellar tendon. After flexibility has been restored, a strengthening program should be instituted, emphasizing the core proximal musculature, including the hip abductors and external rotators, as most patients previously placed too much emphasis on isolated quadriceps strengthening. Quadriceps strengthening, if emphasized, should be performed with closed-chain activities such as elliptical trainer, leg presses, and squats with the knee in less than 30 degrees of flexion from full extension to prevent maximal patellofemoral contact forces. Open-chain resisted quadriceps extensions should be avoided so as not to aggravate patellofemoral pain or cause progression of cartilage damage. Short-arc open-chain quadriceps extensions are performed when the patella is not engaged in the trochlea in the first 0 to 20 degrees of flexion of the knee. Gait training should focus on avoidance of an intoeing gait, which results in functional femoral anteversion. Throughout rehabilitation, it is important to protect the patellofemoral articulation by using isometric and short-arc closed-chain concentric and eccentric muscle strengthening, which is individually designed to avoid specific arcs of pain or loading of cartilage defects. A trial of patellar McConnell taping or patellar bracing to centralize a maltracking patella is worthwhile, especially when symptoms are limited to certain activities, such as athletic endeavors. The patient should understand the comprehensive McConnell approach, which uses taping to allow pain-free rehabilitation (i.e., taping is not an end in itself). Patients should understand that they have mechanical reasons for the imbalance and resultant pain in their extensor mechanism. Therefore, it is important that patients maintain their stretching and strengthening regimen to stay within their envelope of function, their own personal equilibrium. If they are able to experience benefit with physical therapy but have recurrent relapses of discomfort, they should rest, elevate and ice the extremity, and take nonsteroidal antiinflammatory medications until they are able to resume their quadriceps rehabilitation regimen. Only when they fail therapy should they seek definitive surgical intervention for resolution of symptoms and restoration of function.

IMAGING STUDIES

Useful tests that assist in determining the diagnosis are standard radiographs, including standing anteroposterior, 45-degree posteroanterior (Rosenberg), lateral, skyline (Merchant), and standard 54-inch axial alignment x-ray films. Radiographs are useful with any patellofemoral joint to determine joint space narrowing or osteoarthritis on a standard Merchant view. This view is taken at 45 degrees of flexion during which the patella is normally well engaged in the trochlea distally. It is not an effective view for assessing maltracking, which, when it occurs, is usually in the first 0 to 30 degrees of flexion from extension. The dislocated or subluxed patella in full extension travels medially as it travels distally, capturing the trochlea as it reduces. This is the clinical finding of a J-sign. Dejour et al[9] showed the advantages of a true lateral radiograph in assessing trochlear dysplasia and patellar tilt not appreciated on the Merchant view.

Assessment of articular cartilage injury is receiving more attention with newly developed imaging protocols enhanced by intravenous gadolinium as an indirect arthrogram. Although the gold standard for assessing articular injury remains arthroscopy, sensitivity and specificity greater than 90% can be obtained with high-resolution MRI scan using a standard 1.5-T magnet with appropriate orthogonal gantry tilting to surfaces of the trochlea and appropriate sequences.[10,11] This is our preferred method for assessing articular cartilage injury to localize the site and size of chondrosis in the patellofemoral articulation.

To accurately assess patella subluxation, spiral computed tomography (CT) of the patellofemoral joint is performed with the leg in full extension, once with the quadriceps relaxed and again with the muscle maximally contracted (Figure 10–4). It is especially helpful in determining dysplasia of the bony patellofemoral joint (Figures 10–5 and 10–6). CT also allows more precise evaluation of patellar and trochlear anatomy than the Merchant view (Figure 10–7). Accurate documentation of subluxation can be determined with the CT scan with clinical findings are difficult, especially in the obese patient.

The addition of intraarticular gadolinium contrast helps to outline any articular cartilage defects on the patella, trochlea, or both and the exact location and size. My preferred test for patellofemoral maltracking, locating the articular cartilage defect, and assessing dysplasia of the trochlea is a CT arthrogram performed with the quadriceps first relaxed and then contracted in the fully extended knee (Figure 10–8).

Furthermore, superposition of two CT images, one through the patellofemoral articulation and the other through the tibial tubercle, allows calculation of the tibial tubercle to trochlear groove (TT–TG) distance. The center of the trochlear groove and the center of the tibial tubercle are marked, and the medial to lateral distance between the two is measured (Figure 10–9). A TT–TG distance greater than 15 mm is considered normal; values greater than 20 mm are abnormal and should be considered for a tibial tubercle osteotomy (TTO).[12]

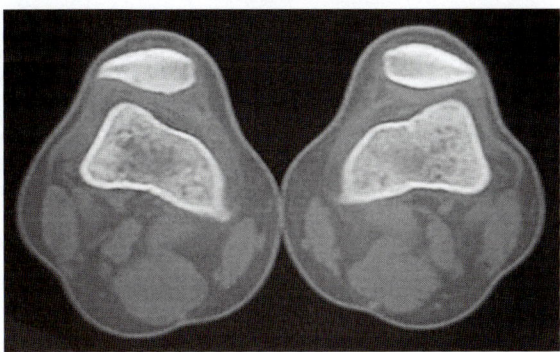

Figure 10–4 Bilateral subluxed patellas noted on CT scan with quadriceps contracted with the knees in full extension.

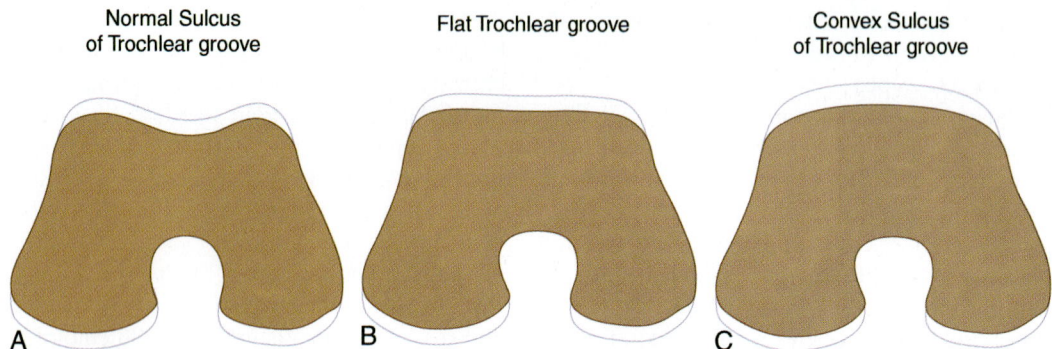

Figure 10–5 *A*, coronal view of a normal trochlea with a central concave groove. Variations of trochlea dysplasia may cause flattening of the groove *B*, or a convex groove *C*, When this occurs developmentally the sesamoid patella articulation is congruent to the dysplastic trochlea and is also abnormally shaped.

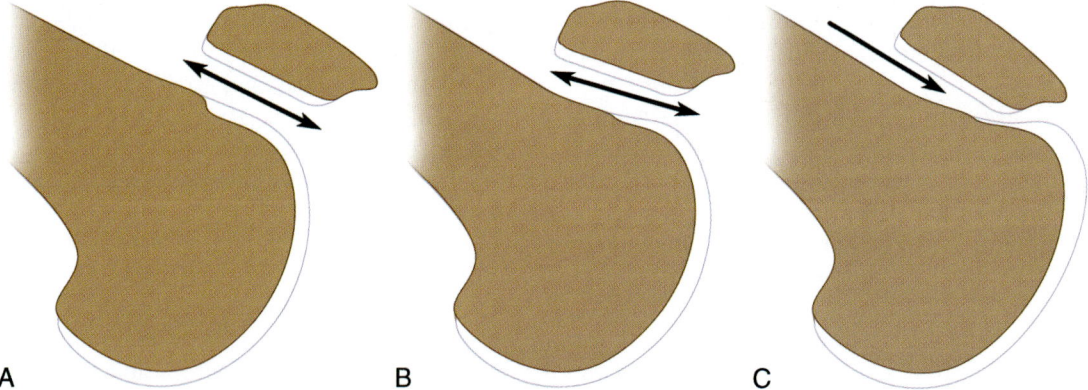

Figure 10–6 *A-D*, Trochlea dysplasia in the sagittal view may exhibit a smooth entry sulcus *A*, or a prominence *B*, which drives the patella inferior pole into a "Speed Bump." Severe changes *C*, or a trochlea "Spur" as noted by Dejour. *(Dejour H, et al: Dysplasia of the femoral trochlea. Rev Chir Orthop Reparatrice Appar Mot 1990;76:45-54)* if there is a commonly associated patella alta, predisposing to abnormal forces to subluxation and premature articular cartilage wear.

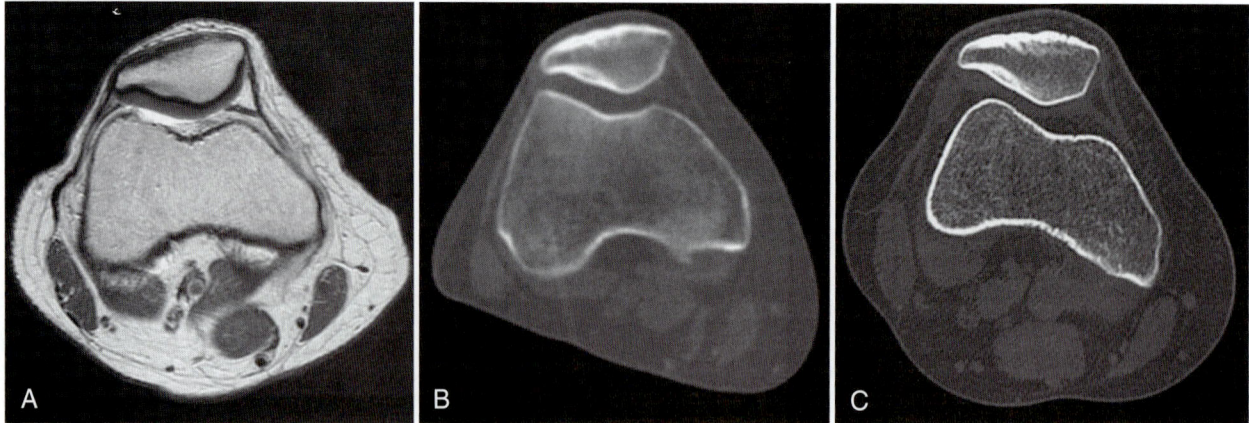

Figure 10–7 *A*, A high-resolution MRI scan with intravenous gadolinium utilized as an indirect arthrogram effect. Notice the intact full thickness nature of the lateral patellar articular cartilage. This 32-year-old woman has had a history of "chondromalacia" since the age of 12 years old. She has undergone multiple courses of physical therapy, taping, and bracing. She has been offered a patellar lateral arthroscopic release and has sought another opinion. *B*, This is a CT scan of the patella in a well reduced to position. Notice the thickening of the subchondral bone to the lateral patellar facet. This is indicative of chronic lateral maltracking, overload with remodeling of the subchondral bone. *C*, The patient contracting her quadriceps with the leg in extension. Notice the lateral subluxation of the patella. The patient requires isolated medial translation of the tibial tubercle accompanied by a patellar lateral retinacular release. The articular cartilage demonstrated in Figure 10–7*A* was normal, therefore there was no need for anterior translation of the tubercle.

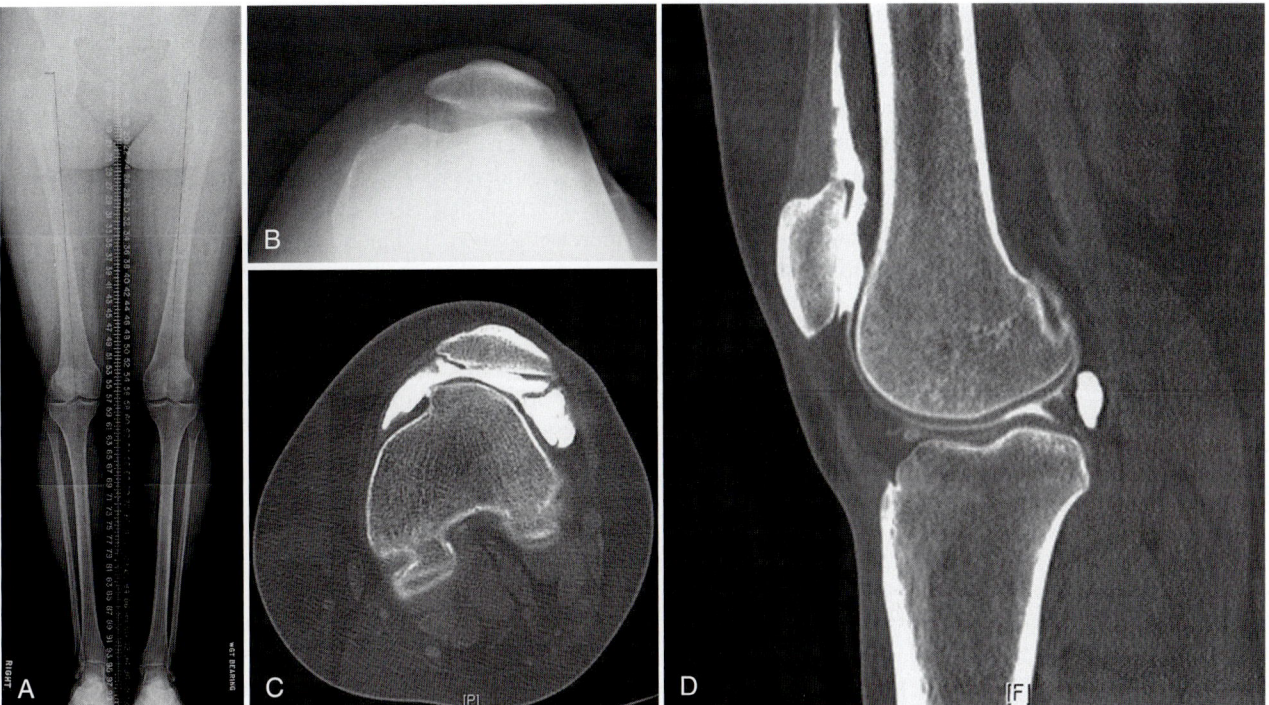

Figure 10-8 *A*, Long alignment x-ray in a young woman with patellofemoral pain demonstrating a neutral mechanical axis. *B*, A merchant or skyline x-ray demonstrates patellar subluxation with intact articular surfaces. *C*, A coronal CT arthrogram with the quadriceps contracted demonstrating subluxation of the patella as it is perched on the superior lateral dysplastic trochlea. A full-thickness articular cartilage loss is noted on the patella central and laterally. A spiral CT arthrogram as a single test is the preferred study for patellofemoral disease. The dye outlines clearly the localization of the cartilaginous loss. Dysplasia of the trochlea is clearly visualized, and the test can be performed rapidly and can assess the position of the patella with the quadriceps in the contracted and the relaxed position. This is especially helpful in obese patients where clinical exam is less reliable. *D*, The sagittal CT scan arthrogram and demonstrates complete loss of cartilage on the patella lateral facet except for a small rim proximally.

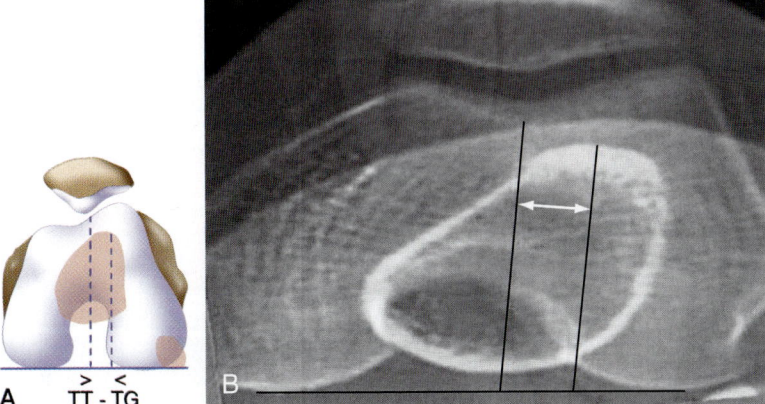

Figure 10-9 *A*, Diagrammatic representation of the tibial groove-tibial tubercle (TG–TT) distance. Anything greater than 20 mm is clearly considered abnormal. This does not take into account the size of the patient, it is absolute number and assists in determining patellofemoral maltracking. *B*, The TT–TG and distance can be measured directly from a CT scan axial cuts that are overlapped at the level of the tibial groove and the level of the tibial tubercle and measured directly.

It is possible to use MRI obtained during routine knee evaluation to measure the TT–TG distance (Schoettle et al[13] demonstrated the equivalency of CT and MRI TT–TG measurements) and the Caton-Deschamps measurement of patellar height (alta, infera, normal), thus providing additional information without added cost.[14]

When the pain pattern arising from the patellofemoral articulation is suspected and other studies are negative, a bone scan may be useful in the difficult patient evaluation to determine increased activity in that part of the joint but rarely is necessary.

IDENTIFY THE PATHOMECHANICS: SUCCESSFUL SURGERY

In a patient with persistent patellofemoral pain and functional disability, certain factors must be determined prior to appropriate treatment. These factors are determined after the history, physical examination, radiography, MRI scan, and CT scan when indicated. The factors include long-leg alignment, patellar tilt, patellar subluxation, location on the patella articular chondrosis, location on the trochlea articular chondrosis, Q angle, and secondary factors; vastus medialis obliquus (VMO) quadriceps hypoplasia or atrophy, patella alta, and dysplasia of the trochlea. Once these factors are accurately determined then an appropriate surgical treatment plan can be recommended.

The primary factors that I have found to guide my treatment algorithm are patellar tilt, subluxation, and localization of the chondrosis (Table 10–1).

Patellofemoral disease represents a spectrum with differing severities of long-leg alignment, patellar subluxation, chondrosis, or arthrosis. This algorithm addresses the different stages of disease in a stepwise fashion of increasing severity depending on the findings.

I assume that the long-leg alignment is in neutral mechanical axis, and the factors at the present time are related to patellofemoral tracking in a neutrally aligned leg. However, the valgus knee with patellofemoral dysplasia and lateral maltracking is a difficult variant to address. An example is shown in Figure 10–10.

ISOLATED PATELLAR TILT: LATERAL RELEASE

The procedure of arthroscopic lateral release is overly used. It is effective for isolated patellar tilt without subluxation of the patella when the lateral retinacular structures of the patella are contracted and mobility of the patella is limited. There may be early grade II Outerbridge chondromalacia associated with a chronically contracted and nonsubluxated patella. The procedure should be performed either arthroscopically or open from the superior lateral pole of the patella to the inferior lateral aspect of the patellar tendon. The superolateral and inferolateral geniculate arteries are cut with this

Table 10–1 Treatment Algorithm for Surgical Management of Patellofemoral Disease

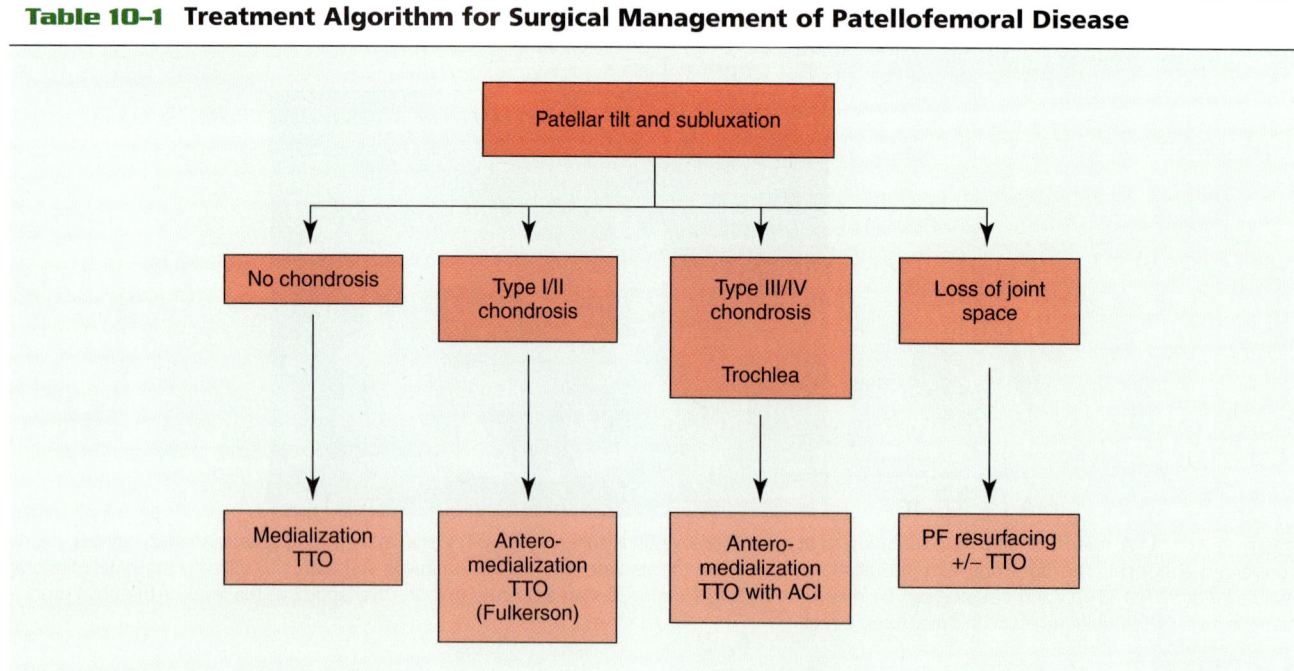

ACI, autologous chondrocyte implantation; *PF*, patellofemoral; *TTO*, tibial tubercle osteotomy.

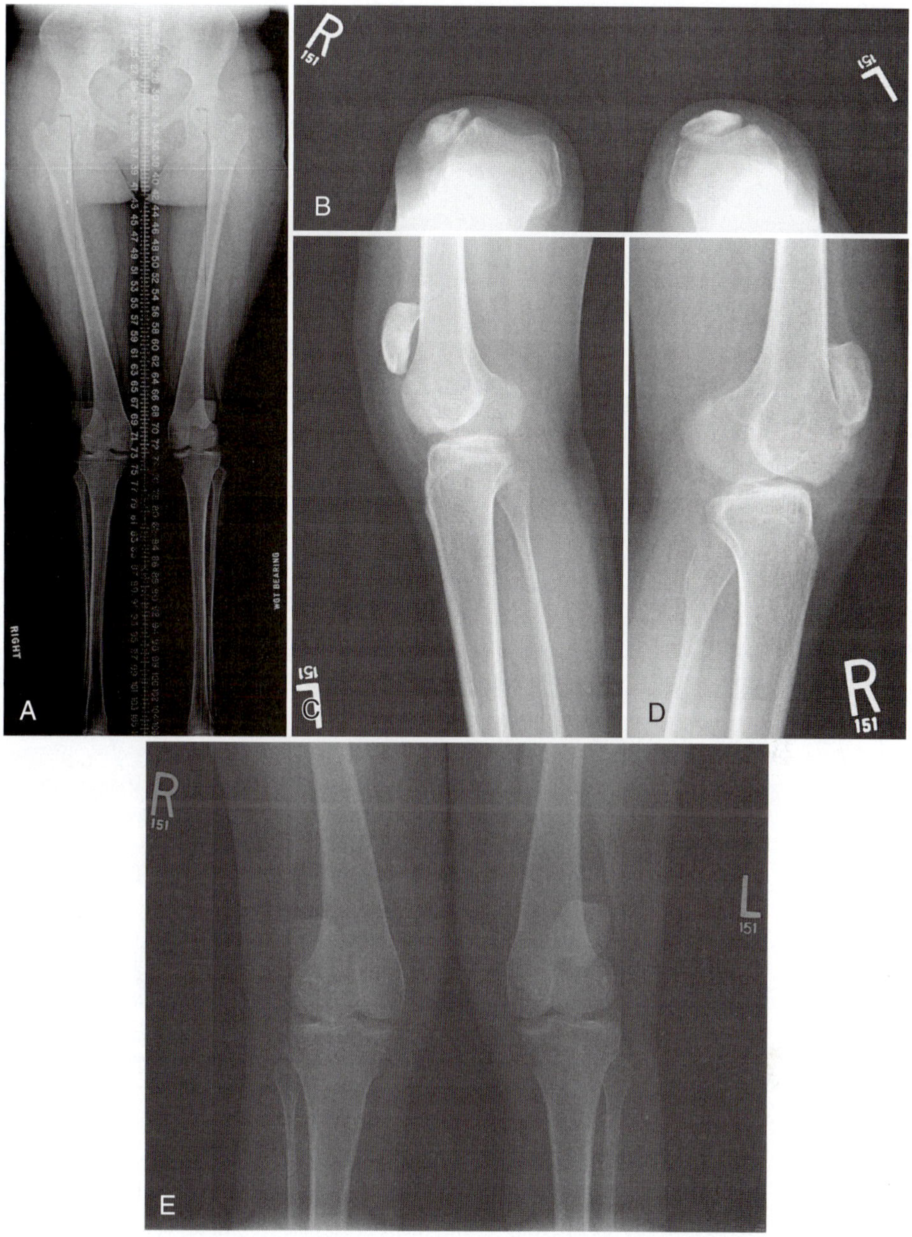

Figure 10–10 *A,* The long alignment x-rays of a 19-year-old woman who has valgus mechanical alignment. She has suffered from anterior knee instability and pain since early adolescence. Valgus malalignment is occasionally associated with trochlea dysplasia, a hypoplastic lateral femoral condyle, and patellar instability as the case here. This is an uncommon variant of trochlea dysplasia, but very difficult to manage because of the combined deformities both which promote patellar instability. *B,* Bilateral skyline x-rays demonstrate dislocation of the patella on the right and medial subluxation of the patella on the left. *C,D,* Lateral x-rays of both knees demonstrating patella alta. *E,* Bilateral AP x-rays demonstrate laterally positioned patellas and intact tibiofemoral joint spaces.

procedure and must be isolated, coagulated, or tied. It is important not to release the tendinous portion of the vastus lateralis muscle from the superior lateral patella because of the ensuing weakness that will develop. Any loose partial-thickness chondrosis flaps should be removed at the time of the lateral release to limit any pain resulting from mechanical causes.

If subluxation is associated with patellar tilt, arthroscopic lateral release should not be performed. Persistent subluxation, mechanical overload with subsequent progressive chondral wear, and pain will remain, resulting in failure of the procedure and unnecessary surgery for the patient (Figures 10–11 and 10–12). The importance of an accurate diagnosis in differentiating tilt and subluxation can be seen in the case shown in Figure 10–7, in which an isolated lateral release would not have been effective. Instead, an isolated medialization of the tibial tubercle with lateral release is indicated and was performed.

PATELLAR TILT AND SUBLUXATION WITH OR WITHOUT CHONDROSIS

Fulkerson Type I and II Chondrosis: Anteromedialization TTO

The usual causes of combination patellar subluxation and tilt include a lateralized tibial tubercle patellar tendon insertion with an abnormally increased Q angle, accompanying soft tissue medial attenuation, and lateral

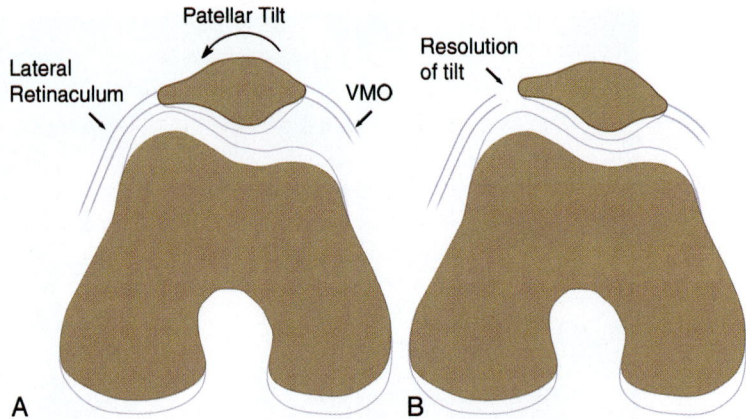

Figure 10-11 Isolated patellar tilt without subluxation is uncommon and due to a tight lateral retinaculum (A), isolated lateral release in this situation from the superior pole of the patella distally will keep attached the insertion of the vastus lateralis muscle to the superior pole of the patella and unload the lateral patellar facet (B). This is an effective but rarely required, and overly performed procedure.

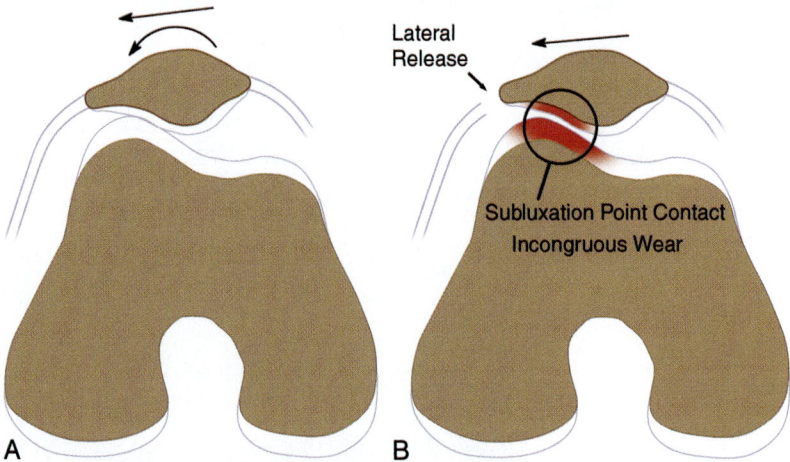

Figure 10-12 The more common situation clinically is a patella that has both lateral patellar tilt and subluxation (A). However a lateral release performed in this situation (B) resolves tilt but not subluxation, and pain often persists. Lateral release in this situation is contraindicated.

retinacular contracture. Chondrosis may have developed, and dysplasia of the trochlea may be present.

Surgical correction of abnormal quadriceps vectors resulting from a lateralized tibial tubercle and lateral retinacular contracture need to be addressed. Various forms of TTO with lateral retinacular release have been performed over the years. Fulkerson anteromedialization TTO[15] has gained popularity in the United States (Figure 10-13) as a modification of the Elmslie-Trillat[16] procedure because it allows more aggressive anterior translation than that provided by the latter. The soft tissue balancing that is required in order to centralize the patella in the trochlea may be performed concomitantly (Figure 10-14). This procedure offloads the lateral and inferior poles of the patella by anterior and medial translation of the tibial tubercle. Therefore it loads the proximal and medial poles of the patella. It has demonstrated successful clinical outcomes when the chondrosis involved with maltracking has been localized to the lateral patella facet or inferior patella pole. Conversely, it has demonstrated poor clinical outcomes in the presence of articular damage to the proximal or medial patella surfaces, or central trochlea involvement.[17] This has led to the classification of articular chondral injury to the patella locations as follows: type 1—chondral injury to the inferior patella pole, type 2—chondral injury to the lateral patella facet, type 3—chondral injury to the medial patella facet, and type 4—chondral injury to the proximal pole or pan-patellar surface (Figure 10-15).

Type III and IV Chondrosis: Anteromedialization TTO plus Autologous Chondrocyte Implantation

In a review of the clinical outcomes of the first 45 patients treated by autologous chondrocyte implantation (ACI) with full-thickness chondral lesions involving the patellofemoral joint, patients reported 70% good and excellent results with type III and type IV articular injuries of the patella.[18] As our experience grew, our clinical results

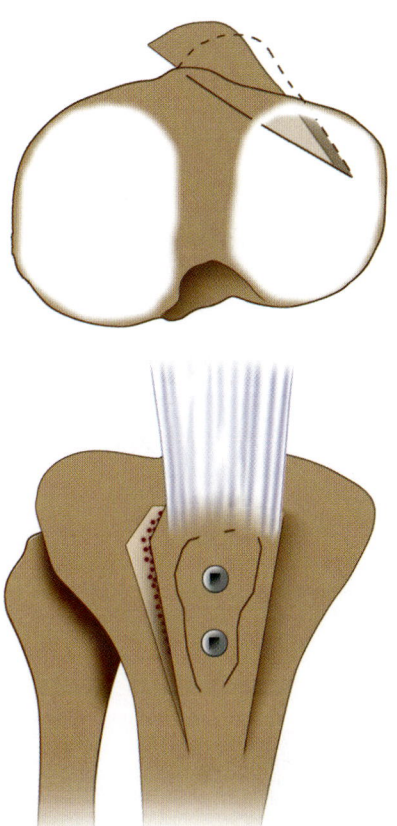

Figure 10-13 A Fulkerson osteotomy is a modification of the Elmslie-Trillat operation. It allows anterior translation of the tibial tubercle along with medial translation dependent on the obliquity of the osteotomy from anterior medial to posterior lateral. This is demonstrated in the diagram.

treating type III and type IV patellar lesions also improved. Including the first cohort of 45 patients, our recent experience with the patella, trochlea, or both articulations in 130 patients noted an 80% good and excellent result reported by patients; 18% of patients noted improved clinical outcomes (fair), and only three patients reported being the same or worse than they were before the surgery (see Chapter 7). ACI presently is our preferred treatment option for articular lesions in the patellofemoral joint when osteotomy alone (type III and IV patellar chondral injury with maltracking) is not indicated and joint preservation is desired.

Modified Surgical Technique of Anteromedialization TTO–Fulkerson[15]

TTO is a well-described treatment for a variety of patellar-related problems, including recurrent instability, maltracking, unloading chondral defects, and arthrosis. Fulkerson[19,20] and Trillat[16,21,22] osteotomy, the most common types, involve some degree of medialization and/or anterior displacement of the tubercle while leaving the distal cortical hinge intact. The amount of anterior and medial displacement can be adjusted based on the steepness of the osteotomy. This is determined by the nature of the pathology. Typically, in cases of instability, the osteotomy is flatter and the translation is more medial than anterior. When treating chondral defects or arthrosis, the purpose of the osteotomy is to decompress and unload the patellofemoral joint. Therefore, a steeper osteotomy is performed, whereby the tubercle is translated more anterior than medial.

When performed for the proper indications, the results of TTO are good. However, a number of possible complications are associated with the procedure.[23] In the past, I have found that patients often complained of a prominent bony ridge along the medial border of the osteotomy. This was seen more commonly after a steeper osteotomy had been performed. Typically, patients complained of tenderness over the area, especially with kneeling. Female patients often complained of difficulty shaving their legs. Some patients also were unhappy about the "knobby" appearance of their knee after an osteotomy. In an attempt to reduce these problems, I have developed a simple and reproducible technique for diminishing the bony prominence along the anteromedial border of the tuberosity after performing a TTO. This has significantly lessened the number of postoperative complaints associated with the procedure.

SURGICAL TECHNIQUE

The patient is placed in the standard supine position. I use a lateral post at the level of the greater trochanter to prevent external rotation of the leg as well as a post at the midcalf in order to maintain the knee in full extension and allow approximately 90 degrees of flexion during the procedure, if necessary. A longitudinal incision is made slightly lateral to midline so that the incision is not directly over the tubercle and the hardware used for fixation is not prominent. Wound breakdown, if it were to occur, would do so over muscle and not bone (Figure 10-16).

Evaluation of the articular pathology to determine the degree of anteriorization versus medialization is performed first, typically a full subvastus lateral release in combination with a TTO. Full-thickness medial and lateral flaps are made. The lateral border of the patellar tendon is identified, and a full-thickness release is made through capsule and synovium into the joint along the lateral border of the patella. The iliotibial band attachment from the iliotibial tract to the lateral superior pole of the patella is released, and the posterior border of the vastus lateralis muscle is identified and released off of synovium and the lateral intramuscular septum. This allows complete mobility to the patella and direct inspection of the trochlea and patella while leaving the

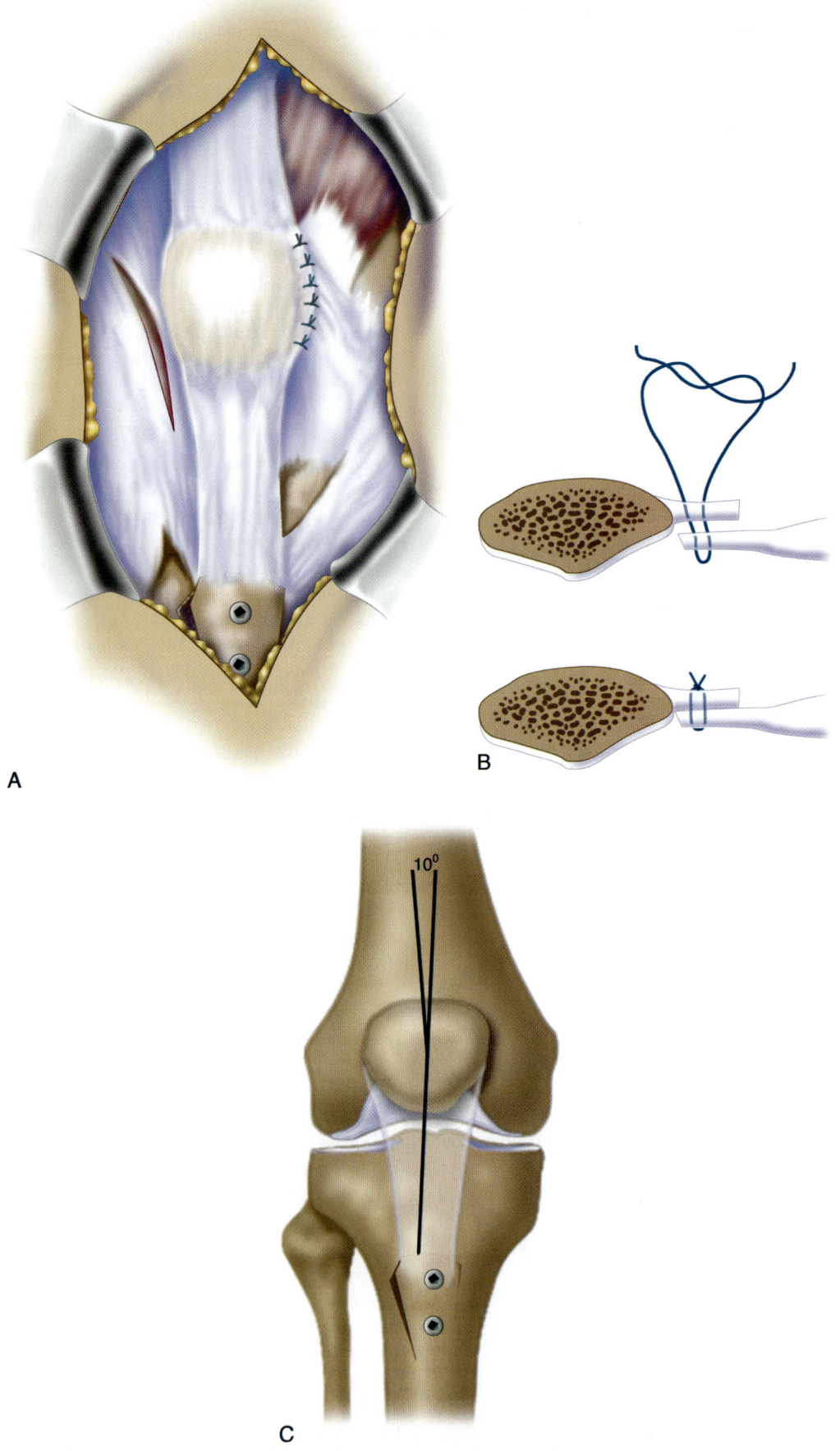

Figure 10-14 In order to translate the patella in response to the direction of translation of the tubercle, a soft tissue balancing must be performed. *A*, Laterally, the lateral capsule and the iliotibial band attachment to the superior pole of the patella are released to the posterior lateral intramuscular septum performing a lateral sub-vastus approach to the joint. This preserves the integrity of the quadriceps and especially the vastus lateralis attachment to the superior pole of the patella. *B*, On the medial side, I prefer a medial parapatellar arthrotomy and a vest–under-pants advancement of the VMO under the patellar retinaculum to further anteriorize the patella away from the trochlea unloading the articular surfaces as shown. *C*, After the procedure is completed the tubercle is usually beneath the tibial spines resulting in a post op Q angle of 0-10 degrees.

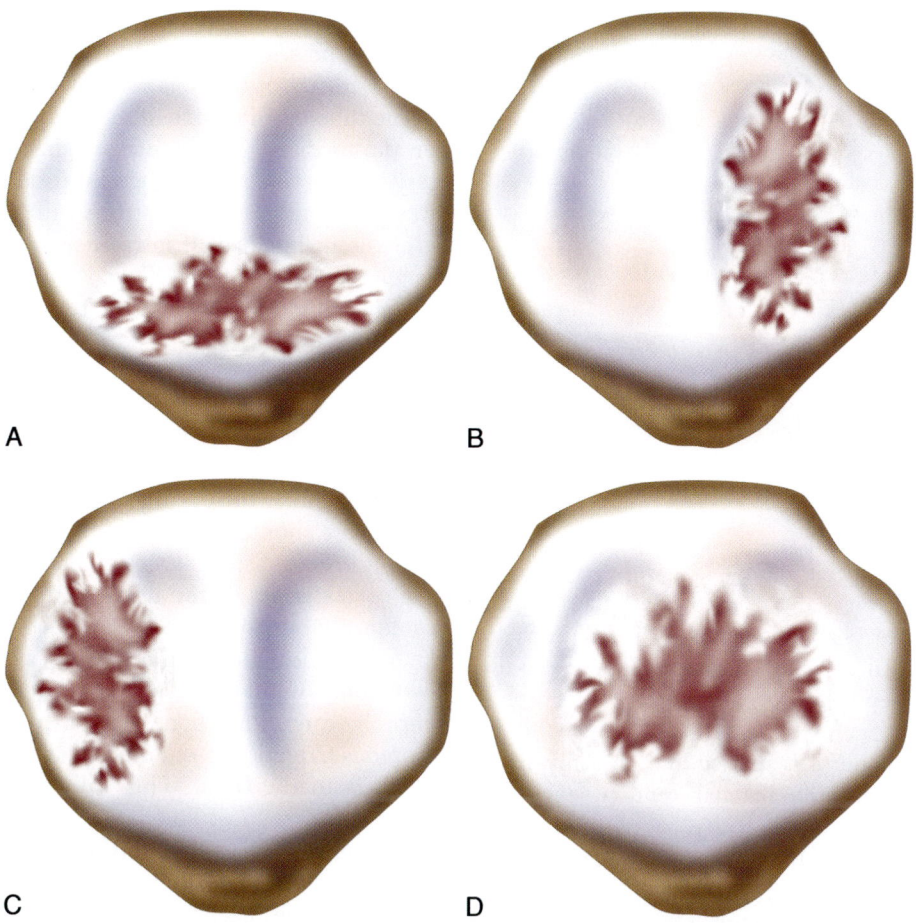

Figure 10–15 Fulkerson Classification of chondral defects to the patella. *A*, Type I – inferior patella pole. *B*, Type II – lateral patella facet. *C*, Type III – medial patella facet (often associated with a trochlea injury). *D*, Type IV – central panpatellar injury.

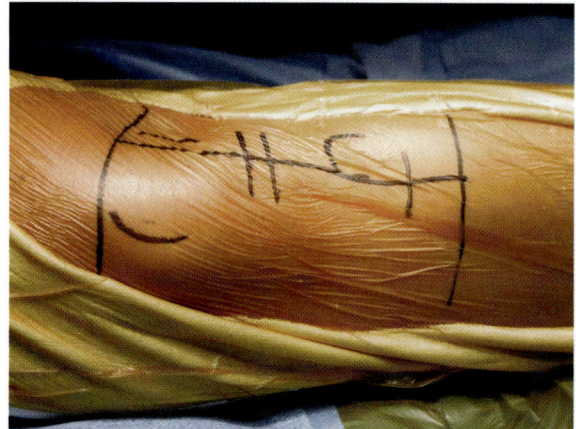

Figure 10–16 Skin incision from superior pole of patella to inferior border of tibial tubercle. Note the incision is slightly lateral to the patella.

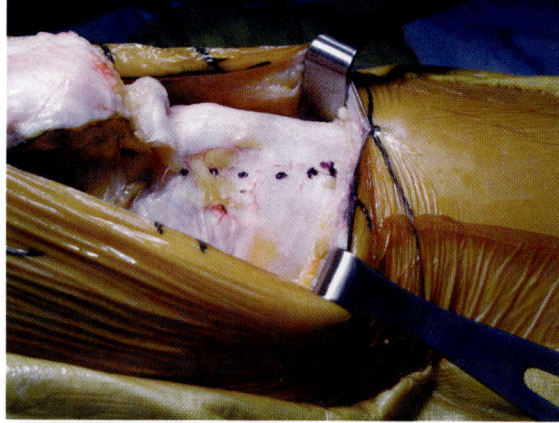

Figure 10–17 Complete exposure of tibial tubercle after creation of full-thickness medial and lateral skin-subcutaneous flaps.

medial sleeve intact. The areas of chondrosis then can be localized and the amount of medialization as well as anteriorization of the tibial tubercle needed to unload the damaged segment determined. The tibial tubercle is exposed in its entirety using full-thickness medial and lateral subcutaneous flaps (Figure 10–17).

An elevator is used from distal to proximal to lift the anterior muscle compartment off the tibia and expose the posterolateral border of the proximal tibia. A small Hohmann or Bennett retractor is placed behind the tibia to protect the neurovascular structures during the osteotomy.

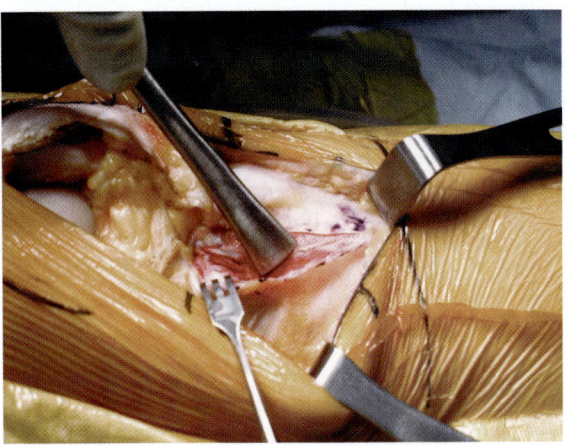

Figure 10–18 Creation of medial subperiosteal flap nearly all the way to the posteromedial border of the tibia including the pes tendon insertions and the superficial MCL.

Medially, an elevator is also used to create a large, full-thickness subperiosteal flap. Dissection is carried nearly to the superficial medial collateral ligament (Figures 10–18 and 10–19). This step is key for later repair to the osteotomized segment.

The retropatellar bursa is incised and an army–navy retractor placed under the patellar tendon, exposing the proximal aspect of the tuberosity.

Next are the bony cuts. Initially, a countercut is made just proximal to the tuberosity, taking care to protect the patellar tendon. This is done with a small sagittal saw from the medial to lateral border of the patellar tendon insertion. An oblique cut is made laterally to prevent propagation of the osteotomy toward the lateral cortex or the joint. The location of the osteotomy on the medial cortex is determined by the desired steepness of the osteotomy. Steeper osteotomies begin more anterior, just adjacent to the tuberosity. Flatter osteotomies begin more posteriorly down the medial face of the proximal tibia. Osteotomy angles vary from 30 degrees for an average steepness to 60 degrees of obliquity to the posterior lateral corner of the tibia for a steep anterior translation of the tubercle. The line of the osteotomy can be marked on the medial cortex with a marking pen or electrocautery. As the osteotomy proceeds distally, the direction of the cut should become flatter so that the distal cortical hinge is maintained. If intraarticular work (e.g., ACI) is required, then the distal hinge is cut obliquely and more steeply to elevate the entire tubercle proximally (see Chapter 7).

A saw is used just to perforate the medial cortex along the entire extent of the osteotomy. The exit point on the lateral cortex is determined and marked. This can be done using a jig (AMZ Tracker, DePuy, Warsaw, IN) or free hand, which is my preference. Again, the level of the cut should become more anterior as the osteotomy proceeds distally. Once the lateral cortex is marked, the cortex is perforated using a small sagittal saw. The osteotomy is completed by connecting the medial and lateral cortical perforations using a sagittal saw. The osteotomy should be deep enough so that it traverses entirely cancellous bone except for the distal hinge. Copious irrigation is required so as to not cause thermal necrosis to the bone. This will lead to rapid healing. However, care must be taken to ensure that the osteotomy is not too deep and perforates the posterior cortex, which can lead to iatrogenic fracture.[23,24] When the osteotomy has been completed, an osteotome can be used at all of the corners to ensure that the tuberosity is mobile. This should not involve a great deal of force.

Once mobile, the tuberosity can be translated into the desired position. I place the tuberosity so that the patellar tendon is directly anterior to the tibial spines. I then temporarily stabilize the tuberosity with large pointed reduction forceps while I range the knee and make sure that I have not overmedialized the tubercle with development of medial subluxation. At 90 degrees with neutral foot rotation, the tubercle–sulcus angle should be collinear or 0 degrees. The tuberosity is then stabilized with large pointed reduction forceps and fixed with two bicortical 3.5-mm fully threaded cortical screws placed using a lag technique orthogonal to the osteotomy site. I have not had loss of fixation with the smaller Synthes screws, do not have prominent hardware and have a tight pitch capture to the posterior cortex with excellent lag effect and compression.

At this point, often a large, sharp edge of bone is overhanging medially (Figure 10–20). This is trimmed vertically flush with the medial cortex of the tibia using a small sagittal saw. It can then be divided and used as bone graft laterally.

Optium DBM (demineralized bone matrix; LifeNet Health, Virginia Beach, VA) is packed tightly along the medial border of the osteotomy site (Figure 10–21). The medial subperiosteal sleeve is closed over the graft

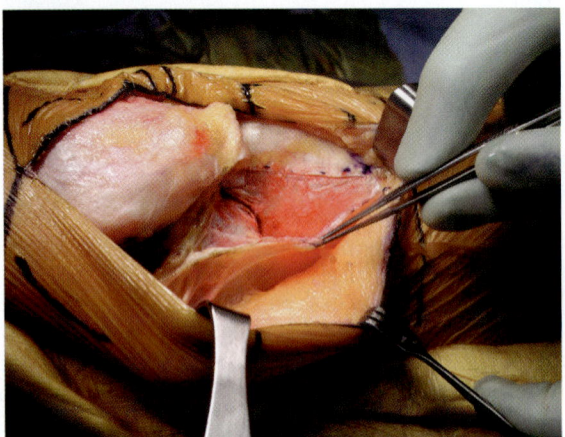

Figure 10–19 Creation of medial subperiosteal flap nearly all the way to the posteromedial border of the tibia including the pes tendon insertions and the superficial MCL.

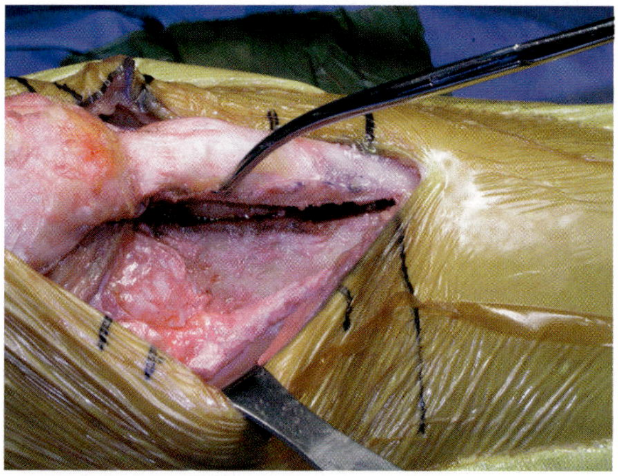

Figure 10-20 Medially overhanging bone after fixation of the osteotomy.

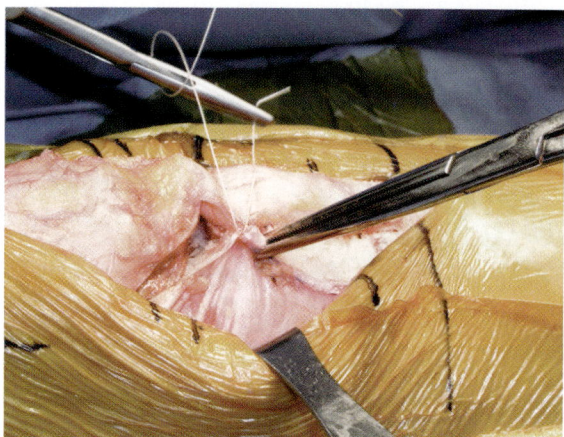

Figure 10-22 Closure of medial periosteal flap to the medial border of the patellar tendon insertion on the mobilized tibial tubercle after fixation over demineralized bone graft without undue tension.

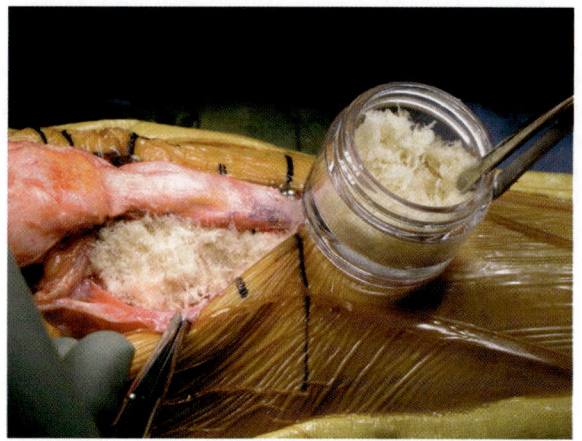

Figure 10-21 Packing of demineralized bone graft under medial periosteal flap.

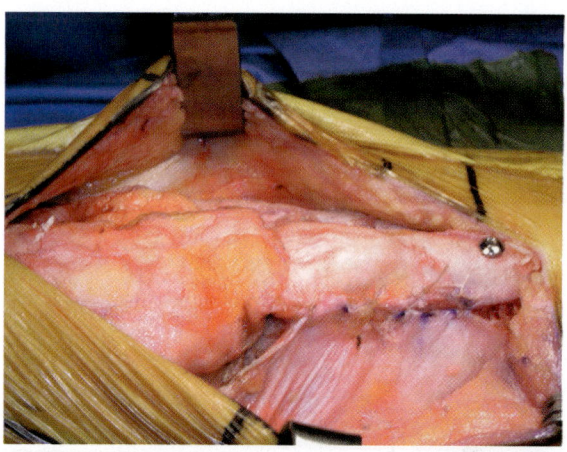

Figure 10-23 Closure of medial periosteal flap to the medial border of the patellar tendon insertion on the mobilized tibial tubercle after fixation over demineralized bone graft without undue tension.

and repaired back to the periosteum on the anterior aspect of the tuberosity (Figures 10–22 and 10–23). This can usually be done with minimal tension if an adequate flap has been raised initially. The envelope contains the superficial medial collateral ligament–pes anserinus insertion with periosteal sleeve to the posterior medial corner of the tibia. I routinely perform a lateral release (Figure 10–24) as part of the initial exposure.

A medial reefing or VMO advancement is performed as necessary depending on the level of insertion of the VMO (Figure 10–25). Normally, the VMO inserts at approximately the midpole of the patella.[25] I use a vest-under-pants technique for performing a medial advancement with the VMO sleeve coming under the patellar retinaculum (Figures 10–26). This advances the VMO as needed while the VMO sleeve is used as a soft tissue interposition[26] to further elevate the patella and not compress posterior the medial patella facet, as is typically performed with a "reefing."

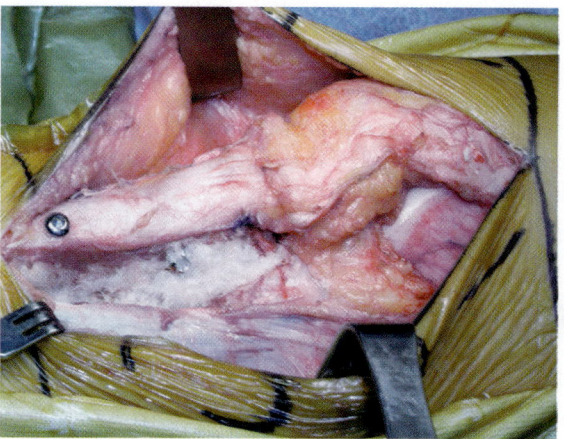

Figure 10-24 Completed osteotomy viewed laterally. Demineralized bone graft has also been added to the cancellous bed of the mobilized tibial tubercle which lessens bleeding and enhances bone union. Note that a full-thickness lateral subvastus release has been performed.

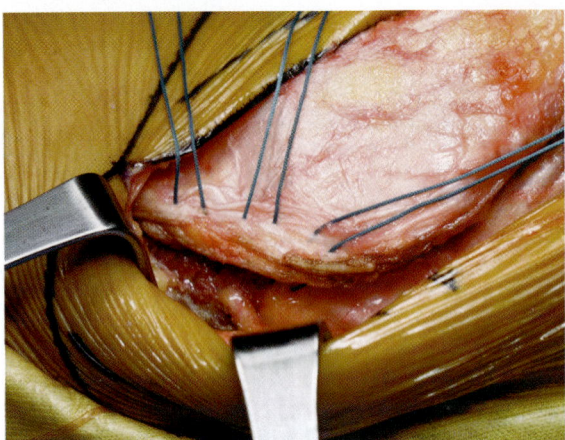

Figure 10-25 Pants-under-vest technique for medial advancement. The VMO insertion is advanced to the mid-pole of the patella and taken under the patellar retinacular sleeve to enhance anterior translation of the patella. Horizontal mattress sutures are used to mid patellar pole and tied. Distal sutures are not used so as to not compress the patella.

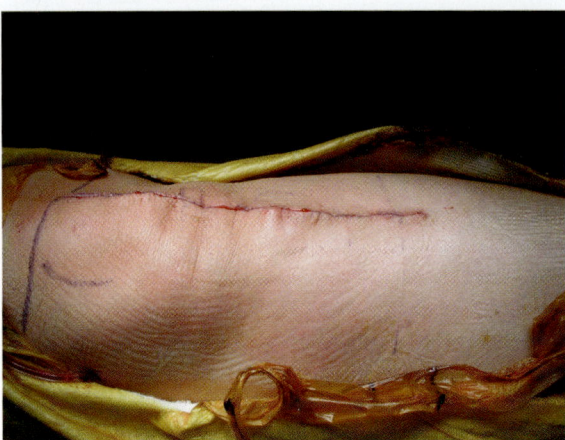

Figure 10-27 Skin closure. Note there is no large prominence of the tuberosity as the medial contour has been restored.

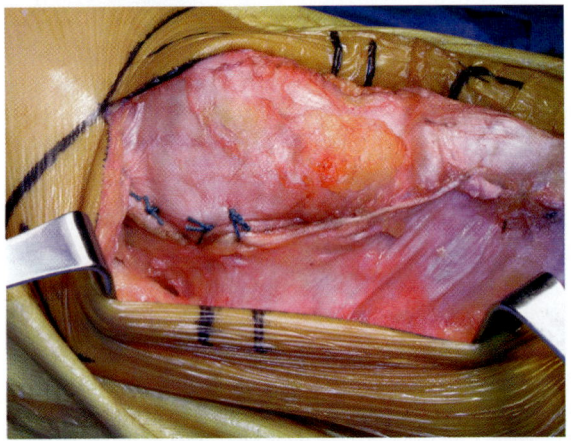

Figure 10-26 Pants-under-vest technique for medial advancement. The VMO insertion is advanced to the mid-pole of the patella and taken under the patellar retinacular sleeve to enhance anterior translation of the patella. Horizontal mattress sutures are used to mid patellar pole and tied. Distal sutures are not used so as to not compress the patella.

Routine closure and postoperative care are then performed (Figures 10-27). Patients are immediately allowed full weight bearing in extension. Passive range of motion is also started on the day of surgery. I have found that these osteotomies generally heal rapidly by 6 to 8 weeks and have not seen any complications directly related to this modification in technique.

TTO is a relatively common procedure with predictable results. The technique differs only slightly from standard descriptions. The careful dissection of the full-thickness medial periosteal sleeve to the posteromedial border of the tibia is the key step in the procedure. Most techniques describe only a limited medial subperiosteal dissection. When only a limited flap is raised, it is difficult to repair at the end of the procedure. Often, a prominent edge of bone remains medially. The subcutaneous tissues are generally very thin in this region, and this prominent edge of bone can be seen and felt by the patient. By excising the prominent bone and repairing the periosteum over allograft bone matrix, a more normal contour can be restored to the proximal tibia. Although this may not affect patient outcomes in terms of restoration of stability or reduction of patellofemoral pain, overall patient satisfaction with the procedure is improved.

TROCHLEA DYSPLASIA

Accurate assessment of patellofemoral maltracking should always include an assessment for trochlea dysplasia in order to have a successful surgical outcome. My assessment for trochlea dysplasia is part of any routine evaluation of patellar instability. However, my treatment for trochlea dysplasia with surgical trochleoplasty is the last part of the decision to stabilize the patella, and I use the technique sparingly. Lateral maltracking secondary to an increased Q angle is the most usual situation that I encounter. The typical surgical algorithm first involves a lateral subvastus arthrotomy to release the tight lateral structures. This allows visualization of articular injury to the patella, trochlea, and dysplasia of the trochlea. TTO is then performed to centralize and possibly unload damaged articular surfaces as assessed intraoperatively. ACI to the patella or trochlea is my preferred method of cartilage repair in the patellofemoral joint because of its excellent clinical outcomes, and the need for this procedure has already been determined prior to the procedure. A VMO advancement is then performed as needed to stabilize the patella. However, at this stage, if the trochlea is dysplastic, ongoing instability issues may be encountered. Slight overtensioning of the VMO may lead to medial subluxation and undertensioning to lateral subluxation if trochlea dysplasia is present. At this point, the last part of the stabilization procedure is a trochleoplasty.

Dysplasia of the trochlea of the distal femur is an uncommon developmental abnormality leading to patellar instability and premature degeneration of the patellofemoral joint. It is occasionally associated with dysplasia of the lateral femoral condyle leading to a valgus deformity accompanied by patellofemoral instability (see Figure 10–10). The degree of dysplasia varies from subtle flattening of the proximal entry site to the trochlea (Figure 10–28) to a bulbous convex entry site leading to severe instability (Figure 10–29). Because the patella is a sesamoid bone that develops secondary to its

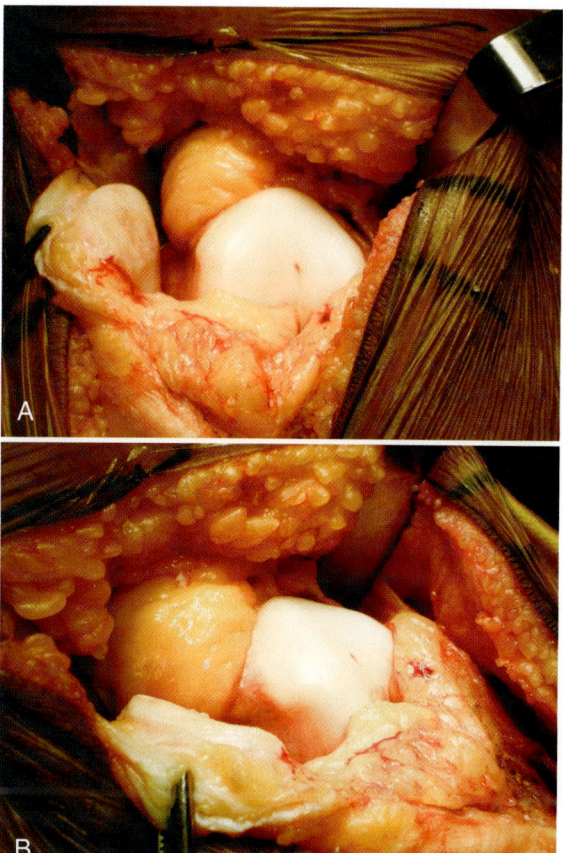

Figure 10–29 *A,* Another case of trochlea dysplasia in a more severe form. Note the prominent bulbous proximal entry site to the trochlea ("trochlea spur" as described by Dejour) that is poorly formed, viewed from below. *B,* The same patient as in 10-30*A*, viewed from lateral noting the prominent anterior spur of the trochlea relative to the anterior femoral cortex. It is associated patella alta is present than severe instability results as the inferior pole of the patella is not engaged in the trochlea sulcus. If early engagement is present in instability it is less severe. Classification of Henri Dejour (see Table 10-2) morphologic variations in Trochlea Dysplasia.

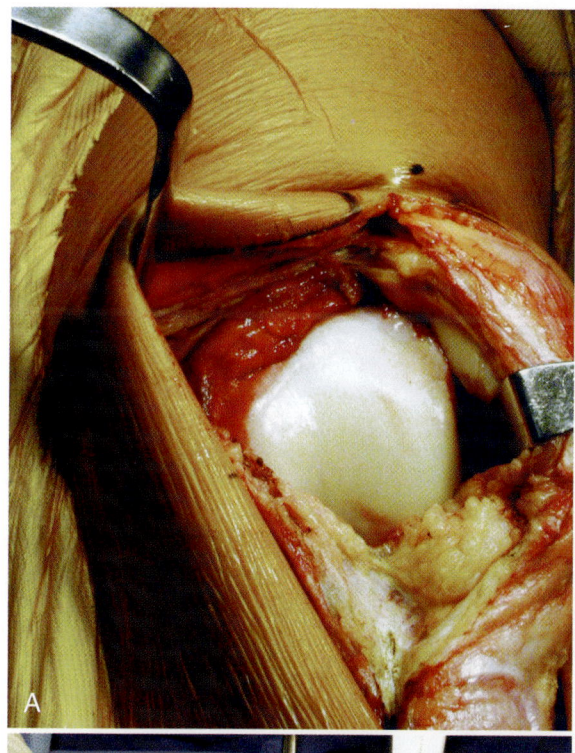

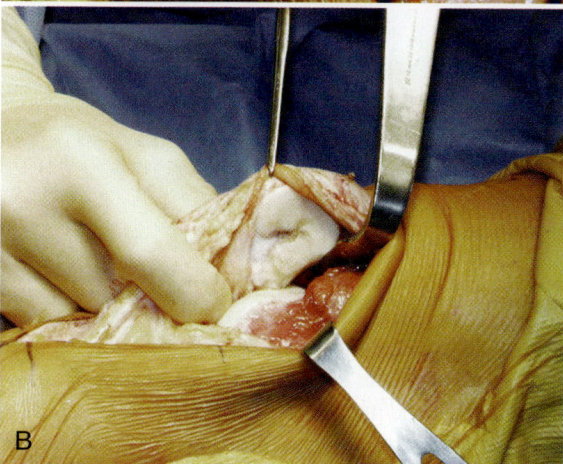

Figure 10–28 *A,* Moderate dysplasia of the trochlea as viewed from below with a superior lateral boss. *B,* Severe patellar damage to the central and inferior pole of the patella secondary to chronic instability and maltracking.

congruity with the trochlea, it is frequently flattened or concave on its large lateral facet to match the shape of the trochlea. Like congenital dislocation of the hip (CDH) in the hip leading to premature osteoarthritis in the fifth decade of life, dysplasia of the trochlea usually presents with instability, anterior knee pain, a diagnosis of "chondromalacia," and end-stage isolated patellofemoral arthritis more commonly in women in the fifth decade of life.

The diagnosis requires attention to the possibility of recurrent patellar instability secondary to dysplasia of the trochlea. If a patient has recurrent instability, a lateral x-ray film may frequently demonstrate a prominent proximal barrel-shaped trochlea as noted by Dejour et al[9] with a "crossing sign" and a trochlea "spur." The Dejour description and classification of dysplasia has been published (Table 10–2).[27] Figure 10–30 shows the morphologic phenotypes described by Dejour that relate

Table 10-2 Henri Dejour Classification Grades of Trochlear Dysplasia

Grade	Conventional Radiography	Computed Tomography
A	Crossing sign	Trochlear morphology preserved
B	Crossing sign supratrochlear spur	Flat or convex trochlea
C	Crossing sign	Asymmetry of trochlear facets
D	Crossing sign supratrochlear spur	Asymmetry of trochlear facets

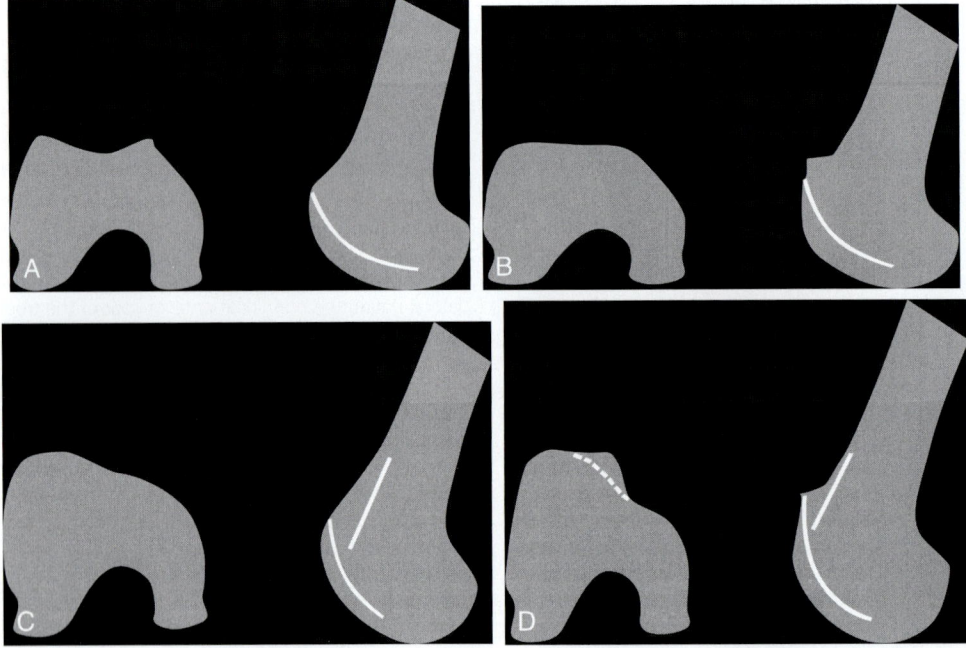

Figure 10–30 *A,* Grade A-dysplasia of the trochlea. *B,* Grade B-dysplasia of the trochlea-Henri Dejour (see Table 10–2). *C,* Grade C-dysplasia of the trochlea-Henri Dejour (see Table 10–2). *D,* Grade D-dysplasia of the trochlea-Henri Dejour (see Table 10-2).

to the radiologic findings listed in Table 10–2. CT scan gives the most accurate diagnosis, but MRI scan is also useful.

Patients frequently have multiple prior failed surgeries, which include proximal soft tissue balancing of the patella along with distal tubercle transfer and a failed clinical outcome with further instability episodes (Figure 10–31). Once the diagnosis is established as instability secondary to trochlea dysplasia, surgical reconstruction is necessary. With trochlea dysplasia in addition to an abnormal shape of the trochlea with flattening or convexity, often too much cartilage is present proximal and centrally. This acts as a type of speed bump over which the patella is misguided away from the central sulcus in flexion. Removing and contouring the proximal entry point to the patella capture is the goal of a synovial interposition trochleoplasty (Figure 10–32). This allows the patellofemoral joint to remain congruent because it does not distort the shape of either articulation. Surgical correction by interposition soft tissue synovial trochleoplasty can be performed with

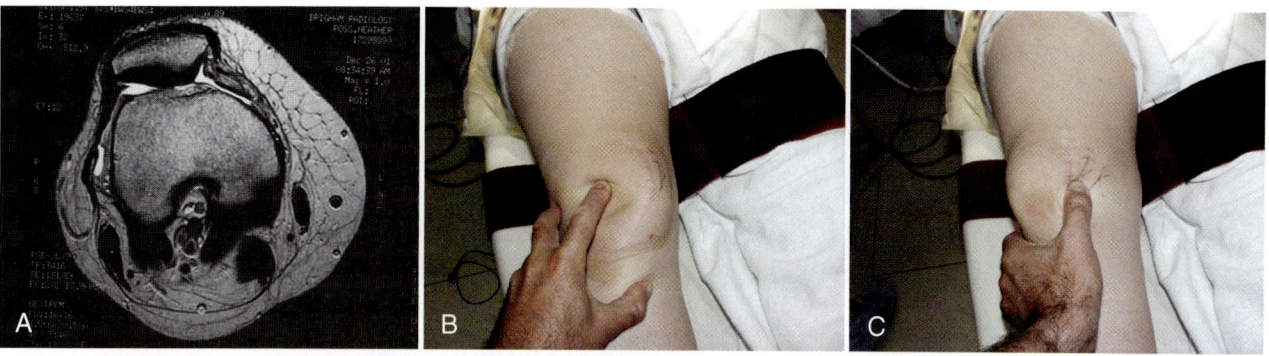

Figure 10–31 *A*, Axial image of a CT scan in a young woman who has had previous proximal and distal realignment surgery that has been unsuccessful with continued recurrent patellar instability. The MRI scan notes a flattened proximal trochlea sulcus. *B,C*, Same patient as in Figure 10–31A, note the marked medial and lateral instability of the patella with previous skin incision noted.

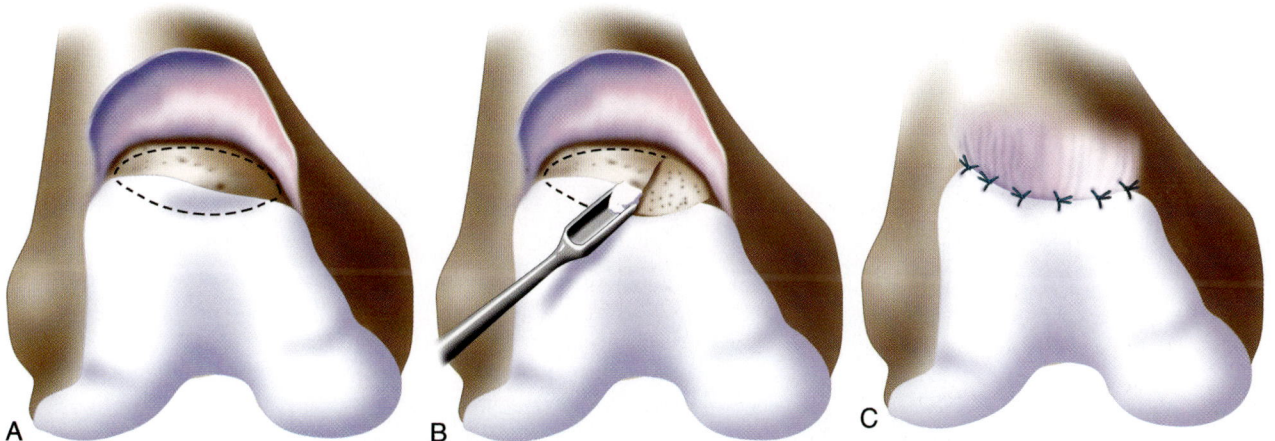

Figure 10–32 *A*, Diagrammatic representation of a Peterson synovial interposition trochleoplasty (as described by Peterson; Peterson L, Karrlson J, Brittberg M, et al: Patellar Instability with recurrent dislocation due to Patellofemoral Dysplasia results after surgical treatment. Bulletin of the Hospital for Joint Disease Orthopaedic Institute 1988;48:130–139). The synovium is reflected proximally from the trochlea attachment. The central proximal one to 1 ½ centimeters of cartilage and bone at the level of the lower patellar pole in engagement to the trochlea is removed in line with the intercondylar notch to allow capture of the lower patellar pole into the trochlea. It is recessed towards the anterior femoral cortex. *B*, Diagrammatic representation of removal of cartilage and bone centrally at the most proximal aspect of the trochlea where the initial instability of the patella occurs when it does not find a central leading sulcus. *C*, Diagrammatic representation of the synovium advanced and sewn through the articular surface to allow a congruent and smooth the entry site for the patella to engage into the trochlea.

good success.[28] Figure 10–33 shows the technique used for the case shown in Figure 10–32. Another example of interposition trochleoplasty as developed and described by Peterson is given in the case studies in Chapter 13.

Bony reconstruction of the trochlea was first described by Albee[29] in 1915. It involved lateral trochlea osteotomy and elevation with a bone block autograft taken from the proximal tibia and fixated with a bony nail. It was performed through a direct lateral approach and was successful in stabilizing the patella; however, because of the increased contact forces on the lateral patella facet, it was prone to develop osteoarthrosis.

Dejour et al[9] described a bony contouring of the trochlea, which has been also successfully performed by others.[30-33] The technique (Figure 10–34) involves an open arthrotomy, recession of the synovium from the attachment of the proximal trochlea to expose the distal femur at the entry site of the trochlea. A bur that has a measured resection from the articular surface then excavates bone deep to the proximal articular surface of the trochlea. The central sulcus is cut with a knife, the medial and lateral trochlea facets are impacted with a bone tamp so as to form a central sulcus, and the osteochondral facets of the trochlea are stabilized with a staple, absorbable screw, or screw that has a countersunk head. Potential complications include delayed or nonunion of the trochlea, chondrolysis, arthrofibrosis, persistent pain because of patellar articular changes, and progression to patellar articular chondrosis secondary to incongruency of the joint. The incongruency of the joint

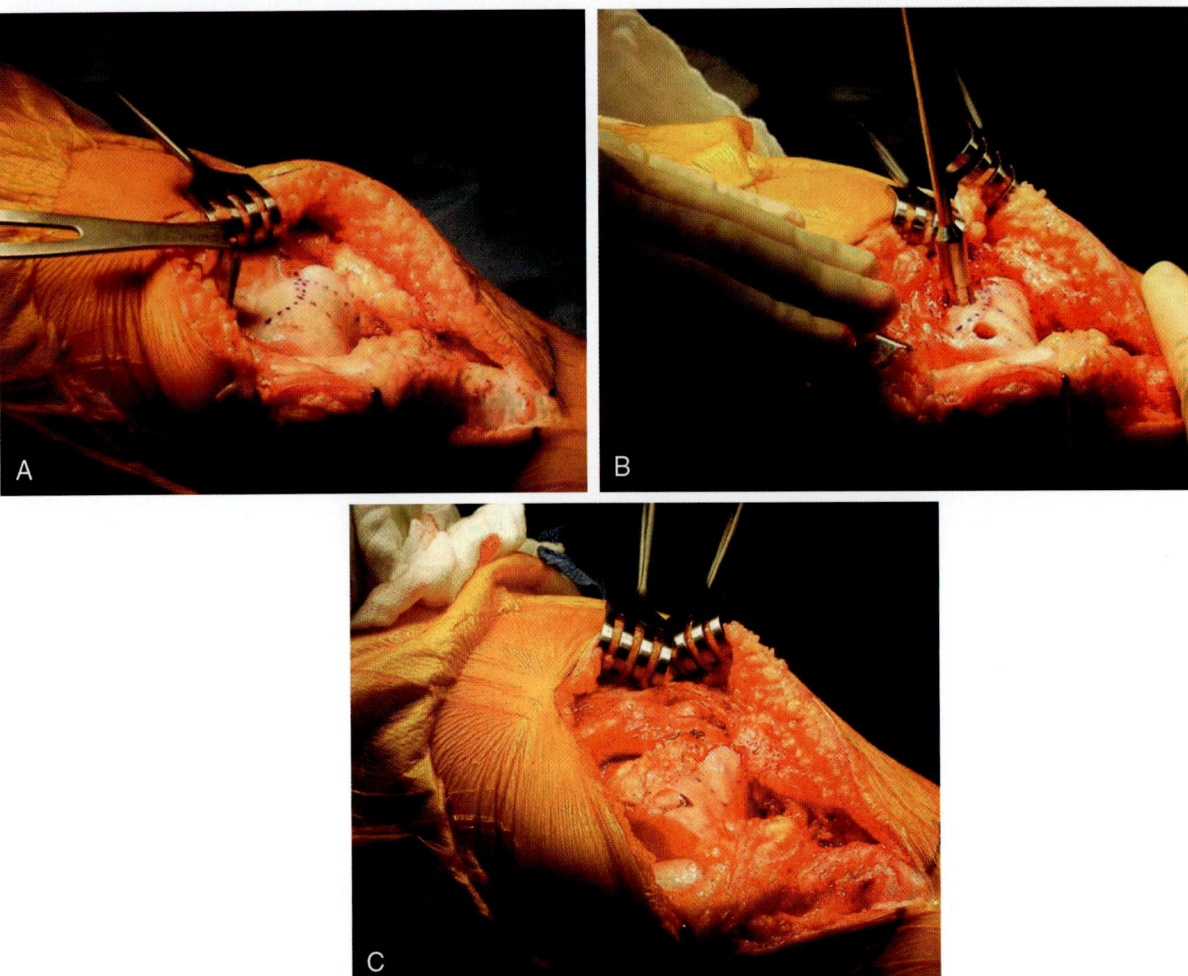

Figure 10-33 *A*, Clinical example of a Peterson Interposition Trochleoplasty-open appearance with central markings towards the intercondylar notch demonstrating the central tracking path of patella. The transverse curvilinear proximal markings represent the cartilage and bone to be removed centering on the distal tracking pathway. *B*, A donor osteochondral plug is being harvested taken from the proposed area of discarded cartilage and bone. The donor osteochondral plug measures 1 mm oversized to ensure a good press fit into the recipient site, noted empty on the lateral trochlea, measured to the same recipient depth. *C*, The final appearance of the joint after the synovium has been advanced to the remaining proximal cartilage and bone. The knee joint is closed with a medial advancement of the VMO. One year postoperatively the patient is asymptomatic with no recurrent instability of the patella and an absence of anterior knee pain. The opposite knee similarity has failed open proximal and distal realignment procedures. It will also undergo open trochleoplasty to ensure stability. Bilateral disease is common in this condition.

specifically concerns me, so I have used the technique described by Lars Peterson with synovial interposition advancement.

Awareness of the importance of the shape of the femoral sulcus as a component of patellar instability has gained more acceptance over the last decade. Consequently, surgical deepening of the sulcus has been introduced. The indications, techniques, rehabilitation, and evaluation of results are still being systematically sought and clarified. However, recurrent patellar instability after surgical treatment should always raise suspicion for dysplasia of the trochlea.

PATELLAR TILT AND SUBLUXATION: RADIOGRAPHIC LOSS OF JOINT SPACE, PATELLOFEMORAL REPLACEMENT WITH OR WITHOUT TTO, AND PATELLOFEMORAL PROSTHETIC ARTHROPLASTY

When collapse of the joint space is seen radiographically by Merchant or skyline view, cartilage repair by ACI is no longer possible. Isolated osteotomy is not possible if parapatellar cartilage loss is present. The procedure relies on intact full-thickness cartilage margins to maintain the

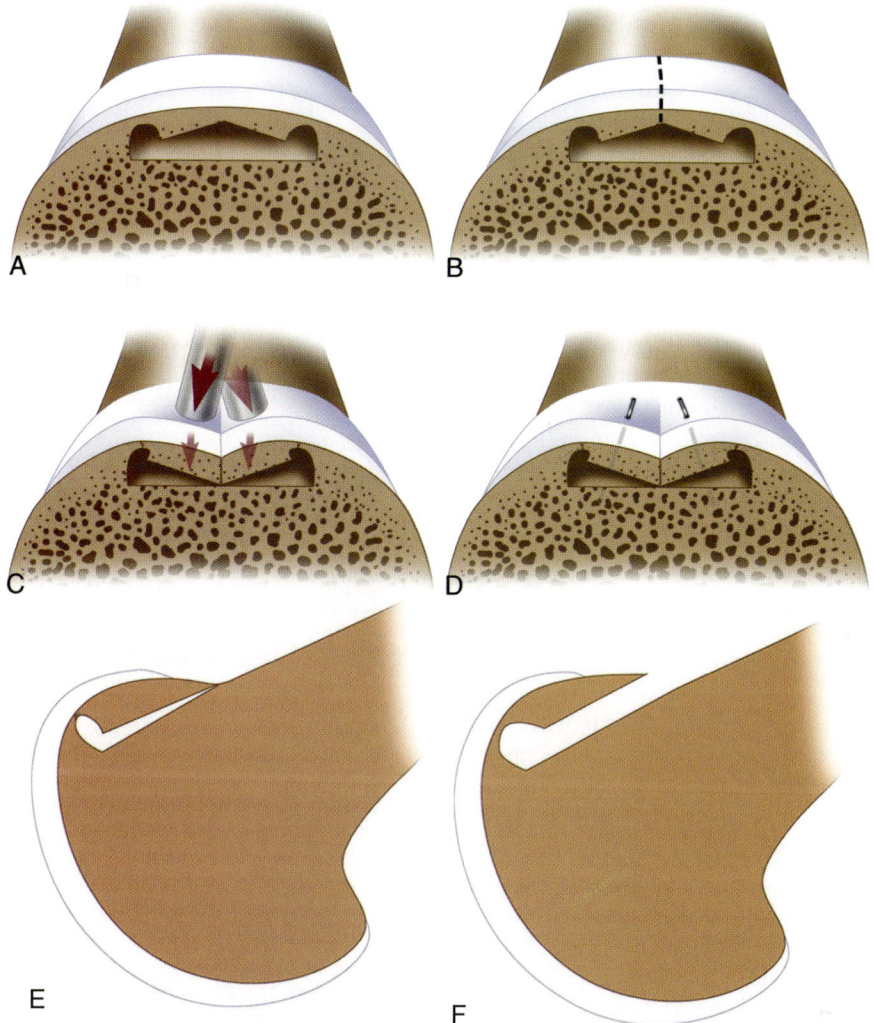

Figure 10–34 The steps in performing a Dejour trochleoplasty. *A*, The anterior femoral cortex is exposed proximal to the trochlea by elevating and moving proximal the synovium and leaving it intact. Using a measured distance micro-bur, removal of bone at a fixed distance posterior to the articular cartilage is performed. It is then thinned out centrally towards the intercondylar notch, and tranversely and distally (see Figure 10–34*E*). *B*, A knife blade is then used centrally to break through where the bone is maximally thinned out. *C*, A bone tamp is then used to implode the medial and lateral trochlea facets to create a central sulcus. *D*, The bone is fixated traditionally with a staple, but presently metal screws with the heads countersunk or bioabsorbable screws are utilized. The synovium is then readvanced to the articular cartilage margin and resutured through it to maintain a soft tissue sleeve to the articular surface and maintain the articular surface flush to the anterior femoral cortical surface. *E*, *F*, Diagrammatic representation of the subchondral bone transversely and distally. At the time of impaction of the medial and lateral trochlea facets the entire articular surface plastically deforms to meet the anterior femoral cortex in the sagittal plane as well.

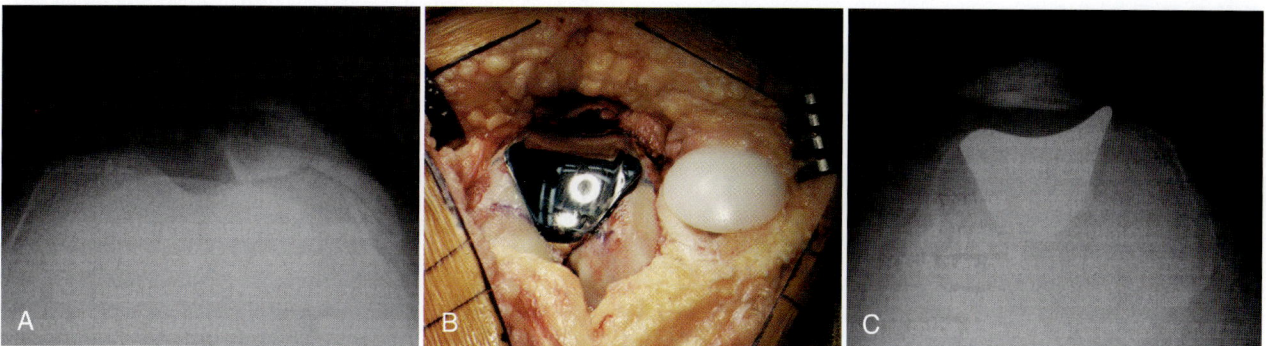

Figure 10–35 *A*, Merchant x-ray view demonstrating obliteration of the articular joint space. *B*, Intraoperative appearance of a patella femoral prosthetic resurfacing using a standard patella from an existing knee system with a custom design inset trochlea metal implant that is 3 mm thick–very bone preserving. *C*, Merchant x-ray view demonstrating postoperative appearance of patellofemoral prosthesis.

joint space so that the growing cartilage repair tissue may fill the defect. If medial or proximal cartilage is absent, then TTO with anterior and medial translation is not effective. In a middle-aged patient with this condition who is too young for a total knee replacement, I have found that patellofemoral prosthesis offers pain relief, improves functionality, and preserves bone stock. Initially, a custom trochlea inset metal prosthesis with a standard polyethylene patella button is used. A standard medial parapatellar arthrotomy is performed with standard patellar resurfacing. The trochlea prosthesis is only 3 mm thick and removes little cartilage and bone (Figure 10–35). It is easily converted to a total knee replacement if the tibiofemoral cartilage degenerates. It does not jeopardize future reconstructions, yet it allows adequate pain relief and functionality for activities of daily living. Several companies presently offer off-the-shelf implants (see Chapter 15 for a description of indications, technique, and results).

SUMMARY

Patellofemoral disease is one of the most problematic management issues for the orthopedist dealing with knee reconstructive surgery. Once nonoperative management has failed in alleviating pain and improving functionality, careful assessment to determine the underlying pathomechanics causing the instability and/or degenerative process is necessary for successful management. These factors include limb alignment and patellar pathomechanics, patella alta, increased Q angle, dysplasia of the trochlea, secondary soft tissue imbalance, and localized chondrosis to the patella and trochlea.

The management algorithm presented attempts to deal with these identified factors and the secondary degenerative processes. When identified carefully, the options of patellar lateral release, anteromedial TTO, trochleoplasty, ACI, and unicompartmental patellofemoral prosthesis will provide improved functionality and pain relief for the young patient suffering with patellofemoral pain.

REFERENCES

1. Aroen A, Loken S, Heir S, et al. Articular cartilage lesions in 993 consecutive knee arthroscopies. *Am J Sports Med.* 2004;32: 211–215.
2. Curl WW, Krome J, Gordon ES, et al. Cartilage injuries: a review of 31,516 knee arthroscopies. *Arthroscopy.* 1997;13:456–460.
3. Hjelle K, Solheim E, Strand T, et al. Articular cartilage defects in 1,000 knee arthroscopies. *Arthroscopy.* 2002;18:730–734.
4. Kaplan LD, Schurhoff MR, Selesnick H, et al. Magnetic resonance imaging of the knee in asymptomatic professional basketball players. *Arthroscopy.* 2005;21:557–561.
5. Nomura E, Inoue M, Kurimura M. Chondral and osteochondral injuries associated with acute patellar dislocation. *Arthroscopy.* 2003;19:717–721.
6. France L, Nester C. Effect of errors in the identification of anatomical landmarks on the accuracy of Q angle values. *Clin Biomech (Bristol, Avon).* 2001;16:710–713.
7. Greene C, Edwards TB, Wade MR, et al. Reliability of the quadriceps angle measurement. *Am J Knee Surg.* 2001;14:97–103.
8. Aglietti P, Insall JN, Cerulli G. Patellar pain and incongruence, I: measurements of incongruence. *Clin Orthop Relat Res.* 1983;176: 217–224.
9. Dejour H, Walch G, Nove-Josserand L, et al. Factors of patellar instability: an anatomic radiographic study. *Knee Surg Sports Traumatol Arthrosc.* 1994;2:19–26.
10. Winalski C, Aliabadi P, Wright R, et al. Enhancement of joint fluid with intravenously administered gadopentetate dimeglumine: technique, rationale, and implications. *Radiology.* 1993;187:179–185.
11. Alparslan L, Winalski C, Boutin R, et al. Postoperative magnetic resonance imaging of articular cartilage repair. *Semin Musculoskelet Radiol.* 2001;5:345–363.
12. Beaconsfield T, Pintore E, Maffuli N, et al. Radiological measurements in patellofemoral disorders. A review. *Clin Orthop Relat Res.* 1994;308:18–28.
13. Schoettle PB, Zanetti M, Seifert B, et al. The tibial tuberosity-trochlear groove distance; a comparative study between CT and MRI scanning. *Knee.* 2006;13:26–31.
14. Caton J, Deschamps G, Chambat P, et al. Patella infera. Apropos of 128 cases. [French]. *Rev Chir Orthop Reparatrice Appar Mot.* 1982;68:317–325.
15. Fulkerson JP. Anteromedialization of the tibial tuberosity for patellofemoral malalignment. *Clin Orthop Relat Res.* 1983;176–181.
16. Trillat A, Dejour H, Couette A. Diagnosis and treatment of recurrent dislocations of the patella. [French]. *Rev Chir Orthop Reparatrice Appar Mot.* 1964;50(Nov-Dec):813–824.
17. Pidoriano AJ, Weinstein RN, Buuck DA, et al. Correlation of patellar articular lesions with results from anteromedial tibial tubercle transfer. *Am J Sports Med.* 1997;25:533–537.
18. Minas T, Bryant T. The role of autologous chondrocyte implantation in the patellofemoral joint. *Clin Orthop Relat Res.* 2005;30–39.
19. Fulkerson JP. Patellofemoral pain disorders: evaluation and management. *J Am Acad Orthop Surg.* 1994;2:124–132.
20. Gomoll AH, Minas T, Farr J, et al. Treatment of chondral defects in the patellofemoral joint. *J Knee Surg.* 2006;19:285–295.
21. Cox J. An evaluation of the Elmslie-Trillat procedure for management of patellar dislocations and subluxations: a preliminary report. *Am J Sports Med.* 1976;4(2):72–77.
22. Barber F, McGarry J. Elmslie-Trillat procedure for the treatment of recurrent patellar instability. *Arthroscopy.* 2008;24(1):77–81.
23. Bellemans J, Cauwenberghs F, Brys P, et al. Fracture of the proximal tibia after Fulkerson anteromedial tibial tubercle transfer. A report of four cases. *Am J Sports Med.* 1998;26(2):300–302.
24. Stetson W, Friedman M, Fulkerson J, et al. Fracture of the proximal tibia with immediate weightbearing after a Fulkerson osteotomy. *Am J Sports Med.* 1997;25(4):570–574.
25. Masri B, Kim W, Pagnano M. Mini-subvastus approach for minimally invasive total knee replacement. *Tech Knee Surg.* 2007;6(2): 124–130.
26. Minas T, Peterson L. Advanced techniques in autologous chondrocyte transplantation. *Clin Sports Med.* 1999;18:13–44, v–vi.
27. Dejour H, Walch G, Neyret P, et al. Dysplasia of the femoral trochlea. *Rev Chir Orthop Reparatrice Appar Mot.* 1990;76(1):45–54.
28. Peterson L, Karrlson J, Brittberg M, et al. Patellar instability with recurrent dislocation due to patellofemoral dysplasia results after surgical treatment. *Bull Hosp Joint Dis Orthop Inst.* 1988;48: 130–139.
29. Albee F. The bone graft wedge in the treatment for habitual dislocation of the patella. *Med Rec.* 1915;88:257–259.
30. von Knoch F, Böhm T, Bürgi M, et al. Trochleoplasty for recurrent patellar dislocation in association with trochlear dysplasia: a 4- to 14-year follow-up study. *J Bone Joint Surg Br.* 2006;88-B: 1331–1335.
31. Verdonk R, Jansegers E, Stuyts B. Trochleoplasty in dysplastic knee trochlea. *Knee Surg Sports Traumatol Arthrosc.* 2005;13: 529–533.
32. Schottle P, Fucentese S, Pfirrmann C, et al. Trochleoplasty for patellar instability due to trochlear dysplasia. *Acta Orthop Scand.* 2005;76:693–698.
33. Donell S. Deepening trochleoplasty for distal femoral dysplasia in patellar instability: thick osteochondral flap technique. *Tech Knee Surg.* 2008;7:19.

Chapter 11

Treatment of Deep Osteochondritis Dissecans Lesions, Avascular Necrosis, and Osteochondral Defects of the Knee Using Autologous Bone Grafting

Tom Minas, MD, MS

INTRODUCTION

OSTEOCHONDRITIS DISSECANS

CLASSIFICATION AND MANAGEMENT

AVASCULAR NECROSIS

CLINICAL RESULTS—CASE SERIES—TECHNIQUE FOR TREATMENT OF DEEP CONTAINED OSTEOCHONDRAL DEFECTS

RESULTS

CONCLUSION

INTRODUCTION

Management of an osteochondral defect in the knee is one of the most difficult conditions for the orthopedist. Although a fresh osteochondral allograft seems to be the treatment of choice for this condition, allografts are not without their own problems. A size match is difficult to obtain, availability is uncertain, and resorption and collapse of the allograft are possible. For these reasons, if an osteochondral defect is well contained, my preferred treatment is autologous bone graft. I reserve use of a fresh osteochondral allograft for a defect that is peripherally uncontained and not suitable for autologous bone grafting or a failed cartilage surgery, such as a failed second-stage autologous chondrocyte implantation (ACI) procedure after bone graft or a failed ACI sandwich technique.

OSTEOCHONDRITIS DISSECANS

Osteochondritis dissecans (OCD) has undergone many treatment strategies, ranging from surgical excision as advocated more than 150 years ago[1] to osteochondral autogenous grafting.[2–4]

The disease is rare in individuals younger than 10 years and in those older than 50 years.[5] The male-to-female ratio has been reported as 2:1[6] or 3:1,[7] with bilateral involvement in up to 33%.[8] The medial femoral condyle is affected approximately 75% of the time (Linden, 1976 incidence study),[5] with three fourths of the lesions affecting the lateral (intercondylar) portion of the medial femoral condyle. Kindreds with clear hereditary patterns have been documented,[9] as has evidence suggesting no clear pattern of familial tendency.[10]

Many etiologies have been proposed, including repetitive microtrauma and impingement of the tibial spine,[11] stress fractures with no identifying trauma,[12] and vascular insult.[13] However, vascular studies of the end the femur have demonstrated a rich vascular plexus to intramedullary cancellous bone, making this etiology unlikely.[14] Histologic evaluation of specimens removed at surgery have demonstrated viable bone and cartilage and not empty lacunae.[15]

CLASSIFICATION AND MANAGEMENT

Categorization of the disease process into a juvenile or adult form is important at the time of diagnosis because the treatment and prognosis may be managed by different treatment algorithms depending on the stage of disease.[16–18]

However, there is consistent agreement that knees treated by removal of OCD fragments that are detached from the weight-bearing femoral condyles do poorly.[19–22] Linden[23] noted that at average 33-year clinical and radiographic follow-up, 38 of 48 patients who had the initial manifestation after closure of the physes (i.e., adult form) had symptomatic and radiographic gonarthrosis. Linden[23] stated that "Symptoms and roentgenographic gonarthrosis become more frequent and approach 100 per cent with time" (Figure 11-1).

Cystic degeneration deep to the lesion in situ may occur, which makes bony healing especially difficult, even in the juvenile form (Figure 11-2).

Treatment by removal of the fragment and drilling to promote fibrocartilage repair is not recommended because the repair tissue is not durable and will break down.[24–26]

Optimal treatment is aimed at assessing the stability of the OCD fragment and obtaining union by casting immobilization in a stable juvenile fragment, or in situ flap, to fixation with or without autogenous bone grafting by open or arthroscopic technique. This is the treatment of choice for the adult form (Figure 11-3). An unstable OCD lesion is assessed for the underlying bony attachment by computed tomographic scan. Fixation to the underlying bony bed by standard AO principles of delayed union with curettage, autologous bone grafting, vascularization of the defect by drilling, and rigid internal fixation gives the best results.

In cases of failed treatment of OCD with an empty defect or fragmented lesion, treatment options are ACI, autologous osteochondral grafting, or osteochondral allografting. ACI has the advantage of being autologous

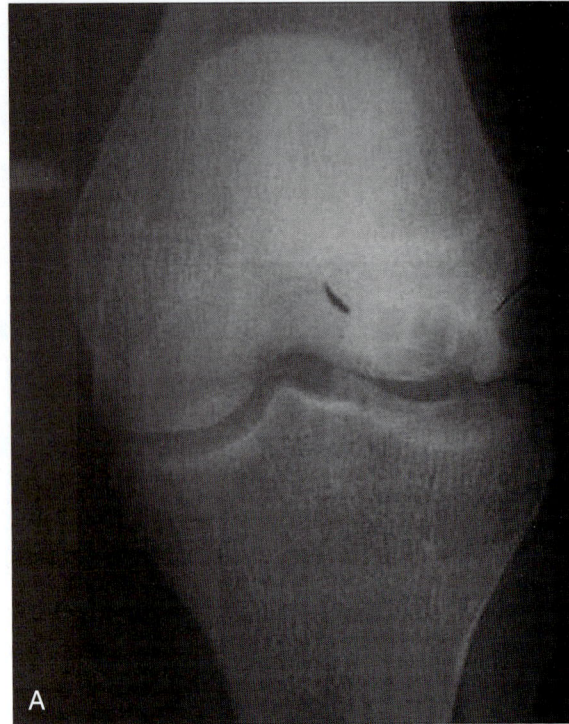

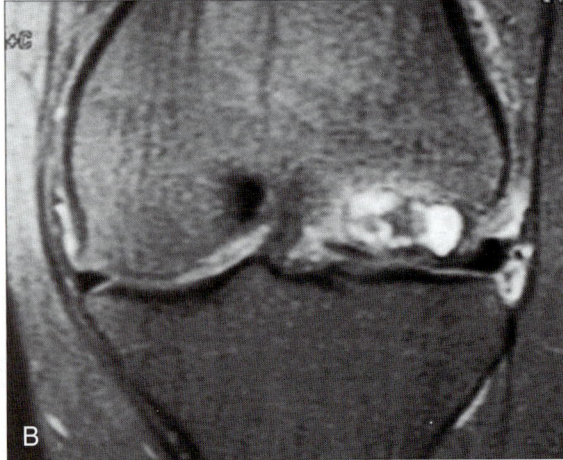

Figure 11-2 *A,* Anteroposterior x-ray film in an 18-year-old woman with lateral femoral condyle osteochondritis dissecans that has not been surgically treated. A degenerative cystic form of the condition is apparent by x-ray film and by magnetic resonance imaging *(B).*

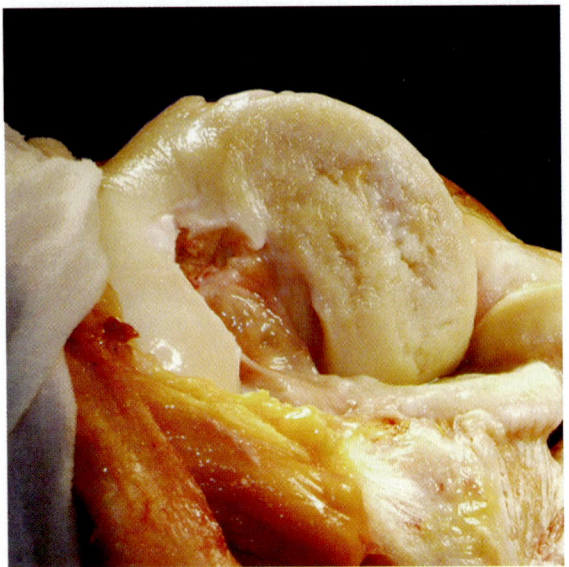

Figure 11-1 A 44-year-old man with typical appearance of an osteochondritis dissecans lesion after the fragment had been removed. Universal progression to osteoarthritis was noted by Linden.[23]

tissue in a young patient, with the potential to resurface large areas without donor site morbidity, as in osteochondral autograft transfers. Most defects can be managed by ACI alone when bone deficiency centrally is less than 6 to 8 mm deep (see Chapter 7).[27]

When cystic changes occur under the defect (see Figure 11-2), the defect has near-vertical walls and is greater than 8 to 10 mm deep, or the defect is very sclerotic due to a chronic lesion that may have undergone drilling, abrasion, or microfracture, it is safer to remove the unhealthy bed and bone graft the defect. The bone grafting technique is much like the preparation

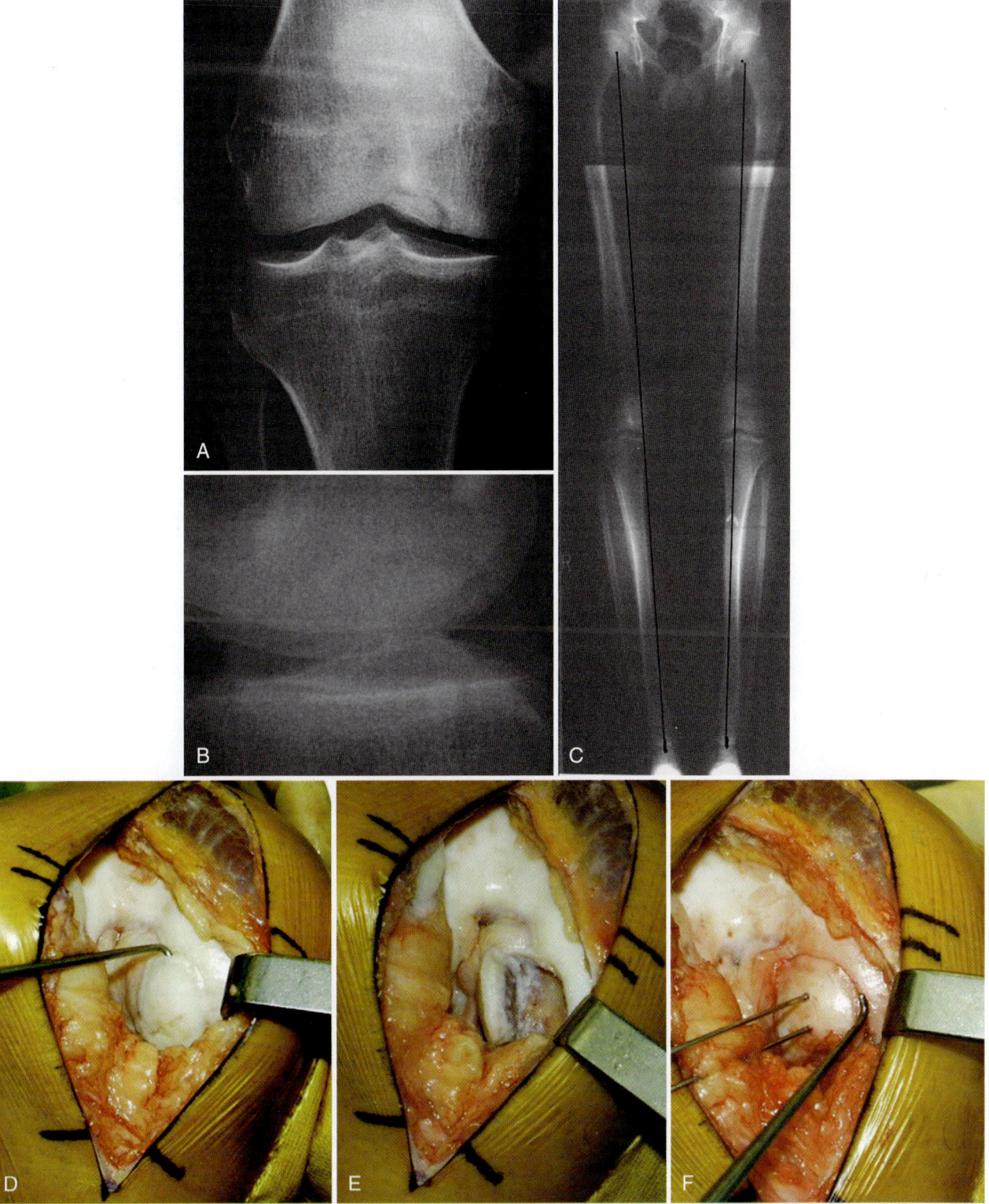

Figure 11-3 A 21-year-old male college hockey player with an unstable painful medial femoral condyle osteochondritis dissecans (OCD) lesion that has failed arthroscopic stabilization with absorbable tack fixation. Persistent catching, swelling, pain, and limp are presenting symptoms. The treatment plan includes open surgical open reduction internal fixation, removal of fibrous tissue at the base of the defect and undersurface of the fragment, drilling of the subchondral bone to promote vascularization of the fragment, and autologous bone grafting with stable internal fixation per classic principles of treatment of a nonunion. Later removal of the internal fixation is performed. *A*, Anteroposterior x-ray film demonstrates classic medial OCD lesion with a large bony fragment.

Continued

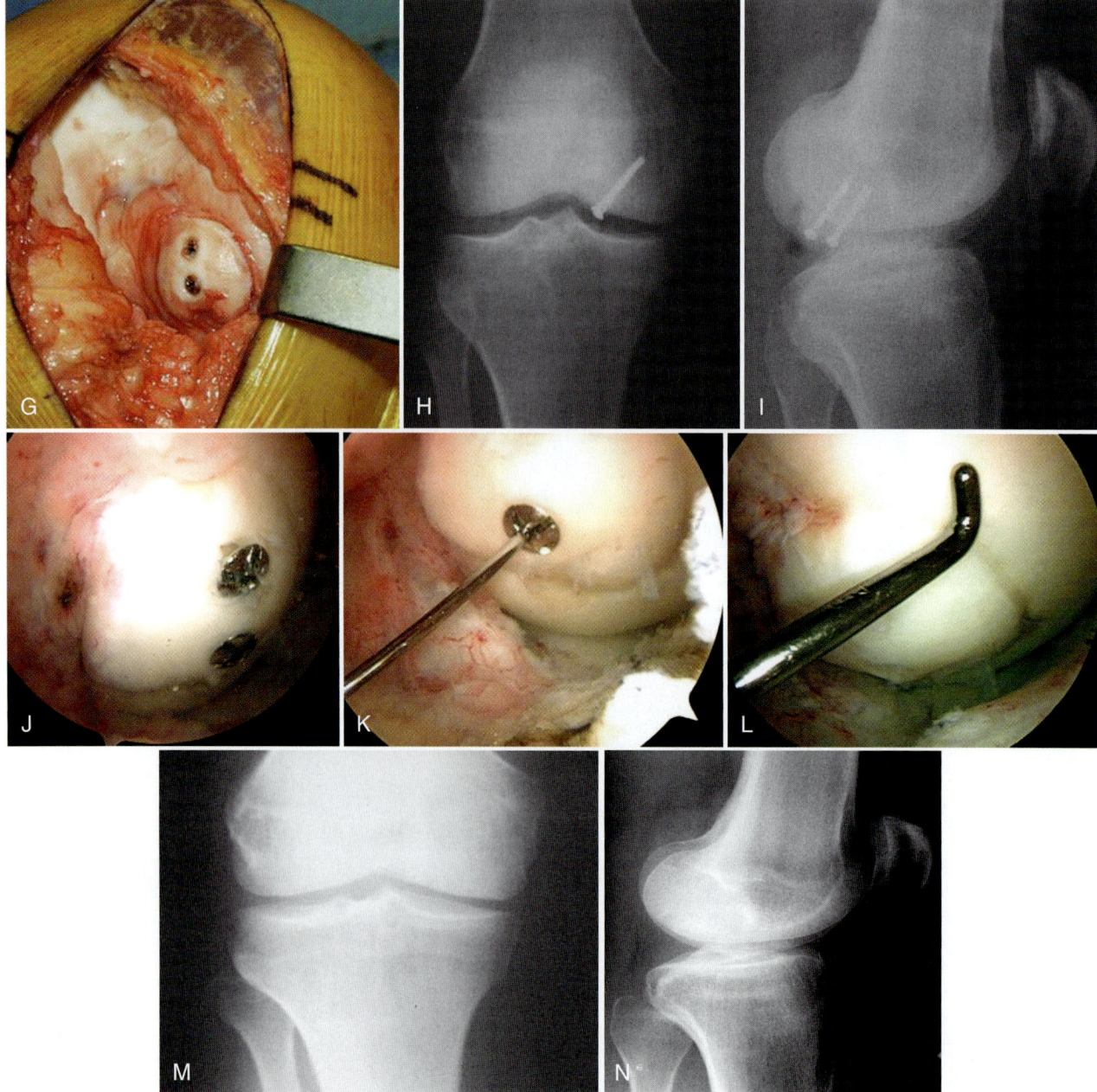

Figure 11-3—cont'd *B*, Lateral x-ray film. *C*, Long alignment x-ray films demonstrate a varus knee with mechanical axis in the medial compartment. *D*, Open appearance of un-united fragment in situ with cracked articular cartilage surface. *E*, The fragment is hinged on its vascular attachment to the posterior cruciate ligament synovium toward the intercondylar notch. This maintains stability of the fragment so that it does not fall out of the wound. Note the chronic appearance of the defect base. The fragment is covered with fibrous tissue and has underlying sclerotic bone. *F*, The underlying fibrous tissue and sclerotic bone are removed, autogenous bone graft from the upper tibia is placed to restore the proper anatomic location of the fragment because they tend to subside, and cannulated screw guidewires are used to check the reduction before screw fixation is performed. *G*, Cannulated screw fixation with anatomic reduction after curettage and bone grafting. The screw heads are buried below the articular surface so as not to damage the tibial surface. *H*, Postoperative anteroposterior x-ray film showing anatomic reduction. *I*, Postoperative lateral x-ray film. *J*, Eight weeks postoperatively, the hardware is removed arthroscopically before weight bearing is permitted. *K*, The cannulated screw guidewires simplify screw removal. *L*, The fragment is probed carefully to assess congruency and stability. Full weight bearing is allowed postoperatively, but sports are restricted for another 4 months to allow solid healing and bone remodeling. Anteroposterior *(M)* and lateral *(N)* x-ray films 1 year after treatment show solid healing of the OCD fragment. The patient returned the following season to varsity-level hockey. He remains asymptomatic after 7 years of follow-up.

of a dental amalgam and is described in detail in Figure 11–4.

In cases with defects requiring bone grafts, a staged bone grafting and later ACI (6–9 months) are recommended (Figure 11–5). A single-stage "sandwich technique" is also a possibility (see Chapter 7). Attention to axial alignment is crucial to success, especially if defects are large (>8–10 cm^2) (Figure 11–6).[27]

If ACI with bone grafting is ineffective, then the last biologic preservation prior to a unicompartmental knee arthroplasty is an allograft. I prefer osteochondral allograft fixation as a salvage option for the management of OCD and not the preferred treatment because a failed allograft is difficult to salvage biologically.

AVASCULAR NECROSIS

Osteonecrosis of the knee classically consists of two distinct entities: spontaneous or secondary osteonecrosis.[28-31] Spontaneous osteonecrosis occurs unilaterally and in one compartment of the knee, and most often in patients older than 55 years. Secondary osteonecrosis could be secondary to corticosteroid therapy, renal and systemic disease, or barotrauma; it occurs most often in younger patients with bilateral multicompartmental disease. For both types of osteonecrosis, the natural evolution without treatment is arthritis.[28,31]

Mont et al[30] described four stages of the radiographic evolution of the lesion. In stage 1, the knee maintains a

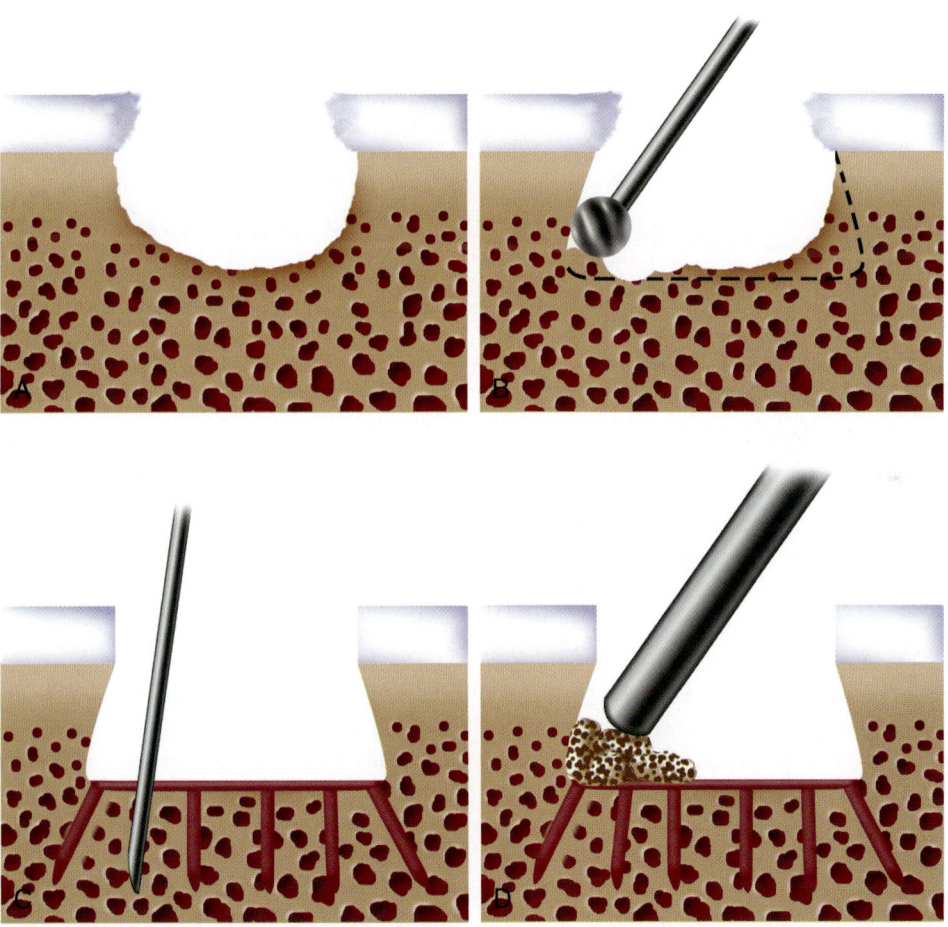

Figure 11–4 Technique for autologous bone grafting of an osteochondral defect. *A,* Defect that is suitable for bone grafting has steep side walls, subchondral cysts, or sclerotic subchondral bone after failed prior marrow stimulation techniques. *B,* The defect is prepared as if it were a dental amalgam preparation. A high speed bur, usually 5-mm diameter, removes all the subchondral sclerotic bone back to healthy-appearing spongy bone. The cartilage margins are undermined so that the deeper area of the defect is larger than the opening to assist in containing the morselized spongy bone after the defect is adequately prepared. *C,* The base of the defect is drilled to assist in vascularizing the bone graft. *D,* Autologous cancellous morselized bone chips are impacted peripherally and then centrally up to the level of the native subchondral bone plate. The autograft is usually harvested from the proximal tibial metaphysic using a 10-mm osteochondral autograft transfer system harvester (OATS, Arthrex, Naples FL), with allograft bone substitute backfill (cadaver cancellous chips preferred).

Continued

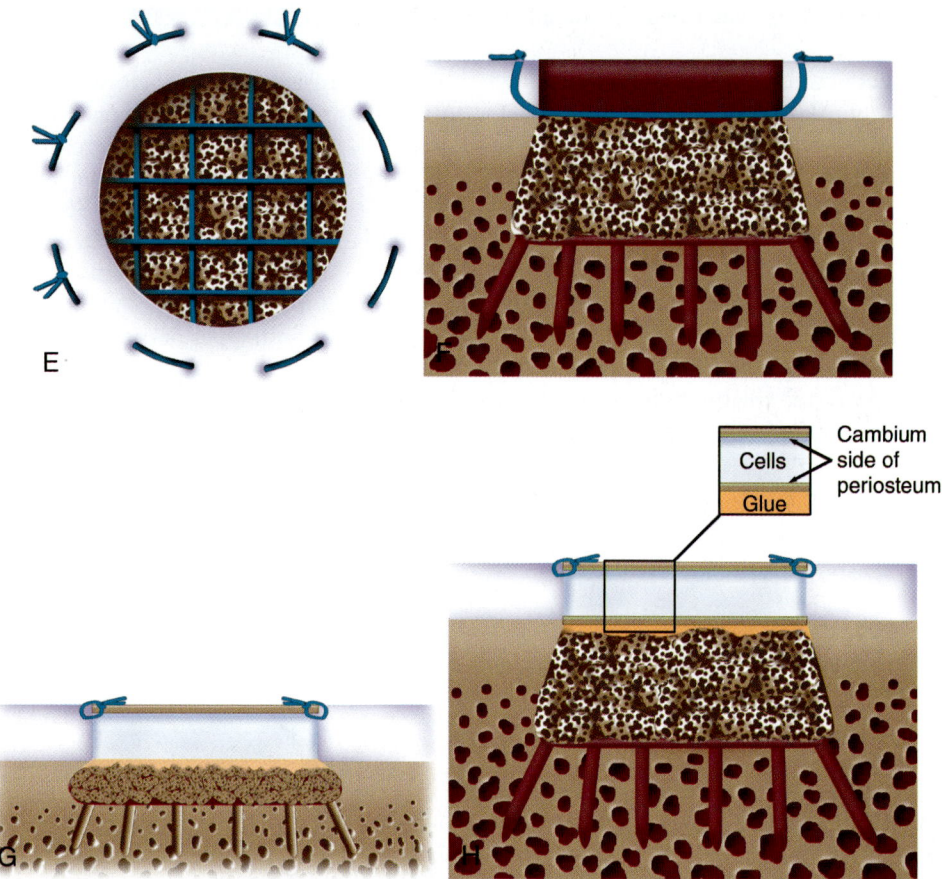

Figure 11-4—Cont'd *E,* To ensure the chips remain in place, an absorbable 5.0 or 6.0 Vicryl suture is woven across the articular surface. This is done only if there is concern about bone graft stability and is required only occasionally. *F,* With the knee joint in full extension to allow the bone grafted area to be further contained by the opposing tibial surface, the tourniquet is let down. The knee is left alone for 3 to 5 minutes to allow the marrow elements to permeate the bone graft to the articular surface and form a "super clot" as in the technique of microfracture. The joint is not irrigated so as not to disturb the "super clot." A drain, if used, is placed away from the treated defect. This marrow-derived clot allows fibrocartilage resurfacing of the bone graft (see panel *H*). *G,* Alternatively, the bone graft and clot can be protected with a membrane of periosteum or synthetic type I to III collagen. *H,* "Sandwich" technique autologous chondrocyte implantation in addition to autologous bone grafting. When periosteum is used, the two cambium layers face each other, and the cells are injected and "sandwiched" between them (see Chapter 7).

normal aspect. In stage 2, cystic or osteosclerotic lesions are observed with normal contour. In stage 3, subchondral collapse is observed. In stage 4, a narrowing of the joint is observed.[30] For stages 1, 2, and 3, core decompression,[30] arthroscopic debridement, and high tibial osteotomy[32] have been used with success. Stage 4 is associated with severe clinical symptoms, and unicompartmental or total knee arthroplasty is recommended in the literature.

I have found that the idiopathic form of osteonecrosis is frequently isolated to the medial femoral condyle in a middle-aged man with a varus knee. My treatment for Ficat stage III and IV disease includes a valgus-producing osteotomy with autologous bone grafting to the necrotic segment. The osteotomy is usually a closing wedge valgus-producing osteotomy that will provide a source of bone for the autograft after excision of the diseased medial osteochondral segment (Figure 11-7). The osteonecrotic bone segment secondary to steroid usage usually involves a more generalized segment of the entire distal femur. In these cases, I have found that fresh osteochondral allografts are more useful because the area of resorption and collapse is more diffuse and is not amenable to a localized autologous bone graft.

CLINICAL RESULTS—CASE SERIES—TECHNIQUE FOR TREATMENT OF DEEP CONTAINED OSTEOCHONDRAL DEFECTS

The study was a prospective, nonrandomized trial of 14 patients, 10 (group 1) with large OCD defects and 4 (group 2) with avascular necrosis of the knee.[33]

Patients were treated with autologous bone grafting after excision of necrotic bone or sclerotic defects. Concomitant realignment procedures of the patellofemoral joint and femorotibial joint were performed if indicated

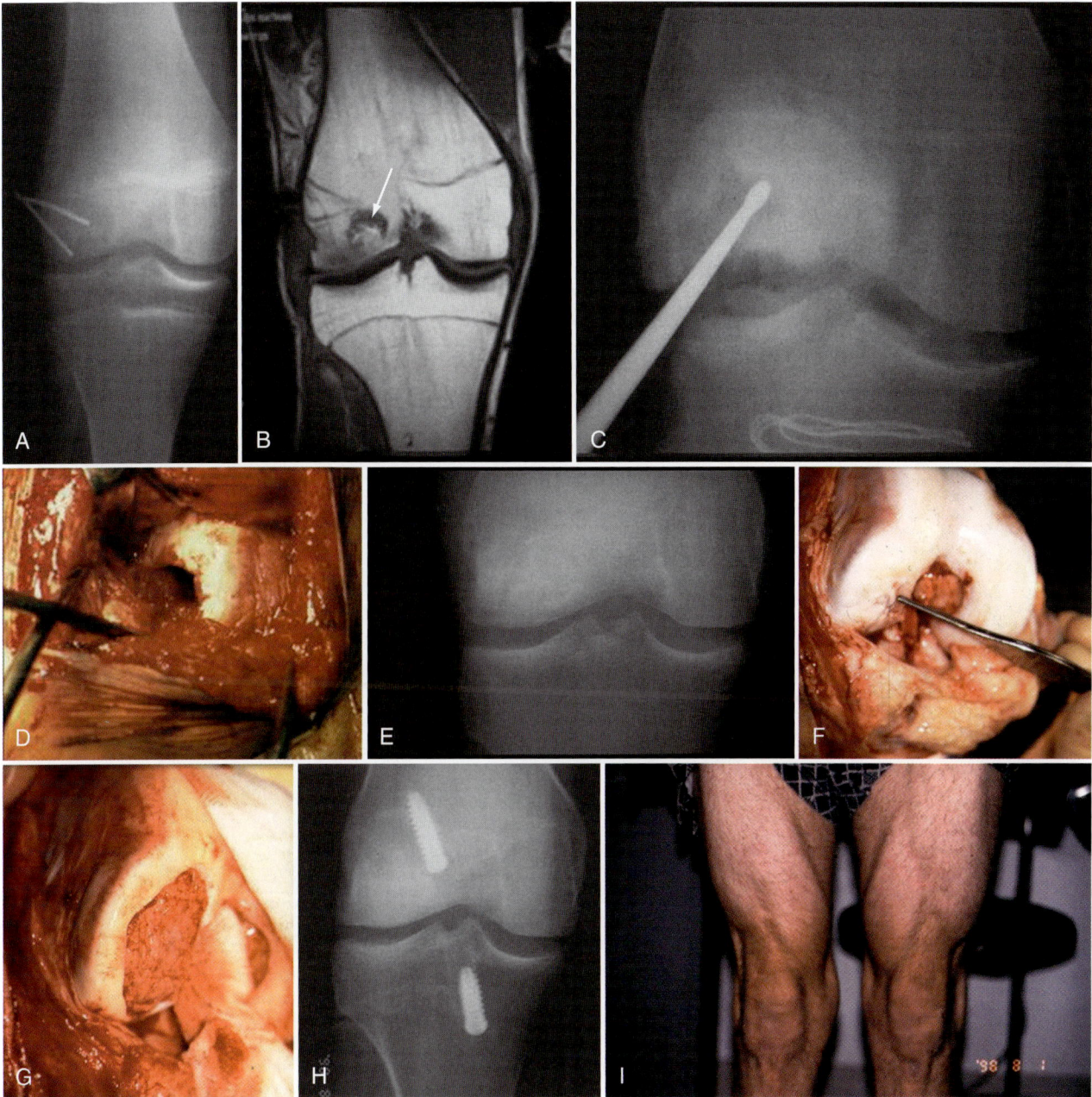

Figure 11-5 Case presentation of a 17-year-old boy with chronic lateral femoral condyle osteochondritis dissecans lesion that has failed open reduction internal fixation and debridement and now has cystic degeneration in addition to anterior cruciate ligament (ACL) insufficiency. He presents with severe leg atrophy, effusions, and laterally based pain and requires double crutch ambulation. *A,* Anteroposterior x-ray film showing failed open reduction internal fixation. *B,* Magnetic resonance imaging demonstrates a large subchondral lateral femoral condyle cyst. *C,* Anteroposterior x-rays of the intraoperative appearance to demonstrate complete removal of the cystic cavity. *D,* Open lateral arthrotomy photo after curettage. Autologous bone grafting (ABG) followed from the ipsilateral iliac crest (performed in 1995). Today ABG would be harvested with osteochondral autograft transfer system harvesters from the proximal tibia with a single-entry corticotomy, and the tibia would be backfilled with allograft freeze-dried cadaver cancellous bone chips. *E,* Anteroposterior radiograph 9 months later demonstrating well-healed lateral femoral condyle. *F,* Intraoperative appearance with fibrous repair over lateral femoral condyles. Some of the condyles have not repaired with fibrous tissue and remain bare bone. *G,* After radical debridement of fibrous repair tissue and autologous chondrocyte implantation (ACI). *H,* Anteroposterior radiograph after ACI to lateral femoral condyles with ACL autogenous bone tendon bone autograft patellar tendon reconstruction and interference screw fixation. *I,* Final clinical appearance 2 years postoperatively shows marked improvement of muscle tone and lessoned atrophy of the right thigh after reconstruction. The patient remains asymptomatic and functioning at a high level 14 years later.

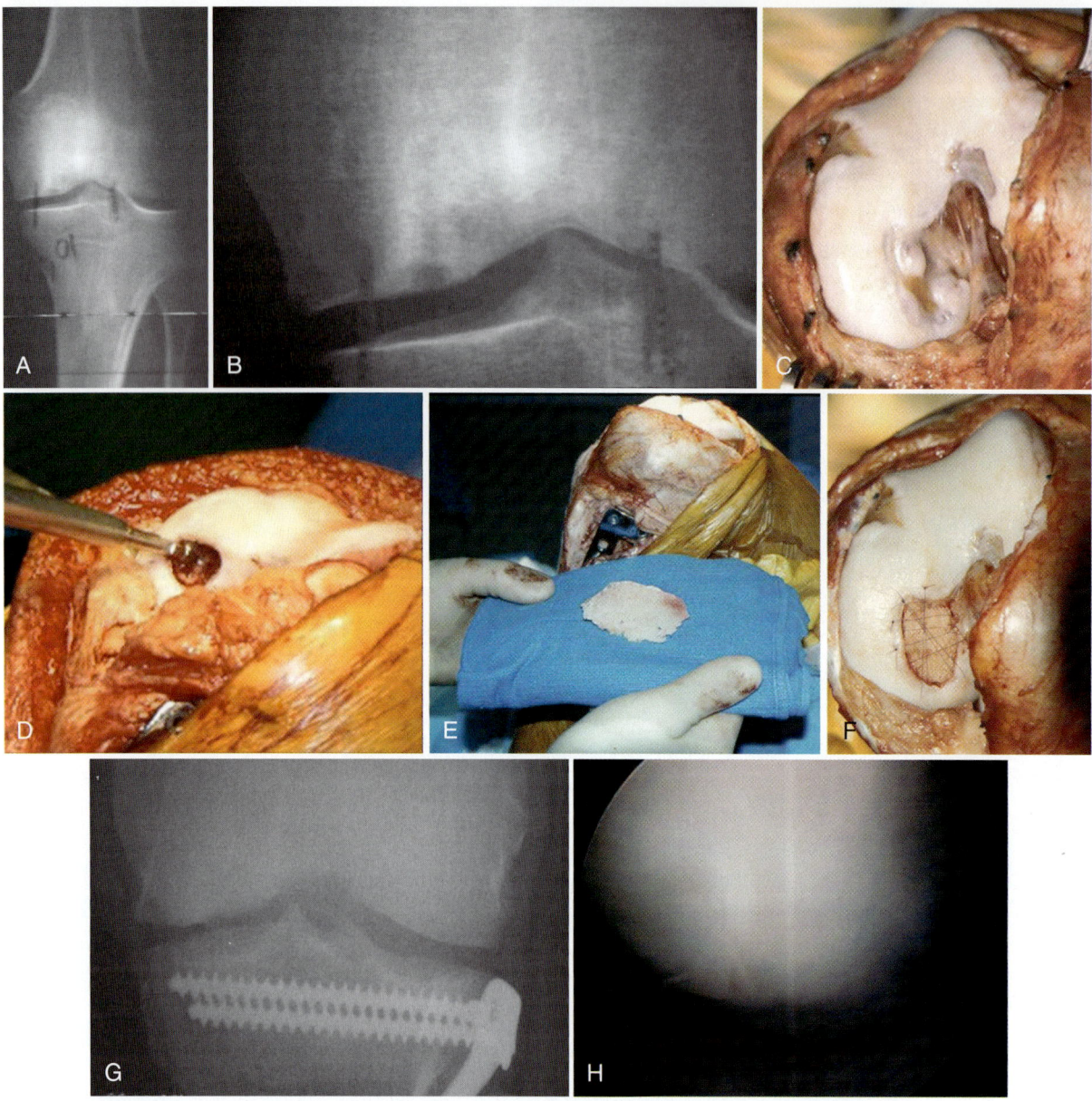

Figure 11-6 Case presentation of a 23-year-old man who has chronic left medial joint pain after arthroscopic removal of loose fragments to the medial femoral condyle osteochondritis dissecans. The patient has varus malalignment with medial compartment pain. He is treated with a closing wedge valgus-producing osteotomy and autologous bone grafting to the medial femoral condyles with an excellent long-term clinical result. *A,* Anteroposterior radiograph demonstrates medial femoral condyle osteochondritis dissecans empty defect. A 10-degree correction is required to place the mechanical axis to the lateral tibial spine. *B,* Close-up radiograph demonstrates the cystic nature of the medial femoral condyle. *C,* Open appearance of the empty defect on the medial femoral condyle adjacent to the intercondylar notch posterior cruciate ligament. *D,* Radical debridement of the sclerotic and cystic changes on the medial femoral condyles requires a high-speed bur to develop an amalgam type of defect for autologous bone grafting and repair of the medial femoral condyle defect. *E,* A 10-degree corrective closing wedge tibial valgus-producing osteotomy is performed. The cancellous bone from the closing wedge osteotomy and the lateral L-plate for the closing wedge osteotomy are shown. This bone is morselized and used to fill the defect, which has been prepared with a high-speed bur to the medial femoral condyle. *F,* The morselized cancellous bone is compacted into the medial femoral condyle until it is flush with the subchondral bone. It is reinforced with absorbable 5.0 Vicryl sutures as a fishnet type of reinforcement to the surface to prevent loss of bone graft. The knee is brought into full extension, the tourniquet is let down, and a marrow clot fills the surface of the bone graft. A rehabilitation program per a marrow stimulation technique with continuous passive motion and protected weight bearing for 6 weeks is followed to allow fibrocartilage repair to the surface of the medial femoral condyle. *G,* Postoperative anteroposterior x-ray film after complete healing of the tibial valgus-producing osteotomy with maintenance of joint space on weight-bearing film. *H,* Second-look arthroscopy 1 year later demonstrates excellent repair tissue fill over the medial femoral condyle. The patient has become completely asymptomatic and requests no further treatment. Twelve years later, this fibrocartilaginous repair tissue remains stable and has not broken down. Careful surveillance postoperatively to ensure a good clinical result with physical examination for crepitus and effusions as well as maintenance of joint space on standing x-ray films is performed. If any symptoms appear, a high-resolution magnetic resonance imaging scan would be performed to assess the status of the repair tissue on the surface of the medial femoral condyle and the possibility of second-stage autologous chondrocyte implantation repair.

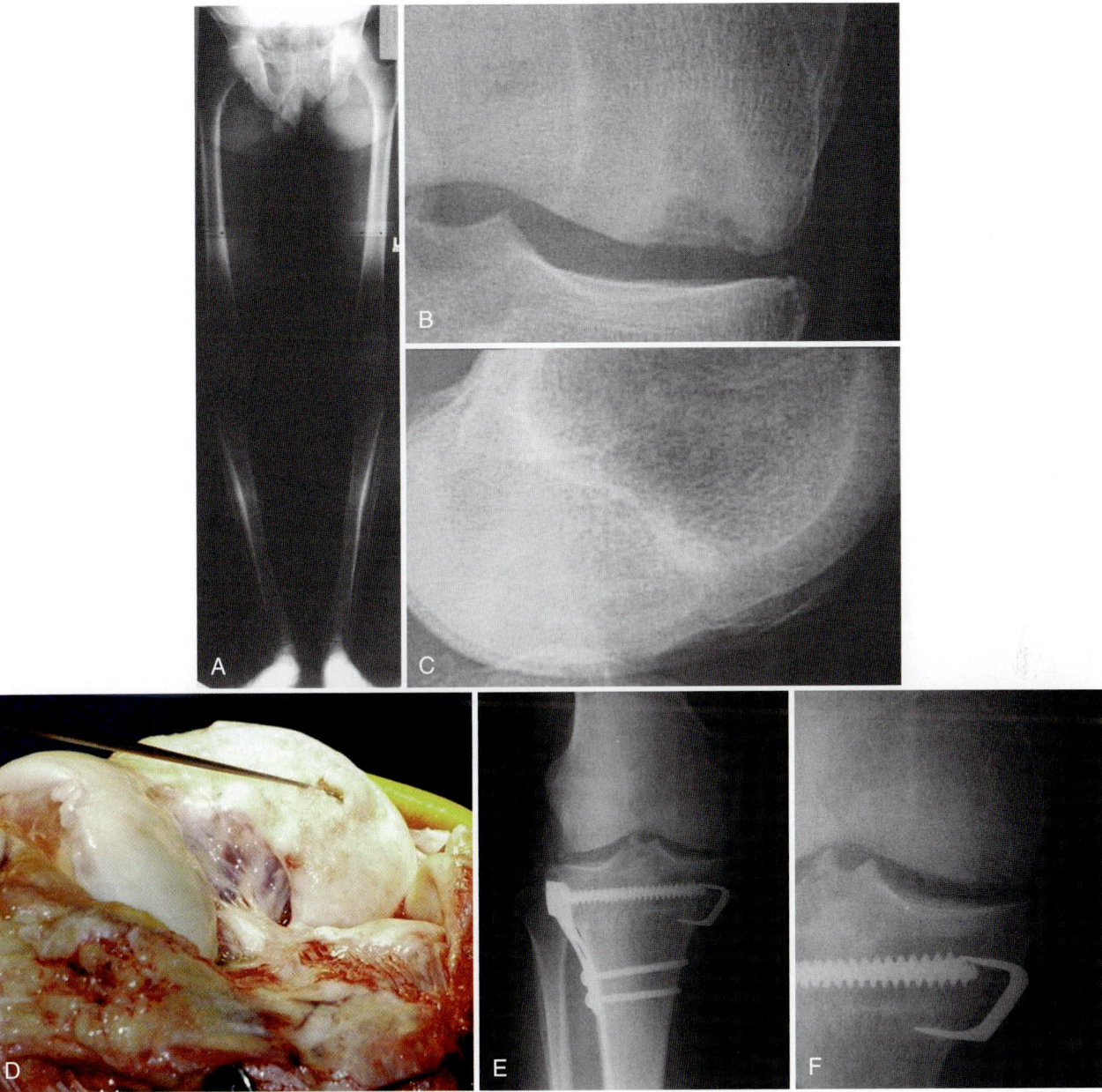

Figure 11–7 Active 54-year-old man presents with medial pain in the right knee. The clinical and radiographic workup is compatible with osteonecrosis of the medial femoral condyle that is idiopathic. A closing wedge tibial valgus-producing osteotomy with curettage and autologous bone grafting of the medial femoral condyle (as in the case shown in Figure 11–6) is performed. At latest follow-up more than 10 years later, he remains asymptomatic and without a prosthesis. *A*, Long alignment x-ray films demonstrate varus alignment of both lower extremities, right greater than left. *B*, Close-up anteroposterior x-ray film demonstrates resorptive cyst formation and flattening of the medial femoral condyle. *C*, Lateral x-ray film demonstrates cyst formation and flattening of the medial femoral condyle. *D*, Intraoperative appearance of the knee with a nerve hook falling into a resorptive cavity to the medial femoral condyle prior to radical debridement and curettage with autologous bone grafting of the medial femoral condyle. *E*, Postoperative anteroposterior x-ray film demonstrating correction of axial malalignment and restoration of bone stock to the medial femoral condyle. *F*, Close-up anteroposterior x-ray film demonstrating restoration of the medial femoral condyle with preservation of the joint space on standing anteroposterior x-ray film 1 year postoperatively.

Continued

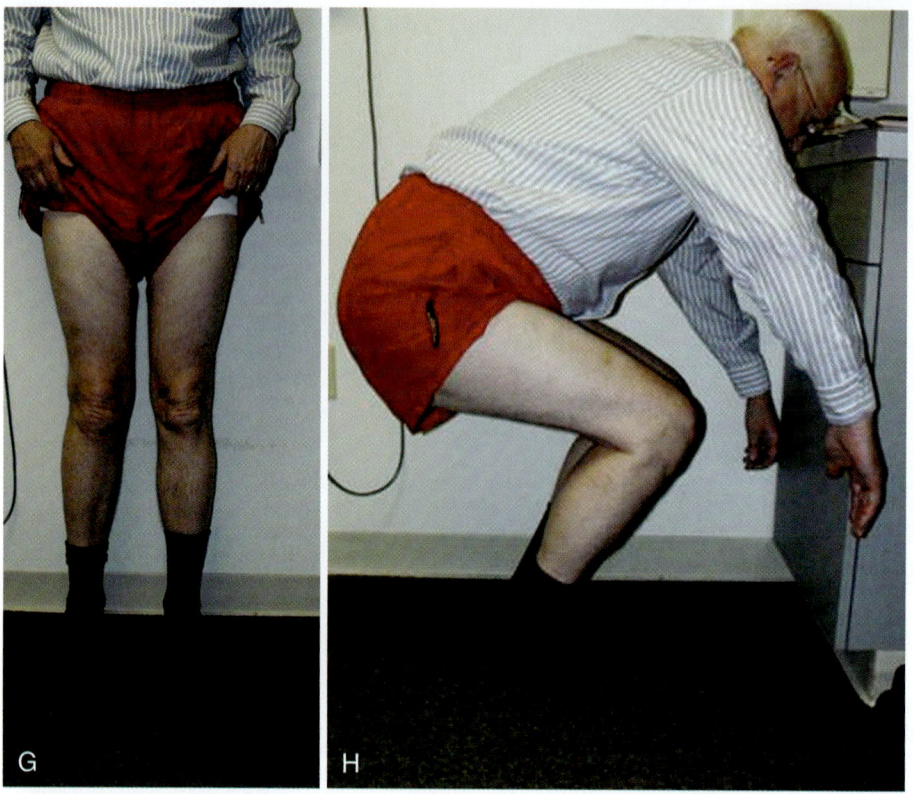

Figure 11-7—cont'd *G,* Clinical appearance 10 years postoperatively. Frontal alignment of the right leg demonstrates mild mechanical valgus, which is cosmetically acceptable to the patient. *H,* Lateral clinical appearance demonstrating good active range of motion with squatting and kneeling. The patient remains asymptomatic.

to correct patellar maltracking or varus deformity with medial joint space narrowing. The autologous bone graft was held in place with a suturing technique or periosteum if autologous bone graft was unstable. Symptoms occurring 6 to 12 months after autologous bone grafting warranted subsequent treatment with ACI in 4 of the 10 group 1 OCD patients and 1 of the 4 group 2 avascular necrosis patients.

The patient group consisted of 8 males and 6 female (average age 34 years, range 14–60 years). Average follow-up was 33 months (range 24–60 months). There were 7 left and 7 right knees. The lateral condyle was affected in 3 patients and the medial condyle in 11 patients. There were 9 high tibial osteotomies (5 from group 1, all 4 from group 2) performed with an average correction of 7.9 degrees. The degree of correction was calculated on longstanding films so that the weight-bearing force went through the lateral intercondylar spine. This resulted in an anatomic overcorrection of 2 degrees.

The average surface area of the group 1 defects was 6.6 cm^2 (range 2–12 cm^2). These lesions had an average depth of 1.5 cm (range 0.8–3.0 cm).

The average surface area of the group 2 defects was 6.7 cm^2 (range 6–8.8 cm^2). These lesions had an average depth of 1.1 cm (range 1–1.5 cm).

Nine of the patients had an intact meniscus in the affected compartment. One patient had a large discoid meniscus. Four patients had a meniscal remnant only in the affected compartment after partial meniscectomy.

Six of the 14 patients had no previous surgeries. Eight of the 14 patients had an average of two prior surgeries (range 1–4). Average preoperative and postoperative femorotibial angles for group 1 was 3.5 degrees and 6.5 degrees, respectively (5/10 had high tibial osteotomy). Average preoperative and postoperative angles for group 2 were 2.3 degrees varus and 8 degrees valgus, respectively (4/4 had high tibial osteotomy). The avascular necrosis group was all in varus prior to surgery, and the correction was believed to be critical to the success.

RESULTS

At 4-year follow-up, autologous bone grafting for OCD (group 1) were effective for 6 of the 10 patients treated. Four of the patients developed recurrent symptoms of weight-bearing pain, catching, and swelling over time that required second-stage ACI. At the time of ACI, the repair tissue over the autologous bone graft was fibrous, gelatinous, and soft. ACI provided excellent pain relief once the subchondral bone had been restored with autologous bone graft.

The other six patients have been followed every 2 years with x-ray films and MRI scans to noninvasively assess the repair tissue. These patients remain asymptomatic today and demonstrate stable repair tissue on MRI.

Three of the four patients in group 2 (avascular necrosis) did well with autologous bone graft and high tibial osteotomy and did not require ACI. The fourth patient was relatively asymptomatic 9 months postoperatively. However, because of his desire to maintain a high level of physical activity at the age of 47 years, he requested a second-stage ACI, which was performed. At the time of open ACI, the repair tissue over the autologous bone graft was of very good quality. There was complete coverage of the bone graft with a white fibrocartilaginous tissue. ACI was performed after the repair tissue was removed. The patient is now 10 years after ACI and remains asymptomatic. Surprisingly, the other three patients who underwent osteotomy with autologous bone graft also remain without symptoms.

Because of our early results with bone grafting for large osteochondral defects (approximately 7 cm^2 in both groups), we recommend that for younger patients with OCD, bone grafting with ACI as a single-stage sandwich technique be performed if the surgeon is skilled in such a technique. Alternatively, a more conservative approach of isolated bone grafting with careful follow-up via clinical examination, magnetic resonance imaging, and radiography to evaluate the repair tissue over the bone graft prior to the possibility of ACI is a very reasonable approach. The defects are large (average approximately 7 cm^2), so the possibility of fibrocartilage breakdown is more likely in this young active population.

In this small case series of males with idiopathic avascular necrosis and varus knees, it appears that a closing wedge osteotomy to correct alignment with autologous bone grafting to an osteonecrotic Ficat stage III or IV lesion leads to an excellent clinical result and is our recommended treatment of choice.

CONCLUSION

Osteochondral defects include OCD, osteochondral cysts, and avascular necrosis. In the adult form of OCD with an unstable fragment, the optimal treatment is open reduction internal fixation with autologous bone grafting to allow revascularization and healing of the fragment.

In cases of an empty defect after failed fixation techniques or spontaneous fragmentation of an OCD fragment, assessment of the defect by computed tomographic arthrogram is recommended. If no subchondral bone cysts are found and the defect is relatively shallow (6–8 mm centrally at its deepest, which is typical), then ACI in isolation is recommended. However, if the margins of the defect are steep and the subchondral bone is thickened and sclerotic after repeated surgeries or if deep subchondral bone cysts are present, then restoration of the osteochondral unit by cartilage and bone grafting with an ACI sandwich technique is optimal. Alternatively, isolated autologous bone grafting and rehabilitation per marrow stimulation techniques with clinical follow-up provide a safe and effective method for restoration of the osteochondral unit. The surgical technique with autologous bone grafting uses local bone graft when available and a dental amalgam type of preparation of the osseous defect. However, the repair tissue at the surface is less predictable and requires surveillance and possibly second-stage ACI.

An osseous defect secondary to idiopathic avascular necrosis generally occurs in combination with varus alignment in a middle-aged man. Closing wedge valgus-producing osteotomy with autologous bone grafting of the osteonecrotic fragment via the same surgical technique of autologous bone grafting of an osseous defect usually provides good to excellent results in Ficat stage III and IV disease.

Secondary forms of avascular necrosis often have multiple necrotic segments and are more amenable to osteochondral allograft treatment or total knee replacement.

REFERENCES

1. Pare A. *Ouevres completes*. vol. 3:. Paris: J.B.Balliere; 1840–1841:32.
2. Yamashita F, Sakakida K, Suzu F, Takai S. The transplantation of an autogeneic osteochondral fragment for osteochondritis dissecans of the knee. *Clin Orthop Relat Res*. 1985;201:43–50.
3. Muller W. Osteochondrosis Dissecans. In: Hastings DE, ed. *Progress in Orthopedic Surgery*. vol. 3:. Berlin: Springer Verlag; 1978:135.
4. Outerbridge HK, Outerbridge AR, Outerbridge RE. The use of a lateral patellar autologous graft for the repair of a large osteochondral defect of the knee. *J Bone Joint Surg Am*. 1995;77:65–72.
5. Linden B. The incidence of osteochondritis dissecans of the femur. *Acta Orthop Scand*. 1976;47:664–667.
6. Pappas AM. Osteochondritis dissecans. *Clin Orthop Relat Res*. 1981;158:59–69.
7. Nagura S. The so-called osteochondritis dissecans of Konig. *Clin Orthop Relat Res*. 1960;18:119–121.
8. Green WT, Banks HH. Osteochondritis dissecans in children. *J Bone Joint Surg Am*. 1953;35:26–47.
9. Mubarick SJ, Carrol NC. Familial osteochondritis dissecans of the knee. *Clin Orthop Relat Res*. 1979;140:131–136.
10. Petrie PWR. Aetiology of osteochondritis dissecans. Failure to establish a familial background. *J Bone Joint Surg Br*. 1977;59:366–367.
11. Fairbank HA. Osteo-Chondritis dissecans. *Br J Surg*. 1933;21:67–82.
12. Cahill BR, Berg BC. 99m-Technetium phosphate compound joint scintigraphy in the management of juvenile osteochondritis dissecans of the femoral condyles. *Am J Sports Med*. 1983;11:329–335.
13. Enneking WF, ed. *Clinical Muskulo-Skeletal Pathology*. 3rd ed. Gainesville Florida University of Florida Press; 1990:166.
14. Rogers WM, Gladstone H. Vascular foramina and arterial supply of the distal end of the femur. *J Bone Surg Am*. 1950;32-A:867–874.

15. Chiroff RT, Cooke III CP. Osteochondritis dissecans: a histologic and microradiographic analyses of surgically excised lesions. *J Trauma.* 1975;15:689–696.
16. Cahill BR. Osteochondritis dissecans of the knee: treatment of juvenile and adult forms. *J Am Acad Orthop Surg.* 1995;3:237–247.
17. Pappas AM. Osteochondritis dissecans. *Clin Orthop Relat Res.* 1981;158:59–69.
18. Cahill BR, Phillipsw MR, Navarro R. The results of conservative management of osteochondritis dissecans using joint scintigraphy: A prospective study. *Am J Sports Med.* 1989;17:601–606.
19. Almgard LE, Wikstad I. Late results of surgery for osteochondritis dissecans of the knee joint. *Acta Chir Scand.* 1964;127:588–596.
20. Cahill B. Treatment of juvenile osteochondritis dissecans and osteochondritis dissecans of the knee. *Clin Sports Med.* 1985;4:367–384.
21. Green JP. Osteochondritis dissecans of the knee. *J Bone Joint Surg Br.* 1966;48:82–91.
22. Hughston JC, Hergenroeder PT, Courtenay BG. Osteochondritis dissecans of the femoral condyles. *J Bone Joint Surg Am.* 1984;66:1340–1348.
23. Linden B. Osteochondritis dissecans of the femoral condyles. A long-term follow-up study. *J Bone Joint Surg Am.* 1977;59:769–776.
24. Landells JW. The reactions of injured human articular cartilage. *J Bone Joint Surg Br.* 1957;39:548–562.
25. Mitchell N, Shepard N. The resurfacing of adult rabbit articular cartilage by multiple perforations through the subchondral bone. *J Bone Joint Surg Am.* 1976;58:230–233.
26. DePalma AF, McKeever CD, Subin DK. Process of repair of articular cartilage demonstrated by histology and autoradiography with tritiated thymidine. *Clin Orthop Relat Res.* 1966;48:229–242.
27. Peterson L, Minas T, Britterg M, et al. Two–nine year outcome after autologous chondrocyte transplantation of the knee. *Clin Orthop Relat Res.* 2000;374:212–234.
28. Aglietti P, Insall JN, Buzzi R, Deschamps D. Idiopathic osteonecrosis of the knee: aetiology, prognosis and treatment. *J Bone Joint Surg Br.* 1983;65:588–597.
29. Ahlback S, Bauer GCH, Bohne WH. Spontaneous osteonecrosis of the knee. *Arthritis Rheum.* 1968;11:705–733.
30. Mont MA, Baumgarten KM, Rifai A, et al. Atraumatic osteonecrosis of the knee. *J Bone Joint Surg Am.* 2000;82:1279–1290.
31. Muheim G, Bohne WH. Prognosis in spontaneous osteonecrosis of the knee. *J Bone Joint Surg Br.* 1970;52:605–612.
32. Koshino T. The treatment of spontaneous osteonecrosis of the knee by high tibial osteotomy with and without bone-grafting or drilling of the lesion. *J Bone Joint Surg Am.* 1982;64:47–58.
33. Headrick J, Minas T. Treatment of Deep Osteochondritis Dissecans and Avascular Necrosis Lesions of the Knee Using Autologous Bone Grafting and Biologic Resurfacing Arthroplasty. Session 57, ICRS, Toronto 2002, June 15–18th.

Chapter 12

Meniscal Allograft Transplantation

Andreas H. Gomoll, MD and Tom Minas, MD, MS

INTRODUCTION
INDICATIONS
PLANNING
TECHNIQUE
    Special Instrumentation

GRAFT PREPARATION
POSITIONING
SURGICAL ANATOMY
SURGICAL APPROACH

COMPLETION MENISCECTOMY
TIBIAL PREPARATION
GRAFT PLACEMENT AND FIXATION
SUMMARY

INTRODUCTION

Loss of meniscal tissue drastically alters the biomechanical environment of the knee joint, especially in the lateral compartment, where contact stress can increase by 200% to 300% after total meniscectomy. Compartment overload syndrome can ensue, presenting with weight-bearing pain and recurrent effusions. Secondary osteoarthritis is a predictable endpoint,[1,2] which has led to increased awareness among orthopedic surgeons of meniscal transplantation in cases where subtotal or total meniscectomy was unavoidable. In carefully selected patients, meniscal allograft transplantation can provide improved biomechanics and function while providing good pain relief.[3–5]

Several techniques exist for allograft meniscus transplantation, including bone-plug and bone-bridge techniques, with additional variations within these groups based on different proprietary instrumentation sets. Regardless of the specific technique used, the majority of current transplantations are performed with bony fixation rather than relying on soft tissue healing of the meniscal roots to a prepared bed on the recipient tibial plateau.

This chapter discusses the techniques for open and arthroscopic meniscal allograft transplantation.

INDICATIONS

The ideal patient for meniscal allograft transplantation has a history of prior total or subtotal meniscectomy, usually followed by a symptom-free interval of varying duration. This is followed by the onset of weight-bearing pain localized to the involved compartment, frequently with recurrent effusions. The articular surfaces should be without full-thickness chondral defects, ligaments should be stable, and the knee should be normally aligned; otherwise, these comorbidities must be addressed in concurrent or staged fashion. Several reports that investigated the outcomes of concurrent meniscal transplantation and cartilage repair demonstrated results comparable to isolated meniscal transplantation.[6,7] Therefore, repairable, focal chondral defects should not be viewed as a contraindication.

Contraindications include diffuse arthritic changes and significant joint space narrowing, especially when associated with advanced femoral condyle and tibial flattening, history of inflammatory arthritis, or marked obesity.

PLANNING

The preoperative radiographic evaluation includes weight-bearing anteroposterior (AP) and posteroanterior 45-degree flexion radiographs, non–weight-bearing 45-degree flexion lateral view, axial view of the patellofemoral joint, and a long-leg mechanical axis view to evaluate malalignment. Furthermore, we routinely perform magnetic resonance imaging to evaluate the joint for articular comorbidities, such as ligamentous or chondral injury.

Meniscal allografts are size, side, and compartment specific; therefore, they must be individually measured and ordered for each patient. Preoperative measurements are obtained from AP and lateral radiographs with magnification markers placed on the skin at the level of the joint line. After accounting for radiographic magnification, meniscal width is measured on the AP radiograph from the edge of the ipsilateral tibial spine to the edge of the tibial plateau. Meniscal length is calculated by multiplying the depth of the tibial plateau (as measured on lateral radiographs) by 0.8 for medial and 0.7 for lateral meniscal grafts (Figure 12–1).

TECHNIQUE

Special Instrumentation

Based on the surgeon's preferred technique, a meniscal allograft workstation is used to shape the bone block or plugs containing the meniscal root attachment sites and prepare a corresponding recipient site on the tibia. Various proprietary systems are available and are usually provided by the company through which the transplant was ordered. Furthermore, meniscal repair equipment, such as zone-specific cannulas and double-armed needles, are needed for the meniscocapsular repair.

GRAFT PREPARATION

The graft should be prepared before the start of the procedure (e.g., while the patient is being induced) to reduce surgical and tourniquet time.

Depending on the specific system used, the bone bridge or plugs are prepared and sutures are placed. For our preferred technique, pull sutures are placed in the posterior horn (Figure 12–2) to assist in reducing the meniscus under the femoral condyle. Additional sutures can be placed through the bone bridge/plugs and around the meniscal roots to assist in graft fixation. After the graft has been prepared, any residual marrow elements should be removed from the bone using pulse lavage.

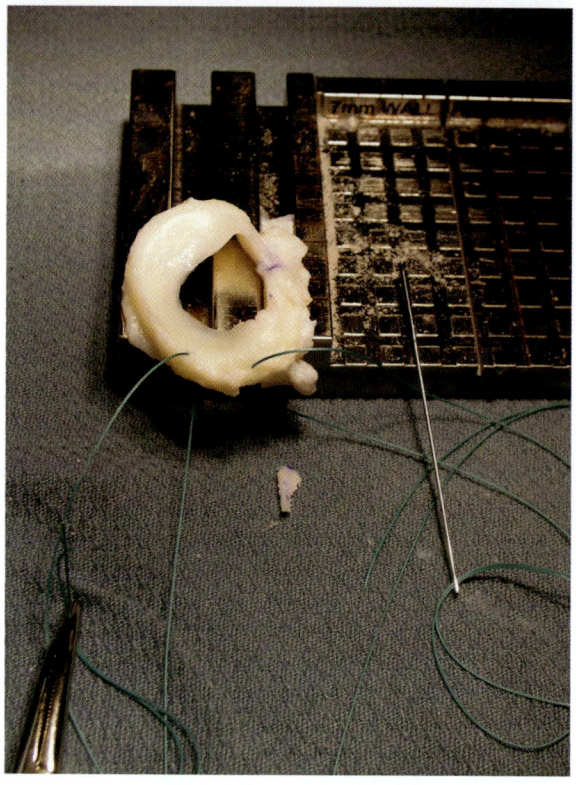

Figure 12–2 Prepared meniscal allograft. A bone bridge has been fashioned from the donor tibial plateau, and two pull sutures have been placed through the posterior horn to assist in reduction and fixation.

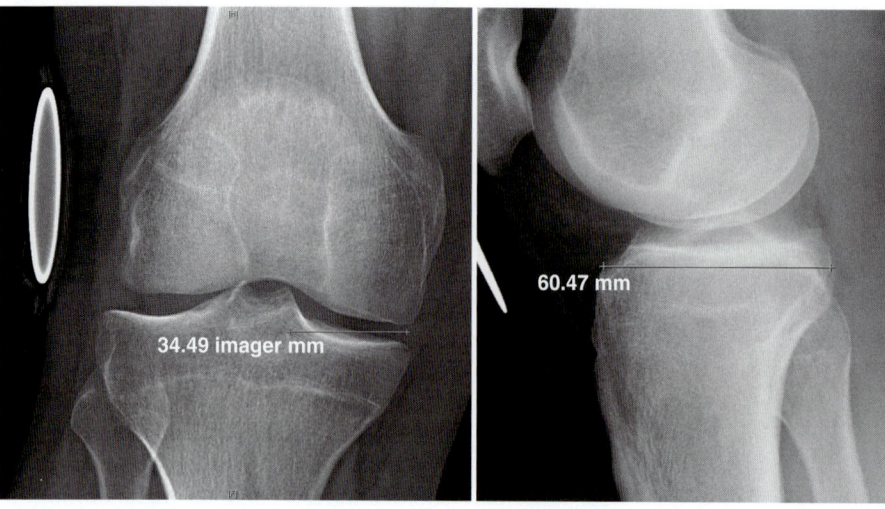

Figure 12–1 Anteroposterior *(left)* and lateral *(right)* radiographs of the knee with sizing disks. The width and length of the medial tibial plateau have been measured.

POSITIONING

The patient is positioned supine on a standard operating room table, with a thigh tourniquet. The posteromedial or posterolateral aspect of the knee must be easily accessible to perform inside–out meniscus suturing. For arthroscopic techniques, it is often helpful to use a thigh holder and drop the foot of the bed. A side post and foot rest can be used for open techniques.

SURGICAL ANATOMY

Useful surgical landmarks include the patella, patellar tendon, tibial plateau, and fibular head. Structures at risk during the procedure include the peroneal nerve, popliteal tendon, and lateral collateral ligament during the posterolateral approach. The posteromedial approach risks injury to the saphenous vein and nerve, potentially resulting in a painful neuroma. Creation of the tibial slot and needle passage during the meniscocapsular repair can injure the popliteal neurovascular bundle.

SURGICAL APPROACH

Arthroscopic techniques use standard medial and lateral portals as well as two accessory incisions: an anterior transpatellar tendon approach to introduce the meniscus into the joint and a posteromedial or -lateral approach to the knee for inside–out meniscocapsular repair. The transpatellar tendon approach is made with spinal needle localization in line with the anterior and posterior meniscal root attachments and extends from the inferior pole of the patella down to the tibial tubercle. Care should be taken to cut in line with the fibers of the patellar tendon so as not to detach a portion of the tendon. Resection of the fat pad just anterior to the anterior root attachment is helpful to visualize the root and facilitate graft insertion, passage, and fixation. The accessory posteromedial and -lateral incisions are standard per meniscal repair techniques.

For open meniscal transplantation, a longitudinal incision is made shifted slightly from the midline toward the respective compartment. Medially, a full-thickness fasciocutaneous flap is raised around the side of the knee to allow posteromedial access to the capsule through a triangle between the semimembranosus inferiorly, the medial head of the gastrocnemius posteriorly, and superiorly, and the joint capsule anteriorly. Laterally, first a full-thickness fasciocutaneous flap is raised around the lateral side of the knee (Figure 12–3A). The iliotibial band (ITB) overlies the capsule and either is split in line with its fibers, or the patellar contribution of the ITB is divided, allowing the ITB to slide posteriorly with knee flexion. The plane between the ITB and capsule is developed to allow suturing (Figure 12–3B). This plane is followed posteriorly past the lateral collateral ligament, which is embedded in capsular tissue. The interval between the biceps femoris inferiorly and the lateral head of the gastrocnemius posteriorly is developed to provide access to the posterior capsule. For both approaches, the surgeon should be able to palpate the area of the tibial posterior cruciate ligament insertion as well as the popliteus tendon during a lateral approach. A spoon is placed in this interval to protect the posterior neurovascular bundle (Figure 12–3C).

An anterior arthrotomy is performed by incising the capsule just medial or lateral to the border of the patellar tendon, and the fat pad is transected. A retractor is placed into the notch to displace the patellar tendon toward the other compartment. The anterior meniscal root is divided, and a full-thickness capsular flap with the anterior meniscal horn attached is raised around the side of the knee toward the medial or lateral midline by subperiosteal dissection of the tissues from the proximal tibia. Medially, this flap includes the superficial and deep medial collateral ligament; laterally it includes the ITB insertion on Gerdy's tubercle. Another retractor is placed around the medial or lateral femoral condyle, providing full exposure (Figure 12–3D).

COMPLETION MENISCECTOMY

The meniscal remnant must be removed in order to prepare a vascularized bed for the transplant. However, leaving a thin shell of meniscal tissue at the meniscocapsular junction (Figure 12–4) is thought to help reduce the risk of meniscal extrusion by providing more mechanical support than the thin capsular tissue alone. The meniscal roots should be left in place at this point because they represent an important landmark for later placement of anatomically correct attachment sites.

TIBIAL PREPARATION

Depending on the specific instrumentation used, a recipient slot for bony fixation of the meniscal roots is prepared on the tibia. An inferior notchplasty as well as limited soft tissue debridement of the most inferior aspects of the anterior cruciate ligament or posterior cruciate ligament fibers can assist in visualization of the posterior root attachment site. In a line connecting the two root attachment sites (Figure 12–5A), the tibial plateau is cleared of cartilage (Figure 12–5B), and a slot

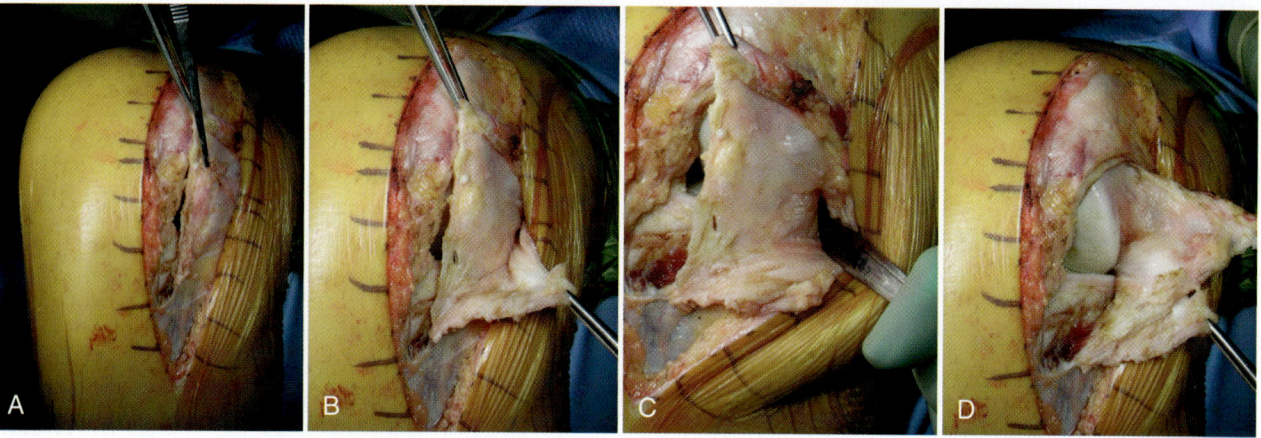

Figure 12-3 Exposure for open lateral meniscal transplantation: *A*, Full-thickness fasciocutaneous flap has been raised. The two forceps hold the capsule and iliotibial band, respectively. *B*, The plane between the iliotibial band (reflected) and capsule has been developed. *C*, The interval between the lateral head of the gastrocnemius muscle and the capsule has been developed, and a spoon has been placed to protect the posterior neurovascular bundle. *D*, The capsule and iliotibial band insertion on Gerdy's tubercle have been reflected by subperiosteal dissection from the lateral proximal tibia, exposing the lateral femoral condyle.

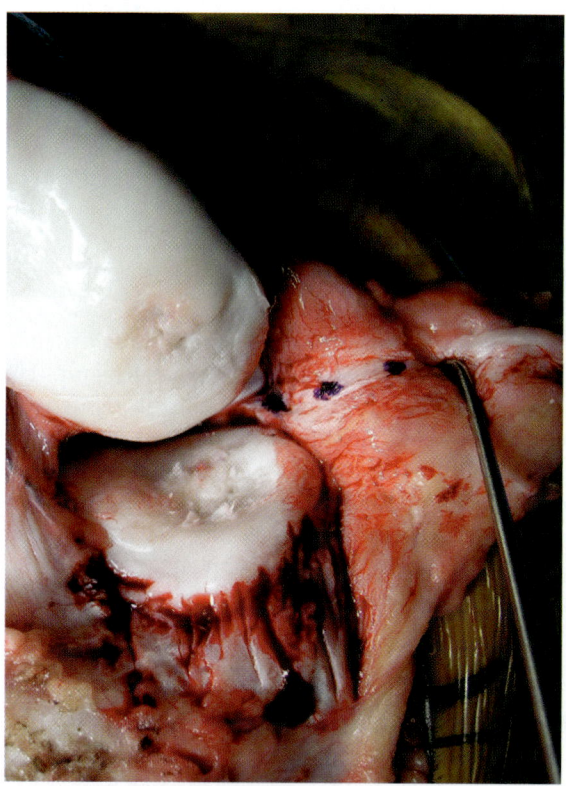

Figure 12-4 Completion meniscectomy has been performed, leaving the sturdier tissue of the meniscocapsular junction *(dots)* intact.

is created with the technique-specific instrumentation (Figure 12-5C). Two bone tunnels for later fixation of the graft can be created in the posterior and anterior aspects of the slot with a standard tibial aiming guide from the anterior cruciate ligament set (Figure 12-6).

GRAFT PLACEMENT AND FIXATION

The previously placed pull suture at the junction of the posterior horn and body of the meniscal graft is shuttled through a corresponding location of the joint capsule. This can easily be performed using zone-specific cannulas and a needle-tip suture passing wire (Figure 12-7). If fixation sutures were placed around the meniscal roots of the graft, then they are shuttled through the tibial bone tunnels at this point. Reduction of the meniscus requires a combination of pulling on the sutures and pushing the bone bridge into the slot while flexing and extending the knee with varus or valgus stress. Once the meniscus is seated under the femoral condyle (Figure 12-8), the knee should be ranged to assess stability.

Fixation of the graft is divided into bony fixation of the meniscal root attachments and soft tissue fixation at the meniscocapsular junction. Some systems create a trapezoidal or keyhole-shaped tibial slot that provides a secure fit for the bone bridge. Others require additional fixation with sutures or a screw. The sutures that were placed around the meniscal roots and pulled through the tibial bone tunnel are tied over a bone bridge on the medial aspect of the tibia for fixation. Alternatively, the bone bridge of the graft can be fixed in the slot with an interference screw or, in open meniscal allograft transplantation, secured to the tibial plateau under direct visualization with heavy, nonresorbable suture.

For arthroscopic techniques, the meniscus is circumferentially repaired to the capsule using standard meniscal repair techniques with inside–out and all-inside techniques for the posterior horn and body and outside–in

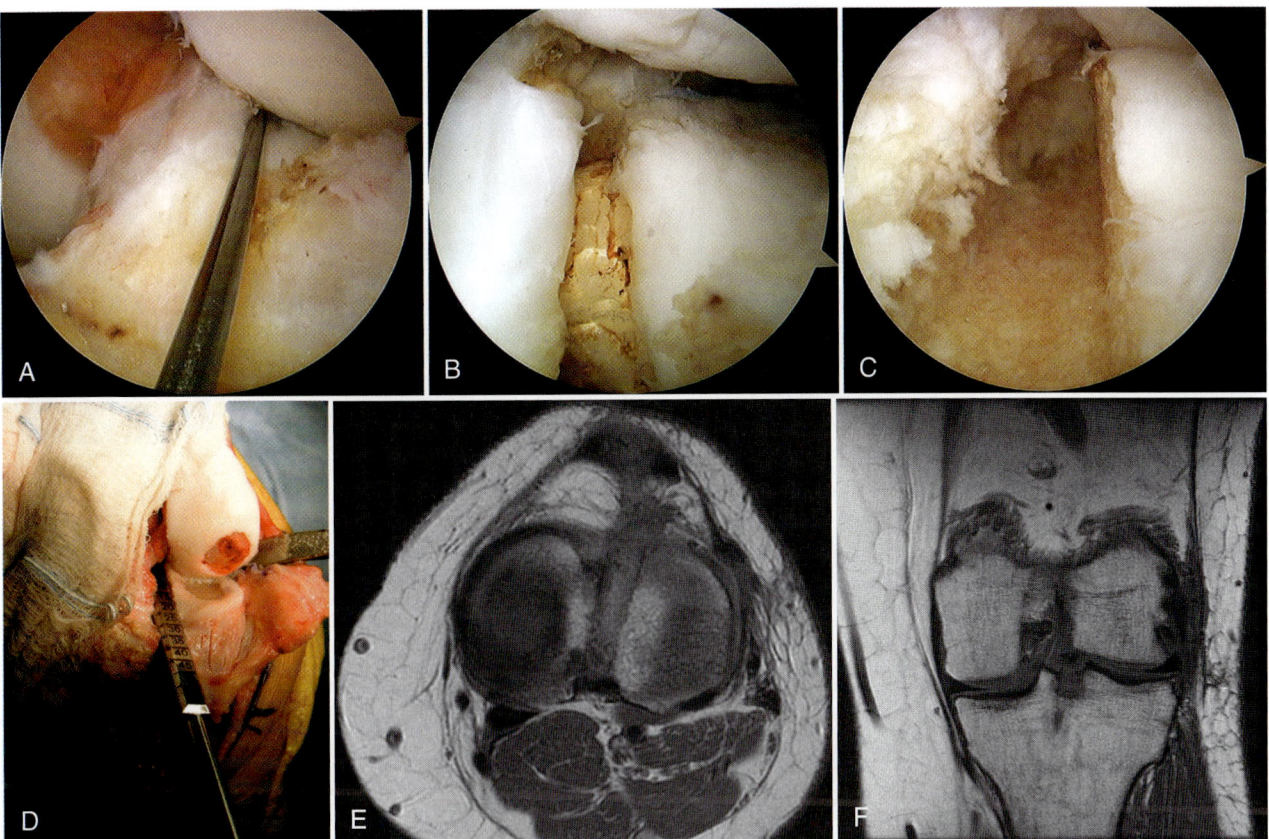

Figure 12-5 Creation of the tibial slot. *A*, A spinal needle is placed connecting the anterior and posterior root attachment sites. *B*, Overlying cartilage is removed with the electrothermal device. *C*, A recipient slot has been created on the tibial plateau. *D*, Using a rasp to finish the tibial slot in an example of open meniscal allograft transplantation. *E*, Postoperative axial magnetic resonance imaging after arthroscopic lateral meniscal allograft transplantation showing the orientation of the tibial slot and surgical changes in the fat pad. *F*, Postoperative coronal magnetic resonance imaging showing the position of the tibial slot.

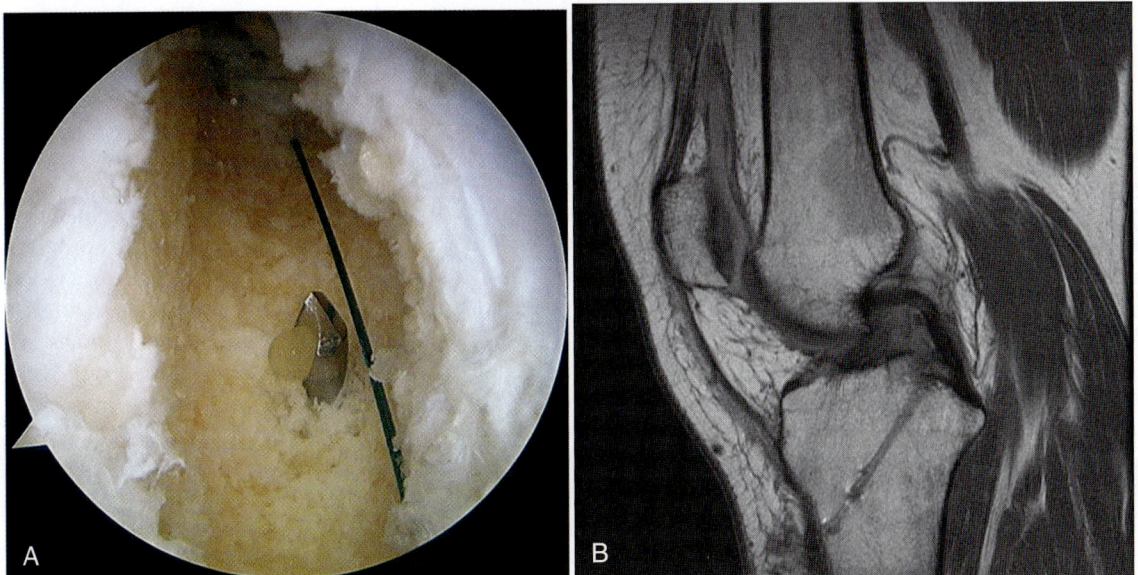

Figure 12-6 Suture fixation of the bone bridge by transosseous tunnels. *A*, Arthroscopic anterior view of the tibial slot. A tunnel has already been drilled into the posterior aspect of the slot, and a pull suture been placed. A standard tibial pin (tip visible) as used for anterior cruciate ligament reconstruction has been drilled into the anterior aspect of the slot using the standard tibial anterior cruciate ligament guide (removed). *B*, Postoperative sagittal magnetic resonance imaging view showing the oblique bone tunnel used for suture fixation of the posterior aspect of the bone bridge. The second, anterior bone tunnel is not visible on this cut.

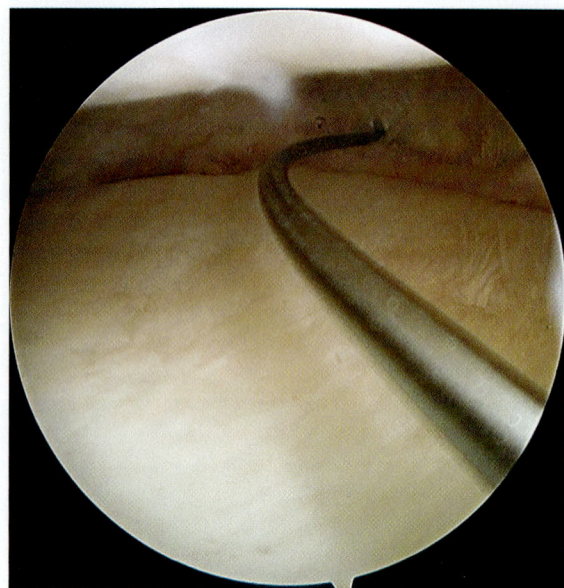

Figure 12–7 Arthroscopic view of a nitinol suture passing wire that has been placed through the capsule.

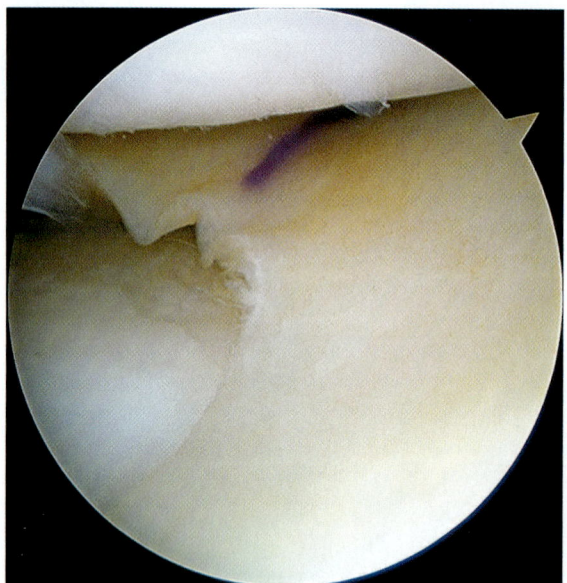

Figure 12–8 The meniscus has been reduced under the femoral condyle. The junction of the body and posterior horn has been marked to assist in orienting the graft.

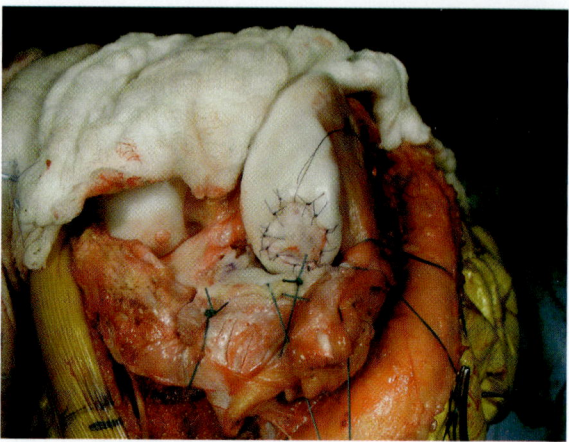

Figure 12–9 Open meniscal allograft transplantation in conjunction with autologous chondrocyte implantation to the lateral femoral condyle and plateau with concurrent tibial tubercle osteotomy. The meniscus has been secured to the tibial plateau with heavy nonabsorbable suture, and additional sutures have been placed through the capsule and meniscus to repair the meniscocapsular junction.

techniques for the anterior horn. For open techniques, the posterior horn is secured with inside–out techniques. The body and anterior horn are repaired with heavy nonresorbable sutures, which are placed through the capsule, meniscus, and tibial plateau sequentially back to front before all sutures are tied at the end (Figure 12–9). This not only repairs the meniscocapsular junction but also secures the previously released capsular flap back to the proximal tibia. If necessary, the medial collateral ligament and ITB can be additionally secured with suture anchors.

Postoperatively, patients are kept on partial weight-bearing restrictions for 2 weeks and then advanced to weight bearing as tolerated. A knee immobilizer is used for 6 weeks during ambulation. Flexion exercises are limited to 90 degrees for 2 weeks, then advanced as tolerated. If meniscal allograft transplantation is performed in conjunction with other procedures such as autologous chondrocyte implantation or osteotomy, the most conservative of the various rehabilitation protocols should be used, usually extending the weight-bearing restrictions for 6 to 8 weeks. Continuous passive motion can be used for 3 weeks for isolated meniscal allograft transplantation and 6 weeks for associated cartilage repair procedures.

SUMMARY

Meniscal allograft transplantation is successful in redistributing joint reactive forces, even though complete normalization does not occur. Patients experience good pain relief and are frequently able to return to higher activity levels, although pivoting and cutting sports are discouraged to reduce the risk of reinjury. Long-term outcomes still demonstrate the development of degenerative changes, possibly due to imperfect size matching with current techniques, which can result in meniscal extrusion.

REFERENCES

1. Alford W, Cole BJ. The indications and technique for meniscal transplant. *Orthop Clin North Am.* 2005;36:469–484.
2. Cameron JC, Saha S. Meniscal allograft transplantation for unicompartmental arthritis of the knee. *Clin Orthop Relat Res.* 1997;337:164–171.

3. Cole BJ, Rodeo S, Carter T. Allograft meniscus transplantation: indications, techniques, results. *J Bone Joint Surg.* 2002;84A:1236–1250.
4. Cole BJ, Dennis MG, Lee SJ, et al. Prospective evaluation of allograft meniscus transplantation: a minimum 2-year follow-up. *Am J Sports Med.* 2006;34(6):919–927.
5. Carter TR. Meniscal allograft transplantation. *Sports Med Arthrosc Rev.* 1999;7:51–62.
6. Rue JP, Yanke AB, Busam ML, McNickle AG, Cole BJ. Prospective evaluation of concurrent meniscus transplantation and articular cartilage repair: minimum 2-year follow-up. *Am J Sports Med.* 2008;36(9):1770–1778.
7. Farr J, Rawal A, Marberry KM. Concomitant meniscal allograft transplantation and autologous chondrocyte implantation: minimum 2-year follow-up. *Am J Sports Med.* 2007;35(9):1459–1466.

Chapter 13

Complex Cases in Cartilage Repair: Tricks and Tips

Tom Minas, MD, MS

CASE 1. MEDIAL SUBVASTUS APPROACH TO THE KNEE
  Introduction
  Surgical Technique
  Discussion

CASE 2. INTRAARTICULAR OSTEOTOMY AFTER TIBIAL PLATEAU FRACTURE

CASE 3. EXTRAARTICULAR SUPRACONDYLAR FEMORAL REVERSE DOME OSTEOTOMY FOLLOWING POSTTRAUMATIC DEFORMITY

CASE 4. REVISION LATERAL TIBIAL PLATEAU ALLOGRAFT FOR FAILED ALLOGRAFT 7 YEARS POSTIMPLANTATION

CASE 5. ACI–SYMPTOMATIC GRAFTING IN A PATIENT WITH LATERAL OSTEOARTHRITIS

CASE 6. ACI FOR END-STAGE PATELLOFEMORAL OSTEOARTHRITIS IN AN ELITE ATHLETE USING COMBINED CARTILAGE REPAIR TECHNIQUES

CASE 7. CARTILAGE REPAIR FOR LATERAL MENISCECTOMY CASCADE WITH VALGUS KNEE IN A YOUNG ATHLETE

CASE 8. CARTILAGE REPAIR WITH ACI SEGMENTAL "SANDWICH TECHNIQUE" AFTER FAILED OBI PLUGS

CASE 9. ACI TO SALVAGE FAILED OSTEOCHONDRAL GRAFTING PLUGS FOR PATELLA CARTILAGE REPAIR

CASE 10. TIBIAL TUBERCLE OSTEOTOMY, TROCHLEOPLASTY, AND PATELLA CARTILAGE REPAIR WITH ADOLESCENT FRESH PRESERVED MORSELIZED ALLOGRAFT
  Summary

My residents and clinical fellows have often asked me where they can find a well-written technique for a medial subvastus exposure as well as the tips and tricks that I use in more complex joint-preserving reconstructions. For this reason, I have included a chapter that demonstrates in detail the technique for a medial subvastus exposure as well as several complex clinical cases that may illustrate differing approaches to joint preservation in more extreme cases.

CASE 1. MEDIAL SUBVASTUS APPROACH TO THE KNEE

Introduction

Recently there has been an emphasis on minimally invasive and muscle-sparing approaches in orthopedic surgery. The subvastus approach to the knee joint has been described as an alternative to traditional approaches, which involve a large arthrotomy with partial division of the quadriceps mechanism. I have found the technique very useful for joint-preserving surgeries as well as prosthesis implantations when the soft tissue mobility of the extensor mechanism is supple. Careful surgical technique is pursued, as described and illustrated here.[1]

The step-by-step surgical technique for the medial subvastus approach to the knee follows. As with any procedure, patient selection is paramount to success, and not all patients are appropriate for this approach. However, in patients who meet our criteria, we believe that this approach offers significant benefit to patients over traditional approaches. These include less postoperative pain and easier, quicker rehabilitation in the early postoperative period. The long-term benefits, if any, are unknown.

Surgical Technique

The author performs a medial subvastus approach whenever possible; however, some patients are better served with a standard medial parapatellar approach.

Suitable candidates for a subvastus approach must have relatively mobile subcutaneous tissues in order to create a "mobile window" for performing the various aspects of the planned procedure. The mobility of the soft tissues can be assessed during a preoperative clinic visit, but the ultimate decision is made on the day of surgery with the patient under anesthesia. Obesity, contractures, and deformity are relative contraindications; however, with experience, the indications can be expanded. Revision surgery is usually a contraindication due to scar tissue formation and obliteration of tissue planes.

The patient is positioned supine in the standard fashion. We generally use employ a lateral post at the level of the thigh tourniquet as well as a post to support the foot, such that the knee can be flexed and maintained at 90 degrees of flexion. The skin incision can be made directly midline or slightly medial to midline, depending on the nature of the pathology. The length of the incision is based on the underlying pathology. Generally, it extends from the superior pole of the patella to the inferior aspect of the tibial tubercle (Figure 13–1*A*). The incision is carried sharply through the subcutaneous tissue down to the retinacular tissue. Full-thickness medial and lateral flaps are then created sharply with careful hemostasis (Figure 13–1*B*). The creation of large, full-thickness flaps is important because it allows the extensor mechanism to be mobilized deep to the subcutaneous tissues.

The distal insertion of the vastus medialis obliquus (VMO) on the patella is exposed (Figure 13–1*C*). The fascia overlying the VMO is released sharply, taking care not to injure any underlying muscle fibers (Figure 13–1*D*). The fascia is released posteriorly toward the attachment of the VMO on the medial intermuscular septum. This exposes the entire distal extent of the VMO (Figure 13–1*E*). Using blunt dissection, a finger can be placed underneath the VMO at its inferior border. The VMO is retracted proximally and laterally while maintaining its attachment to the patella. A Z-retractor is inserted anterior to the distal femur and deep to the muscle to maintain retraction (Figure 13–1*F*).

Two no. 1 Vicryl marking sutures are placed at the level of the VMO attachment to the patella (Figure 13–1*G*). An oblique capsular incision is made just distal to the VMO, beginning posteriorly at the level of the intermuscular septum and extending laterally, parallel to the inferior border of the muscle, toward the medial border of the patella. The incision is made between the marking sutures, which then serve as a guide for later repair. At the medial border of the patella, the arthrotomy is extended distally, taking care to leave a cuff of tissue attached to the patella for closure (Figure 13–1*H*). The arthrotomy incision is carried distally across the joint line and parallel to the medial border of the patellar tendon. Care is taken to avoid damaging the anterior horn of the medial meniscus if a biologic procedure is being performed. If necessary, the retropatellar bursa and fat pad can be incised to gain additional exposure.

Next, attention is turned to the suprapatellar pouch, where the synovial capsular attachments to the undersurface of the quadriceps tendon are released completely from medial to lateral (Figure 13–1*I*). This is the key maneuver that allows full mobilization of the extensor mechanism because it detaches the quadriceps muscle from the anterior femoral synovial supracondylar attachments. The patella can then be subluxed into the lateral gutter. Creating a large, full-thickness, lateral subcutaneous flap during the initial exposure is necessary in order to create a pocket into which the patella can be subluxed. A 90-degree bent Hohman or Z-retractor is placed in the lateral gutter at the level of the quadriceps tendon insertion above the patella to maintain retraction of the patella. Flexing the knee to approximately 90 degrees provides excellent exposure of the entire joint, and the appropriate procedure can be performed (Figure 13–1*J*). A standard closure is performed at the end of the case (Figure 13–1*K*). The closure is quite simple because no muscle needs to be repaired.

Discussion

The medial subvastus approach was originally described in the German literature by Erkes in 1929.[2] A modified version was reintroduced by Hofman in 1991.[3] A so-called "mini" subvastus approach has since been described.[2,4,5] Multiple reports in the literature describe the results with respect to total knee arthroplasty. Although concerns have been raised regarding appropriate component positioning, many studies demonstrate more rapid recovery, better pain scores, less blood loss, and better short-term knee range of motion when comparing the subvastus approach to more traditional approaches.[6–12] Schroer et al[13] reported their results of 600 primary total knee arthroplasties performed through a subvastus approach. Follow-up was short term, averaging 28 months. A historical group of 150 total knee arthroplasties performed through a standard medial parapatellar arthrotomy was used as a control. Overall, 11 (1.8%) major complications required reoperation in the subvastus group and 6 (4.0%) in the traditional group. The rates of both major and minor complications were found to be independent of surgical technique. The rate of major complications in the subvastus group was associated with surgical experience, as the rate was reduced by 16% for each additional 50 procedures performed. Mean knee flexion at 1 year averaged 125 degrees in the subvastus group and 114 degrees in the traditional group. Average operative time was initially higher in the subvastus group but decreased with experience so that it was less than the traditional group in the last 400 subvastus procedures performed. Of note, the authors stated that 99% of total knee arthroplasties performed

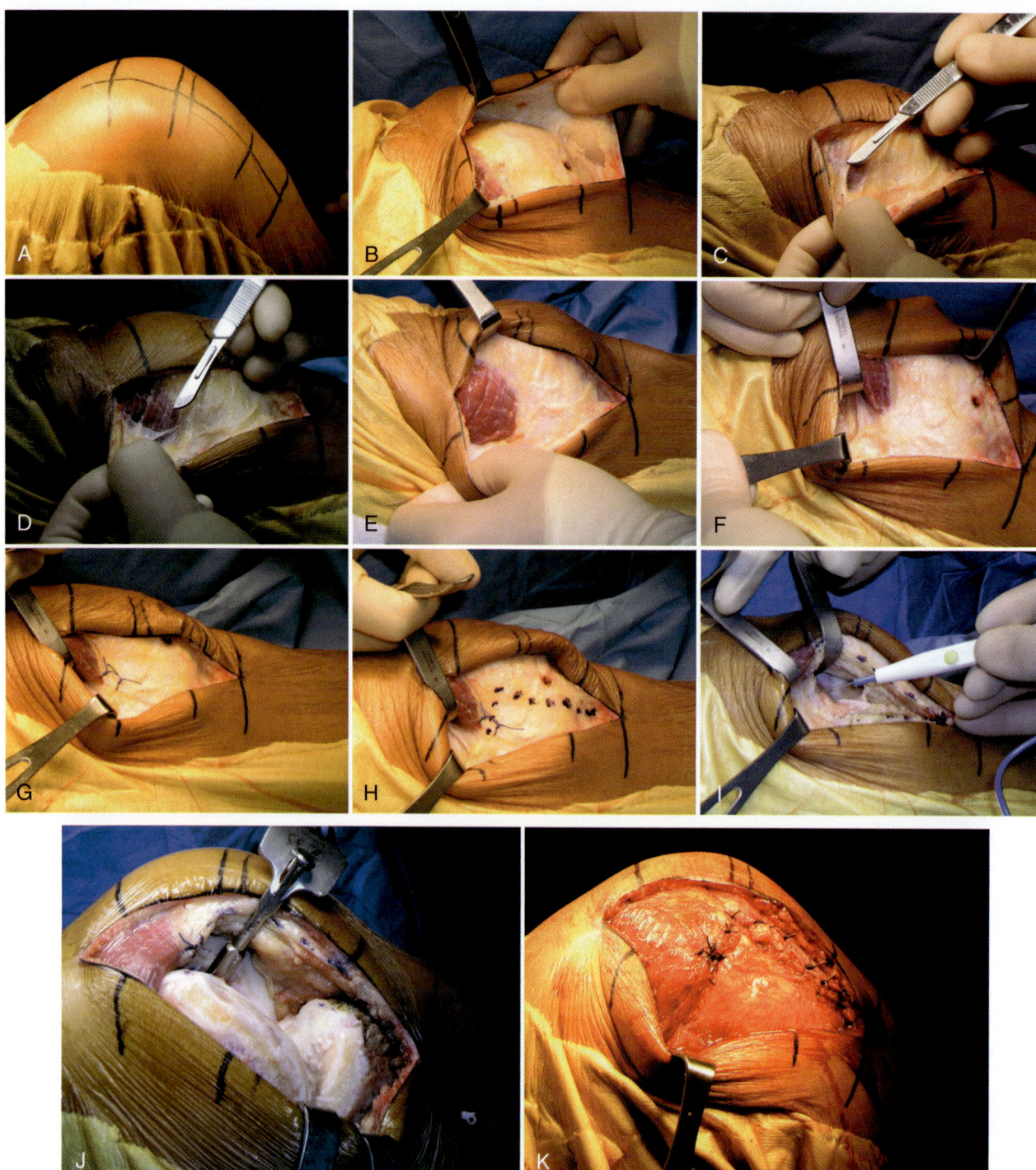

Figure 13-1 *A,* Typical skin incision extending from superior pole of patella to tibial tubercle. *B,* Development of medial and lateral full-thickness subcutaneous flaps. *C,* Exposure of vastus medialis obliquus (VMO) insertion. *D,* Subfascial dissection of VMO. *E,* Complete exposure of distal VMO insertion. *F,* Placement of Z-retractor underneath distal VMO. Note insertion on patella is left completely intact. *G,* Tagging sutures marking distal extent of insertion of VMO on patella. *H,* Proposed line of incision for performing medial arthrotomy. *I,* Release of synovial attachments from femur to undersurface of quadriceps. This is done from medial to lateral. The superior retractor is placed above the synovial attachments, while the inferior retractor is intraarticular. This clearly delineates the synovial tissue that must be released to mobilize the extensor mechanism and expose the joint. *J,* Exposure of articular surfaces. In this example, a medial unicompartmental arthroplasty is being performed. During total knee arthroplasty, we routinely place a knurled pin in the patellar tendon insertion to protect it from detachment during the case. *K,* Standard closure of the arthrotomy. The VMO is left completely intact.

during the study period were done through a subvastus approach, with 91% of patients classified as overweight and 11% as morbidly obese.

We have found that the subvastus approach provides excellent exposure and allows quicker advancement of rehabilitation after knee surgery. As with any procedure, a definite learning curve is associated with the subvastus approach. The author's technique and indications have evolved with time and experience. Less emphasis is placed on the length of the skin incision and more emphasis is placed on careful dissection of large medial and lateral skin flaps and atraumatic mobilization of the muscle. In addition to total knee arthroplasty and medial unicompartmental knee arthroplasty, we have applied the subvastus approach to the treatment of other intraarticular pathologies, primarily chondral defects. Procedures such as autologous chondrocyte implantation (ACI) and osteoarticular allografts can easily be performed through this approach.

CASE 2. INTRAARTICULAR OSTEOTOMY AFTER TIBIAL PLATEAU FRACTURE

A 31-year-old woman is thrown from her horse while riding. She sustains an injury to her left knee, consisting of a comminuted split depression fracture of her lateral tibial plateau. It is treated with external fixation distraction and percutaneous lag screw fixation of the lateral plateau. The procedure results in a malunion of the proximal tibia with valgus deformity. She has instability and pain, and she requires crutch ambulation in order to get around. She has been referred in an attempt to avoid total knee replacement.

Clinical examination demonstrates a valgus alignment to the left lower extremity. She has no effusion of the joint and has full extension and flexion to 135 degrees. She had near full passive correction to neutral alignment of the left knee and an excellent soft tissue envelope. Her distal circulation is intact. Her hardware has been removed.

Radiographic assessment (Figure 13–2A and B) reveals she has mechanical alignment passing through the center of the lateral tibiofemoral compartment. The medial and patellofemoral compartments are intact. Joint-preserving considerations for treatment include corrective realignment osteotomy combined with intraarticular osteotomy through the fracture site versus a lateral tibial plateau allograft.

Radiographic sizing of the opposite intact uninjured knee (Figure 13–2C) allows sizing for both allograft tissue as well as the normal medial to lateral tibial plateau dimensions for restoring the opposite knee if possible through intraarticular osteotomy surgery.

Computed tomographic (CT) scan with sagittal (Figure 13–2D) and coronal (Figure 13–2E) imaging allows assessment of the size of the comminuted fracture fragments to assist in decision making of osteotomy versus allograft. Because several large articular fragments are present, it was believed that osteotomy through the old fracture site would be possible, with elevation of the articular surfaces, autologous and allogeneic bone grafting from the iliac crest, and varus-producing femoral osteotomy to unload the damaged lateral compartment.

Angular correction for the osteotomy is determined by long alignment x-ray films corresponding to an 8-degree angular correction placing the mechanical axis to the medial tibial spine. A longitudinal anterior incision is made along the lateral patellar border distally and proximally. A lateral parapatellar arthrotomy is performed to expose the lateral tibial plateau as well as the distal lateral femur (Figure 13–2F). The anterior to posterior intraarticular osteotomy is made by using small K-wires and sharp wide osteotomes along the K-wires through the prior fracture sites. The comminuted metaphyseal bone is elevated. The articular fragments are reconstructed and temporarily held with K-wires and pointed reduction forceps as the width of the tibia is measured compared to the opposite knee native tibial surface. Intraoperative fluoroscopy (Figure 13–2G) confirms an adequate reduction. Autologous bone grafting from the iliac crest to the elevated tibial plateau articular fragments is performed along with compression buttress plating. Opening wedge femoral osteotomy is performed to correct the alignment and unload the reconstructed lateral tibial plateau. Seven years postoperatively, the patient continues to have minimal or no pain, functions at a high level, and is satisfied with her reconstruction (Figure 13–2H).

CASE 3. EXTRAARTICULAR SUPRACONDYLAR FEMORAL REVERSE DOME OSETOTOMY FOLLOWING POSTTRAUMATIC DEFORMITY

A 38-year-old female attorney has had longstanding deformity of the right knee following a childhood injury to her right knee. As an adolescent she sustained an open supracondylar distal femur fracture, which was treated with debridement, patellectomy, and tibial skeletal traction pin until union of her right knee. This procedure resulted in varus and flexion deformity of her right knee with limited range of motion. She was able to tolerate this situation for many years until now, when she suffers with medial joint pain that is disabling and prevents her from carrying on with her day-to-day activities. She is referred for an assessment to determine options other than total knee replacement in a woman of her age.

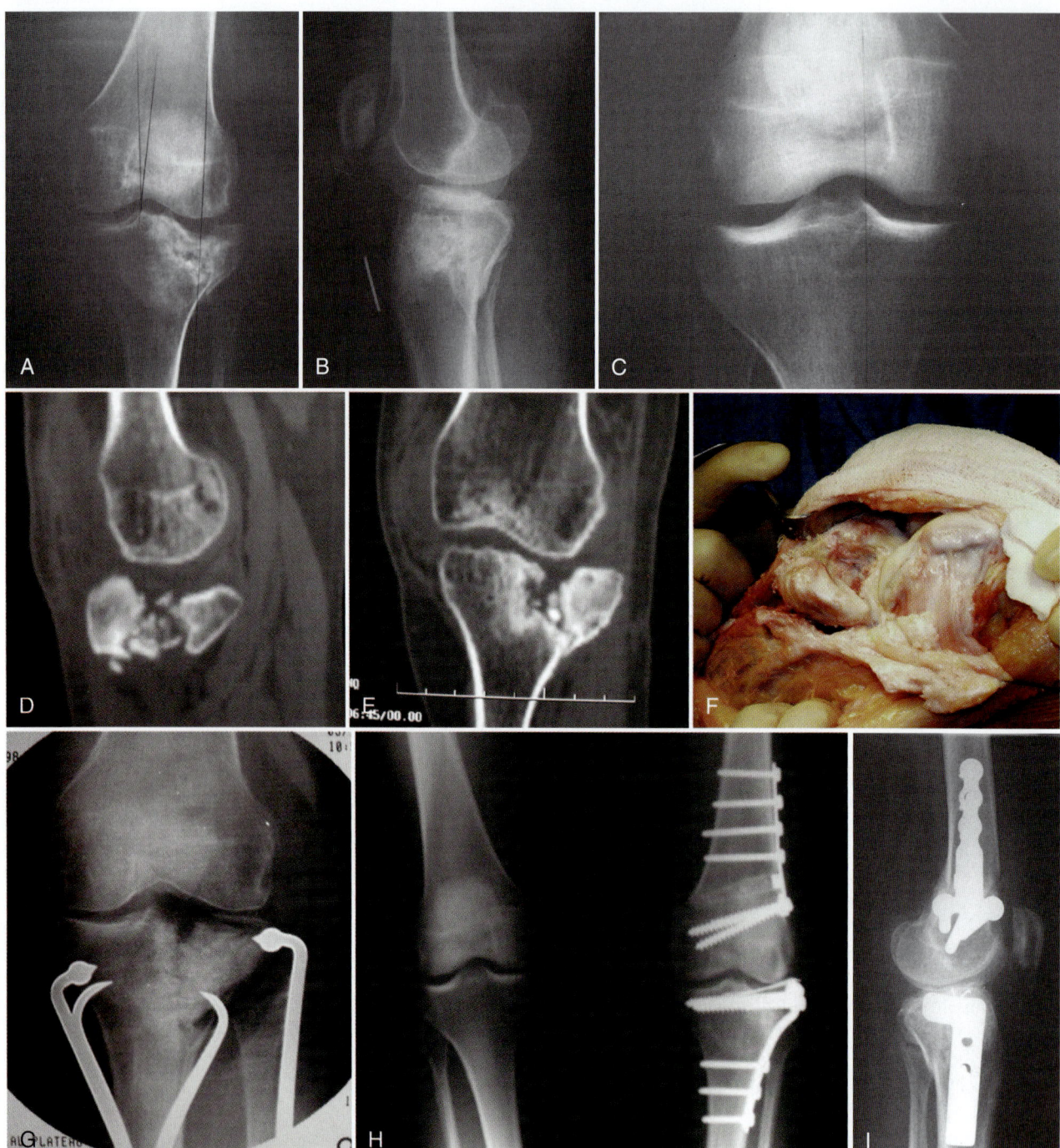

Figure 13-2 *A,* Preoperative anteroposterior (AP) radiograph demonstrating malunion of the lateral tibial plateau. *B,* Preoperative lateral radiograph. *C,* AP radiograph of the opposite right knee. *D,* Sagittal computed tomographic (CT) scan demonstrating central comminution and depression of the lateral tibial plateau. *E,* Coronal CT scan demonstrating lateral displacement through a split depression fracture type. *F,* Intraoperative appearance of the lateral tibial plateau split depression fracture. *G,* Intraoperative fluoroscopic image to assess adequate intraoperative reduction of the lateral tibial plateau fracture after intraoperative intraarticular osteotomy, elevation, medialization, and bone grafting with temporary reduction forceps. *H,* Final AP radiographs after distal femoral varus-producing osteotomy combined with intraarticular tibial plateau osteotomy. *I,* Lateral radiograph.

Clinical examination reveals the patient is healthy, slim, and eager to avoid knee replacement. She has a 10-degree flexion deformity and flexes her knee further to 90 degrees. She has a marked varus deformity to the leg and walks with an antalgic limp with a varus thrust. There is no effusion in the joint and no correction to her varus or flexion deformity.

Long alignment x-ray films (Figure 13–3A) demonstrate that the mechanical axis to her right knee falls outside the medial joint space, requiring a 15-degree angular correction to bring it back to normal mechanical axis. Lateral x-ray films (Figure 13–3B and C) demonstrate that her distal femoral flexion deformity is approximately 20 degrees.

Clinically and radiologically it appears that her lateral tibial femoral compartment is both asymptomatic and without disease. The option of a supracondylar reverse dome osteotomy through the old fracture site with intramedullary fixation is discussed.

An anterior approach to the knee with a medial parapatellar arthrotomy is performed. The intermuscular septum on the medial and lateral sides of the distal femur is released off the distal metaphyseal flare sharply. This allows a blunt finger dissection of the soft tissue structures

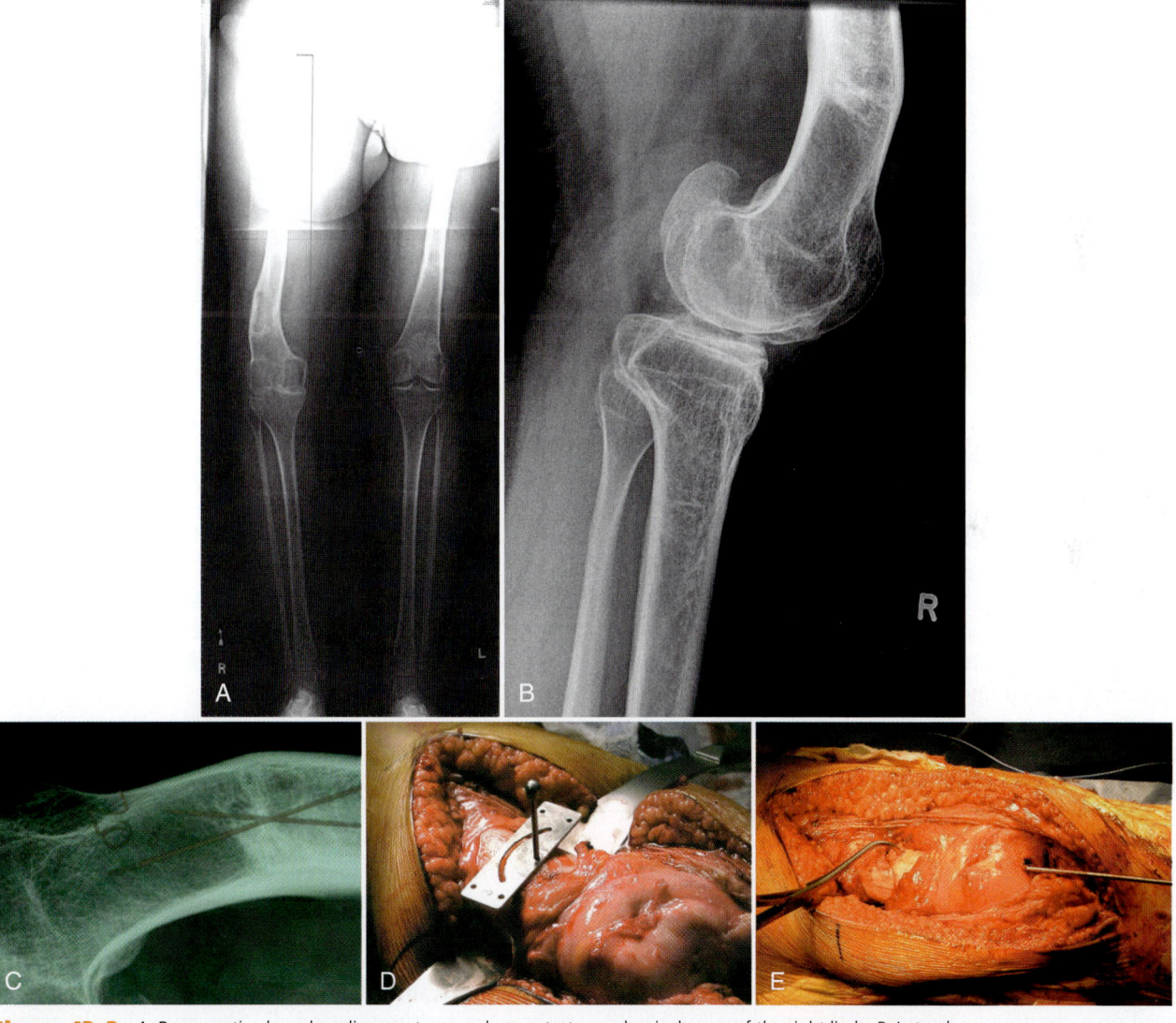

Figure 13-3 *A*, Preoperative long-leg alignment x-rays demonstrate mechanical varus of the right limb. *B*, Lateral radiograph of the right knee demonstrates flexion deformity of the distal femur and deformity of the proximal tibia, absence of the patella is noted. *C*, 20 degree flexion deformity of the distal femur is present in addition to the varus deformity at the level of the prior supracondylar femoral fracture. *D*, Anterior exposure to the right distal femur with retractors protecting the posterior neurovascular structures after packing the back of the femur with small wet sponges. An appropriately sized supracondylar reverse dome jig is applied at the level of the correction in preparation for multiple drilling, and small chisel osteotomy of the distal femur. *E*, Intramedullary alignment rod for retrograde reaming after osteotomy and correction.

Continued

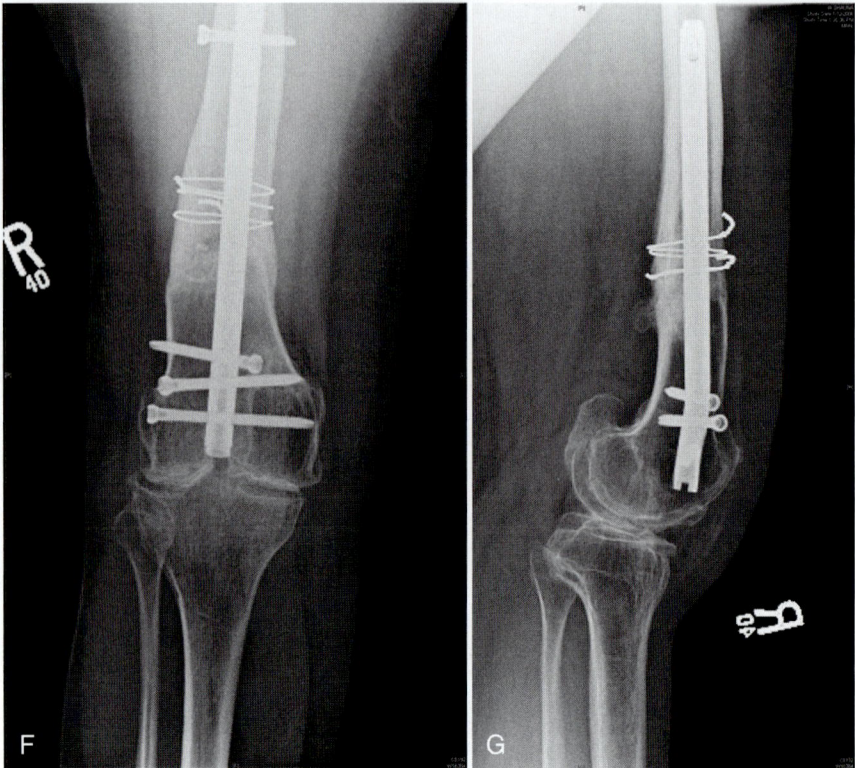

Figure 13-3—cont'd *F,* Anteroposterior radiograph 3 years after osteotomy. *G,* Lateral radiograph.

and neurovascular structures off the back the distal femur with the knee flexed. Small sponges and retractors can be placed to protect the neurovascular structures. A curved jig (Figure 13-3D) can then be applied at the level of the proposed osteotomy site, which fits the radius of curvature at that level. Small 2-mm drill bit holes are made across the femur from anterior to posterior, perforating both cortices. Small drill holes are connected with a fine sharp 0.25-inch osteotome from anterior to posterior. The distal fragment is rotated upon the proximal fragment until the desired angular correction is obtained in both the medial lateral and anteroposterior (AP) planes to correct both deformities. A K-wire and pointed reduction forceps hold the two fragments in apposition until a guidewire can be placed from the distal fragment into the proximal metaphyseal canal under image intensification (Figure 13-3E). Retrograde reaming is performed, and a appropriately sized retrograde intramedullary femoral rod is locked proximally and distally, maintaining the osteotomy correction. The fixation is stable, and the patient is immediately placed on a continuous passive motion machine for a full range of motion and touch weight-bearing until solid osteotomy union is obtained. Radiographs obtained at 3-year follow-up (Figure 13-3F and G) demonstrate a well-healed osteotomy with well-preserved joint spaces. Six years later, the patient remains pain free and very satisfied with her realignment osteotomy. Reconstruction to a total knee replacement at this time would be technically much easier once the intramedullary (IM) rod is removed because minimal extraarticular deformity is present as she approaches a more suitable age for prosthetic arthroplasty if her symptoms worsen.

CASE 4. REVISION LATERAL TIBIAL PLATEAU ALLOGRAFT FOR FAILED ALLOGRAFT 7 YEARS POSTIMPLANTATION

Seven years after undergoing reconstruction of her right knee with femoral osteotomy combined with lateral tibial plateau allograft, a 35-year-old woman sustains recurrent injury to her right knee. The initial reconstruction was performed for a lateral tibial plateau malunion after fracture with valgus instability. Following her reconstruction, she had excellent clinical use of her right leg. Her recent injury occurred when she was pitching at a softball game and was hit directly in the right knee by the struck ball. She immediately experienced pain and collapsed to the ground.

She was seen at the local emergency room, where she was noted to have a large tense effusion of the right knee. The knee was aspirated for hemarthrosis, immobilized, and x-rayed (Figure 13-4A and B). The radiographs demonstrated collapse of the lateral tibial plateau allograft. Radiographic markers were used during the x-ray

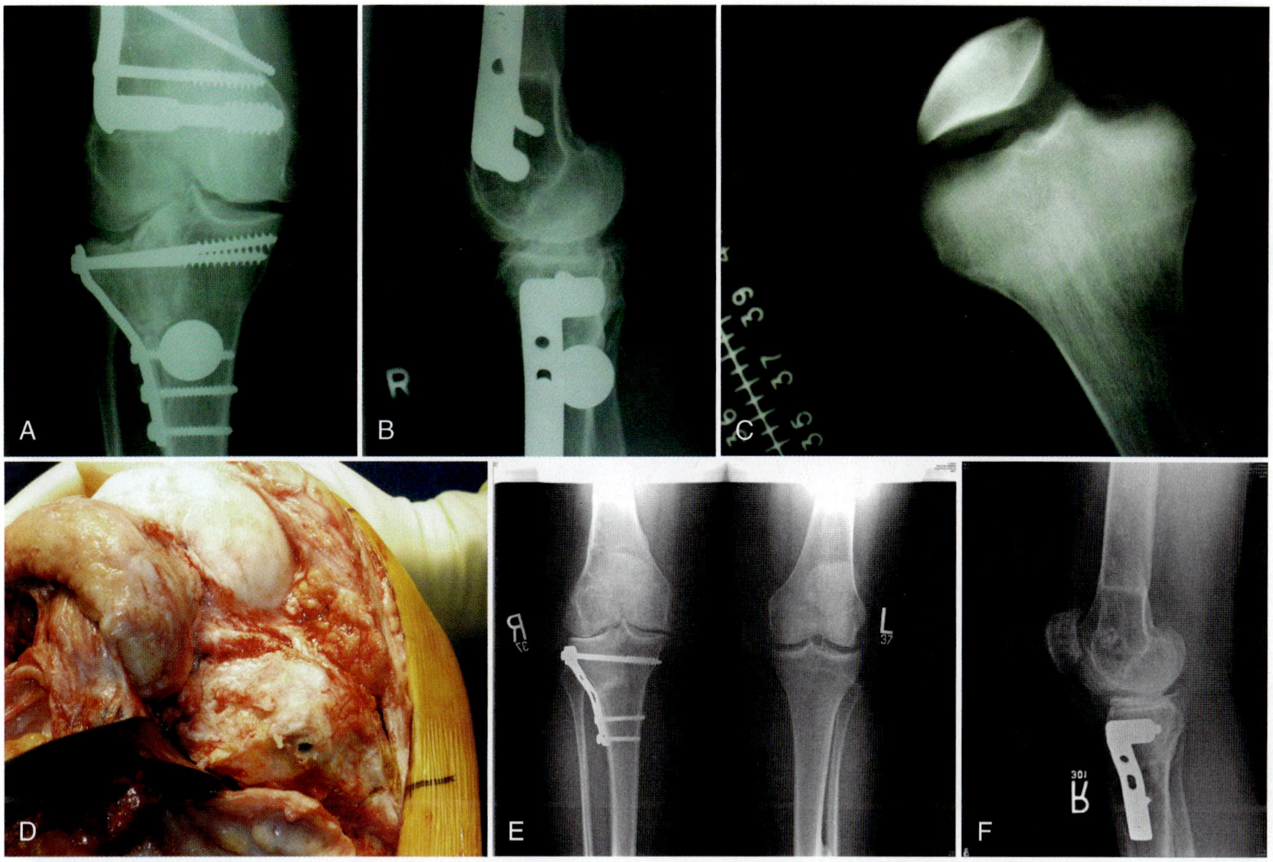

Figure 13-4 *A,* Anteroposterior (AP) radiograph with radiographic sizing marker showing collapse of lateral tibial plateau allograft 7 years after femoral osteotomy with lateral tibial plateau allograft. *B,* Lateral radiograph. *C,* Matched fresh osteoarticular bulk allograft. *D,* Intraoperative appearance of collapsed lateral tibial plateau allograft 7 years after implantation following traumatic collapse with removal of hardware. *E,* AP x-ray films, bilateral knees, 5 years after revision lateral tibial plateau osteoarticular allograft. *F,* Lateral x-ray film 5 years after revision allograft.

process to remeasure the medial lateral width of the tibial plateau as well as the AP dimensions for repeat reconstruction with osteoarticular bulk allograft to the lateral tibial plateau. A match became available (Figure 13-4C), and reconstruction was performed. The previous lateral parapatellar arthrotomy was reopened, and the hardware from the distal femur and lateral tibial plateau were removed. The joint canal demonstrated disease through the lateral femoral condyles as well as the collapsed lateral tibial plateau (Figure 13-4D). A total knee replacement cutting guide was used to make the transverse cut at right angles to the longitudinal axis of the tibia and a sagittal cut along the top of the lateral tibial spine. The posterior capsule was dissected in order to pass sutures through the lateral meniscal allograft attachment to the tibial plateau insecure the posterior capsular structures. The tibial plateau allograft was fashioned appropriately to fit in position and then fixated with a buttress plate. Despite radiographic evidence of loss of articular joint space to the lateral tibiofemoral compartment (Figure 13-4E and F), the patient continues to remain asymptomatic 5 years later.

CASE 5. ACI–SYMPTOMATIC GRAFTING IN A PATIENT WITH LATERAL OSTEOARTHRITIS

A 40-year-old police officer is at risk of losing his job. Every time he attempts to walk distances while on patrol, his left knee becomes swollen and globally painful. He has a history of a prior subtotal lateral meniscectomy.

On physical examination, he is fit and healthy appearing. He walks with a slight antalgic gait on the left side with valgus alignment of the left knee. He has full extension and flexion limited by a large effusion in the left knee. Most of his pain is felt retropatellar and lateral. He has minimal medially based pain.

Standing AP and posteroanterior (PA) radiographs demonstrate well-preserved tibiofemoral joint space (Figure 13-5A). Long alignment x-ray films demonstrate mechanical axis to fall to the lateral tibial spine. After discussing the options available to him after having failed conservative treatment, the patient agrees to arthroscopic assessment of the left knee for the possibility of ACI.

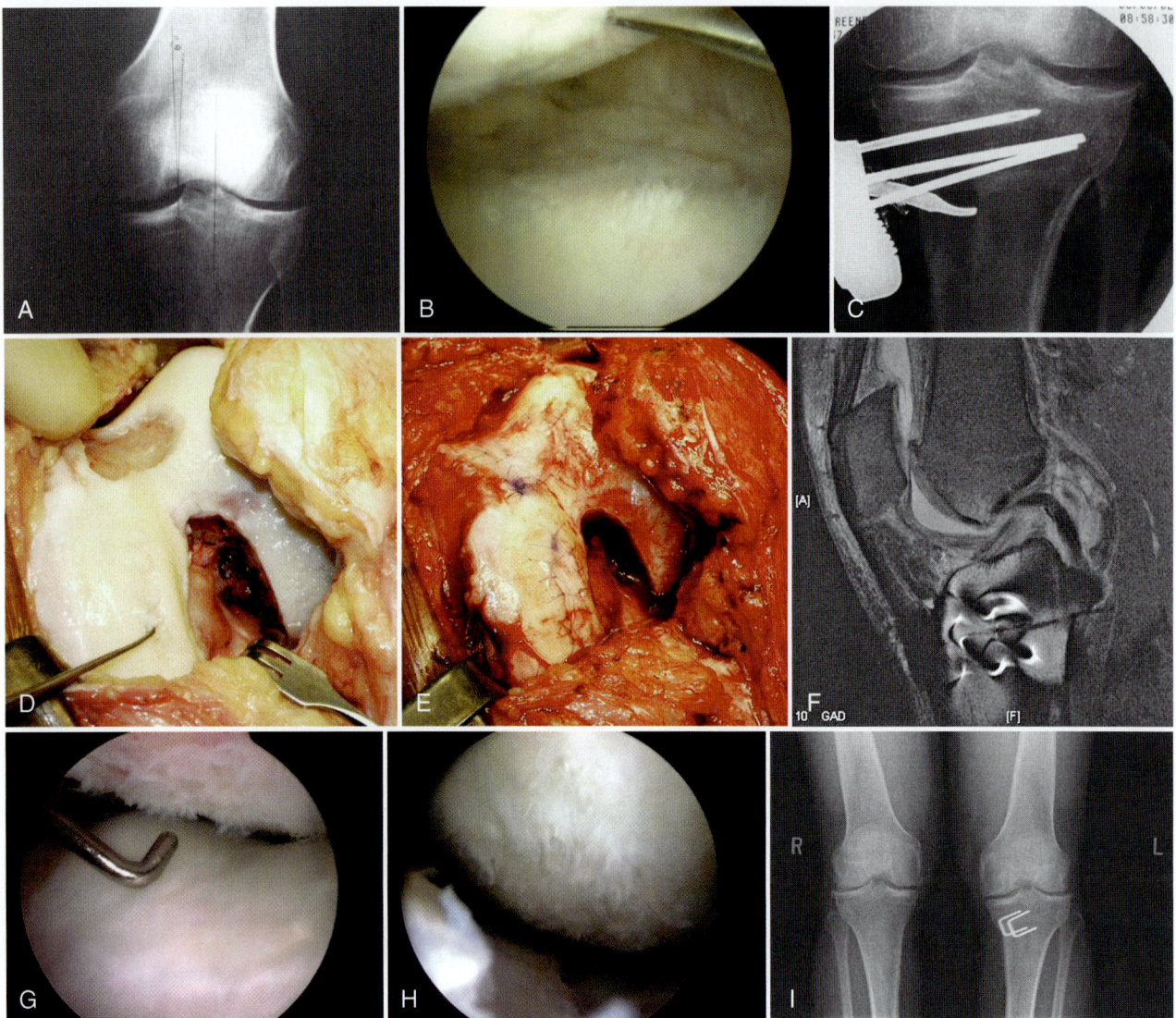

Figure 13-5 *A,* Standing anteroposterior (AP) radiograph. *B,* Arthroscopic appearance of lateral compartment, absent lateral meniscus with grade 4 changes to posterior lateral tibial plateau and femoral condyles. *C,* AP fluoroscopic intraoperative image demonstrating closing wedge tibial varus-producing osteotomy of 6 degrees using a calibrated jig. *D,* Open appearance of left knee after debridement of trochlea defect with probe at the level of grade 3 changes to the medial femoral condyle. *E,* Open appearance of left knee after autologous chondrocyte implantation (ACI) performed to the trochlea and medial femoral condyle. *F,* Sagittal magnetic resonance imaging scan of left knee 1 year postoperative demonstrating adhesions from Hoffa fat pad to anterior cruciate ligament as well as excellent repair tissue fill of trochlea ACI graft. *G,* Arthroscopic appearance of trochlea ACI graft 1 year after transplantation at the time of arthroscopic lysis of adhesions at Hoffa fat pad. *H,* Arthroscopic appearance of medial femoral condyles ACI graft after removal of periosteal hypertrophy with intact underlying cartilage repair tissue. *I,* Standing AP radiographs 7 years after transplantation. The patient remains without symptoms and without evidence of arthritic progression to the left knee radiographically.

At the time of arthroscopy, the patient is noted to have complete absence of the lateral meniscus and grade 4 changes to the lateral tibial plateau and lateral femoral condyles (Figure 13–5B). He also has a localized large grade 4 defect to the trochlea and a small grade 3 lesion to the medial femoral condyle. A biopsy for cultured articular chondrocytes is performed for second-stage ACI.

A proposed reconstruction to alleviate the patient's symptoms and preserve his joint so that he can continue working as a police officer includes a varus-producing osteotomy to unload the lateral tibiofemoral compartment in combination with ACI to the trochlea and medial femoral condyle. This procedure may halt the progression of continued cartilage breakdown and stop the recurrent effusions. Because the patient does not have hypoplasia of the lateral femoral condyle accounting for the valgus alignment and he only requires a small angular correction (6 degrees), a closing wedge tibial varus-producing osteotomy (Figure 13–5C) with ACI to the trochlea and medial femoral condyles (Figure 13–5D and E) is proposed. The lateral compartment will not be treated by ACI but rather just the unloading effect of the osteotomy in isolation. Hence, a selective treatment of the most symptomatic chondral defects will be performed.

One year after surgery, the patient has mild stiffness and medial joint compartment catching. Magnetic resonance imaging (MRI) scan (Figure 13–5F) demonstrates adhesions from Hoffa fat pad to anterior cruciate ligament (ACL), a well-filled ACI graft to the trochlea, and hypertrophy of the periosteum to the medial femoral condyle.

Arthroscopic appearance of the trochlea ACI graft demonstrates excellent repair tissue fill (Figure 13–5G). After hypertrophy to the medial femoral condyle ACI graft is removed, the underlying tissue demonstrates excellent quality and fill (Figure 13–5H). The patient becomes asymptomatic, is able to return to his previous position as a police officer, and remains asymptomatic 7 years later, with healthy-appearing joint spaces on radiograph (Figure 13–5I).

CASE 6. ACI FOR END-STAGE PATELLOFEMORAL OSTEOARTHRITIS IN AN ELITE ATHLETE USING COMBINED CARTILAGE REPAIR TECHNIQUES

A 42-year-old elite female athlete has a 1-year history of rapidly worsening anterior knee pain with recurrent effusions. It limits her from activities of daily living, such as climbing up and down stairs and walking on uneven ground, and limits her from participating in any sports or lower-extremity resisted weight training. She seeks surgical consultation for treatment what will allow her to participate comfortably in activities of daily living and possibly return to competitive swimming.

She has undergone arthroscopic debridement of the affected left knee for loose articular fragments and the patellofemoral joint, with minimal improvement. She has undergone aspirations and steroid injections as well as plasma-rich protein injections, with no improvement.

Clinical examination shows a fit 42-year-old woman who appears younger than her stated age. She has atrophy of her left thigh musculature. A large intraarticular effusion and a Baker cyst are present in the left knee. Flexion of the left knee is limited secondary to the intraarticular effusion and Baker cyst. She has an increased quadriceps angle clinically. Due to the large effusion, crepitations within the knee cannot be palpated. The collateral and ligamentous examinations are normal.

AP, lateral, and skyline x-ray films (Figure 13–6A through C) demonstrate erosive changes to the retropatellar surface of the left knee with intact tibiofemoral joint spaces. CT scan in full extension with the quadriceps relaxed (Figure 13–6D) and then contracted (Figure 13–6E) demonstrate subluxation of the patellofemoral joint, subchondral bony cysts on the median ridge and lateral facet of the patella, complete loss of joint space of the lateral patellofemoral articulation, and a tibial tubercle–trochlear groove distance (TT–TG) of 19 mm. Arthroscopic assessment of the left knee joint demonstrates intact tibiofemoral articulations with evidence of partial medial and lateral meniscectomies, advanced loss of articular cartilage to the patella with only a median ridge of articular cartilage remaining, and near complete loss of articular cartilage to the entire lateral trochlea are facet surface. A biopsy for cultured articular chondrocytes is performed at the time of arthroscopy.

Options for biologic reconstruction of the patient's damaged left knee patellofemoral surfaces include tibial tubercle osteotomy combined with kissing matched fresh osteoarticular allografts of the patella and trochlea or ACI to the patella and trochlea. However, treatment with ACI also requires dealing with the subchondral bone cysts, sclerotic subchondral bone surface, and near complete loss of articular surface to the entire patella. Because ACI is a surface treatment to articular surfaces that can be salvaged with a fresh osteoarticular allograft, if it were to fail, this option was chosen.

The surgery consists of a lateral subvastus arthrotomy with inspection of the articular surfaces that are damaged. The damaged patellar surfaces can be assessed, and tracking and tibial tubercle osteotomy can be performed to medialize and normalize the tracking of the extensor mechanism. The osteotomy is performed with a transverse proximal cut, a length of 6 cm with a sloping distal cut, and anteromedialization that centralizes and minimally unloads the lateral facet of the patella. The entire extensor mechanism can then be reflected proximally and medially. This allows excellent exposure to the patellofemoral joint without filing the quadriceps extensor mechanism. The appearance of the patella reveals only a small rim of medial facet cartilage (Figure 13–6G) and proximal pole cartilage. The trochlear lateral facet demonstrates vertical ridging of the remaining proximal cartilage with central erosive full-thickness cartilage loss (Figure 13–6H). Radical debridement of both defects requires removal of all subchondral bone cysts to the patella with a high-speed bur while attempting to retain a thin margin of articular cartilage for sewing peripherally circumferentially on both trochlea and patella. The sclerotic subchondral bone is deepened and thinned out with a high-speed bur. The peripheral synovium around the patella that is well attached to its margins is incised and reflected 5 mm circumferentially to assist in suture anchorage of the membrane that will cover the transplanted surface (Figure 13–6I). The area of subchondral cysts removed with the high-speed bur is bone grafted

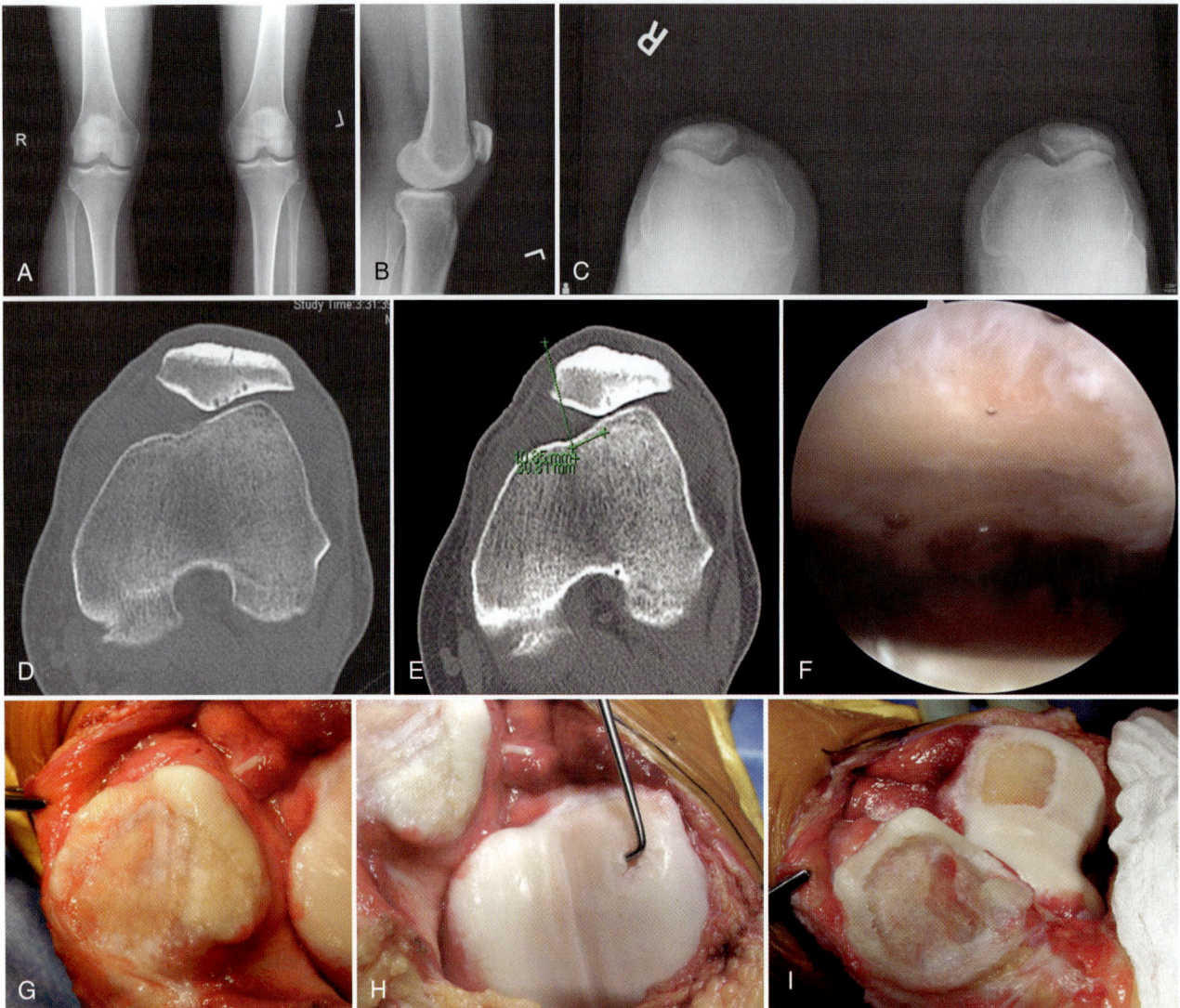

Figure 13–6 *A,* Anteroposterior (AP) radiograph. *B,* Lateral radiograph demonstrating retropatellar subchondral erosive changes. *C,* Skyline radiograph demonstrating left patellar subchondral bone changes with tilt and subluxation. *D,* Computed tomographic (CT) scan with the quadriceps relaxed demonstrates subchondral bone cysts on the median ridge lateral facet of the patella with loss of lateral facet articular space. *E,* CT scan of the quadriceps contracted demonstrates further subluxation of the patella laterally. *F,* Arthroscopic appearance of patella demonstrates near pan patellar cartilage loss with bare bone exposed. *G,* Open appearance of patella demonstrates only a small rim of median ridge cartilage remaining, with complete loss of articular surface to the lateral facet and median ridge. *H,* Open appearance of trochlea demonstrates global thinning of lateral trochlea facet and breakdown as demonstrated by a nerve hook with bare bone exposed and undermining of articular cartilage and with. *I,* Open appearance of trochlea and patella after radical debridement of damaged articular cartilage with removal of subchondral bone cysts using high-speed bur to the patella.

Continued

with proximal tibial cancellous bone taken from the osteotomy site. The median ridge in this area is maintained centrally with a 10-mm osteochondral graft harvested from the distal pole sulcus terminalis and transplanted into the osseous-deficient region centrally (Figure 13–6*J*). The donor site for the 10-mm osteochondral graft taken from the sulcus terminalis of the distal lateral trochlea set is backfilled with a TruFit plug (Smith & Nephew, Andorer, MA) (Figure 13–6*K*). The patella is resurfaced with type I–III collagen porcine membrane (Biogide-Geischich Industries, Wolhusen, Switzerland). Microsuturing is performed with 6—*zero*. Vicryl sutures circumferentially in a manner that restores the V-shaped articular surface to the patella anchoring specifically at the osteochondral graft median ridge centrally (Figure 13–6*L* and *M*). Fifty million autologous articular chondrocytes are injected underneath the membranes and sealed. The tibial tubercle osteotomy is

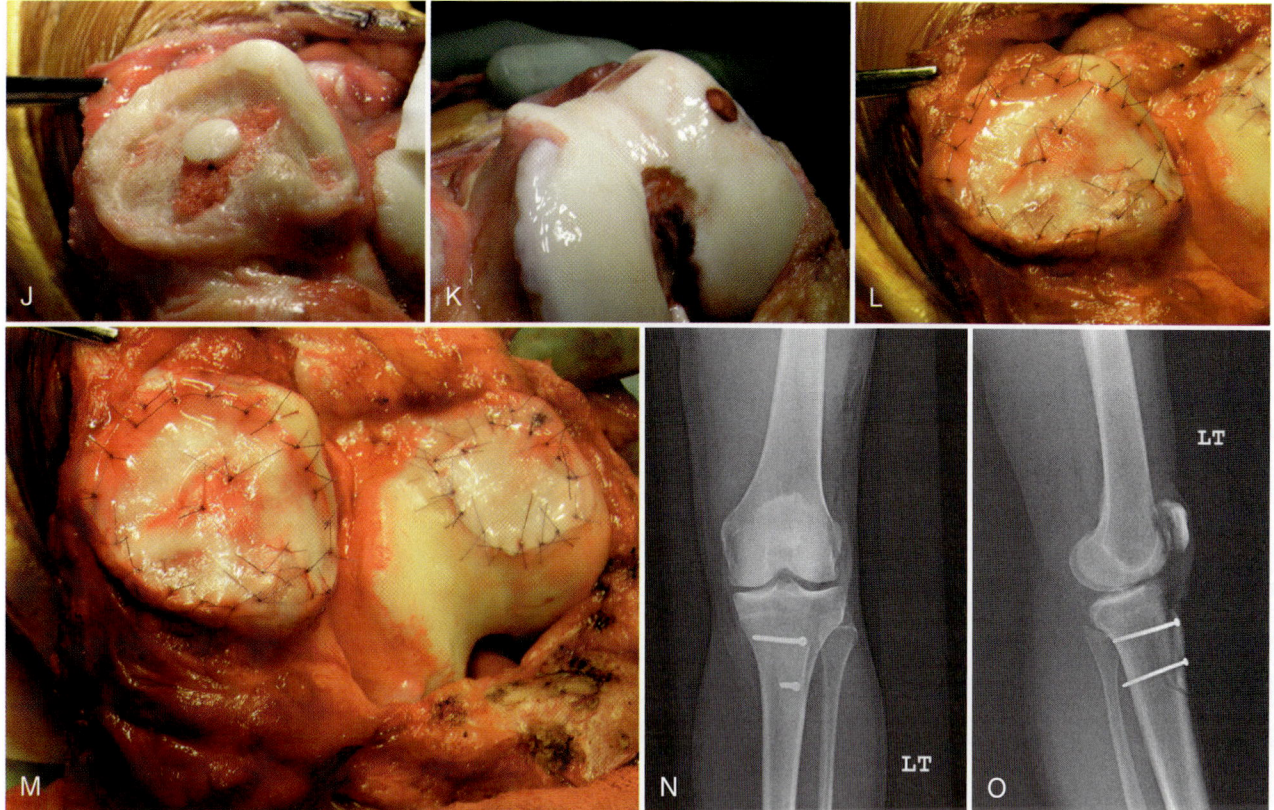

Figure 13-6—cont'd *J*, Appearance of patella with osteochondral graft placed at the area of the central median ridge in order to restore the volume of the articular surface of the patella after membrane microsuturing and bone grafting of the subchondral bone loss. *K*, TruFit plug to sulcus terminalis of the distal lateral trochlea for backfill of the osteochondral dowel used to repair the patella. *L*, Appearance of patella after autologous chondrocyte implantation (ACI). *M*, Open appearance of patella and trochlea after ACI. *N*, AP radiograph after tibial tubercle osteotomy. *O*, Lateral radiograph after tibial tubercle osteotomy.

repositioned centrally and held with two interfragmental compression screws (Figure 13–6*N* and *O*).

A gentle rehabilitation program emphasizing patellar mobility in the proximal–distal, medial, and lateral directions to prevent retropatellar adhesions, lower-extremity muscle tone to the quadriceps, hamstrings, and gluteal muscles, and functional rehabilitation results in an excellent early functional return. The patient's goals of pain-free quality of life with activities of daily living are restored, and further athletic endeavors are pursued.

CASE 7. CARTILAGE REPAIR FOR LATERAL MENISCECTOMY CASCADE WITH VALGUS KNEE IN A YOUNG ATHLETE

A 16-year-old girl sustains a lateral meniscus tear to the left knee while playing soccer. Arthroscopy is performed, and the meniscus is completely removed. Within 12 to 18 months of subtotal lateral meniscectomy, she develops recurrent effusions, laterally based joint pain, and inability to participate in sports as well as limitations of activities of daily living.

A second arthroscopy demonstrates cartilaginous loss throughout the weight-bearing surface of the lateral femoral condyle and lateral tibial plateau. A biopsy for ACI is taken. She is referred for definitive reconstruction of her left knee.

Long alignment x-ray films demonstrate that the mechanical axis falls to the lateral compartment of her left knee (Figure 13–7*A*). Standing PA radiographs (Figure 13–7*B*) demonstrate that, at age 17 years, she already has 50% loss of the articular space of the lateral compartment of her left knee. Skyline x-ray film (Figure 13–7*C*) demonstrates tilt and subluxation of the patella of the left knee. Lateral x-ray film demonstrates a normal patellar height (Figure 13–7*D*).

The planned reconstruction involves tibial tubercle anteromedialization to centralize the extensor mechanism with a lateral subvastus approach to expose the distal lateral femur and lateral tibiofemoral joint surfaces (Figure 13–7*E*). After radical debridement of the damaged articular cartilage to the distal femur and lateral tibial plateau (Figure 13–7*F*), a trough is prepared in anticipation of the lateral meniscus allograft. The lateral meniscus is prepared on the back table with type 0 Ethibond sutures through the posterior horn of

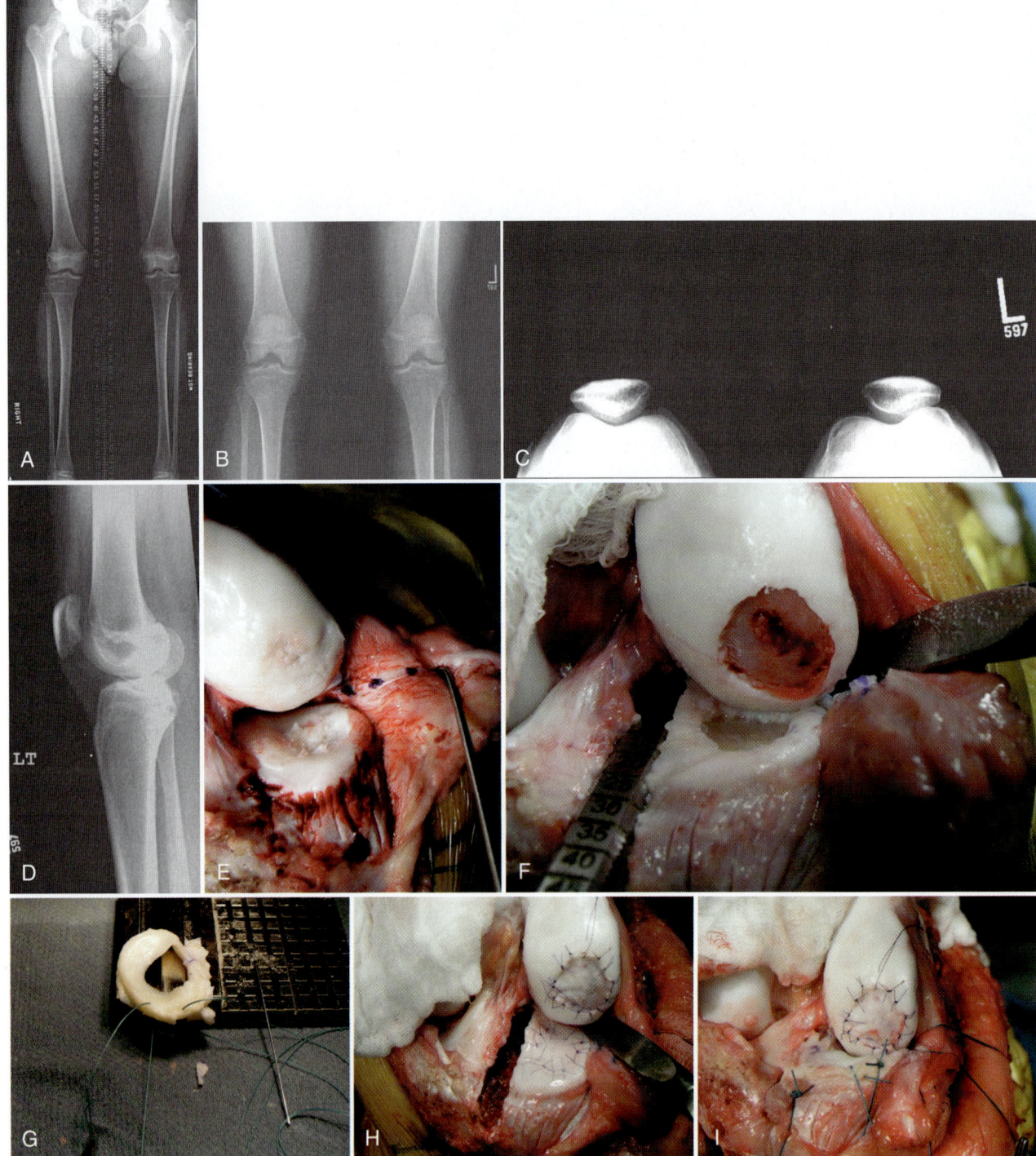

Figure 13–7 *A,* Long alignment x-ray films. *B,* Standing posteroanterior radiographs demonstrate 50% cartilage loss to the left knee lateral tibiofemoral joint. *C,* Skyline x-ray films demonstrate lateral tilt and subluxation to the left patella. *D,* Lateral x-ray film. *E,* Central cartilage loss grade 3 and grade 4 changes to lateral tibial plateau and lateral femoral condyles. *F,* Lateral tibial femoral compartment after radical debridement to damaged articular cartilage surfaces and trough preparation for lateral meniscus allograft passage. *G,* Lateral meniscus allograft preparation on back table with sutures through the posterior horn of the lateral meniscus. *H,* Autologous chondrocyte implantation grafts sutured in position. *I,* Lateral meniscus allograft passed into lateral compartment.

Continued

Figure 13-7—cont'd *J,* Postoperative anteroposterior radiograph of left knee following femoral osteotomy with tibial tubercle osteotomy. *K,* Lateral radiograph. *L,* Skyline radiograph.

the lateral meniscus (Figure 13-7*G*) to allow passage of the lateral meniscus allograft through the posterior capsule, which has been carefully dissected off the posterior aspect of the knee joint. ACI grafts are microsutured and prepared (Figure 13-7*H*). Prior to performing the opening wedge distal femoral varus osteotomy, the lateral meniscus allograft is passed and repaired (Figure 13-7*I*), which tightens up the lateral column of the knee (Figure 13-7*J* and *K*). The tibial tubercle osteotomy is repositioned, centralized, and fixated at the end of the surgery (Figure 13-7*L*).

Postoperatively, the patient undergoes continuous passive motion, touch weight-bearing, and isometric quadriceps contractions for the first 6 weeks. She is then fit with a custom lateral compartment unloader brace and progresses with weight bearing as comfort allows based on pain in the lateral tibiofemoral compartment. A stationary bicycle is also permitted at 6 weeks postoperatively, along with isometric quadriceps straight leg raises. She is off her crutches by postoperative week 10.

The unloader brace is worn for 6 months, at which time she is pain free. She resumes normal activities of daily living and gradually resumes nonimpact sports 9 to 12 months after reconstruction.

CASE 8. CARTILAGE REPAIR WITH ACI SEGMENTAL "SANDWICH TECHNIQUE" AFTER FAILED OBI PLUGS

A 23-year-old young woman sustains an ACL tear with an articular cartilage injury to the medial femoral condyle. This is treated by an ACL reconstruction with allograft patellar bone tendon bone and TruFit plug (Smith & Nephew) to the medial femoral condyle. Her medial pain persists, as does persistent effusions and anterior knee pain. She undergoes repeat arthroscopy by her treating surgeon, who notes a large trochlea defect, lateral femoral condyles defect, and harvests cartilage for ACI. She is referred for definitive treatment.

Clinical examination demonstrates neutral alignment to the right lower extremity, a large effusion in the right knee, and antalgic gait pattern. She has a stable ligamentous examination, mild retropatellar crepitus, and medial joint line tenderness.

Standing PA x-ray film demonstrates an intralesional osteophyte to the lateral femoral condyle and well-preserved tibiofemoral joint spaces (Figure 13-8*A*). Lateral x-ray film (Figure 13-8*B*) demonstrates an increased tibial posterior slope with hardware intact from previous ACL reconstruction. Skyline x-ray film demonstrates a well-preserved joint space (Figure 13-8*C*).

At the time of open ACI procedure, a large intralesional osteophyte to the lateral femoral condyle, a large trochlea defect, and evidence of a TruFit plug to the medial femoral condyle that is in situ but is not incorporated with surrounding cartilage degradation are noted (Figure 13-8*D*). The TruFit plug is easily removed with forceps, with no evidence of incorporation or healing (Figure 13-8*E*). The osseous defect to the medial femoral condyle is filled with autologous bone harvested from the proximal femoral metaphysis with a core harvester. The autologous cancellous bone graft is morselized and fills in the bony deficiency to the medial femoral condyle (Figure 13-8*F*). It is then covered with a collagen membrane (Figure 13-8*G*). The other defects are radically debrided, and the tourniquet is let down (Figure 13-8*H*). The ACI grafts are microsutured into place over the defects in the usual fashion (Figure 13-8*I*). The patient undergoes standard rehabilitation for ACI to the weight-bearing Codell with trochlea defect. Six months postoperatively, MRI scan (Figure 13-8*J*) demonstrates minimal bone marrow edema, excellent bone graft incorporation to the osseous defect from the previous TruFit plug, and good cartilage repair development. Three years postoperatively, the patient remains symptom free.

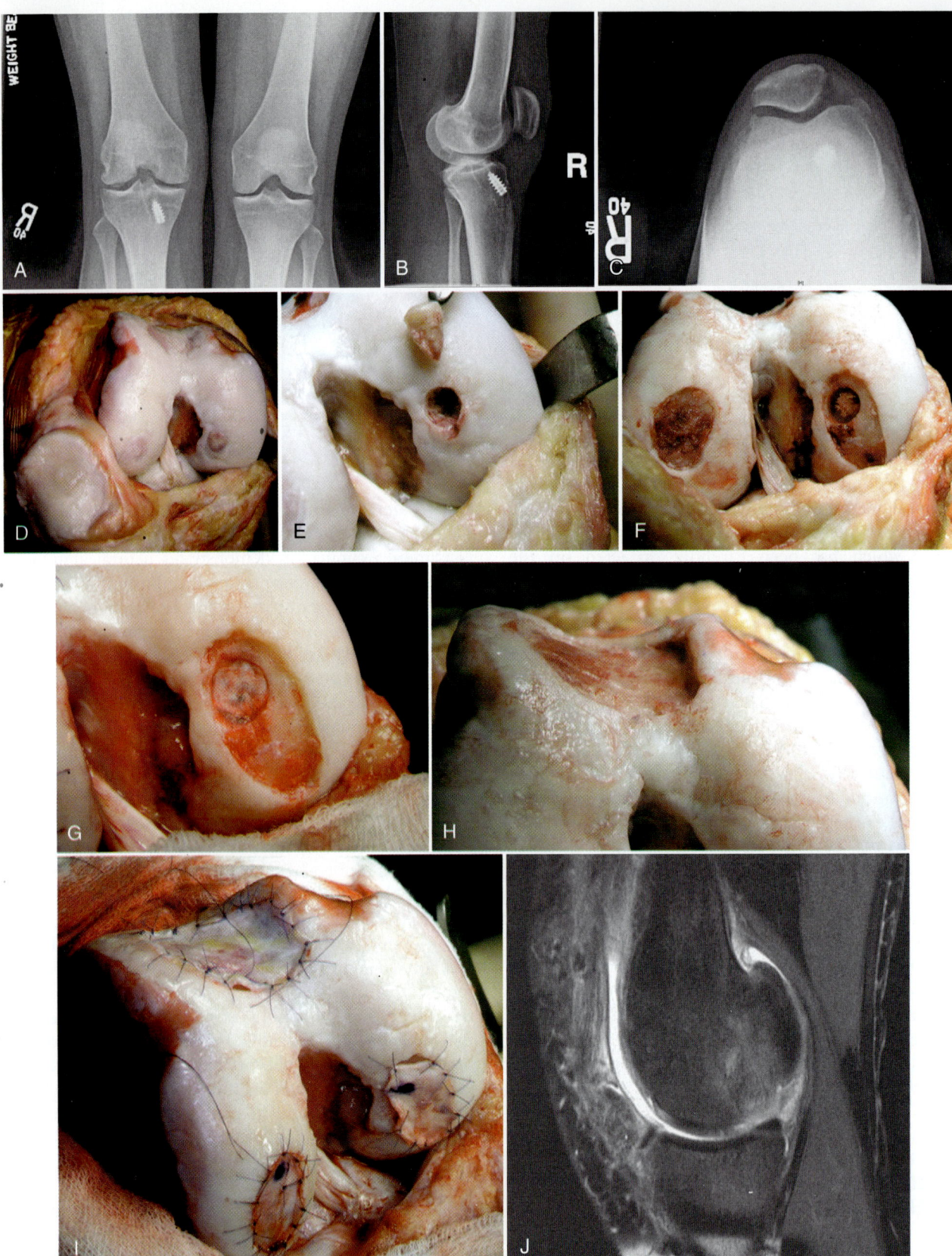

Figure 13-8 *A,* Posteroanterior radiograph demonstrates intralesional osteophyte to lateral femoral condyles with well-preserved tibiofemoral joint. *B,* Lateral x-ray film. *C,* Skyline x-ray film. *D,* Medial parapatellar arthrotomy. Intralesional osteophyte to lateral femoral condyles, large trochlea defect, and TruFit plug to medial femoral condyle with surrounding cartilage thinning are evident. *E,* TruFit plug to medial femoral condyles is easily removed with forceps and unincorporated. *F,* Open appearance of knee after radical debridement. Intralesional osteophyte to lateral femoral condyles is removed. Autologous bone grafting to medial femoral condyle TruFit plug recipient site is performed. *G,* Medial femoral condyle, after collagen cover, to autologous bone graft to recipient site for failed TruFit plug. *H,* Trochlea defect. *I,* Autologous chondrocyte implantation defects prepared. *J,* Sagittal fat-suppressed magnetic resonance imaging scan 6 months postoperative demonstrating incorporated autologous bone graft and cartilage repair to surface of the medial femoral condyle.

CASE 9. ACI TO SALVAGE FAILED OSTEOCHONDRAL GRAFTING PLUGS FOR PATELLA CARTILAGE REPAIR

A 42-year-old man has undergone bilateral staged tibial tubercle osteotomies and has intractable anterior knee pain. The left knee has also undergone cartilage repair with osteochondral graft transfers from the lateral trochlea to the patella, with worsening of symptoms. The patient presents with severe bilateral anterior knee pain, left worse than right, and inability to work. He wishes to pursue biologic preservation of his knee joints if possible.

Physical examination reveals an overweight 42-year-old man who appeared his stated age. He walks with a stiff-legged antalgic bilateral lower-extremity gait pattern. He has severe palpable and audible patellofemoral crepitus on the left knee with a large effusion and mild to moderate palpable crepitus on the right. He has anterior midline incisions bilaterally. The soft tissue envelope is healthy bilaterally.

Standing AP x-ray film (Figure 13–9A) demonstrate well-preserved tibiofemoral joints with mild varus alignment of both knees. There is evidence of bilateral tibial tubercle elevation with a synthetic bone substitute used for elevation on the left (Figure 13–9B). Skyline x-ray films (Figure 13–9C) demonstrate well-preserved patellofemoral joint spaces. Further evaluation with CT arthrogram demonstrates loss of patellar articular surface (Figure 13–9D) and lateral trochlea articular surface (Figure 13–9E), and thinning of the medial femoral condyle cartilage surface (Figure 13–9F).

At the time of open reconstruction with ACI, it is evident that the cartilage cap for two of the three osteochondral graft transfers to the patella have delaminated (Figure 13–9G), and only one remains intact for further reconstructive advantage after radical debridement (Figure 13–9H). Patella ACI graft is performed, incorporating the osteochondral graft transfer that has remained intact (Figure 13–9I). Repair tissue fill to the donor sites of the lateral trochlea is poor (Figure 13–9J). After radical debridement (Figure 13–9K), the donor sites in the trochlea and medial femoral condyle can be transplanted with ACI in usual fashion (Figure 13–9L).

Postoperative rehabilitation per ACI to the patella, with a focus on patellar mobility, quadriceps tone, and functional recovery, resulted in an excellent clinical outcome to the patient.

This case illustrates donor site complications when osteochondral grafts are harvested from the proximal lateral trochlea facet. Crepitation and pain are common when this high-contact area is used. Second, osteochondral autografting to the patella is a relative contraindication. Resorption and collapse of grafts are common in the patella because cartilage surface thickness of the donors is only 2 to 3 mm compared to 5 to 7 mm normally found in the patella cartilage surface. This mismatch leads to poor vascularity to the prominent bone of the donor osteochondral dowel, which undergoes creeping substitution resorption and collapse.

CASE 10. TIBIAL TUBERCLE OSTEOTOMY, TROCHLEOPLASTY, AND PATELLA CARTILAGE REPAIR WITH ADOLESCENT FRESH PRESERVED MORSELIZED ALLOGRAFT

A 27-year-old woman presents with severe bilateral anterior knee pain greater on the right than the left. She has undergone bilateral tibial tubercle realignment osteotomies with proximal soft tissue realignment. She continues to have a sense of bilateral knee patellar instability and severe anterior pain.

Clinical examination demonstrates a healthy 27-year-old woman who walks with a stiff-legged, circumducting gait pattern. She is very apprehensive to clinical examination. She is able to actively flex and extend her knees on her own with a positive J-sign bilaterally, audible patellofemoral crepitus worse on the right than the left, and a tremendous sense of instability with a fear of dislocation, especially on the right side. She comments that her surgeries have not helped her sense of instability or lessened her pain.

Preoperative CT arthrography (not shown) demonstrates patellar subluxation, near pan patellar cartilage loss, and dysplasia of the trochlea. Based on the severe degree of dysplasia noted at the time of CT arthrography, trochleoplasty with the possibility of revision tibial tubercle osteotomy, soft tissue realignment, and cartilage repair with adolescent minced allograft tissue is discussed. The patient is in agreement.

At the time of open medial arthrotomy, severe erosive change to the concave patella (Figure 13–10A) and reciprocal convex dysplasia to the trochlea are noted (Figure 13–10B). Radical debridement to the patella is performed per ACI. Minced allograft adolescent cartilage (DeNovo NT, Zimmer–ISTO Technologies) is applied to the base of the defect and sealed with fibrin glue. A collagen membrane is circumferentially microsutured per ACI technique to the surrounding rim and synovial tissue is present (Figure 13–10C). After the tibial tubercle osteotomy is revised to centralize the tubercle underneath the tibial spines, instability persists. It is believed that a trochleoplasty is necessary in order to allow the patella to centralize without subluxation medially or laterally. The center of the trochlea is marked with dots by sterile marking pen (Figure 13–10D and E). The proximal-most portion of the trochlea cartilage and bone is removed and contoured toward the anterior femoral cortex (see Chapter 10), synovial advancement trochleoplasty. The synovium is then advanced and sutured

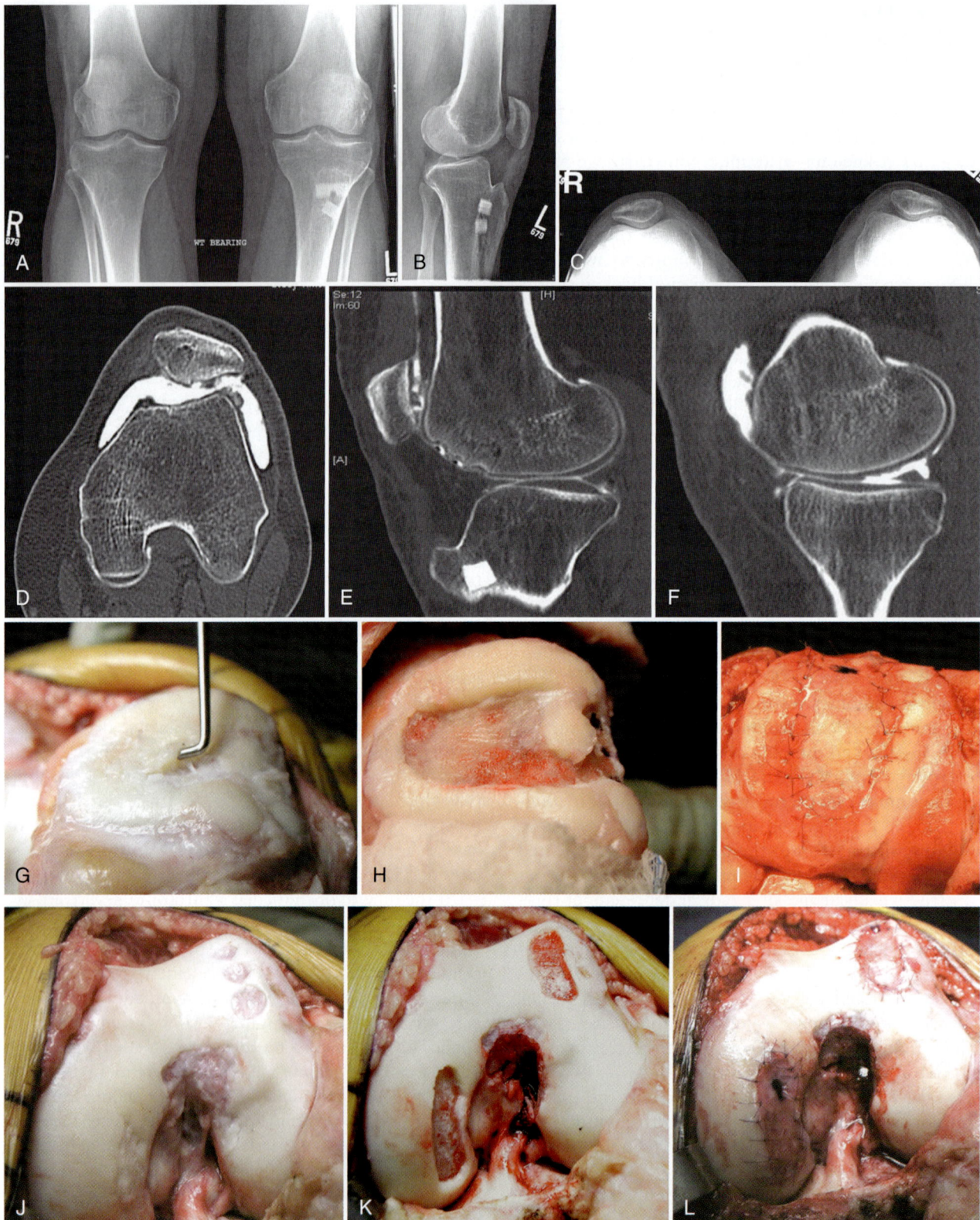

Figure 13–9 *A*, Anteroposterior radiograph. *B*, Lateral radiograph of left knee, with tibial tubercle elevation using synthetic bone substitute. *C*, Skyline x-ray films demonstrate intact patellofemoral joint spaces. *D*, Computed tomographic (CT) arthrogram axial view. *E*, CT arthrogram sagittal view over donor sites. *F*, CT arthrogram sagittal view over medial femoral condyle. *G*, Failed osteochondral graft to lateral patella facet. *H*, Radical debridement of patella with only one of three osteochondral grafts remaining intact to the patella. *I*, Patella autologous chondrocyte implantation (ACI). *J*, Donor sites to lateral trochlea incompletely filled with repair tissue and medial femoral condyles grade 3 defect. *K*, Radical debridement of lateral trochlea donor sites and medial femoral condyles in preparation for ACI. *L*, ACI to medial femoral condyle and lateral trochlea facet.

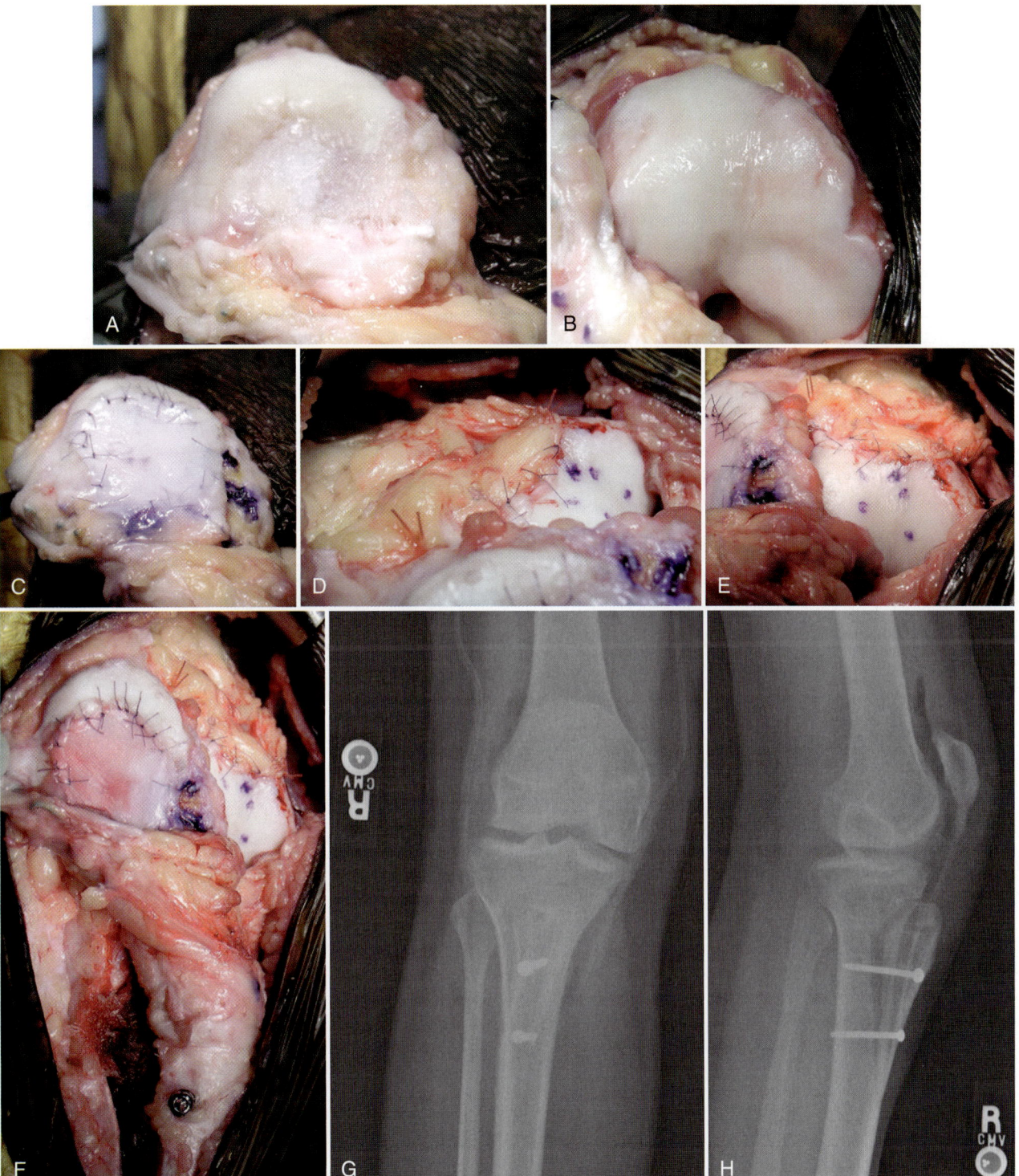

Figure 13-10 *A,* Open appearance of patella with articular damage. *B,* Open appearance of dysplastic trochlea. *C,* Cartilage repair to patella with morselized adolescent allograft cartilage (DeNovo NT, Zimmer-ISTO Technologies) with collagen cover membrane. *D,* Lateral view of synovial interposition advancement trochleoplasty. *E,* Frontal view of synovial interposition advancement trochleoplasty. *F,* Frontal view of final reconstruction, which includes revision tibial tubercle osteotomy, lateral patellar release, cartilage repair to patella, synovial advancement trochleoplasty, and vastus medialis obliquus quadriceps plasty. *G,* Anteroposterior x-ray film. *H,* Lateral x-ray film.

through the articular surface. The final appearance of the reconstruction with tibial tubercle osteotomy, cartilage repair to the patella, and synovial interposition trochleoplasty is shown in Figure 13–10F. The wound is closed, and the medial and lateral retinacula are balanced through a range of motion.

Rehabilitation consists of continuous passive motion, patellar mobilizations, isometric quadriceps contractions, and progression to full weight bearing with functional activities as described in Chapter 7 for ACI to the patella. Postoperative radiographs are shown in Figure 13–10G and H.

This case demonstrates the difficulty encountered when standard techniques are used for stabilizing patellofemoral maltracking in the presence of trochlea dysplasia. The history is classic. Recurrent instability episodes are unresponsive to conservative measures, and proximal and distal realignment procedures have failed. Trochlea dysplasia should be considered the major cause of recurrent instability in the case presented in Figure 13–10.

Summary

The previous case presentations are meant to assist the surgeon in dealing with the more complex situations that are encountered occasionally in practice. Although total knee replacement is an excellent operation for the low-demand patient, it is fraught with problems in young active patients and has a satisfaction rating less than 50%, in contrast to biologic reconstruction with satisfaction among patients greater than 90% in my experience. Attention to the principles of assessing background factors and meticulous technique and follow-up after care for patients will result in excellent clinical outcomes in the majority of patients. I hope that the previous cases have helped to alert the surgeon as to the breadth of possibility for joint preservation.

REFERENCES

1. Enders NK, Minas T. Medial subvastus approach to the knee: Surgical technique. *The Orth J at Harvard Med School*. 2008;10(2): 64–67.
2. Masri BA, Kim WY, Pagnano M. Mini-subvastus approach for minimally invasive total knee replacement. *Tech Knee Surg*. 2007; 6(2):124–130.
3. Hofmann AA, Plaster RL, Murdock LE. Subvastus (Southern) approach for primary total knee arthroplasty. *Clin Orthop Relat Res*. 1991;(269):70–77.
4. Pagnano MW, Meneghini RM. Minimally invasive total knee arthroplasty with an optimized subvastus approach. *J Arthroplasty*. 2006;21(4 suppl 1):22–26.
5. Sporer SM. The minimally invasive subvastus approach for primary total knee arthroplasty. *J Knee Surg*. 2006;19(1):58–62.
6. Aglietti P, Baldini A, Sensi L. Quadriceps-sparing versus mini-subvastus approach in total knee arthroplasty. *Clin Orthop Relat Res*. 2006;452:106–111.
7. Berth A, Urbach D, Neumann W, Awiszus F. Strength and voluntary activation of quadriceps femoris muscle in total knee arthroplasty with midvastus and subvastus approaches. *J Arthroplasty*. 2007;22(1):83–88.
8. Boerger TO, Aglietti P, Mondanelli N, Sensi L. Mini-subvastus versus medial parapatellar approach in total knee arthroplasty. *Clin Orthop Relat Res*. 2005;440:82–87.
9. Chang CH, Chen KH, Yang RS, Liu TK. Muscle torques in total knee arthroplasty with subvastus and parapatellar approaches. *Clin Orthop Relat Res*. 2002;(398):189–195.
10. Dalury DF, Dennis DA. Mini-incision total knee arthroplasty can increase risk of component malalignment. *Clin Orthop Relat Res*. 2005;440:77–81.
11. Roysam GS, Oakley MJ. Subvastus approach for total knee arthroplasty: a prospective, randomized, and observer-blinded trial. *J Arthroplasty*. 2001;16(4):454–457.
12. Weinhardt C, Barisic M, Bergmann EG, Heller KD. Early results of subvastus versus medial parapatellar approach in primary total knee arthroplasty. *Arch Orthop Trauma Surg*. 2004;124(6):401–403.
13. Schroer WC, Diesfeld PJ, Reedy ME, LeMarr AR. Evaluation of complications associated with six hundred mini-subvastus total knee arthroplasties. *J Bone Joint Surg Am*. 2007;89(suppl 3):76–81.

Chapter 14

Emerging Technologies

Tom Minas, MD, MS

INTRODUCTION
MARROW STIMULATION TECHNIQUE
AUGMENTATION
　BST–CarGel
　　Background
　　Nonclinical Studies
　　Clinical Experience
SCAFFOLDS
　MaioRegen
　Chondro-Gide
　　Autologous Chondrocyte Implantation
　　　Preclinical Results for Chondro-Gide in ACI
　　　Clinical Results for Chondro-Gide in ACI
　　Autologous Matrix-Induced Chondrogenesis
　　　Preclinical Results for AMIC
　　　Clinical Results for AMIC
　　　AMIC Registry
　Kensey Nash Corporation Cartilage Repair Device
　　Implant Description
　　Preclinical Studies

TRUFIT CB for Cartilage Repair
　Properties of TRUFIT CB
　Preclinical Study Using an Ovine Osteochondral Model
　Clinical Case Series
MINCED CARTILAGE
　One-Stage Autologous Procedure for Cartilage Regeneration
　Cartilage Autograft Implantation System
　DeNovo Natural Tissue Graft
SECOND-GENERATION CELL-BASED ACI
　Matrix-Induced Autologous Chondrocyte Implantation
　　Background
　　Manufacturing Process
　　Commercial Availability
　　Clinical Outcomes
　Hyalograft C Autograft
　　Preclinical Findings
　　Clinical Development
　ChondroCelect
　　Introduction

　　Translational Research Background
　　Refining Predictive Power: Development of the ChondroCelect Score
　　Developing the ChondroCelect Manufacturing Process
　　Proof of Concept in a Large Animal Model
　　Clinical Development: The TIGACT01 Study
　CaReS Cartilage Regeneration System
　BioCart II
　Cartipatch
　　Second-Generation Autologous Chondrocyte Transplantation Technique
THIRD-GENERATION CELL-BASED THERAPIES
　NeoCart System
　　The Concept
　　The Procedure
　　Preclinical Animal Studies
　　Clinical Trials
　DeNovo Engineered Tissue Graft
CONCLUSION

INTRODUCTION

New biologic options are being developed throughout the world to enhance existing techniques, offer new off-the-shelf options, and provide reproducible structural repair.

I contacted several companies worldwide and asked them to share their core technologies, preclinical development, clinical trial outcomes, and postmarketing surveillance outcomes, as available. The following list is by no means complete but offers a sampling of what potentially may be available to our patients in the United States after regulatory approval.

The categories of technology roughly translate to marrow stimulation improvement using gels or scaffolds to enhance marrow stimulation techniques; use of minced autograft and allograft cartilage; second-generation autologous chondrocyte implantation (ACI) techniques, which use scaffolds of different biomaterials precultured with cells to deliver the cells to the injury site; and third-generation tissue-engineered cartilage, which is preformed histologically and physically.

MARROW STIMULATION TECHNIQUE AUGMENTATION

BST-CarGel

Background
BST-CarGel (BioSyntech Canada, Laval, Quebec, Canada), a new medical device for cartilage repair, was developed to improve outcomes of bone marrow stimulation procedures

while preserving the intrinsic low cost and simple arthroscopic approach. With traditional marrow stimulating techniques, clot shrinkage and detachment from lesion surfaces occur. BST-CarGel was designed to stabilize the blood clot in the cartilage lesion by dispersing a soluble and adhesive chitosan scaffold throughout autologous, fresh whole blood. Chitosan, a cationic linear polysaccharide composed predominately of polyglucosamine, is derived from the deacetylation of chitin, the structural component of crustacean shells.[1,2] By dissolving chitosan in an aqueous glycerol phosphate buffer, BST-CarGel is uniquely obtained as a liquid chitosan solution having physiologic pH and osmolarity, intrinsic cytocompatibility, and biodegradability.[2,3] When mixed with blood (BST-CarGel-to-blood ratio of 1:3), the viscous mixture can easily be applied to cartilage lesions that have been prepared by bone marrow stimulation (microfracture, drilling), where it permits normal clot formation while simultaneously reinforcing the clot and impeding clot retraction. Furthermore, the cationic nature of the chitosan increases the adhesivity of the mixture to cartilage lesions, ensuring longer clot residency. This maintenance of critical blood components above the marrow access holes allows activation of the tissue repair process, while chitosan itself brings an intrinsic ability to stimulate wound repair.[4] Box 14–1 summarizes the primary mode of action for BST-CarGel, an approach that has been termed *scaffold-guided regenerative medicine*, where BST-CarGel provides in situ chondroinduction for cartilage repair.[5]

Nonclinical Studies

The efficacy and underlying mechanisms of action of BST-CarGel were examined in several animal studies. A skeletally mature (8–15 months) rabbit model that used drilling of surgically prepared bilateral trochlear defects elucidated BST-CarGel early reparative events and compared them with drilled controls.[6,7] Box 14–2 summarizes the key findings of BST-CarGel–mediated cartilage repair.

In another large study in adult (3–6 years) sheep, repair of surgically prepared 1-cm^2 condylar and trochlear defects was investigated by measuring the quantity and quality of BST-CarGel repair tissue after 6 months compared with microfracture-only defects.[8] Box 14–3 summarizes the efficacy of BST-CarGel treatment for cartilage repair. Figure 14–1 shows a best case repair from a sheep condylar lesion treated with BST-CarGel. After 6 months of repair, a relatively mature articular cartilage containing superficial, transitional, and radial zones with a reestablished tidemark was observed.

Overall, the BST-CarGel device has been shown to statistically increase the volume and hyaline character of repair tissue compared to microfractured or microdrilled controls. The chondrogenic foci observed resemble endochondral processes and are believed to be responsible for the synthesis of cartilaginous repair tissue. Notably, the specific mechanisms underlying BST-CarGel–mediated repair (see Boxes 14–2 and 14–3) were independent of species or bone marrow stimulation technique.[7]

Clinical Experience

In 2003 and 2004, 33 human subjects were treated with BST-CarGel under Health Canada's Special Access Program for medical devices (compassionate use on a case-by-case basis; not considered a clinical trial). Treated patients encompassed the spectrum of both traumatic and degenerative lesions, along with other pathologies. Lesions ranged in size from 0.5 to 12 cm^2 (mean 4.3 cm^2). In 16 cases, opposing tibial lesions (kissing lesions) were

---

BOX 14–1 BST-CarGel Primary Mode of Action

Physical biomaterial scaffold for natural cartilage repair
Stabilizes blood clot
Impedes clot retraction, providing a space-filling provisional matrix
Generates an adhesive bond between clot and cartilage lesion
Provides structural framework for subsequent repair processes

---

BOX 14–2 BST-CarGel Stabilized Blood Clots

Mechanisms of Action for Cartilage Repair

Chitosan clearance via neutrophil phagocytosis after approximately 1 month
Chemotaxis of marrow stromal cells toward the lesion
Transient increase in vascularization in subchondral bone
Greater porosity, remodeling, and vascularization of subchondral bone
Induction of chondrogenic foci from repair tissue near 1 month
Increased quality of hyaline cartilage repair arising from subchondral bone
Improved integration of repair cartilage within the lesion

All comparisons were made to drilled-only contralateral controls (n = 49).[11,12]

BOX 14–3 BST-CarGel Stabilized Blood Clots

Six-Month Efficacy in Sheep

Greater adhesion of CarGel blood clot to bone and cartilage
Increased volume of repair tissue
Improved hyaline character of repair tissue
Increased GAG and collagen content of repair tissue
Reduced incidence of subchondral cyst formation
No treatment-specific safety issues

All comparisons were made to microfracture-only control group. BST-CarGel (n = 8), microfracture only (n = 6).

Figure 14-1 Best case cartilage repair of 1-cm² defects in adult sheep treated with BST-CarGel. At 6 months, uniform cartilage resurfacing was observed. Safranin O/fast green–stained section from this block reveals relatively mature articular cartilage containing superficial *(SZ)*, transitional *(TZ)*, and radial *(RZ)* zones with a reestablished tidemark *(TM)* above an actively remodeling bone bed.

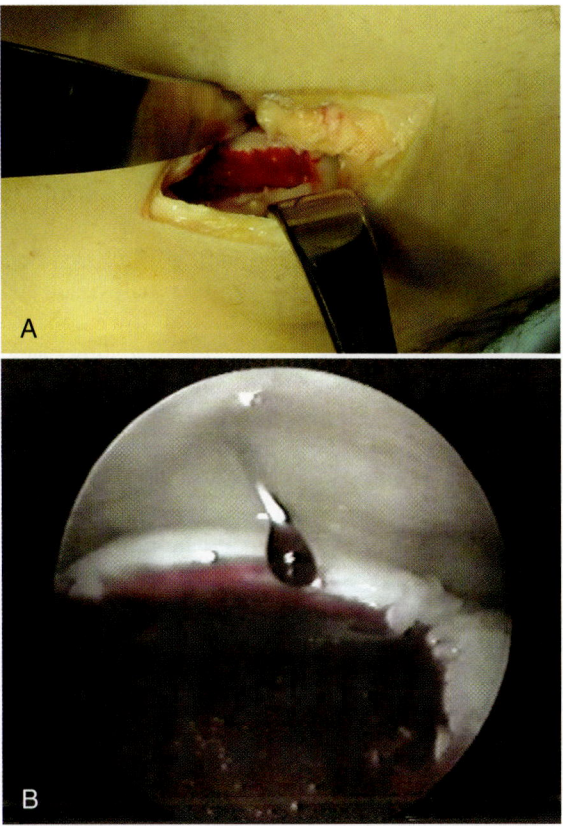

Figure 14-2 *A*, BST-CarGel open surgical technique includes a mini-arthrotomy to facilitate visualization of the horizontal lesion and delivery of BST-CarGel. Using a syringe, the BST-CarGel/blood mixture is applied in a controlled dropwise manner over all of the bone marrow access holes and then into the entire lesion, taking care not to overfill. *B*, Arthroscopic delivery of BST-CarGel is performed when the entire lesion can be observed within the arthroscopic field of view. Prior to BST-CarGel application, the joint and lesion are fully suctioned of perfusion liquid and blood to create a "dry field" in the horizontal lesion. The delivery needle is positioned directly perpendicular and central to the lesion, and the BST-CarGel/blood mixture is delivered in dropwise fashion, being sure not to overfill. Both approaches A and B require a 15-minute solidification period, followed by incision closure.

debrided and treated with microfracture only. One case of osteochondritis dissecans and one exposed subchondral cyst were treated; two concomitant anterior cruciate ligament replacements were performed. BST-CarGel delivery by arthroscopic (22 patients) as well as mini-open approaches (11 patients) was confirmed (Figure 14–2). Physiotherapy follow-up was standardized and required 6 weeks of non–weight-bearing exercise and early passive range of motion by physiotherapists (i.e., no continuous passive motion). Western Ontario McMaster (WOMAC)[9] osteoarthritis index questionnaires were administered preoperatively and again postoperatively after 3, 6, and 12 months. WOMAC scores for pain, stiffness, and function improved substantially over preoperative baseline scores, although the absence of a control group and the wide-ranging patient demographics and lesion types prevent overinterpretation of outcomes.[5]

In 2005, BioSyntech initiated a multicenter randomized level 1 clinical trial in Canada and Europe comparing treatment with BST-CarGel to microfracture in the repair of grade 3 or 4 articular cartilage lesions on the femoral condyles in the knee. The study was designed to measure repair tissue structure at 12 months as the primary endpoint through quantitative magnetic resonance imaging (MRI) of repair tissue volume and quality (T2, delayed gadolinium-enhanced magnetic resonance imaging of cartilage [dGEMRIC]) and microscopic analysis of biopsies (when available). The secondary endpoint assessed clinical benefit (Visual Analog Scale [VAS], WOMAC, Medical Outcomes Study 36-Item Short-Form Health Survey [SF-36]) and safety. The trial enrolled 80 patients, and an interim histologic analysis of 22 available biopsies (13 BST-CarGel and 9 microfracture patients) using International Cartilage Repair Society Histological Scoring systems I and II[10] provided statistically significant evidence that BST-CarGel improved the quality and quantity of repair tissue compared to microfracture. The International Cartilage Repair Society (ICRS) II overall score, which assimilates all the parameters listed in the grading system and generates an overall assessment of tissue repair, was significant ($P < .05$), as were individual parameters of cell morphology, cell viability, and superficial zone morphology on the biopsies. Macroscopic grading of the cartilage repair by the surgeon at the time of biopsy, which included the extent of lesion filling, tissue surface characteristics, and integration with surrounding tissue, also was statistically significant. Full study analysis on all 80 patients after 12-month follow-up will be conducted in the spring of 2010, followed by Canadian and European submissions for device marketing approval. A similar pivotal study will be conducted in the United States for Food and Drug Administration (FDA) approval.

SCAFFOLDS

MaioRegen

Because the intrinsic ability of articular cartilage to self-repair is poor due to the lack of blood support and lymph and nervous systems, the development of effective therapies for articular cartilage and subchondral bone regeneration is an important goal in orthopedic surgery. After achondral damage, the repair tissue shows histologic and mechanical properties lower than the native tissue, which may lead to impaired functionality of the joint itself. Many treatment options have been proposed, but no optimal long-lasting solutions have been achieved, particularly for deep cartilaginous and osteochondral defects.

MaioRegen (Fin-Ceramica Faenza S.p.A., Faenza, Italy) is a novel composite osteochondral monolithic scaffold. It is a multilayered structure that reproduces the chemical gradient naturally found inside osteocartilaginous compartment.[13,14] MaioRegen is composed of equine tendon-derived type I collagen on the upper side, which mimics the cartilaginous layer, and a blending of type I collagen and magnesium-enriched nonstoichiometric hydroxyapatite (Mg-HA) on the bottom side, which mimics the subchondral bone (Figure 14–3). Due to its high similarity with the anatomic osteocartilaginous portion to be replaced, in terms of chemical, biologic, and structural composition, the scaffold is defined as a biomimetic device, able to be recognized as self by the recipient connective tissues. Toxicologic profile, performed in compliance to EN ISO 10993–1 European regulation on class III medical devices, showed high biocompatibility and tolerability.

An in vivo, randomized controlled study has been performed to assess the safety and efficacy of MaioRegen in an osteochondral reconstruction sheep model.[15] An osteochondral lesion was induced in the right knee, either on the medial or lateral condyle, of each animal (n = 8). Animals were then randomly assigned to three treatment groups. The objective of the study was to demonstrate a substantial equivalence (in terms of effectiveness) between the acellular approach using MaioRegen alone (group A) and chondrocytes cultured on the scaffold (cell-engineered scaffold, group B). Comparisons were made with an untreated control group (group C). No adverse events were observed in all groups, and the device was completely tolerable and fully biocompatible. At 6 months postoperative, animals were euthanized, and macroscopic and histologic investigations showed complete absorption of MaioRegen. The newly formed tissues in the treated groups were well integrated, whereas a gap on the defect was still

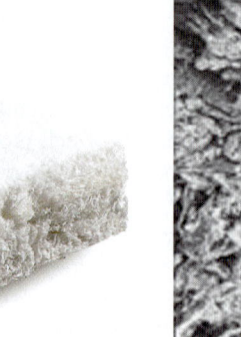
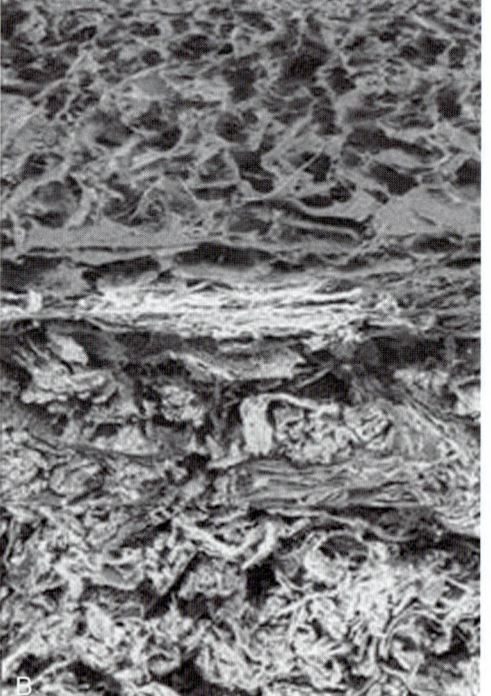

Figure 14–3 *A*, MaioRegen osteochondral scaffold. Scanning electron micrograph of inner structure of MaioRegen. *B, A*, Cartilaginous layer (100% type I collagen); *B*, tidemark (60% type I collagen, 40% Mg-HA); bone layer (30% type I collagen, 70% Mg-HA).

noticeable in the control group. Applying a Fortier score (0–15),[16] no statistical differences in average score values were seen between scaffold alone (2.63 ± 0.71) and cell-engineered scaffold (4.00 ± 0.53), whereas both groups exhibited statistical difference ($P < .05$) versus the control group (12.88 ± 0.95). Histologic evaluation showed newly formed tissue that was well organized and characterized by chondrocytes with tangential orientation in the upper part. In the two treated groups, tissues were differentiated at either the chondral or subchondral bone level, whereas fibrous tissue was evident in the control group (Figure 14–4).

The hypothesis of a scaffold-guided tissue regeneration process is that mesenchymal and progenitor cells from subchondral bone marrow blood after surgical curettage are able to migrate inside and wholly colonize the scaffold, then differentiate along either a chondrogenic or osteogenic lineage based on the peculiar physical–chemical gradient composition found. Therefore, MaioRegen itself promoted osteoblast differentiation and bone regeneration in the deepest portions while restoring the tidemark in the intermediate portion and hyaline cartilage formation in the upper surface (chondrogenic differentiation). After the preclinical and toxicologic studies, a pilot, uncontrolled, prospective clinical trial of 30 patients has been designed and approved by an institutional review board to investigate the performance and safety of MaioRegen. Inclusion criteria for study admission were patients ranging in age from 15 to 60 years who were affected by traumatic, posttraumatic, or degenerative osteochondral defects of the knee (grade III and IV Outerbridge classification) sizing 1–9 cm^2. After arthrotomy, a curettage of the defect was made, and scaffold was implanted dry by simple press fit, without fixation with suture or surgical glue (Figure 14–5). Early stability of MaioRegen assessed 30 days postoperative by MRI revealed neither migration from the implant site nor delamination. With regard to the safety outcome,

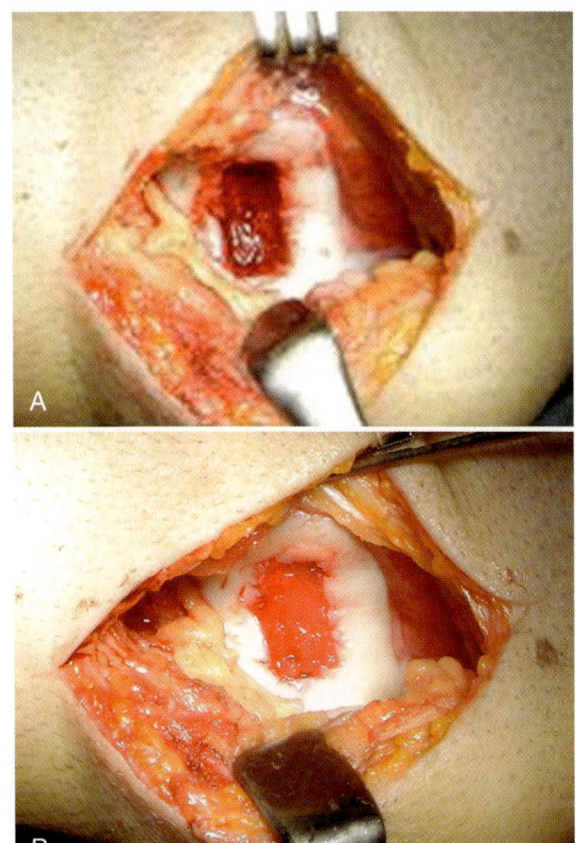

Figure 14–5 *A*, ostochondral (OC) defect curettage. *B*, OC defect filled with MaioRegen.

patients were monitored for the onset of any adverse events. Most of the episodes reported were considered related to surgery and not to the device itself, and most occurred within the immediate postoperative period. In addition, clinical assessment by MRI performed 6 and 12 months postoperative evaluated the quality of regenerated osteochondral tissue and integration with recipient

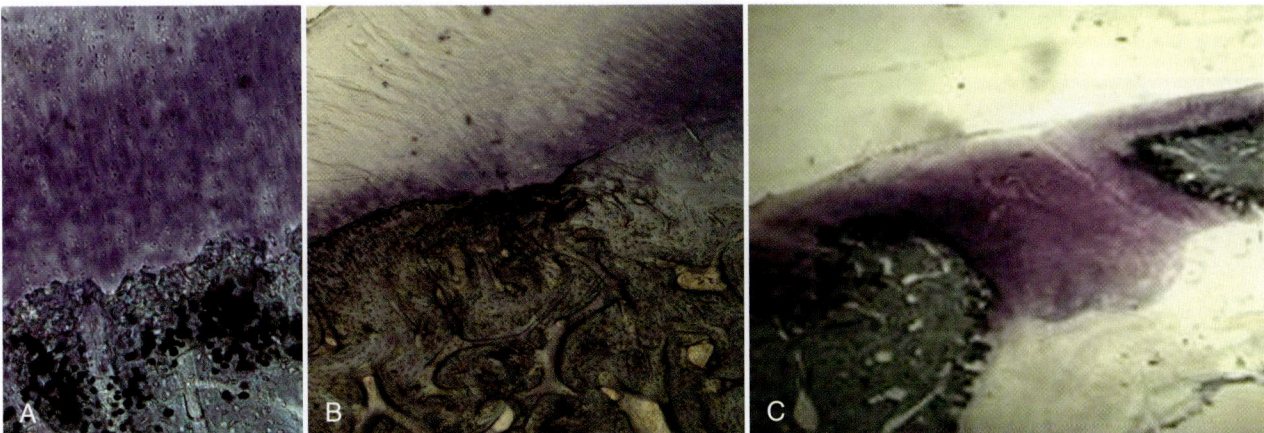

Figure 14–4 *A*, MaioRegen alone group (hematoxylin–eosin/fast green stain). *B*, Autologous chondrocyte-engineered MaioRegen group. *C*, Control group.

tissues applying the MRI MOCART Scoring System. Functional joint recovery, improvement of patient's quality of life, and return to normal sport activity were further evaluated by applying ICRS evaluation package questionnaires and Kujala and Tegner scores. Results of statistical data analysis highlighted positive results for each observed variable with respect to both surgeon and patient evaluations at each follow-up visit. Modifications of the result for each examined variable, comparing 6- and 12-month postsurgery scores to the preoperative score, were statistically significant ($P < .05$). Upon study planning, the modification of study variables between preoperation and postoperation was identified as a success index. Because modifications in the study were reported as positive (i.e., sustained by statistical relevance), they were considered indexes of study success. Moreover, all of the parameters evaluated improved significantly after 12 months compared to 6 months, confirming good progression and enhancement of quality of life.

The preliminary results of the clinical trial at intermediate follow-up appear promising.[17,18] MaioRegen may be considered a potential innovative surgical treatment of severe osteochondral lesions; however, longer follow-up would be essential to fully validate this one-step acellular approach.

Chondro-Gide

Chondro-Gide (Geistlich Pharma AG, Wolhusen, Switzerland) is a CE-marked product for covering articular cartilage defects that are treated with either ACI or bone marrow stimulation techniques (autologous matrix-induced chondrogenesis [AMIC]).

The proprietary manufacturing process of Chondro-Gide involves several steps before the unique bilayer design consisting of a compact side and a porous side is achieved (Figure 14–6). Standardized processes under clean room conditions and rigorous in-process and end controls guarantee a high-quality natural product. Chondro-Gide consists of porcine type I and III collagen, which is naturally resorbed. Collagenases, gelatinases, and proteinases are responsible for the breakdown of Chondro-Gide into oligopeptides and finally single amino acids.

The compact layer consists of a smooth, cell-occlusive surface that prevents cells, chondrocytes, and mesenchymal stem cells from diffusing into the joint space and protects them from mechanical stress. The porous layer of the matrix consists of loose collagen fibers that support cell invasion and attachment. The arrangement of the fibers provides high tensile strength and resistance to tearing.

Thorough biocompatibility safety testing according to international standards proves that all elements that possibly could cause an undesirable local or systemic response are removed during the manufacturing process and that the immunogenic potential of the matrix is reduced to a minimum.

The Chondro-Gide matrix is available in sizes of 20×30 mm, 30×40 mm, and now up to 60% thicker than the largest size 40×50 mm.

Autologous Chondrocyte Implantation
Preclinical Results for Chondro-Gide in ACI
Ovine animal models and preclinical culture condition studies have validated the proof of concept that a porcine collagen membrane may be successfully used in cartilage repair with good tissue repair and no rejection response.[19–24]

Clinical Results for Chondro-Gide in ACI
Chondro-Gide used in several human ACI studies has demonstrated clinical results equal to periosteum without hypertrophy.[21,25–32] Ease of handling, lessened operative time, and arthroscopic delivery are possible.

Autologous Matrix-Induced Chondrogenesis
AMIC as an enhanced microfracture technique combining microfracturing with the collagen I/III matrix Chondro-Gide has become a recognized cartilage repair technique. Studies evaluating the performance of this new treatment option are ongoing.

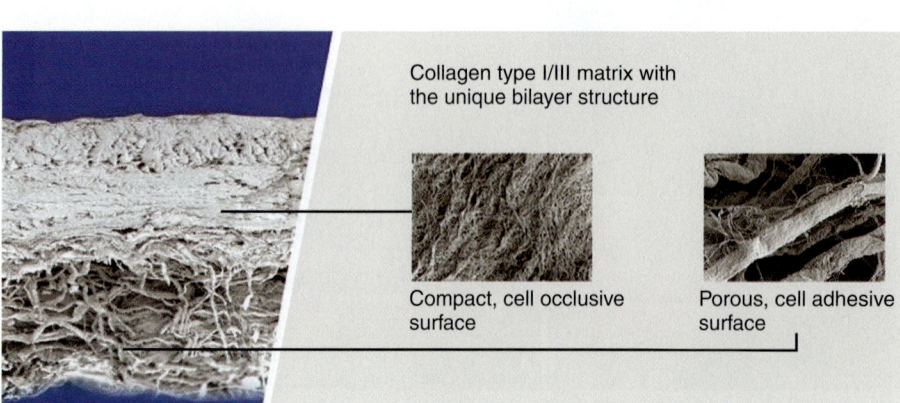

Figure 14–6 Bilayer structure of Chondro-Gide porcine type I–III membrane.

An initial study by Behrens et al[33] showed that costs were significantly reduced by AMIC compared to ACI, and immediate cartilage repair was possible in a single procedure. Improved tissue repair to ACI has not yet been studied.

Preclinical Results for AMIC

Preclinical animal work confirms that marrow clot is contained and repair tissue develops.[34,35]

Clinical Results for AMIC

Numerous early reports on the femoral condyles support positive short-term clinical results.[36–41]

AMIC Registry

In the beginning of 2007, Geistlich Surgery successfully launched the AMIC Registry online database "to offer surgeons worldwide an easy platform to collect and share their AMIC data." Data entry is standardized, simple, and rapid. Patient evaluation is based on the Lysholm knee score, VAS pain scale, and magnetic resonance testing (MRT) analysis. All data can be easily exported and graphically illustrated. By October 2008, 179 patients (67 female and 112 male, age 14–64 years, mean 36.8 years) with focal cartilage defects (Outerbridge grade II–IV) of the knee in the medial or lateral condyle (62%), patella (29%), and/or trochlea (9%) underwent AMIC and were included in the AMIC Registry.

Excellent 2-year results (n = 57) showed improvement of knee function as assessed by the Lysholm score from an average of 50 to 85 points and pain reduction from 6.7 to 2.0 (VAS). After 3 years (n = 28), the mean Lysholm score improved from 56.6 to 87.0 points. Pain on a VAS diminished from 6.2 to 2.3. During the 3-year observation period, the AMIC technique resulted in a considerable increase in knee function, with 75% reporting good to excellent results and 10% satisfactory results and exceptional pain reduction.

Kensey Nash Corporation Cartilage Repair Device

The Kensey Nash Corporation (Exton, PA) cartilage repair device (CRD) has been designed to address many of the concerns regarding current cartilage repair procedures. Significant preclinical research and development has yielded a bioresorbable, acellular, biphasic scaffold for cartilage repair. This technology uses an implant design that contains two phases, each specifically engineered to favor the growth of the histologically distinct tissues of articular cartilage and subchondral bone.

Implant Description

The Kensey Nash CRD is a porous biphasic scaffold comprised of type I collagen, β-tricalcium phosphate (β-TCP), and polylactic acid (PLA), three well-known biomaterials with a long history of use in orthopedics. The implant (Figure 14–7) has 100% interconnected porosity that enables movement of cells and biologic fluids throughout the entire implant. The chondral phase of the implant consists of a type I collagen formulation. The collagen provides a malleable, biocompatible scaffold for repair of cartilage tissue that can be contoured to the surrounding joint surfaces. The implant's

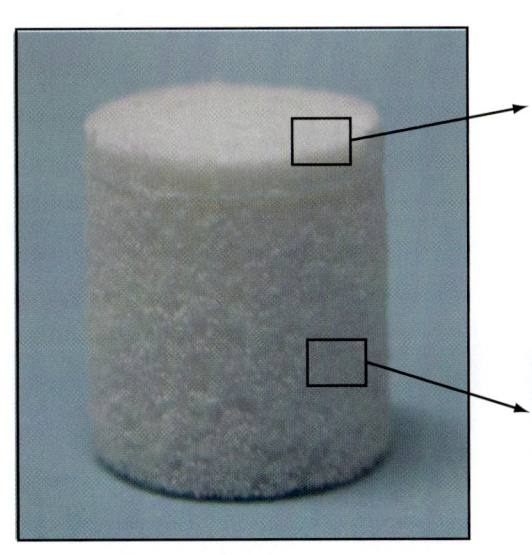
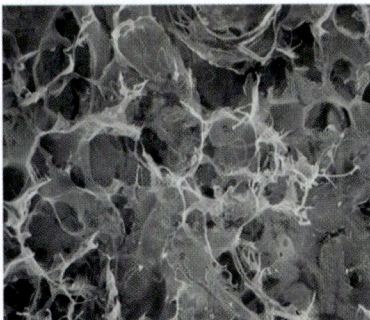
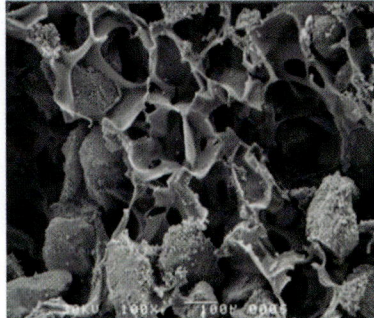

Figure 14–7 The Kensey Nash cartilage repair device implant is a biphasic plug, designed as a resorbable scaffold for the repair of articular cartilage and subchondral bone. The chondral region is composed of type I collagen *(top)*, with a subchondral bone region of β-tricalcium phosphate suspended within a polylactic acid lattice *(bottom)*. Scanning electron micrograph (magnification ×100).

subchondral bone phase contains 80% β-TCP and 20% PLA by mass. The ceramic provides an osteoconductive element to the subchondral phase of the CRD implant while supplying a source of calcium and phosphorous ions necessary for natural bone mineralization.[42,43] The PLA scaffold provides biomechanical support and three-dimensional structure for this region and ultimately breaks down into natural body metabolites via the Krebs cycle.[44,45] As a result of Kensey Nash's proprietary process, the ceramic granules are suspended within, not coated by, the polymer scaffold so that the ceramic is immediately available to the host upon implantation. The implant is available in a range of diameters and is loaded in an insertion tool that facilitates implant hydration and arthroscopic placement.

Preclinical Studies

Kensey Nash conducted a caprine study that evaluated the performance of the CRD in a 6-mm × 6-mm defect on the medial femoral condyle of 38 Nubian Cross goats at 6-, 12-, and 18-month time points (Figure 14–8). Histology, biomechanical testing, immunohistochemistry, MRI, gross evaluations, and radiographs were the evaluation methods used. The study concluded that, by 6 months, CRD-treated defects displayed a rapid repair that was sustained through the 12-month[46] and 18-month time points. Repair tissue at each time point appeared hyaline, stained positively for type II collagen, and was biomechanically similar to healthy articular cartilage. The repair tissue also displayed excellent integration not only with the host cartilage but with the host bone as well.

Kensey Nash is also studying the performance of the CRD in healing a 10-mm × 10-mm osteochondral defect on the lateral trochlear ridge of 12 horses (Figure 14–9). The repair of CRD-treated defects will be evaluated over a 2-year study, with interim arthroscopies at 4- and 12-month time points. Interim arthroscopies are scored using a modified ICRS system for safety and efficacy.

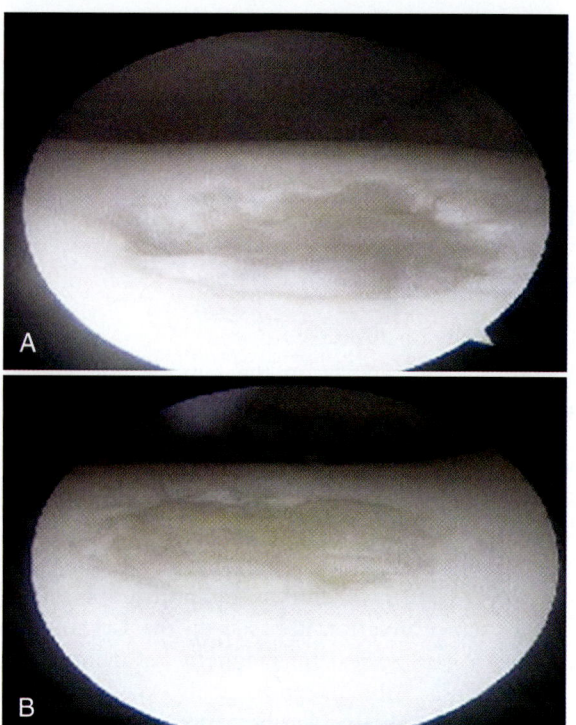

Figure 14–9 Four-month interim arthroscopy images for microfracture control *(A)* and Kensey Nash cartilage repair device (CRD)–treated defect *(B)* in equine lateral trochlear ridge. CRD treatment group scored significantly higher than microfracture in terms of efficacy and equivalent to microfracture in terms of safety using a modified International Cartilage Repair Society scoring system.

At time of sacrifice, histology, biomechanical testing, immunohistochemistry, MRI, gross evaluations, and radiographs will be used to evaluate the repair compared to a microfracture control. Four-month interim arthroscopy showed equivalency to microfracture in terms of safety scores and a significant improvement over microfracture in efficacy scoring.[47]

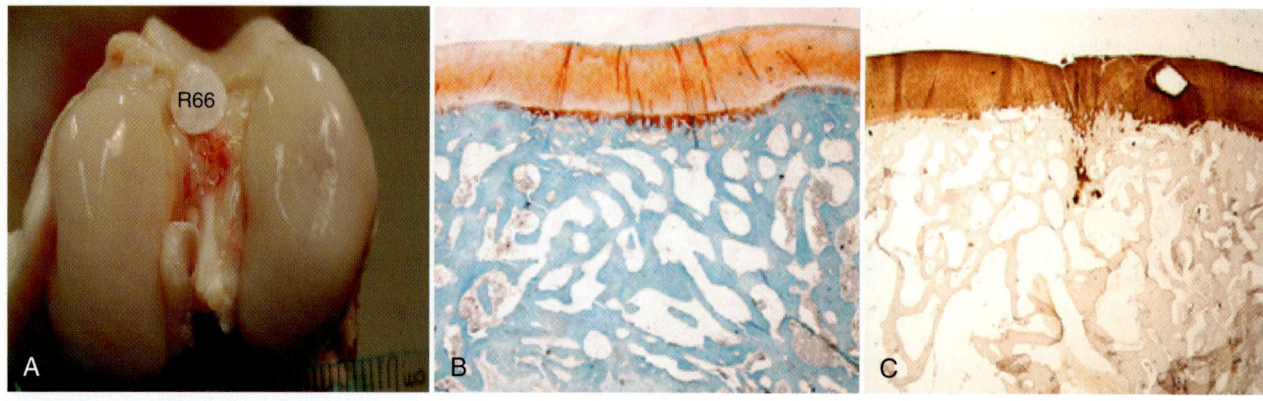

Figure 14–8 Caprine stifles treated with cartilage repair device at 12 months. *A,* Grossly, the defects were well filled with smooth resurfacing. *B,* Histologically, safranin O staining showed the presence of proteoglycan within the repair tissue. *C,* Repair tissue also stained strongly positive for type II collagen.

Together, these studies are being used to support an Investigational Device Exemption application to commence clinical investigation of the CRD in the United States. Kensey Nash is pursuing regulatory approvals for the CRD in both the United States and Europe.

TRUFIT CB for Cartilage Repair

Properties of TRUFIT CB

The TRUFIT CB scaffold (Smith & Nephew, Andover, MA) is a cartilage repair option for small chondral or osteochondral lesions. It comes in preformed cylindrical plugs with diameters ranging from 5 to 11 mm. This synthetic resorbable scaffold has two phases to mimic the critical portions of osteochondral healing. Each phase is designed to initially approximate the physical and mechanical properties of the adjacent cartilage and bone (Figure 14-10). TRUFIT CB is made of Polygraft, a porous material composed of 85:15 poly(d,l-lactide-co-glycolide) copolymer, polyglycolide (PGA) fibers, calcium sulfate, and a trace amount of surfactant. Slivka et al[48] showed that PGA reinforcement fibers improved the early structural integrity of the scaffold and provided a mechanically stable environment for cell migration and tissue repair. Calcium sulfate in the bone phase releases calcium ions, which are known to enhance osteoconductivity,[49,50] whereas the top phase is malleable to allow contouring with the adjacent articular surface after implantation. At the surgery, the original chondral/osteochondral defect is cored out with TRU-KOR instrumentation to create a uniform circular defect. The implant is press fit into the defect site using the preloaded delivery device. Because the TRUFIT CB scaffold is hydrophilic, fluids such as blood and marrow containing nutrients, proteins, and cells can be easily wicked up into the pores. TRUFIT CB then acts as a scaffold for microfracture to hold the blood and marrow cells from subchondral bleeding. Its 70% porosity and interconnected pores promote cell infiltration across the scaffold and provide a mechanically stable environment for tissue repair. TRUFIT CB is currently sold in Europe, Canada, and Australia but is not available in the United States and its territories.

Preclinical Study Using an Ovine Osteochondral Model

In an ovine study assessing cartilage repair by TRUFIT CB implants in osteochondral defects at 18 months, a unilateral circular (5.1 mm diameter × 5 mm) osteochondral defect was created in the medial femoral condyle of skeletally mature sheep.[51] The defects were repaired by TRUFIT CB (5.3 mm diameter × 5 mm; n = 6) press fit into the site or left empty in the empty defect control group (n = 3). Outcome of cartilage repair was assessed 18 months after surgery. None of the sheep showed any lameness and had regained a full range of motion. The medial condyle of all animals in the TRUFIT CB group had no abnormalities. By 18 months, the material of TRUFIT CB had predominantly resorbed, and the defect sites were filled with repair tissue. Cartilage restoration was evident in all TRUFIT CB specimens. The repaired cartilage was well integrated with the adjacent tissue and had a similar thickness and contour (Figure 14-11). Safranin O staining revealed a highly cellular tissue in the repair by TRUFIT CB with the same intensity of proteoglycan staining as the adjacent hyaline cartilage. The organized collagen patterns of the mid and deeper levels of TRUFIT CB repair were similar to those of normal cartilage (Figure 14-12).

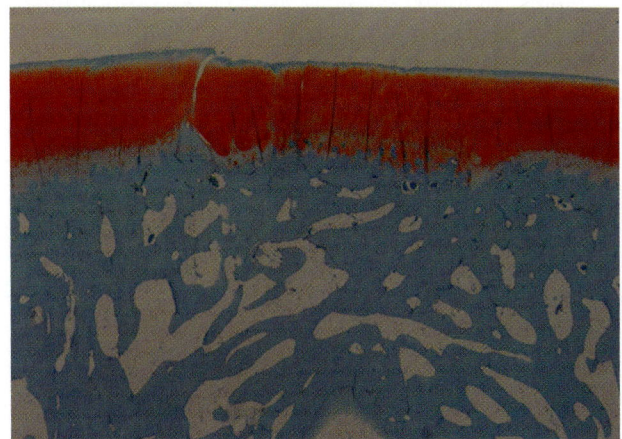

Figure 14-11 Safranin O–stained sections of TRUFIT CB–treated defect and empty osteochondral defect.

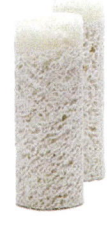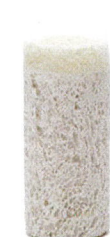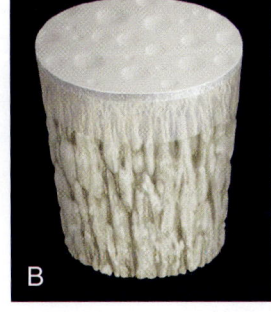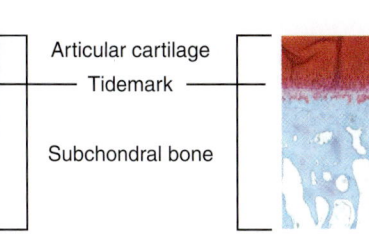

Figure 14-10 *A,* TRUFIT CB scaffolds. *B,* TRUFIT CB mimics cartilage, tidemark, and subchondral bone in osteochondral healing.

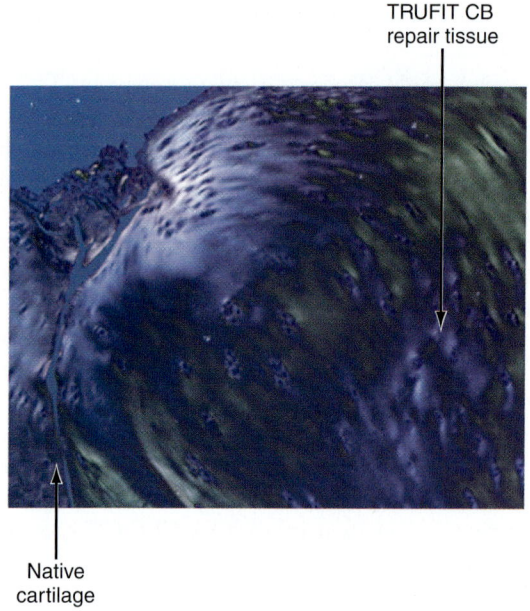

Figure 14-12 Polarized light photomicrograph (hematoxylin–eosin stain, magnification ×100) of TRUFIT CB repair tissue at 18 months. The pattern of collagen is organized, similar to that of normal cartilage.

In contrast, repair cartilage in the empty defect control was thinner than normal cartilage tissue, and the adjacent cartilage showed signs of degeneration, including proteoglycan loss (see Figure 14–11). The subchondral bone portion of the defect repaired by TRUFIT CB was replaced by bone with a statistically similar bone volume as the untreated contralateral control (66.4% and 63.0%, respectively). Areas of new bone growth with active osteoblasts, increased cellularity, and nonlamellar structure were observed in the repair, indicating that subchondral bone remodeling was ongoing and expected to continue to completely remodel to mature bone over time.

Clinical Case Series

A prospective series by the Spalding group reported the outcome of 24 patients (mean age 34 years, range 19–50 years) with 12- to 36-month follow-up for treatment of chondral or osteochondral lesions in the knee with TRUFIT CB implants.[52] There were 13 primary procedures and 11 revision procedures (microfracture 7, osteochondral grafting 1, matrix-induced autologous chondrocyte implantation [MACI] 1, and failed fixation osteochondritis dissecans 2). Mean lesion size was 1.8 cm^2, 14 of which were on the medial femoral condyle, 4 on the lateral femoral condyle, and 6 on the lateral or central trochlea. Up to four implants were used in the repair. After surgery, patients who had undergone repair on the weight-bearing femoral condyle surface were allowed partial weight bearing at 2 weeks and full weight bearing at 4 weeks.

Lysholm score, International Knee Documentation Committee (IKDC) score, and Knee Injury and Osteoarthritis Outcome Score (KOOS) showed statistically significant improvement ($P < .001$) at 12 months compared to preoperatively (Figure 14–13). Activity levels and hence the mean Tegner activity score ($P = .05$, see Figure 14–4) improved after 12 months when return to sport was allowed. MRI showed maintenance of the thickness of the new articular surface, gradual differentiation of the implant, and remodeling of the bony component over time (Figure 14–14). Subchondral lamina formation also was evident. Five patients underwent second-look arthroscopy, which showed that although

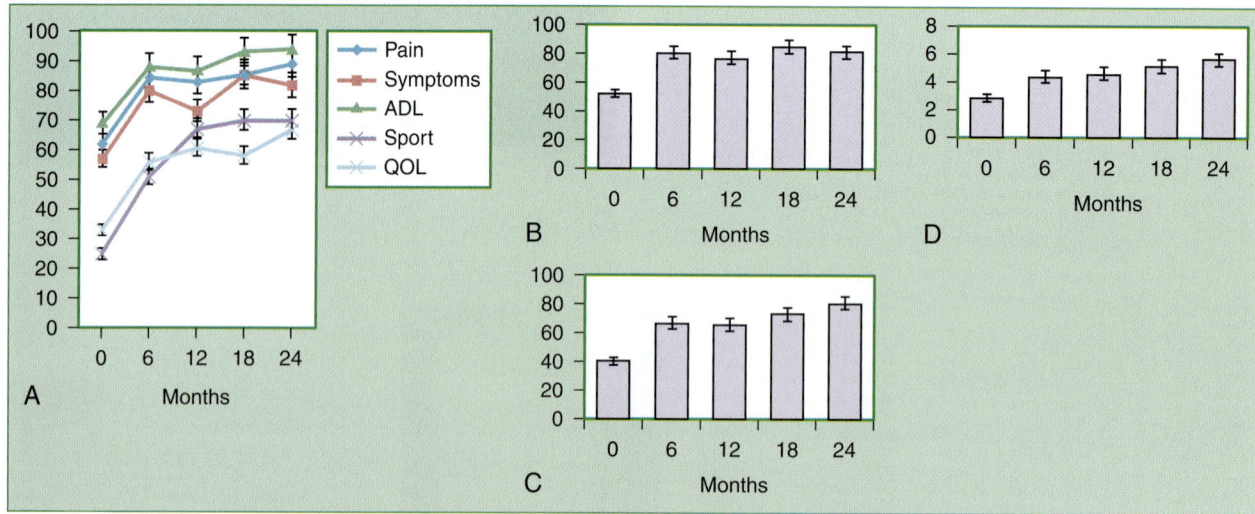

Figure 14-13 Knee Injury and Osteoarthritis Outcome Score (KOOS) (A), Lysholm score (B), International Knee Documentation Committee score (C), and Tegner activity level score (D). Mean KOOS pain, symptom, activities of daily living, sport, and quality-of-life scores increased 21, 16, 18, 42, and 28 points at 12 months from baseline, respectively (all $P < .004$).

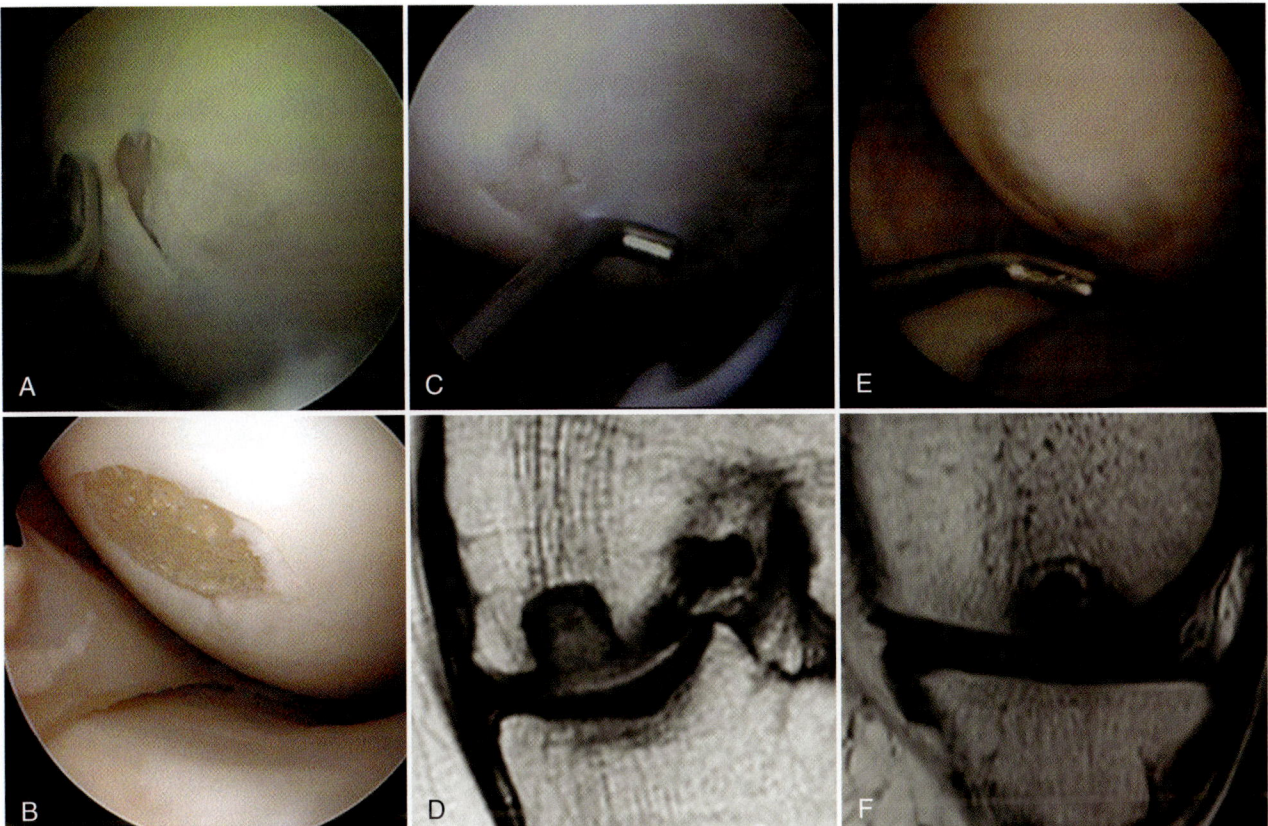

Figure 14-14 A 37-year-old patient in the series undergoing repair of defect on medial femoral condyle. *A,* Initial operative view showed delamination. *B,* Repair with a 9-mm TRUFIT CB implant. *C,* Second-look arthroscopy at 8 months showed soft area of repair. *D,* Magnetic resonance imaging (MRI) at 8 months. *E,* Arthroscopy at 3 years postoperative showed a smooth articular surface. *F,* MRI showed reformation of the subchondral lamina and well-integrated articular cartilage.

TRUFIT CB stayed soft up to 8 months or more, excellent defect fill and integration with surrounding cartilage were seen. In one patient with slow incorporation of the plugs, patience and perseverance with rehabilitation allowed full resolution of symptoms and return to semiprofessional soccer.[53]

Following the treatment of chondral or osteochondral lesions in the knee with TRUFIT CB, the most active patients in the series returned to semiprofessional sports; the remainder returned to their previous level of activity by 12 months, with no deterioration to date. This series of patients demonstrated outcome comparable to microfracture at 12 months. The improvement of KOOS (see Figure 14-13) was similar to Saris' report on patients who received microfracture at 12 months (mean KOOS pain, symptom, activities of daily living [ADL], and quality-of-life [QOL] scores increased 13, 11, 12, and 16 points, respectively, from baseline).[54] TRUFIT CB provides a stable scaffold for early mobilization of the knee postoperatively, avoiding the prolonged period of limited weight bearing in microfracture. Other benefits of TRUFIT CB include its availability as an "off-the-shelf" product, the avoidance of donor site morbidity associated with osteochondral grafting, and the ease of the procedure. The results from this case series indicate that TRUFIT CB provides a one-step solution in managing small (<2-cm diameter) areas of chondral or osteochondral injury, particularly in patients who require rapid rehabilitation and a high level of activity.

MINCED CARTILAGE

One-Stage Autologous Procedure for Cartilage Regeneration

One-stage and two-stage surgical therapies to repair or restore articular cartilage in the treatment of focal chondral defects have been explored. Point-of-care techniques include marrow stimulation (e.g., microfracture) and osteochondral autografting and allografting; two-stage therapies include ACI and MACI. Each therapy has clinical advantages and limitations in terms of applicable defect size and location, patient age, and long-term durability of the repair tissue. Although ACI-based procedures have demonstrated promising clinical results, the requirement for multiple surgical exposures and ex vivo cell expansion can impact rehabilitation time, surgical/anesthesia risk, and health care costs. As a result, several emerging technologies are being studied to either improve existing single-stage therapies or enable point-of-care chondrocyte-based implantation.

Cartilage Autograft Implantation System

The CAIS cartilage autograft implantation system (DePuy Mitek, Raynham MA) has been developed as a point-of-care therapy composed of mechanically fragmented autologous cartilage implanted on a bioresorbable scaffold. (*Note:* CAIS is an investigational device limited by federal and local regulations to investigational use only.) This one-stage approach uses a customized harvester device to morselize donor tissue from an unaffected, low-weight-bearing region of the knee (intercondylar notch, trochlear ridge or other minor load-bearing site) into small fragments to promote cell outgrowth from the dense cartilaginous matrix (Figure 14–15A). These cartilage fragments are overlaid onto a bioresorbable scaffold that provides both structural integrity and a defined three-dimensional architecture to support cell outgrowth, proliferation, and matrix deposition in the repair site. The CAIS scaffold is a synthetic composite matrix composed of polycaprolactone-co-glycolide polymeric foam reinforced with a polydioxanone mesh. Cartilage fragments are uniformly distributed over the scaffold surface using a custom dispersion device and subsequently coated with a layer of fibrin sealant to promote fragment retention during implant templating and fixation (Figure 14–15B). Following debridement of the cartilage lesion to healthy margins, the implant is cut to size (Figure 14–15C) and rigidly affixed in the repair site using bioresorbable polydioxanone staples (Figures 14–15D and 14–16). Cyclic testing (10,000 cycles at 1 Hz) of this staple-based fixation in human cadaveric knees demonstrated robust scaffold retention with no detectable wear of adjacent cartilage or meniscus.[55]

In vitro studies have demonstrated chondrocyte viability as well as time-dependent cellular outgrowth into the CAIS scaffold following tissue fragmentation and seeding. In a subcutaneous implantation model, outgrowth cells from morselized cartilage exhibit

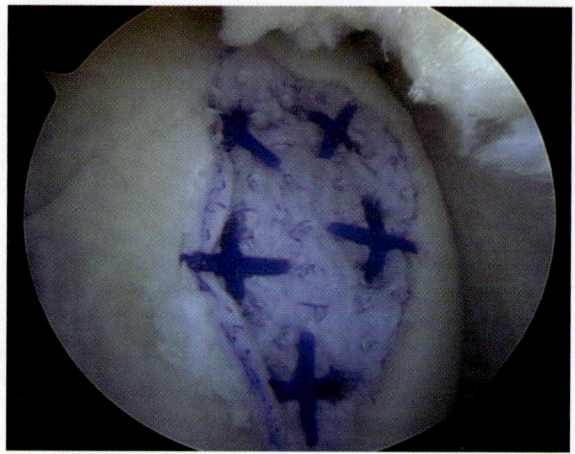

Figure 14–16 Cartilage autograft implantation system implant affixed with bioresorbable staples.

more prominent neocartilaginous tissue formation than subculture-expanded chondrocytes, as revealed by safranin O staining.[56] These studies indicate that morselized cartilage fragments are a viable repository of chondrocytes capable of outgrowth and synthesis of a cartilaginous repair tissue.

Large animal cartilage repair models implementing this one-stage technique demonstrated safranin O–positive, hyaline-like tissue repair that was well integrated with adjacent cartilage and subchondral bone as early as 6 months postsurgery.[56] Empty defects or those treated with scaffold alone typically resulted in repair tissue of inferior quality and staining intensity compared to lesions treated with morselized cartilage fragments (Figure 14–17A–C). In addition, results from a 12-month equine study suggested that this one-step approach may provide similar or improved healing progression and hyaline-like tissue repair compared to a modified ACI technique (Frisbie et al, unpublished data). Human clinical studies evaluating the safety and efficacy of CAIS compared to microfracture are ongoing in North America and Europe.

In summary, CAIS, a one-stage cartilage regeneration therapy, potentially offers several practical advantages

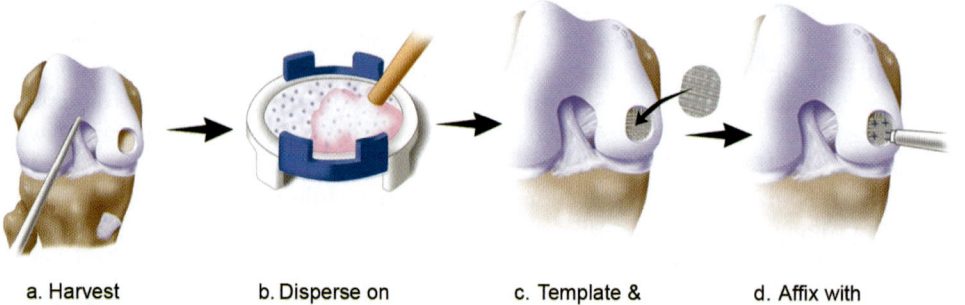

a. Harvest Cartilage

b. Disperse on Scaffold & Apply Fibrin Sealant

c. Template & Implant

d. Affix with Staples

Figure 14–15 Procedural steps of the cartilage autograft implantation system surgical technique, including harvest of donor cartilage *(A)*, dispersion and fixation of cartilage fragments using fibrin sealant *(B)*, sizing of the implant *(C)*, and fixation with bioresorbable staples *(D)*.

Emerging Technologies CHAPTER 14

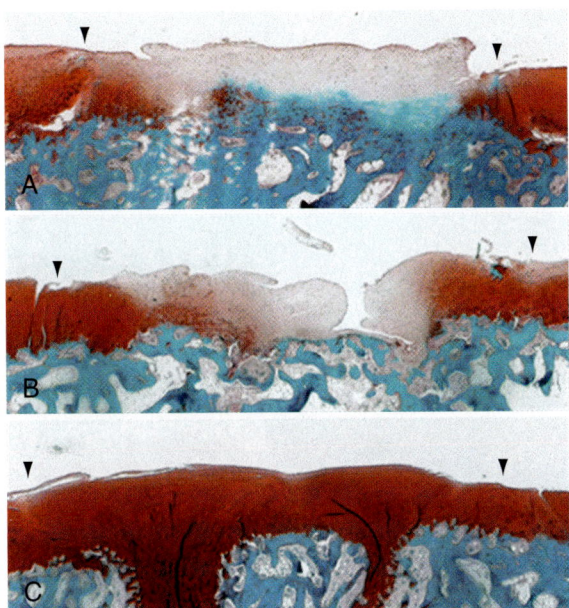

Figure 14–17 Representative histology micrographs (safranin O staining) showing chondral defect repair in a goat model at 6 months: empty defects (A), scaffold only (B), and scaffold with morselized cartilage tissue fragments (C).

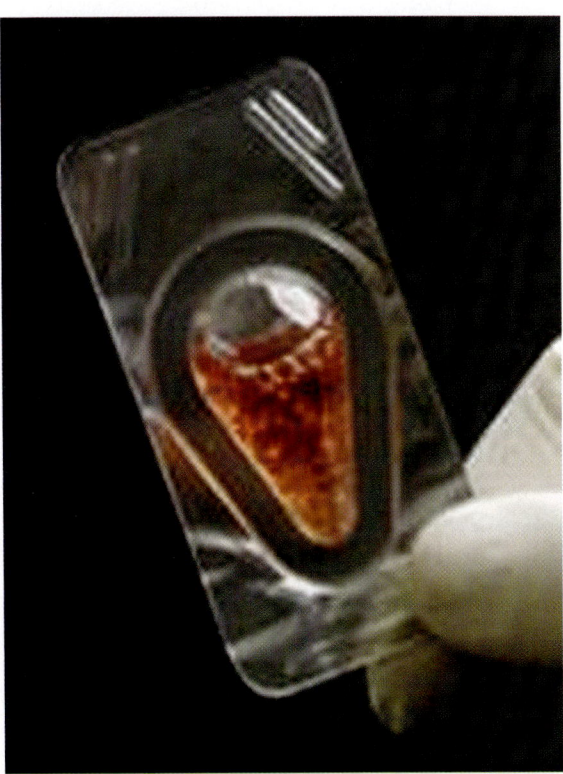

Figure 14–18 DeNovo natural tissue (NT) graft.

over other cell-based techniques. Delivery of morselized cartilage provides a direct source of primary autologous chondrocytes to the site of repair as opposed to a heterogeneous population of marrow-derived cells resulting from marrow stimulation procedures. The incarcerated chondrocytes subsequently outgrow and proliferate in vivo, thereby reducing the time, cost, and multiple procedures required for two-step ACI-based techniques. Morselized cartilage-derived chondrocytes may retain a more potent chondrogenic phenotype than culture-expanded cells because they are not exposed to the environmental trauma associated with ex vivo expansion. CAIS is a promising first-line cartilage regeneration therapy for the treatment of focal chondral defects in a single surgical procedure.

DeNovo Natural Tissue Graft

DeNovo natural tissue (NT) graft (Zimmer, Warsaw, IN/ISTO Technologies, St. Louis, MO) is composed of aseptically processed particulated cartilage tissue recovered from donated juvenile human knee joints (Figure 14–18). No biologic manipulation or chemical processing is performed. The tissue pieces are packaged in a sterile blister package filled with a proprietary nutrient medium. The cartilage pieces are implanted into articular cartilage defects using fibrin adhesive for graft fixation. In an equine study in which human juvenile cartilage pieces were implanted to repair chondral defects of horse knee joints, no inflammation/immune rejection due to the xenograft transplantation was observed (D. Frisbie, unpublished data). The DeNovo NT graft is considered to be human tissue per section 361 of the Public Health Service (PHS) Act and therefore is regulated solely under 21 CFR 1271 in the same way as many other allograft products, such as fresh osteochondral allografts and bone–tendon–bone allografts. Since May 2007, this product has been implanted to repair cartilage defects in more than 300 patients in various anatomic locations (knee, ankle, shoulder, hip, elbow, and great toe). Early clinical data on patients receiving DeNovo NT graft treatment have been encouraging.[57] Patients who were implanted with DeNovo NT Graft more than 2 years ago are reporting good clinical outcomes.

SECOND-GENERATION CELL-BASED ACI

Matrix-Induced Autologous Chondrocyte Implantation

Background
MACI is a second-generation ACI therapy for repair of full-thickness cartilage defects. Developed by Verigen and later acquired by Genzyme Biosurgery (Cambridge, MA), MACI was designed to overcome the surgical complexity and invasiveness associated with first-generation ACI, Carticel (cultured ACI). For Carticel, cells are delivered in a liquid suspension, implanted in the defect, and secured with an autologous periosteal cover that is harvested from the proximal tibia. MACI is a surgically convenient delivery method in which cells are implanted

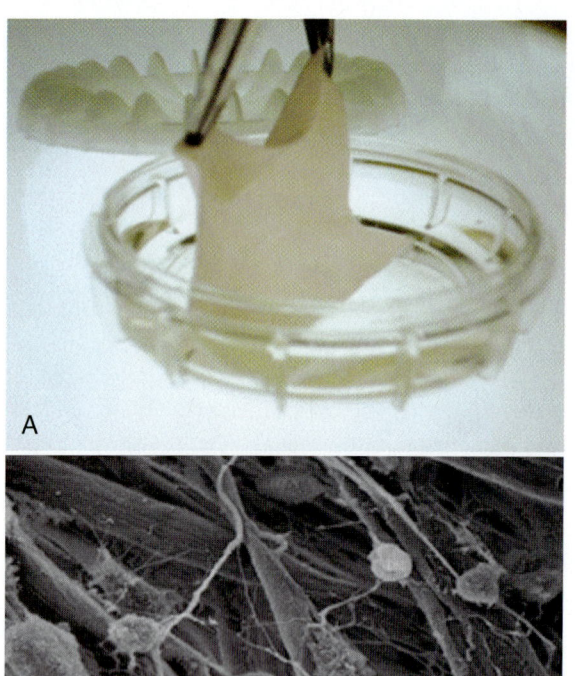
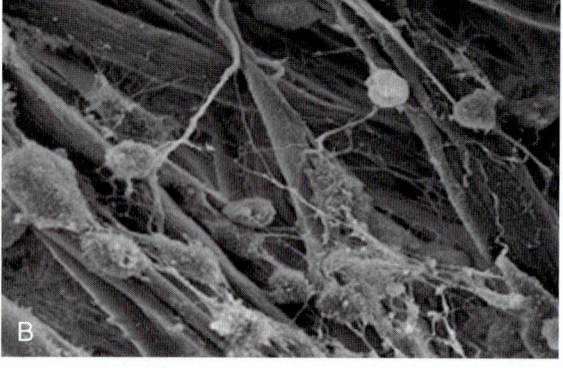

Figure 14–19 *A*, Matrix-induced autologous chondrocyte implantation (MACI). Collagen type I–III membrane is preseeded with autologous cultured chondrocytes and cultured, then is ready for surgical implantation. *B*, Scanning electron micrograph of autologous chondrocyte seeded MACI. *(Courtesy Dr. Ming-Hao Zheng, School of Surgery and Pathology, University of Western Australia, Perth, Australia.)*

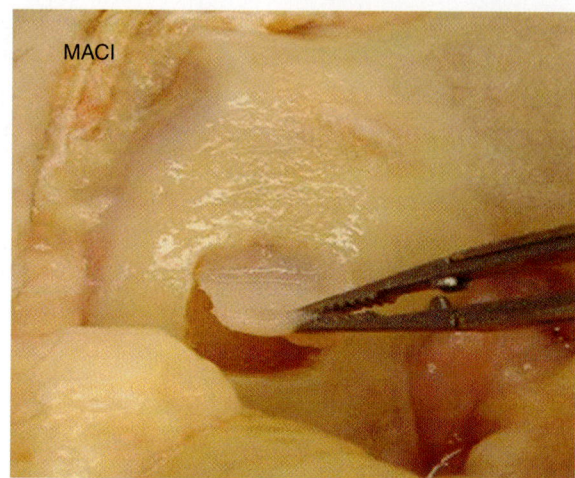

Figure 14–20 Matrix-induced autologous chondrocyte implantation of a femoral condyle with fibrin glue fixation.

attached or "seeded" onto the surface of a purified porcine biodegradable type I/III collagen membrane (Figure 14–19). MACI typically is secured in the defect with fibrin sealant, and sutures are used if supplemental fixation is deemed necessary (Figure 14–20). Patients are not exposed to a second incision that is needed to harvest the periosteum and a large arthrotomy that is required to accommodate periosteal fixation. Arthroscopic delivery of MACI has been reported.[58]

Manufacturing Process

For MACI, chondrocytes are isolated from a cartilage biopsy using an enzymatic process, expanded in a monolayer cell culture, and seeded onto an absorbable purified type I/III collagen membrane. When cells are grown in monolayer cell culture, they dedifferentiate; that is, they change their phenotype and down-regulate expression of cartilage matrix genes. To ensure proper cell expression and phenotype within final product, MACI implants are characterized for cell potency, identity, and viability using proprietary assays that were designed to meet regulatory guidelines. MACI also undergoes extensive quality control release testing, including sterility, mycoplasma, and endotoxin assays.

Commercial Availability

MACI has been commercially available in several European member states and Australia since 1998. Because of the EU Advanced Therapy Medicinal Products regulation, commercial availability of MACI after December 2012 will require formal approval of MACI by the centralized European Medicines Agency (EMEA) process. In response to this regulation, Genzyme is conducting a phase III prospective, randomized, open-label, parallel-group, multicenter study, known as SUMMIT (Superiority of MACI vs Microfracture Treatment), to demonstrate the superiority of MACI versus arthroscopic microfracture for the treatment of symptomatic articular cartilage defects of the femoral condyle, including the trochlea. The endpoints of SUMMIT include patient-reported assessments of pain and function, MR assessments, and histology assessments. MACI currently is not available in the United States.

Clinical Outcomes

Results from several studies demonstrate significant reductions in pain and functional impairment at early follow-up (2 years). Although longer-term data are limited, results from two studies demonstrate significant improvement from baseline out to 5-year follow-up.[59,60] Although no comparative ACI and MACI studies have been published, comparable rates of good/excellent results have been reported. After treatment with MACI, 70% to 89% of patients reported good/excellent results.[61-63] Overall, results of MRI, histology, and arthroscopic (macroscopic) assessments of the repair tissue demonstrate that treatment with MACI can yield repair tissue with hyaline-like cartilage (Figure 14–21),[64-66] complete defect fill,[67] complete integration with surrounding cartilage,[68] and ICRS score of grade I/II.[64] Some studies have reported that MACI repair tissue was fibrocartilage and failed to completely integrate or fill the defect, findings that may

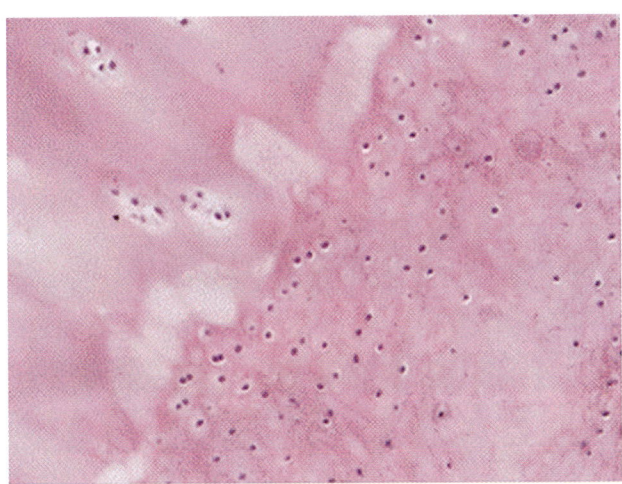

Figure 14–21 Integration of native and regenerative cartilage (with appearance of hyaline-like cartilage) by matrix-induced autologous chondrocyte implantation. *(Courtesy Dr. Ming-Hao Zheng, School of Surgery and Pathology, University of Western Australia, Perth, Australia.)*

be due to the negative bias associated with limiting objective assessments to patients with only postoperative complications and not a representative sample of patients in the entire study.[62,67] The reported incidence of postoperative complications associated with the MACI procedure is low (range 0%–6.3%).[62,64,68,69] Reported postoperative complications include tissue hypertrophy, partial graft detachment, infections, and subsequent surgical procedures. The reported incidence of treatment failure, defined as graft detachment or bone to bone contact, also is low (range 0%–6.3%).[62,64,68,69]

Hyalograft C Autograft

Preclinical Findings

Hyalograft C autograft (Fidia Advanced Biopolymers, Abano Terme, Italy) is a second-generation ACI product.[70,71] It is a graft composed of autologous chondrocytes grown on a three-dimensional hyaluronan-based scaffold. The scaffold is a nonwoven pad composed of HYAFF 11, a hyaluronic acid benzyl ester polymer.[72]

Chondrocytes can be easily isolated from small biopsies and expanded in vitro; however, when cultured in two dimensions they tend to lose their characteristic phenotype, namely, collagen type II and aggrecan expression.[73] In vitro characterization studies confirmed that maintenance of a differentiated phenotype is favored by the use of a three-dimensional scaffold. Studies have clearly demonstrated that Hyalograft C scaffolds not only allow chondrocyte attachment but also provide adequate support to permit expression of the differentiated chondrocytic phenotype.[74,75] Excellent functional integration of Hyalograft C seeded with chondrocytes with the surrounding native bone and cartilage was demonstrated via the assessment of structure, biochemical composition, and mechanical behavior of the construct in an ex vivo model.[76] Moreover, an in vitro study has been conducted in order to analyze the growth and differentiation behavior of human articular chondrocytes on Hyalograft C scaffold compared to a porcine collagen scaffold and a gelatin gel matrix.[77] Results demonstrated that Hyalograft C scaffold was superior to the other scaffolds in terms of supporting rapid redifferentiation of chondrocytes after monolayer culture, as shown by electron microscopic evaluation of cell phenotype and the differentiation index (calculated as collagen II/I ratio), which was ~1 and stable during the observation period. The same index was only 10^{-3} for the collagen and gelatin scaffolds. Only Hyalograft C scaffold enabled the formation of a relatively large amount of cartilage-like differentiated cells, indicating that the nature of the matrix greatly influences the differentiation behavior of dedifferentiated human chondrocytes.

Expanded human chondrocytes cultivated on Hyalograft C scaffold and then subcutaneously implanted in the athymic mice for up to 3 months confirmed that this scaffold is an adequate support for cartilage formation. Explants examination after implantation showed formation of hyaline-like cartilage.[78] Moreover, study using a functional animal model verified that chondrocyte transplantation using Hyalograft C induces the regeneration of injured articular cartilage.[79] Nonclinical protocols in small and large animal models have also been performed to assess the biocompatibility and feasibility of Hyalograft C autograft in view of its use in a clinical setting.[80–84]

Based on the nonclinical findings, Hyalograft C autograft was evaluated in clinical settings for the treatment of full-thickness articular cartilage defects.

Clinical Development

Since Hyalograft C autograft became available in clinical practice, more than 4,800 patients have been treated with this technology. Of these patients, 230 have been evaluated in investigator-initiated clinical studies, and the results of more than 900 patients have been reported in published literature.

Preliminary clinical experience derived from pilot clinical studies indicated that the Hyalograft C autograft was well tolerated. The studies also showed that the surgical technique was substantially simpler compared to ACI (Figure 14–22) because the product could be shaped to fit the lesion and could be applied by mini-invasive arthrotomy without the need for a periosteal flap, thus significantly reducing operation times and morbidity.

Consequently, in 2001, an Italian investigator initiated a multicenter observational study of more than 200 consecutive patients (mean age 37.4, mean lesion size 3.7 cm^2) who were treated with the Hyalograft C autograft and prospectively followed for 5 years, with 4-year follow-up data available to date.[71,85–87] The durability results suggest that clinical improvements obtained 2 years

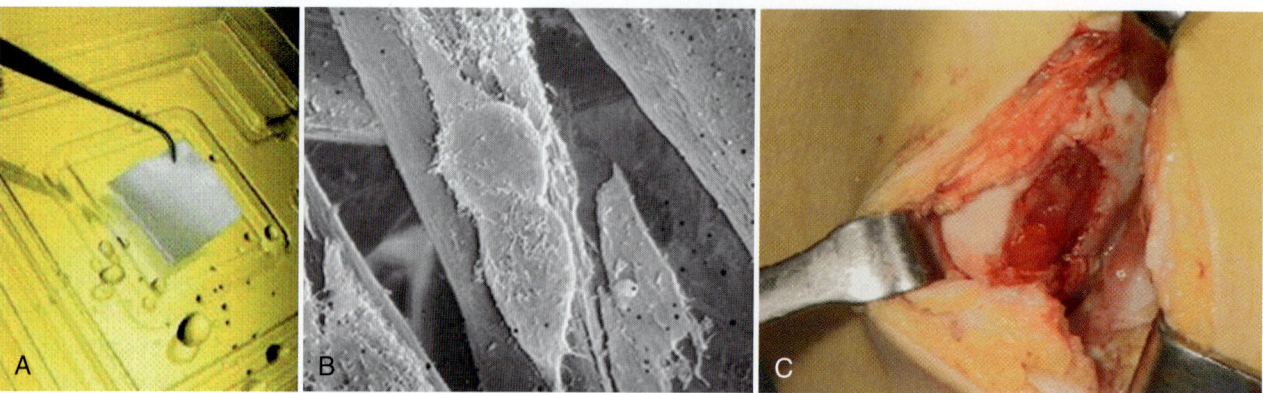

Figure 14–22 *A,* Hyalograft C. Membrane seeded with cultured autologous chondrocytes ready for surgical implantation. *B,* Scanning electron micrograph of chondrocyte attachment to hyaluronan-based scaffold. *C,* Mini-arthrotomy for delivery of Hyalograft C with fibrin glue fixation.

after implantation are maintained at 5-year follow up. After an average of 4 years (n = 179) from implantation, 86% of patients had a significant benefit in knee symptoms and function. A mean IKDC subjective score of 78.6 points was obtained postoperatively, reflecting high levels of function and sports activities and low level of symptoms, compared to a mean IKDC preoperatively of 39.9 ($P < .0001$). After clinician-performed examination, 95.7% of the knees were rated as normal and nearly normal based on objective IKDC score. Significant improvements (86.4%, $P < .0001$) were obtained for health-related quality of life (EuroQol EQ-5D), particularly for pain and mobility aspects that overlap those obtained in an age- and gender-matched reference population.

In 2009, Kon et al[88] reported a prospective, comparative, nonrandomized study with 5-year follow-up. In their study, the clinical outcome of patients treated with Hyalograft C autograft was compared with the microfracture technique. Eighty active symptomatic patients (mean age 29.8 years) with grade III to IV chondral lesions of femoral condyles or trochlea (mean defect size 2.4 cm^2) were enrolled and treated with arthroscopic Hyalograft C autograft (40 patients; Figure 14–23) or microfracture (40 patients) techniques. More patients who had undergone previous surgery (47.5% vs 25%, respectively, $P < .05$) and had fewer traumatic cartilage lesions (45% vs 67.5%, respectively, $P < .05$) were enrolled in the Hyalograft C autograft group than in the microfracture group.

Both groups showed statistically significant improvement of all clinical scores from preoperative to 5-year follow-up ($P < .001$). In the microfracture group, the IKDC objective score increased from 2.5% normal and nearly normal knees before surgery to 75% at 5-year follow-up, and the subjective score increased from 41.1 preoperatively to 70.2 at 5-year follow-up. In the group treated with Hyalograft C autograft, the IKDC objective score increased from 15% normal and nearly normal before surgery to 90% at 5-year follow-up, and the subjective score increased from 40.5 preoperatively to 80.2

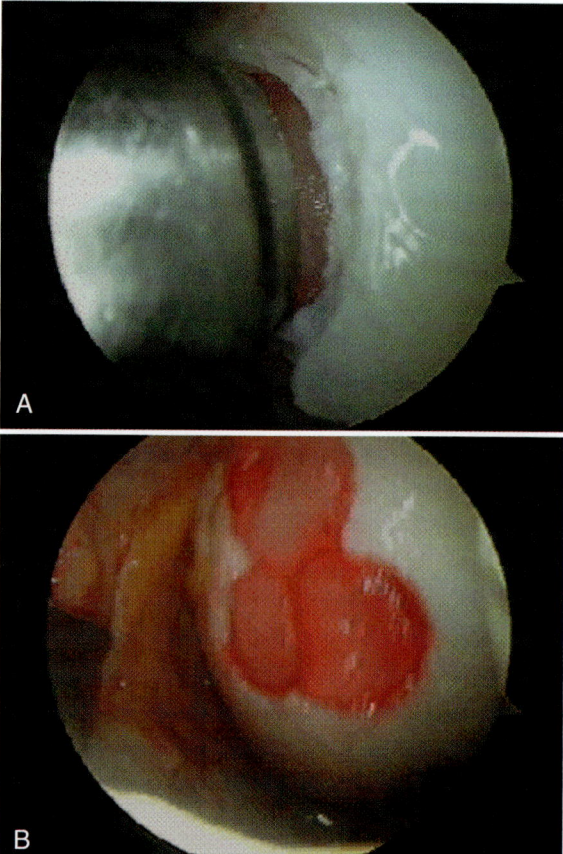

Figure 14–23 *A,* Arthroscopic delivery of Hyalograft C in an air environment after preparation of the defect in a mosaic pattern. Debridement of the chondral defect is performed in a saline environment using specially sized and cannulated guide instruments that facilitate the technique. *B,* Final arthroscopic appearance of arthroscopically transplanted chondral defect in a mosaic pattern with Hyalograft C.

at 5-year follow-up. When comparing the groups, better clinical results assessed with objective ($P < .001$) and subjective ($P = 0.003$) IKDC scores at 5-year follow-up were found in the group treated with arthroscopic Hyalograft C autograft transplantation. Also, no decrease in the resumption of sports activities evaluated with the Tegner score from 2- to 5-year follow-up was observed in patients treated with Hyalograft C autograft transplantation versus a decrease in sports activity in the group treated with microfracture.

These findings confirming the clinical superiority and durability of Hyalograft C autograft over microfracture in treating large articular cartilage defects.

Since Hyalograft C autograft became available in clinical practice, a total of 70 biopsies have been harvested from consenting patients from 5 to 33 months (mean 14.1 months) after Hyalograft C autograft implantation, both for purely investigative and for diagnostic purposes (i.e., in symptomatic patients).[89,90] The data were analyzed as a function of time from implantation, and biopsies taken after a longer follow-up time appeared to show a significantly ($P = .0042$) higher percentage of hyaline cartilage (45.4% in hyaline specimens vs 23.7% in biopsies taken within the first 18 months). Evidence of cartilage maturation over time was confirmed by analysis of the third-look biopsies. Hyaline tissue was present in all third-look specimens (mean time from implantation 30.6 months) but not in second-look biopsies (mean time from implantation 13.6 months) of the same patients. Taken together, these data indicate that after Hyalograft C autograft implantation, cartilage resurfacing is achieved, with consistent integration with subchondral bone, tidemark formation, and clear evidence of hyaline-like maturation over time. Evidence of cartilage maturation over time using Hyalograft C autograft has also been reported in studies using high-resolution MRI techniques, which confirmed stability of the implant postimplantation and analyzed the in vivo kinetics of defect filling.[91–93]

Other clinical reports have confirmed these observations in both the knee (Table 14-1) and the ankle.[94] Table 14-1 summarizes some of the findings of clinical studies on the use of Hyalograft C autograft in the knee.[95–101]

The population treated is uniform in terms of age, lesion etiology, and lesion size and severity and is very similar to the demographics of first-generation ACI patients. Candidates for Hyalograft C autograft treatment were relatively young, active, and clinically challenging patient population that presented, on average, with severe pain and functional impairment resulting from moderate to large chondral defects.

The 2- to 5-year follow-up data demonstrate that following Hyalograft C autograft treatment, the improvements in pain and mobility are durable and that patients have resumed their preinjury levels of activity.

These findings support algorithms that recommend cell-based therapies for treatment of large, disabling, articular cartilage lesions of traumatic origin or consequent to osteochondritis dissecans.

Taken together, the long-term clinical evidence available on Hyalograft C autograft indicates that, following treatment, the improvements in pain and mobility are durable and that patients have resumed their preinjury levels of activity, suggesting that Hyalograft C autograft is a safe and effective cartilage substitute for the indication proposed.

ChondroCelect

Introduction

ChondroCelect (TiGenix N.V., Leuven, Belgium) is a characterized cell therapy product (according to the European regulatory framework for Advanced Therapy Medicinal Products) that consists of autologous cartilage cells that are expanded ex vivo via a highly controlled and consistent manufacturing process.

In order to culture cells with the best potential to generate stable cartilage, it is critical that the cell culture

Table 14-1 Clinical Studies on Use of Hyalograft C Autograft in the Knee

	Marcacci (2006)	Marlovits and Nehrer (2004)	Kon et al (2009)	Ferruzzi et al (2008)	Nehrer (2008)	Marlovits et al (2006)	Gobbi et al (2009)
No. of patients treated	206	24	40	50	53	13	32
Mean age (years)	37.4	32.4	29.8	31.0	32	34	30.5
Mean defect size (cm^2)	3.7	5.98	2.4	5.9	4.4	5.3	4.7
Outerbridge defect grade	III–IV	III–IV	III–IV	III–IV	III–IV	III–IV	III–IV
Previous surgeries (%)	45.6	87.5	47.5	—	77.8	—	59.4
Previous failed cartilage treatment (%)	33	29.1	20	—	32	—	21.9
Patients improved after minimum 2-year follow-up (%)	86	70.8	90	77	84.6	81.6	90.7

Clinical demographics and outcomes from studies by Marcacci,[96] Marlovits and Nehrer,[98] Kon et al,[100] Ferruzzi et al,[99] Marlovits et al,[97] and Gobbi et al.[101]

process not cause the cells to lose their cartilage phenotype.[73] Maintaining the ability of the cells to maximally conserve their preculture phenotype and high-quality cartilage-forming capacity was the key element for product development.

The initial research conducted by Dell'Accio et al[102,103] was used as the basis to develop both the ChondroCelect process and the ChondroCelect score, which is used as a quality measure before the release of each cell batch.

Translational Research Background

Dell'Accio et al[102,103] tested different mesenchymal cell populations (including precursor cells, chondrocytes, primitive cells, stem cells) in nude (immunosuppressed) mice for their basic ability to form stable cartilage. This research led to the development of an in vivo model: the ectopic cartilage formation assay (ECFA). This assay tests the potency and capacity of a cell population to form a cartilage implant in an in vivo environment. It is now used as one of the pillars in the ChondroCelect research and development process.

The ECFA potency test consists of the following steps (Figure 14–24):
- The cells are injected into the thigh of a nude mouse.
- The cells are allowed to grow in this ectopic site (i.e., in vivo) for a period of 3 to 4 weeks.
- The tissue, which has developed at the injection site, is removed for histologic examination, including scoring using toluidine blue and safranin O staining.

In this model, the cells' intrinsic capability to form cartilage is tested in a stringent, noncartilaginous environment. Hence, it provides a direct measure of the relevant biologic properties of the cells in regenerating hyaline cartilage. This is accomplished by assessing some of the main characteristics of cartilage formation, such as extracellular matrix (ECM) deposition leading to tissue formation, absence of vascular invasion, and absence of pathologic mineralization.

The following insights were gained through these initial experiments:
- Identification of cell populations that retain their ability (their phenotype) to form cartilage implants in vivo and those that either had no potential or had lost that capability (laying the foundation for the ChondroCelect score)
- Development of a cell culturing process with the goal of preserving the chondrocyte phenotype in cells (the precursor of the ChondroCelect process)

Refining Predictive Power: Development of the ChondroCelect Score

Although the ECFA is a powerful assay for demonstrating a cell population's ability to regenerate stable

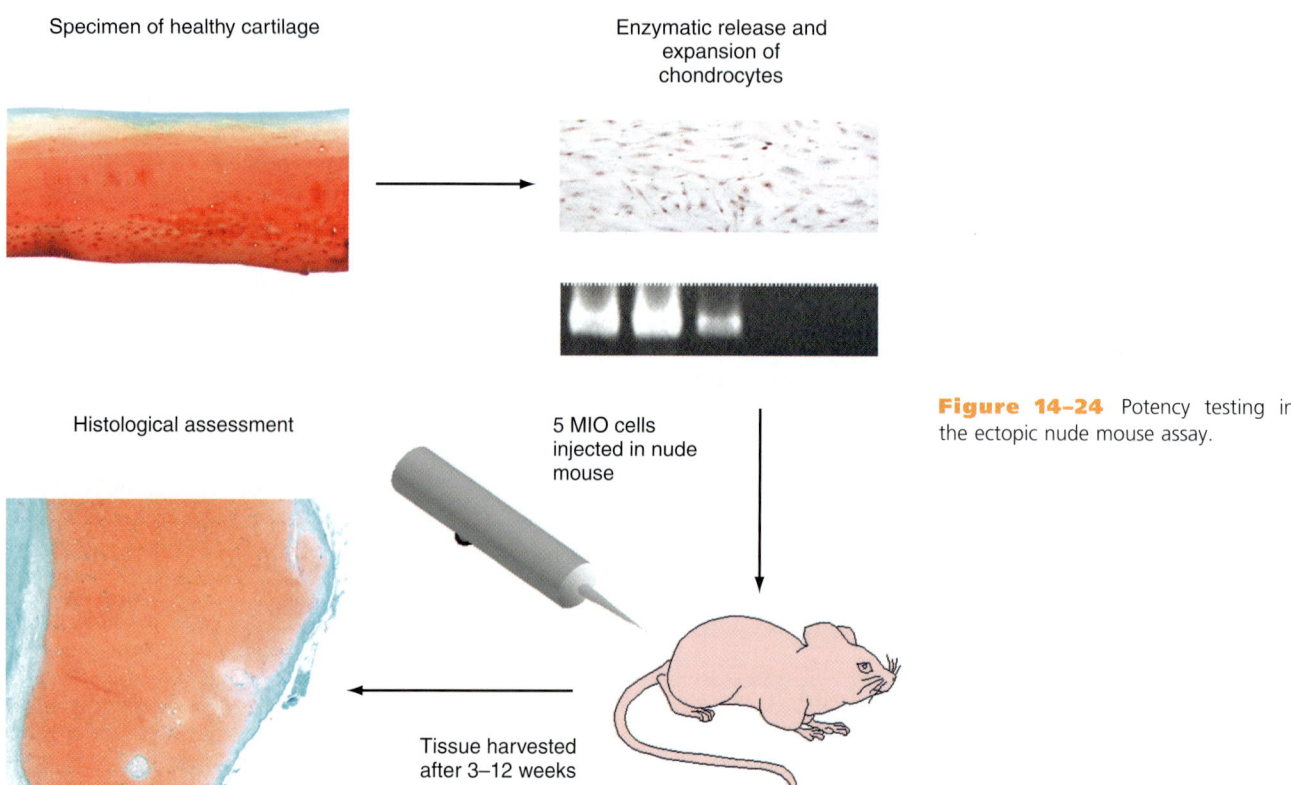

Figure 14–24 Potency testing in the ectopic nude mouse assay.

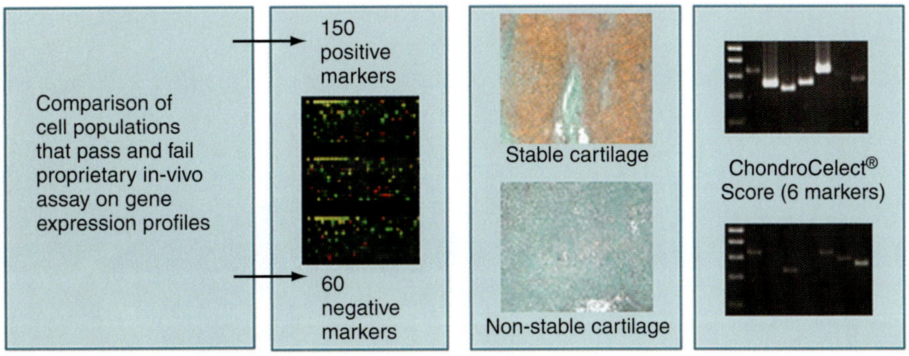

Figure 14–25 Development of surrogate marker assay.

cartilage, it is not practical for use as a quality test in a routine manufacturing setting. A quicker, less cell consuming, preferably in vitro assay was needed.

In order to develop an in vitro assay, the same cell populations tested in the ECFA were analyzed in a comparative microarray analysis (Figure 14–25). This assay looks at the expression of a large number of genes with the goal of identifying both positive and negative markers relevant for cartilage formation.

Through this assay, 150 positive markers (genes that are highly expressed in the cells that produced a cartilage implant in the ECFA and are not or are very lowly expressed in the cells that have no ability to form cartilage) and 60 negative markers (genes that are highly expressed in cells that have no ability to form cartilage in the ECFA) were identified.

Of these 210 markers, six markers were selected (four positive and two negative) based on their capacity to generate cartilage tissue in the ECFA. These markers form the basis of the ChondroCelect score.

To determine the prediction threshold of the score in cartilage formation, a correlation was drawn between the score and the outcome of the ECFA histology score. The histology score is based on the presence and brightness of staining of the ECM of cartilage cells.

When analyzing the results between the in vitro assay of cells and the in vivo capacity of cells to form cartilage in the ECFA implants, a clear correlation was noted between cells having a good score and a good histology score.

In routine manufacturing, the marker gene expression profile of these six markers can be measured using reverse transcriptase polymerase chain reaction (RT-PCR) methodology. Each of the individual markers can be scored based on its overall expression level in the assay. The combination of these individual scores gives the ChondroCelect score.

Developing the ChondroCelect Manufacturing Process

The second major development push and product differentiation was through the creation of the ChondroCelect process. As stated in the scientific rationale, the goal during cell culture is for the cells to maintain their phenotype. For proper cartilage defect filling, one million cells per centimeter squared are required and must be cultured from the original biopsy material. The problem is the well-documented issue of gradual cell dedifferentiation during routine cell culturing.

In order to develop the process, factors influencing the cell culture process were varied in a controlled manner. The expanded cells obtained from each of these batches were qualified for their ability to produce cartilage in vivo. The goal of these tests was to identify which factors during the cell culture process influenced the cells' ability to maintain their chondrocyte phenotype.

The ChondroCelect process strictly controls the different factors during the culturing process that support the multiplication of chondrocyte cells while preventing these cells from becoming too dedifferentiated.

At the end of each individualized patient batch production, the potency is measured to verify that the cultured cells have retained their ability to grow cartilage. By using this controlled and consistent culturing process, an optimal quality product is obtained.

Proof of Concept in a Large Animal Model

In order to evaluate the validity of the process, a preclinical experiment in a large animal model was initiated. The experiment compared autologous goat cells cultured according to the ChondroCelect process versus dedifferentiated and fibroblast cells.

Stable chondrocyte cells (obtained through the ChondroCelect culturing method) showed good filling of the defect at 10 weeks. In contrast, the dedifferentiated cells gave only limited filling at the edges and little or no filling at the center of the defect.

Consequently, the cells cultured by the ChondroCelect process had a higher overall modified O'Driscoll Score (MODS) and much higher integration score than the dedifferentiated cells, which had scores only slightly better than the negative control fibroblast cell group at 10 weeks. In addition, the cells cultured by the ChondroCelect process gave a high-quality overall filling of the defect with superior integration into the surrounding tissue.

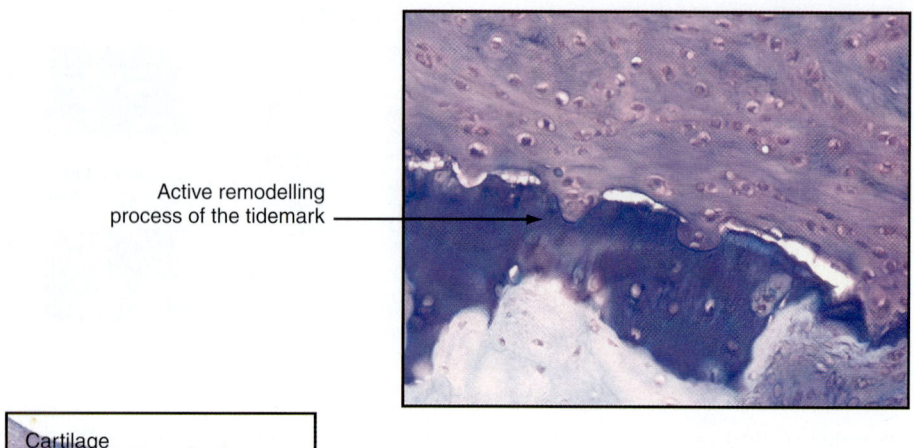
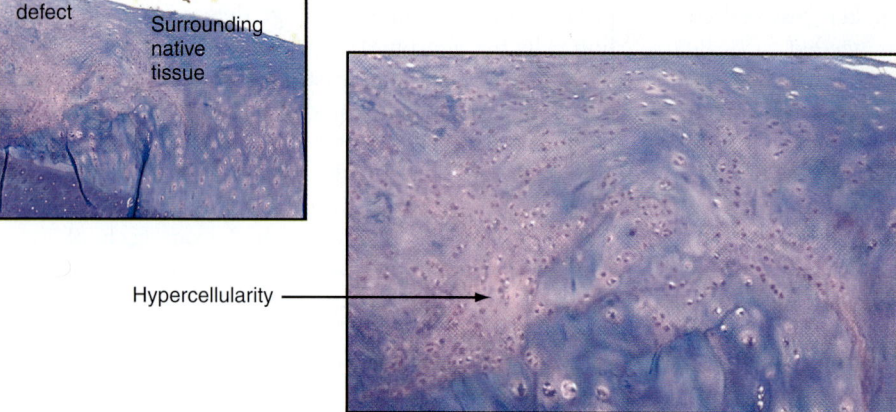

Figure 14–26 Mode of action studies in goat.

Further research demonstrated that the cells cultured by the ChondroCelect process were capable of resorbing and then reforming the calcified layer and were signaling to the environment, thereby recruiting cells from the surrounding tissues (Figure 14–26). This led to better filling of the defect and superior basal and lateral integration in the ChondroCelect process cell group.

In contrast, the dedifferentiated cells did not demonstrate any reforming of the calcified layer or signaling capabilities to surrounding cells.

This experiment confirmed the original rationale that differentiated cells are needed in order to form cartilage. The dedifferentiated cells, as well as the fibroblast negative control group, did not yield good cartilage implants.

Clinical Development: The TIGACT01 Study

The objective of the TIGACT01 study was to evaluate the efficacy and safety of ChondroCelect (CC) versus microfracture (MF) in the repair of symptomatic full-thickness cartilage defects of the femoral condyles.

CC (N = 51) was compared to MF (N = 61) in patients with grade III to IV symptomatic cartilage defects of the femoral condyles in a prospective, multicenter, randomized controlled trial. Structural repair was assessed at 1 year by histopathologists blinded to the treatment using computerized histomorphometry and the Overall Histology Assessment Score (item 1 of the ICRS II score).

CC resulted in better structural repair than MF at 1 year as assessed by histomorphometry ($P = .003$) and Overall Histology Assessment Score ($P = .010$) (Figure 14–27). Structural repair parameters relating to chondrocyte phenotype and tissue structure also were superior with CC.[54]

Mean improvement in overall KOOS at 36 months compared to baseline was higher in the CC group versus the MF group (21.65 ± 3.05 vs 15.27 ± 3.07, respectively).

When applying a mixed linear model analysis, statistically significantly greater improvement was shown for the CC group versus the MF group with regard to change from baseline in overall KOOS as well as in four of five KOOS subdomains (ADL, pain, symptoms/stiffness, and QOL).

Two failures (defined as need for reintervention) occurred in the CC group versus seven in the MF group at 36 months (Figure 14–28).

Patients treated within 3 years of symptom onset had a better clinical outcome (as measured by overall KOOS) than did patients treated beyond 3 years of symptom onset (and compared to MF).

MRI scans were performed at 12, 24, and 36 months and were assessed using the Magnetic resonance Observation

Figure 14–27 Superior structural repair at 12 months.

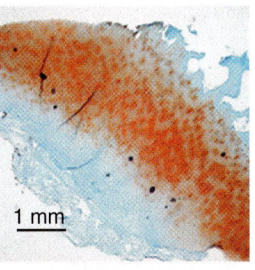
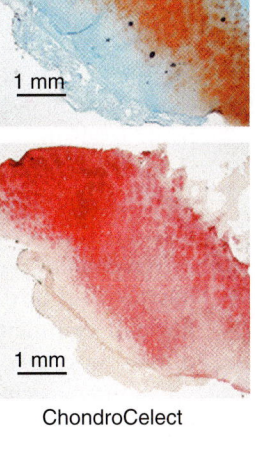

ChondroCelect

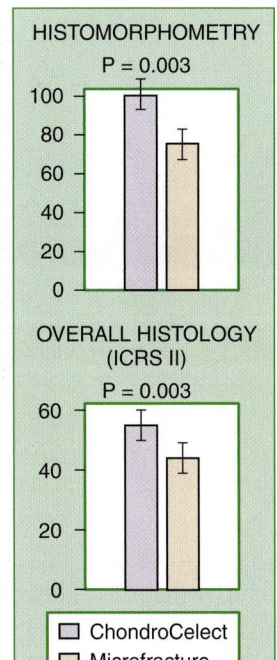

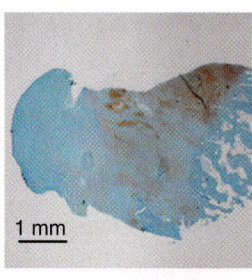
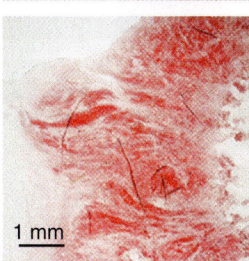

Microfracture

Figure 14–28 Superior clinical outcome at 36 months.[54]

Longitudinal analysis: treatment effect at 36 months (mixed linear model)

KOOS	P-value***
Overall*	0.018
Pain	0.028
Symptoms	0.020
Activity (ADL)	0.035
Sports	0.200
Quality of life	0.041

Treatment failures (reinterventions)
CC: 2   MF: 7

*Average of all KOOS domains, except Sports
**FAS without imputation for missing data of failures
***Between group KOOS changes from baseline

of Cartilage Repair Tissue (MOCART) score and nine additional items.

On MRI, several parameters (e.g., filling of the defect) were comparable between the two treatment groups. However, more patients in the MF group than in the CC group reported having subchondral bone reaction and enhanced elevation of the subchondral bone plate at 36 months. This resulted in a thinner "covering" layer of cartilage, which could potentially explain failure after MF.

ChondroCelect is currently under regulatory review for EU market authorization. It is not approved for use in the United States.

CaReS Cartilage Regeneration System

The CaReS cartilage regeneration system (Arthro Kinetics, Esslingen, Germany) is a minimally invasive method for treating large cartilage defects in the knee. Using the patient's own cartilage cells and a biologically purified collagen type I matrix derived from rat tail collagen, CaReS is a cartilage transplant with ease of application.

With the cartilage regeneration system, isolated autologous cultured chondrocytes (passage 0) are embedded in the purified collagen type I matrix, which then solidifies within 25 minutes at room temperature.

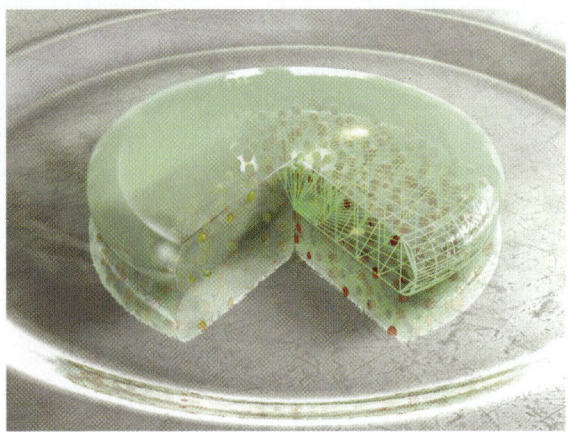

Figure 14-29 Schematic representation of cellular suspension in a three-dimensional collagen–gelatin matrix ready for implantation.

The construct is then incubated for 8 to 13 days and then implanted. The cell count is that of healthy cartilage, and the cells are outside of their accustomed three-dimensional matrix environment for only a few hours (Figure 14–29). The size and thickness of the transplant are variable during manufacture of the transplant and also may be sized during the operation with the cutting instruments provided (Figure 14–30A–C). The operative time is significantly reduced because microsuture of a cover to secure the implant is not required. The transplant is fixated using standard fibrin glue.

The transplant is manufactured by Arthro Kinetics under an extensive total quality management system (QMS). The manufacturing is based on pharmaceutical law (German drug law Arzneimittelgesetz [AMG]) and Good Manufacturing Practices (GMP), internationally established.

Requirements for the surgery are grade III or IV Outerbridge chondral defects measuring 2.5 to 10 cm^2. Intact and healthy surrounding cartilage is necessary in order for the graft to remain stable within its implanted bed. A maximum of two defects is allowed. Contraindications include joint stiffness, ligamentous instability, infectious disease, and background factors that have not been addressed, such as varus or valgus malalignment.

BioCart II

Optimal repair of focal articular cartilage lesions requires physiologically active chondrocytes delivered in biocompatible, self-instructive scaffolds. Such integrated products should result in the deposition of authentic cartilage matrix, duplicating both the structure and function of the native tissue. A novel approach combining growth factor driven chondroprogenitors that do not proliferate but rapidly produce cartilage matrix in a true three-dimensional, fibrin–hyaluronan scaffold has enabled successful repair of full-thickness cartilage defects.

Mature articular cartilage is composed primarily of postmitotic cells separated from each other by a thick and dense matrix (ECM); as a result, it has a highly restricted ability for self-repair. Chondrocyte cell functions are primarily regulated through specific cell–matrix interactions mediated by both integrin and nonintegrin receptors as well as mechanosensitive ion channels with direct implications for the expression and deposition of physiologic, hyaline-type cartilage.

In tissue culture the cells can be expanded, but their proliferation is frequently accompanied by dedifferentiation in which where their "chondrocytic" phenotype is lost and their ability to produce high-quality ECM upon reimplantation is compromised. Therefore, despite pioneering successes, the regeneration of physiologic hyaline cartilage, the goal of tissue regeneration, is not reproducibly attained.

An optimal scaffold for implantation should be both highly porous and permeable, facilitating homogeneous cell seeding, cell attachment, and diffusion of nutrients and instructive molecules. It should have the ability to support the deposition of authentic cartilage matrix until the cells have produced sufficient ECM and then be

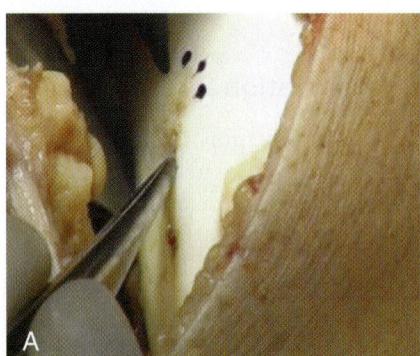
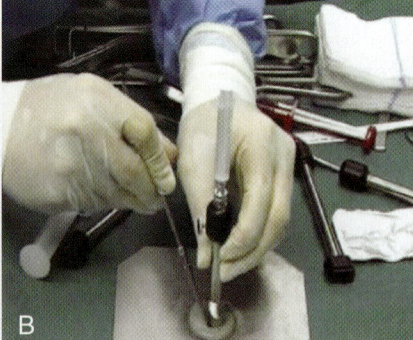
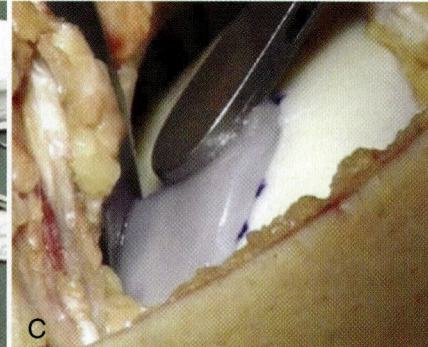

Figure 14-30 A, Chondral defect being outlined for radical debridement. B, The cartilage regeneration system transplant being cut precisely to the defect on the back table. C, The cartilage regeneration system transplant being glued with fibrin sealant to the chondral bed after it has been cut precisely to the defect. Pressure is maintained for up to 5 minutes to allow the collagen gel implant to mold to the defect and become secure.

biodegradable, allowing for the replacement of scaffold with cartilage.

BioCart II (ProChon Biotech, Ness Ziona, Israel) is a growth factor–directed autologous chondrocytes in a fibrin–hyaluronan matrix for enhanced focal articular cartilage repair. In designing BioCart II, the conditions for ex vivo expansion of primary human chondrocytes are used, consisting of autologous serum supplemented with a recombinant variant of fibroblast growth factor 2 (rFGF2v) in cultures that promote rapid expansion of the cells while preserving their chondrogenic potential. Chondrocytes cultured for 10 days with FGF2v yield 10 times as many cells as cultures without the growth factor and, most importantly, can generate, in mass cultures, extensive, highly differentiated, cartilage-like structures (Figure 14–31A). The cells are subsequently seeded throughout a three-dimensional scaffold composed of human plasma–derived fibrin and hyaluronic acid.

Fibrin is the naturally occurring matrix through which healing occurs in the human body. However, in marked contrast to a fibrin clot environment, this particularly designed scaffold does not support chondrocyte proliferation; rather, it provides the correct microenvironment for the embedded chondrocytes to express a mature chondrocyte phenotype and build up of ECM.

The scaffold is a highly porous structure (Figure 14–31B) that allows for even cell distribution (Figure 14–31C). This semisolid construct is unique because it combines the tensile, resistant, cross-linked fibrin fibers with the viscoelastic properties of an intercalated fibrinogen hyaluronan hydrogel. Such a unique composite provides enough mechanical resilience to support cell attachment and mechanical loads combined with a highly conductive microenvironment optimized to support cell survival and matrix deposition. Indeed, static mechanical testing demonstrated a dramatic increase in tensile strength a few days after cell seeding contributed by deposition of ECM, giving the implant distinct mechanical properties that allow it to be easily handled and cut to a defined shape during the implantation procedure.

The clinical experience with BioCart II has extended to the almost 100 BioCart II implantations performed to date. The majority of the recipients of the BioCart II have significantly improved by most measurable clinical parameters,[104] in good agreement with radiologic evidence by MRI demonstrating complete filling of defects after 1 and 2 years of follow-up in most implanted cases.[105] Most interesting is the very high rate of success in highly active individuals and athletes. This may be a result of the unique combination of a differentiation supportive environment with the mechanotransduction features of the BioCart II scaffold responding to the mechanical stimuli exerted during the enhanced and highly disciplined rehabilitation program of these particular patients.

It is rather ambitious to try and recapitulate the stepwise progression that occurs during normal chondrogenesis. However, understanding and successfully implementing some of the key necessary signals may guide the direction of cells along physiologic routes of differentiation, thereby dramatically improving the quality of the derived tissue and the clinical outcome.

Cartipatch

Second-Generation Autologous Chondrocyte Transplantation Technique

TBF Tissue Engineering Company (Mions, France) developed and validated Cartipatch, an autologous chondrocyte transplantation technique that includes a biomaterial scaffold designed according to the three following criteria:

1. Ability to obtain differentiated cells as a result of a three-dimensional environment
2. Ease of handling and implantation
3. Potential to make the transplanted chondrocytes evolve into an osteochondral functional tissue

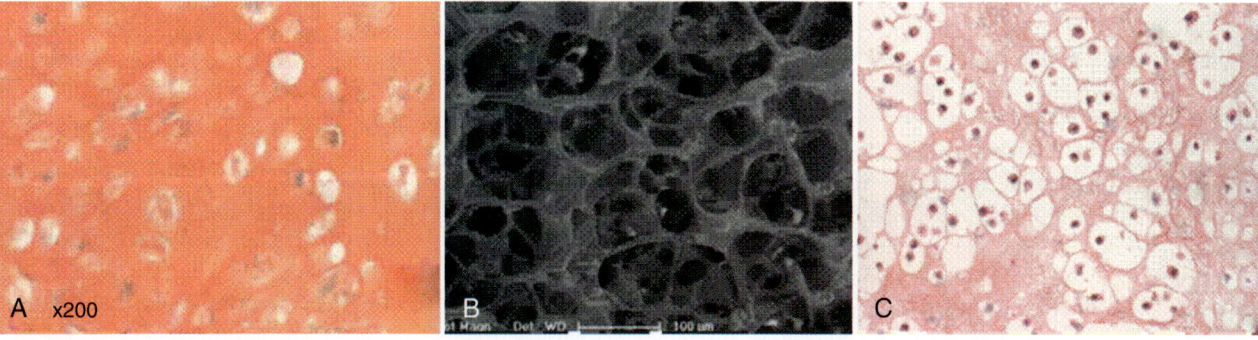

Figure 14–31 *A,* Standard mass pellet culture of chondrocytes cultured in vitro with FGF2v showing cartilage structure formed during the culture. *B,* Scanning electron micrograph of BioCart scaffold showing the porous structure of the matrix. *C,* Cross section of scaffold loaded with cells and stained with hematoxylin-eosin stain showing the cells distributed throughout the pores of the scaffold.

The combination of agarose and alginate was selected based on their safety and performance.[106-108] They both are of nonanimal origin, show high biocompatibility properties when properly purified, and can be steam sterilized. Once mixed with a cell suspension, the gel can be molded (at 37° C) into complex shape implants, which solidify at approximately 25° C in conditions that do not stress the cells. Even cell distribution is obtained by quick gelation. Hydrogel porosity allows culture medium diffusion, ensuring good cell viability. Alginate provides matrix elasticity,[109] improving ease of handling during production and surgery. Because the implant is not porous to cells once implanted, the biomaterial can protect the chondrocytes from immunogenic cells and allows cells maturation through protein synthesis. The hydrogel is patented in Europe (1 355 981), and a patent was submitted in the United States (2004-0047912).

Dedicated instrumentation was developed in order to press fit one or several premolded implants in the debrided lesion during an open knee surgical procedure. One or several cylindrical implants of various diameter, with a conical bottom, can be used to obtain adequate coverage of the lesion (Figure 14-32). The Cartipatch surgical procedure is easy, reproducible, and precise and can be performed within 1 hour.[110]

Chondrocyte viability and distribution in Cartipatch were validated in vitro. Cell potency and functionality were assessed after 14 days of incubation using both real-time quantitative PCR and immunostaining techniques. Real-time quantitative PCR showed a positive evolution of the ratio between type II and type I collagen when the expansion phase was compared with the incubation phase. Immunostaining showed that more than 50% of the chondrocytes included in the matrix were marked positively for both type II collagen and aggrecan.[111]

An in vivo proof of concept on agarose gel implanted in sheep condyles allowed development of a surgical procedure and evaluation of biocompatibility. At 6 months, a hyaline-type cartilaginous repair was observed. An in vivo safety and efficacy study on the final gel formulation is in progress, including condyle and trochlear implantation in 11 sheep up to 12 months. The preliminary results obtained after 6 months showed good cartilage repair.

The Cartipatch phase II prospective, multicenter clinical study (sponsored by TBF, main investigator Philippe Neyret, CHU de Lyon, period January 9, 2002, to January 6, 2006) enrolled 20 patients and was completed in 2006 after 2 years of follow-up.[112] The evaluation included clinical, radiologic, arthroscopic, and histologic parameters and allowed demonstration of the following:
1. Surgical feasibility of the Cartipatch technique
2. Absence of serious unexpected adverse events
3. First clinical encouraging results: significant improvement ($P < .001$ by t-test) of mean subjective IKDC score at 1 and 2 years (+39 and +41, respectively)

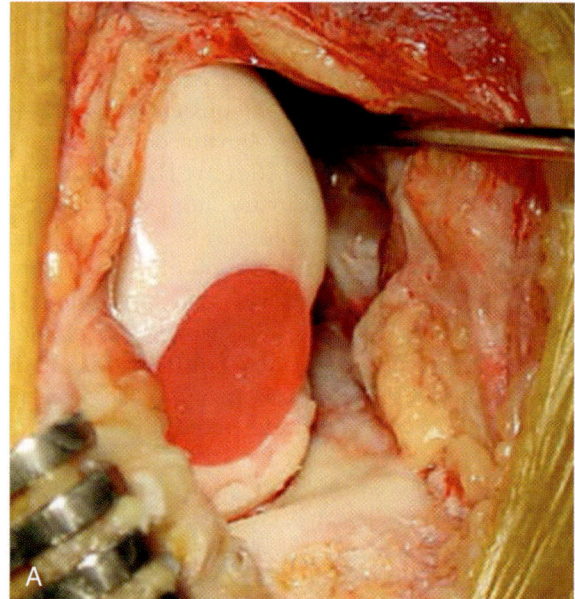
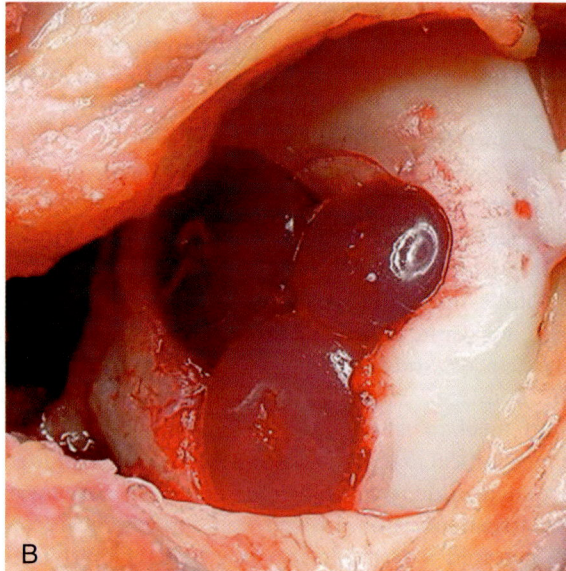

Figure 14-32 *A*, Cartipatch implantation: single implant. *B*, Cartipatch implantation: mosaic pattern.

4. Significant decrease of mean defect size measured by MRI, from 2.7 cm² preoperatively to 0.4 cm² at final follow-up ($P < .001$ by t-test)
5. Reconstruction of predominant hyaline-like cartilage observed in 8 of 13 biopsied patients and reconstruction of hyaline-like cartilage mixed with fibrocartilage in 3 of 13 patients
6. Both chondral and osteochondral reconstruction of the cartilage

Two separate phases III clinical multicentric studies comparing Cartipatch to mosaicplasty or microfracture are in progress.

THIRD-GENERATION CELL-BASED THERAPIES

NeoCart System

The Concept

The NeoCart autologous cartilage implant (Histogenics Corporation, Waltham, MA) is designed to restore articular cartilage of chondral lesions. The NeoCart system applies concepts of cell biology, materials science, and tissue engineering to develop, ex vivo, a regenerated tissue with the characteristics of hyaline neocartilage, that is, the NeoCart implant, when newly placed in the lesion, actively produces ECM components. At the same time, individual cells are continuing to divide and are free to migrate and exchange with the surrounding tissue. By simulating the biophysical and biochemical conditions in the joint environment, the chondrocytes retain their phenotype and respond with increased ECM production.

The NeoCart implant is produced by seeding autologous chondrocytes into a type I collagen honeycomb-type scaffold with through pores that permit diffusion of nutrients throughout the construct. This construct is placed in a tissue processor that regulates the hydrostatic pressure and oxygen levels to mimic the physiologic stresses experienced by chondrocytes in native articular cartilage within the joint.[113-123] This process results in a neocartilage with well-distributed chondrocytes in lacunae and ECM containing sulfated glycosaminoglycans and type II collagen. Implantation of this neocartilage will result in accelerated repair of the lesion site and continued maturity of the tissue into hyaline cartilage.

Fixation of the implant into the chondral lesion without adversely affecting adjacent tissue or underlying bone is a concern that has prompted investigation into alternatives to current techniques, such as sutures. In the NeoCart system, fixation is accomplished using a bioadhesive that is strong, biodegradable, biocompatible, and easy to use. It is composed of methylated collagen and polyethylene glycols (PEGs) that, when combined, polymerize to form a clear viscous solution that effectively seals the implant in the lesion, is an order of magnitude stronger than fibrin glue, and is more benign.

The Procedure

NeoCart uses non–weight-bearing cartilage retrieved by arthroscopic biopsy and digested with collagenase to isolate the chondrocytes. Once the cells have attained the desired expansion index in two-dimensional culture, they are transferred to the NeoCart type I collagen scaffold and placed in a tissue processor under hydrostatic pressure and low oxygen to promote ECM production (Figure 14–33).

Six to eight weeks after biopsy, the NeoCart implant, approximately 3 cm in diameter and 2 mm thick, is returned to the surgeon for implantation, which is performed via mini-arthrotomy. The lesion is debrided of all damaged tissue, and the calcified cartilage layer is removed carefully to avoid penetration of the subchondral plate and osseous bleeding into the site. The lesion site then is templated, and the NeoCart is cut to size using the template. NeoCart is secured by applying a thin layer of the proprietary bioadhesive CT3 onto the lesion bed prior to positioning the implant and then across the top of the NeoCart overlaying the adjacent cartilage.

Preclinical Animal Studies

In the porcine chondral defect model, NeoCart constructs, produced from autologous chondrocytes retrieved from the contralateral knee and grown in culture as described, were secured to 4-mm defect sites using the

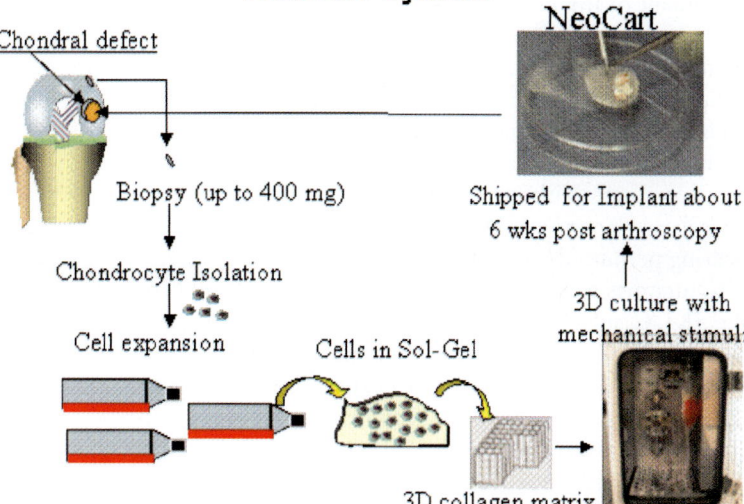
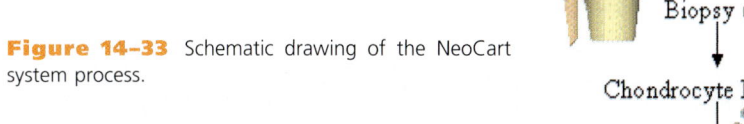

Figure 14–33 Schematic drawing of the NeoCart system process.

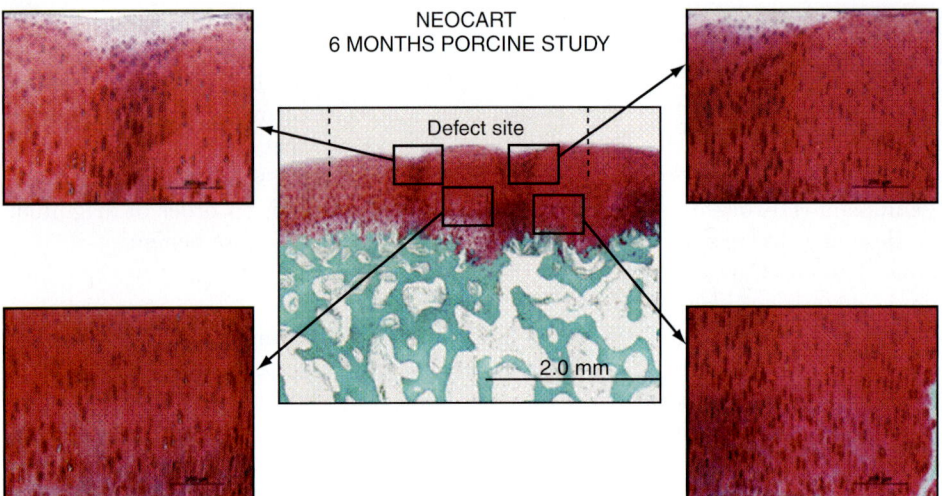

Figure 14-34 Photomicrograph of histologic section (stained with safranin O) of porcine chondral defect site 6 months after implantation with NeoCart. The NeoCart implant has integrated with the host tissue and has sulfated glycosaminoglycans (S-GAG) content and chondrocyte organization similar to that of the host.

bioadhesive. At 3 and 6 months after implantation, the NeoCart system demonstrated biocompatibility, with no inflammation or other adverse effects. Histologic evaluations of the defect sites at 6 months showed that chondrocytes in the defect site were oriented in a columnar fashion throughout the newly formed matrix and that the autologous implant was integrated well with the adjacent cartilage and subchondral bone. The chondrocytes in the NeoCart construct continued to produce ECM that, by 6 months, was equivalent to the host tissue (Figure 14-34).

Clinical Trials

A phase I clinical trial enrolled 10 patients and reported results up to 24 months for eight patients.[124] The first two of the 10 implantation procedures were unsuccessful because sutures that were used to augment the bioadhesive damaged the NeoCart implant when it was subjected to intraoperative range of motion. All subsequent procedures were sutureless, and intraoperative motion was limited to full extension for closure of the incision and placement of the knee immobilizer.

The rehabilitation program was analogous to that used after microfracture and ACI-type procedures and included use of a continuous passive motion machine for 6 hours per day during the 6 weeks after removal of the immobilizer approximately 10 days postsurgery.[2,125-129] In accordance with the protocols mentioned, the first 6 weeks were non-weight-bearing with unrestricted weight bearing permitted thereafter.

Outcomes were assessed using the VAS pain scale and the IKDC subjective score and by measuring range of motion. Clinical evaluations were performed at 6 and 12 weeks after surgery, at 6 and 12 months after surgery, and annually thereafter. As a secondary outcome, analysis of cartilage repair quality was evaluated by MRI obtained at 12 weeks after surgery, 6 and 12 months after surgery, and annually thereafter.

No serious adverse events associated with the NeoCart implant occurred, and the implant remained stable within the lesion site. A second-look arthroscopy performed on one patient 3 months after NeoCart implantation showed uniform fill with good integration to adjacent cartilage (Figure 14-35). By 12 months, all patients had decreased pain scores (average 0.9 ± 1.5) compared to baseline (average 3.3 ± 2.8). At 24 months, pain scores remained statistically significantly lower than baseline, and IKDC scores increased in 7 of 8 patients to 76 ± 17 from 57 ± 25 at baseline.

MRI evaluations showed that 7 of 8 patients had good to complete fill of the defect site and improved integration with the adjacent cartilage at 1 year, and 6 of 8 subjects had good to complete fill of the defect at 2 years. T2 mapping also was performed to assess the

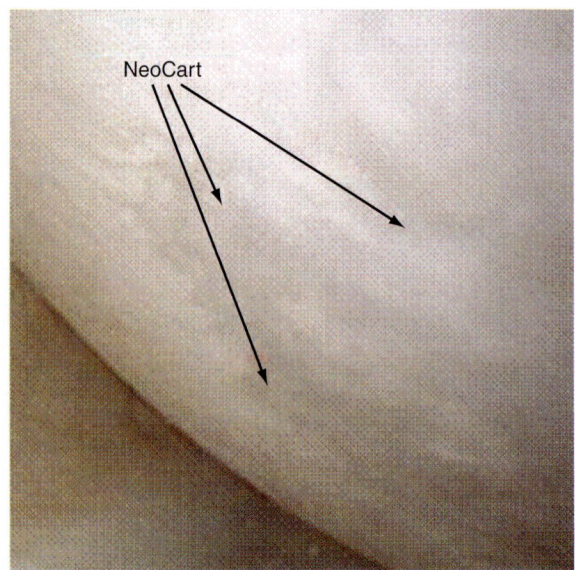

Figure 14-35 Second-look arthroscopy performed on a phase I patient 3 months after NeoCart implantation. Note excellent integration and fill throughout the lesion.

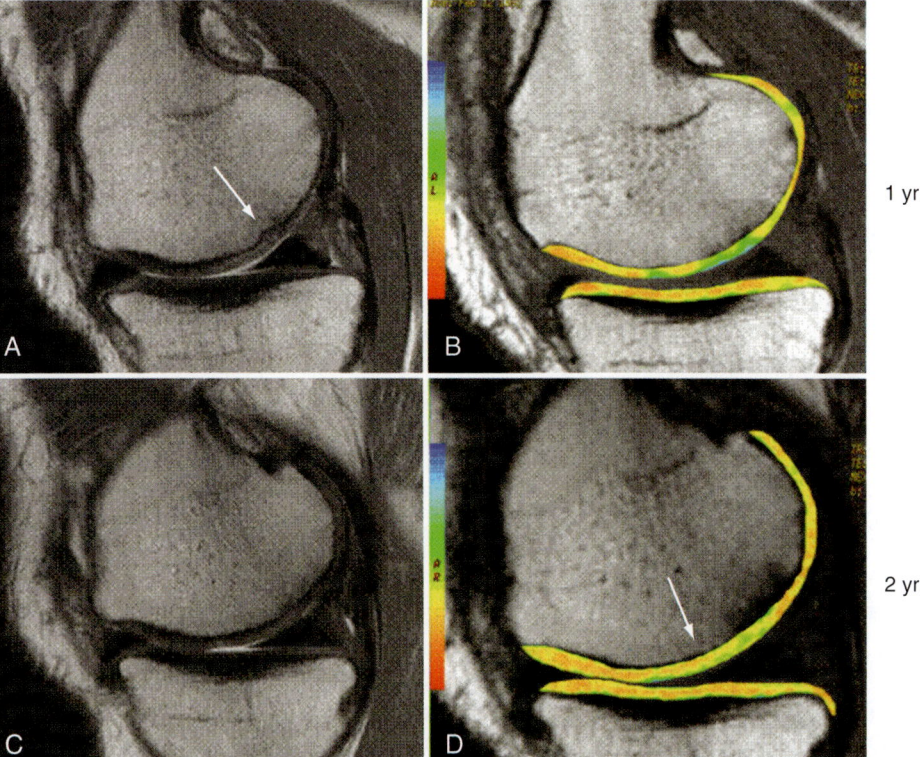

Figure 14–36 Sagittal magnetic resonance images taken 1 year (A, B) and 2 years (C, D) after NeoCart implantation. Fast spin-echo images (A, C) show good fill and progressive decrease in signal intensity. Corresponding T2 mapped images (B, D) show progressive matrix organization with partial stratification or layering at 2 years.

collagen matrix content and organization. Normal cartilage, when perpendicular to the magnetic field, has a laminar appearance or stratification.[130] At 24 months, 4 of 8 patients had stratification of T2 values similar to the adjacent cartilage (Figure 14–36).

These promising results led to a 30-patient prospective, randomized phase II trial that compared NeoCart to microfracture (2:1). Although patient enrollment and treatment have been completed, the 12-month data are still being collected and collated. Early results indicate similar trends to those seen in phase I with the NeoCart system.

The NeoCart System provides a biocompatible, neocartilage implant that remains stable within the site and matures in situ as the autologous chondrocytes within the construct continue to synthesize cartilage-specific ECM.

DeNovo Engineered Tissue Graft

DeNovo engineered tissue (ET) graft (Zimmer/ISTO Technologies) is a three-dimensional articular cartilage tissue (Figure 14–37) grown with cultured human juvenile chondrocytes. DeNovo ET graft is currently in a phase I/II clinical trial in the United States. After undergoing a phase III clinical trial, a Biologics License Application (BLA) will be submitted to the FDA for approval to commercialize the product. The primary chondrocytes used to produce DeNovo ET graft are obtained

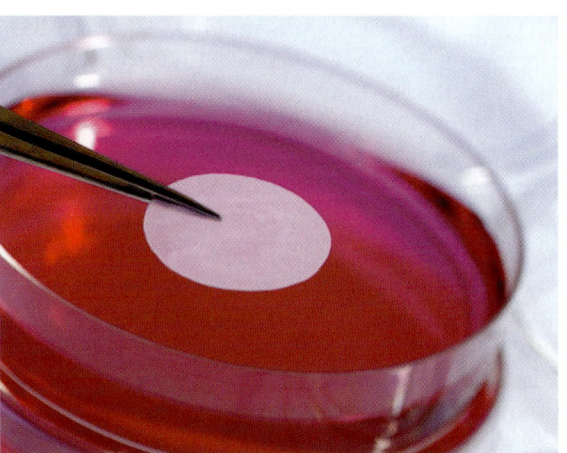

Figure 14–37 DeNovo engineered tissue (ET) graft can be handled with forceps and trimmed to required sizes to fill cartilage defects. A fibrin adhesive is applied to fix the graft in the defect.

by enzymatic digestion of donated juvenile cartilage. No fetal cartilage tissue is used. A proprietary cell expansion technology is then used to increase the number of cells. These expanded cells are subsequently cultured by a proprietary process to produce a large number of grafts for implantation. This process uses a defined serum-free medium *without* a scaffold, and the resulting engineered tissue can be physically handled with forceps and trimmed to required sizes to fill cartilage defects. A fibrin adhesive is used to fix the graft in the defect.

CONCLUSION

The field of cartilage repair is rapidly advancing. Many of the new techniques offer simplicity of application with less arduous rehabilitations and excellent clinical outcomes. They may offer improvements to existing techniques and have unique profiles that potentially could fill in the voids in existing treatment algorithms.

Assessment of procedural cost effectiveness will be difficult. Head-to-head comparative, randomized, blinded, multicenter clinical trials may be necessary. However, this has proved problematic in the past in obtaining homogeneous populations of injuries treated, surgical skill, and numbers.

The future of cartilage repair is bright. We now are able to treat and cure a problem that for centuries has been known to "be a troublesome thing."[2]

ACKNOWLEDGMENTS

I thank the following companies and their representatives for their contributions to this chapter: Matthew Shive, PhD (BioSyntech, Laval, Quebec, Canada); Claudio De Luca, PhD, and Daniele Presato (Fin-Ceramica Faenza S.p.A., Faenza, Italy); K. Martin, MD (Geistlich Pharma AG, Wolhusen, Switzerland); Gino Bradica, PhD (Kensey Nash Corp., Exton, PA); Ada Au, PhD (Advanced Biomaterials Group, Smith & Nephew Endoscopy, Andover, MA); Ben Byers, PhD, and Chris Kilburn-Peterson (DePuy Mitek, Raynham, MA); Jian Yao, PhD (Zimmer, Warsaw, IN); Steve Duguay, PhD, and Prudence Roaf (Genzyme Corp., Cambridge, MA); Alessandra Pavesio, PhD, Manuela Minto, PhD, and Cristina Longinotti, PhD (Fidia Advanced Biopolymers, Abano Terme, Italy); Micheline Wille (TiGenix N.V., Leuven, Belgium); Arthro Kinetics (Esslingen, Germany); ProChon (Ness Ziona, Israel); Laurence Barnouin and Gaelle Regeur (TBF Tissue Engineering Company, Mions, France); and Sonya Shortkroff, PhD (Histogenics Corp., Waltham, MA).

REFERENCES

1. Kumar M, Muzzarelli R, Muzzarelli C, et al. Chitosan Chemistry and Pharmaceutical Perspectives. *Chem Rev.* 2004;104:6017–6084.
2. Hunter W. On the structure and diseases of articulating cartilage. *Phil Trans R Soc Lond B Biol Sci.* 1743;9:267.
3. Chenite A, Chaput C, Wang D, et al. Novel injectable neutral solutions of chitosan form biodegradable gels in situ. *Biomaterials.* 2000;2155–2161.
4. Mattioli-Belmonte M, Muzzarelli B, Muzzarelli R. Chitin and chitosan in wound healing and other biomedical applications. *Carbohydrate Eur.* 1997;30–36.
5. Shive M, Hoemann C, Restrepo A, et al. BST-CarGel: In situ chondroinduction for cartilage repair. *Oper Tech Orthop.* 2006; 271–278.
6. Chevrier A, Hoemann C, Sun J, et al. Chitosan-glycerol phosphate/blood implants increase cell recruitment, transient vascularization and subchondral bone remodeling in drilled cartilage defects. *Osteoarthr Cartil.* 2007;316–327.
7. Buschmann MD, Hoemann CD, Hurtig M, Shive MS. Cartilage repair with chitosan/glycerol-phosphate stabilised blood clots. In: Williams RJ, ed. *Cartilage Repair Strategies.* Totowa, NJ: Humana Press; 2007:85–104.
8. Hoemann C, Hurtig M, Rossomacha E, et al. In situ chitosan-glycerol phosphate/blood implants significantly improve hyaline cartilage repair in ovine microfracture defects. *J Bone Joint Surg Am.* 2005;2671–2686.
9. Bellamy N, Buchanan W, Goldsmith C, et al. Validation study of WOMAC: a health status instrument for measuring clinically important patient relevant outcomes to antirheumatic drug therapy in patients with osteoarthritis of the hip or knee. *J Rheumatol.* 1988;1833–1840.
10. Mainil-Varlet P, Aigner T, Brittberg M, et al. Histological assessment of cartilage repair: a report by the Histology Endpoint Committee of the International Cartilage Repair Society (ICRS). *J Bone Joint Surg Am.* 2003;85-A:45–57.
11. Chevrier A, Hoemann C, Sun J, et al. Chitosan-glycerol phosphate/blood implants increase cell recruitment, transient vascularization and subchondral bone remodeling in drilled cartilage defects. *Osteoarthr Cartil.* 2005 in revision.
12. Hoemann C, Sun J, McKee M, et al. Chitosan-glycerol phosphate/blood implants elicit hyaline cartilage repair integrated with porous subchondral bone in microdrilled rabbit defects. *Osteoarthr Cartil.* 2007;15:78–89.
13. Tampieri A, Sandri M, Landi E, et al. Biomimetic hybrid composites to repair osteo-chondral lesions. *Key Eng Mater.* 2008;361–363: 927–930.
14. Tampieri A, Sandri M, Landi E, et al. Design of graded biomimetic osteo-chondral composite scaffolds. *Biomaterials.* 2008;29: 3539–3546.
15. Kon E, Delcogliano M, Filardo G, et al. Orderly osteochondral regeneration in a sheep model using a novel nano-composite multilayered biomaterial. *J Orthop Res.* 2010;28:116–124.
16. Fortier L, Mohammed H, Lust G, et al. Insulin-like growth factor-I enhances cell based repair of articular cartilage. *J Bone Joint Surg Br.* 2002;276–288.
17. Kon E, Delcogliano M, Filardo G, et al. Novel nano-composite multi-layered biomaterial for osteo-chondral regeneration: early stability evaluation. *Injury.* (Submitted).
18. Kon E, Delcogliano M, Filardo G, Altadonna G, Marcacci M. Novel nano-composite multi-layered biomaterial for the treatment of multifocal degenerative cartilage lesions. *Knee Surg Sports Traumatol Arthrosc.* Published online 26 May 2009.
19. Russlies M, Behrens P, Ehlers EM, et al. Periosteum stimulates subchondral bone densification in autologous chondrocyte transplantation in a sheep model. *Cell Tissue Res.* 2005;319:133–142.
20. Fuss M, Ehlers EM, Russlies M, Rohwedel J, Behrens P. Characteristics of human chondrocytes, osteoblasts and fibroblasts seeded onto a type I/III collagen sponge under different culture conditions. A light, scanning and transmission electron microscopy study. *Ann Anat.* 2000;182:303–310.
21. Gille J, Meisner U, Ehlers EM, et al. Migration pattern, morphology and viability of cells suspended in or sealed with fibrin glue: a histomorphologic study. *Tissue Cell.* 2005;37:339–348.
22. Russlies M, Behrens P, Wünsch L, Gille J, Ehlers EM. A cell-seeded biocomposite for cartilage repair. *Ann Anat.* 2002;184: 317–323.
23. Russlies M, Rüther P, Köller W, Stomberg P, Behrens P. Biomechanical properties of cartilage repair tissue after different cartilage repair procedures in sheep. *Z Orthop Ihre Grenzgeb.* 2003;141:465–471.
24. Scherer K, Schünke M, Sellckau R, Hassenpflug J, Kurz B. The influence of oxygen and hydrostatic pressure on articular chondrocytes and adherent bone marrow cells in vitro. *Biorheology.* 2004; 41:323–333.
25. Steinwachs M, Kreuz PC. Autologous chondrocyte implantation in chondral defects of the knee with a type I/III collagen membrane: a prospective study with a 3-year follow-up. *Arthroscopy.* 2007;23:381–387.
26. Niemeyer P, Kreuz PC, Steinwachs M, et al. Technical note: the "double eye" technique as a modification of autologous chondrocyte implantation for the treatment of retropatellar cartilage defects. *Knee Surg Sports Traumatol Arthrosc.* 2007;15:1461–1468.

27. Haddo O, Mahroof S, Higgs D, et al. The use of Chondro-Gide membrane in autologous chondrocyte implantation. *Knee*. 2004;11:51–55.
28. Steinwachs M, Kreuz PC. *Clinical Results of Autologous Chondrocyte Transplantation Using a Collagen Membrane, in Cartilage Surgery and Future Perspectives*. Berlin: Springer Verlag; 2003:37–47.
29. Bentley G, Biant LC, Carrington RW, et al. A prospective, randomised comparison of autologous chondrocyte implantation versus mosaicplasty for osteochondral defects in the knee. *J Bone Joint Surg Br*. 2003;85:223–230.
30. Briggs TW, Mahroof S, David LA, et al. Histological evaluation of chondral defects after autologous chondrocyte implantation of the knee. *J Bone Joint Surg Am*. 2003;85:1077–1083.
31. Steinwachs M. New technique for cell-seeded collagen matrix-supported autologous chondrocyte transplantation. *Arthroscopy*. 2009;25:208–211.
32. Niemeyer P, Pestka J, Kreuz M, et al. Characteristic complications after autologous chondrocyte implantation for cartilage defects of the knee joint. *Am J Sports Med*. 2008;36:2091–2099.
33. Behrens P. Matrixgekoppelte mikrofrakturierung. *Arthroskopie*. 2005;193–197.
34. Kramer J, Bohrnsen F, Lindner U, et al. In vivo matrix-guided human mesenchymal stem cells. *Cell Mol Life Sci*. 2006;63:616–626.
35. Steck E, Fischer J, Lorenz H, et al. Mesenchymal stem cell differentiation in an experimental cartilage defect: restriction of hypertrophy to bone-close neocartilage. *Stem Cells Dev*. 2009;18:969–978.
36. Kusano T, Jacobi R, Jakob P. AMIC: Treatment of chondral and osteochondral defects of the knee. *Leading Opin Orthop*. 2007.
37. Wendler NO, et al. Ein neues Therapiekonzept zur Knorpeldefektbehandlung. *Med Rev*. 2006;7:2.
38. Wendler NO, et al. *Autologous Matrix-Induced Chondrogenesis (AMIC) mid-term results*. Universitätsklinikum Schleswig-Holstein; 2008.
39. Anders S, et al. Autologous matrix induced chondrogenesis (AMIC) for focal chondral defects of the knee—first results. In: EFFORT 2007. Florence, Italy: 2007.
40. Steinwachs MR, Guggi T, Kreuz PC. Marrow stimulation techniques. *Injury*. 2008;39(suppl 1):S26–S31.
41. Valderrabano V, et al. The AMIC technique: new option for osteochondral defects of the Talus. *Leading Opin*. 2008;04/2008:34–36.
42. Cameron H. Tricalcium phosphate as a bone graft substitute. *Contemp Orthop*. 1992;25:506–508.
43. Vaccaro A. The role of the osteoconductive scaffold in synthetic bone graft. *Orthopedics*. 2002;571–578.
44. Bostman O. Absorbable implants for the fixation of fractures. *J Bone Joint Surg Br*. 1991;73:148–153.
45. Hollinger J, Battistone G. Biodegradable bone repair materials: Synthetic polymers and ceramics. *Clin Orthop Relat Res*. 1986;290–305.
46. Ahern BJ, Engiles J, Underwood C, et al. *Single site osteochondral resurfacing – an in vivo caprine study*. Paper presented at: International Cartilage Repair Society 2009 Meeting; Miami, FL: May 26, 2009.
47. Fortier LA, McCarrel TM, Bradica G, et al. *Evaluation of a biphasic graft for osteochondral repair in an equine model*. Paper presented at: International Cartilage Repair Society 2009 Meeting; Miami, FL: May 26; 2009.
48. Slivka M, Leatherbury N, Kieswetter K, et al. Porous, resorbable, fiber-reinforced scaffolds tailored for articular cartilage repair. *Tissue Eng*. 2001;767–780.
49. Gao C, Gao J, You X, et al. Fabrication of Calcium Sulphate/PLLA Composite for Bone Repair. *J Biomed Mater Res A*. 2005;244–253.
50. Pecora G, De Leonardis D, Ibrahim N, et al. The use of calcium sulphate in the surgical treatment of a "through and through" periradicular lesion. *Int Endod J*. 2001;189–197.
51. Advanced Biomaterials Group. *Cartilage/bone repair using TRUFIT CB implants*. Technical white paper, Andover, MA: Smith & Nephew Endoscopy; 2009.
52. Spalding T. *TRUFIT CB plugs for articular cartilage repair in the knee: Early experience and important considerations*. Presentation at the 28th Annual Meeting of the Arthroscopy Association of North America; 2009.
53. Carmont M, Carey-Smith R, Saithna A, et al. Delayed incorporation of TRUFIT plug: perseverance is recommended. *Arthroscopy*. 2009;25:810–814.
54. Saris D, Vanlauwe J, Victor J, et al. Characterized chondrocyte implantation results in better structural repair when treating symptomatic cartilage defects of the knee in a randomized controlled trial versus microfracture. *Am J Sports Med*. 2008;236–246.
55. Zheng, et al. *J Musculoskel Res*. 2008;11:151–159.
56. Lu Y, Dhanaraj S, Wang Z, et al. Minced cartilage without cell culture serves as an effective intraoperative cell source for cartilage repair. *J Orthop Res*. 2006;24:1261–1270.
57. Farr J. DeNovo NT Natural Tissue Graft. 8th World Congress of International Cartilage Repair Society. Miami, FL: May 2009:182.
58. Abelow S, Guillen P, Ramos T. Arthroscopic technique for matrix-induced autologous chondrocyte implantation for the treatment of large chondral defects in the knee and ankle. *Oper Tech Orthop*. 2006;16:257–261.
59. Zilko S, Woodhouse J, Smith A, et al. *A prospective clinical evaluation of Matrix-Induced Autologous Chondrocyte Implantation (MACI) at five years*. Paper presented at: 8th World Congress of the International Cartilage Repair Society, Miami, Florida: 2009.
60. Behrens P, Bitter T, Kurz B, et al. Matrix-associated autologous chondrocyte transplantation/implantation (MACT/MACI)-5-year follow-up. *Knee*. 2006;13:194–202.
61. Bartlett W, Gooding C, Carrington R, et al. Autologous chondrocyte implantation at the knee using a bilayer collagen membrane with bone graft. A preliminary report. *J Bone Joint Surg Br*. 2005;87:330–332.
62. Bartlett W, Flanagan A, Gooding C, et al. Autologous chondrocyte implantation versus matrix-induced autologous chondrocyte implantation for osteochondral defects of the knee: A prospective, randomised study. *J Bone Joint Surg Br*. 2005;87:640–645.
63. Amin A, Bartlett W, Gooding C, et al. The use of autologous chondrocyte implantation following and combined with anterior cruciate ligament reconstruction. *Int Orthop*. 2006;30:48–53.
64. Cherubino P, Grassi F, Bulgheroni P, Ronga M. Autologous chondrocyte implantation using a bilayer collagen membrane: a preliminary report. *J Orthop Surg (Hong Kong)*. 2003;11:10–15.
65. Ronga M, Grassi F, Bulgheroni P. Arthroscopic autologous chondrocyte implantation for the treatment of a chondral defect in the tibial plateau of the knee. *Arthroscopy*. 2004;20:79–84.
66. Ronga M, Grassi F, Montoli C, et al. Treatment of deep cartilage defects of the ankle with matrix-induced autologous chondrocyte implantation (MACI). *Foot Ankle Surg*. 2005;11:29–33.
67. Bachmann G, Basad E, Lommel D, et al. MRI in the follow-up after MACI(R) or microfracture [German]. *Radiologe*. 2004;44:773–782.
68. Marlovits S, Striessnig G, Kutscha-Lissberg F, et al. Early postoperative adherence of matrix-induced autologous chondrocyte implantation for the treatment of full-thickness cartilage defects of the femoral condyle. *Knee Surg Sports Traumatol Arthrosc*. 2005;13:451–457.
69. D'Anchise R, Manta N, Prospero E, et al. Autologous implantation of chondrocytes on a solid collagen scaffold: clinical and histological outcomes after two years of follow-up. *J Orthop Traumatol*. 2005;6:36–43.
70. Marcacci M, Kon E, Zaffagnini S, et al. New cell-based technologies in bone and cartilage tissue engineering. II. Cartilage regeneration. *Chir Organi Mov*. 2003;42–47.
71. Marcacci M, Zaffagnini S, Kon E, et al. Second generation ACI technique. *Am Acad Orthop Surg*. 2003;49–58.
72. Campoccia D, Doherty P, Radice M, et al. Semisynthetic resorbable materials from hyaluronan esterification. *Biomaterials*. 1998;2101–2127.
73. Benya P, Shaffer J. Dedifferentiated chondrocytes reexpress the differentiated collagen phenotype when cultured in agarose gels. *Cell*. 1982;30:215–224.
74. Grigolo B, Lisignoli G, Piacentini A, et al. Evidence for redifferentiation of human chondrocytes grown on a hyaluronan-based biomaterial (HYAFFs11): molecular, immunohistochemical and ultrastructural analysis. *Biomaterials*. 2002;1187–1195.

75. Grigolo B, Roseti L, Fiorini M, et al. Cathepsin B as a soluble marker to monitor the phenotypic stability of engineered cartilage. *Biomaterials.* 2003;1751–1757.
76. Tognana E, Chen F, Padera R, et al. Adjacent tissues (cartilage, bone) affect the functional integration of engineered calf cartilage in vitro. *Osteoarthr Cartil.* 2005;129–138.
77. Schlegel W, Nürnberger S, Hombauer M, et al. Scaffold-dependent differentiation of human articular chondrocytes. *Int J Mol Med.* 2008;691–699.
78. Aigner J, Tegeler J, Hutzler P, et al. Cartilage tissue engineering with novel nonwoven structured biomaterial based on hyaluronic acid benzyl ester. *J Biomed Mater Res.* 1998;(Part A):172–181.
79. Grigolo B, Roseti L, Fiorini M, et al. Transplantation of chondrocytes seeded on a hyaluronan derivative (hyaff-11) into cartilage defects in rabbits. *Biomaterials.* 2001;22:2417–2424.
80. Solchaga L, Dennis J, Goldberg V, et al. Hyaluronic acid-based polymers as cell carriers for tissue-engineered repair of bone and cartilage. *J Orthop Res.* 1999;205–213.
81. Solchaga L, Yoo J, Lundberg M, et al. Hyaluronan-based polymers in the treatment of osteochondral defects. *J Orthop Res.* 2000;773–780.
82. Solchaga L, Temenoff J, Gao J, et al. Repair of osteochondral defects with hyaluronan- and polyester-based scaffolds. *Osteoarthr Cartil.* 2005;297–309.
83. Buma report, data on file 1999, internal Fidia files.
84. Busetto report, data on file 2001, internal Fidia files.
85. Pavesio A, Abatangelo G, Borrione A, et al. Hyaluronan-based scaffolds (Hyalograft C) in the treatment of knee cartilage defects: preliminary clinical findings. *Novartis Found Symp.* 2003;249:203–217.
86. Marcacci M, Zaffagnini S, Kon E, Viscellari A. Second generation ACI technique. *Am Acad Orthop Surg.* 2003;6:49–58.
87. Marcacci M, Berruto M, Brocchetta D, et al. Articular cartilage engineering with Hyalograft C: 3-year clinical results. *Clin Orthop Relat Res.* 2005;96–105.
88. Kon E, Gobbi A, Filardo G, et al. Arthroscopic second-generation autologous chondrocyte implantation compared with microfracture for chondral lesions of the knee: prospective nonrandomized study at 5 years. *Am J Sports Med.* 2009;37:33–41.
89. Hollander A, Dickinson S, Sims T, et al. Maturation of tissue engineered cartilage implanted in injured and osteoarthritic human knees. *Tissue Eng.* 2006;1787–1798.
90. Brun P, Dickinson S, Zavan B, et al. Characteristics of repair tissue in second-look and third-look biopsies from patients treated with engineered cartilage: relationship to symptomatology and time after implantation. *Arthritis Res Ther.* 2008;10:R132.
91. Trattnig S, Pinker K, Krestan C, et al. Matrix-based autologous chondrocyte implantation for cartilage repair with Hyalograft C: two-year follow-up by magnetic resonance imaging. *Eur J Radiol.* 2006;9–15.
92. Marlovits S, Striessnig G, Resinger C, et al. Definition of pertinent parameters for the evaluation of articular cartilage repair tissue with high-resolution magnetic resonance imaging. *Eur J Radiol.* 2004;310–319.
93. Marlovits S, Singer P, Zeller P, et al. Magnetic resonance observation of cartilage repair tissue (MOCART) for the evaluation of autologous chondrocyte transplantation: determination of interobserver variability and correlation to clinical outcome after 2 years. *Eur J Radiol.* 2006;16–23.
94. Giannini S, Buda R, Vannini F, et al. Arthroscopic autologous chondrocyte implantation in osteochondral lesions of the talus: surgical technique and results. *Am J Sports Med.* 2008;873–880.
95. Marcacci M, Berruto M, Brocchetta D, et al. Articular cartilage engineering with Hyalograft C: 3-year clinical results. *Clin Orthop Relat Res.* 2005;435:96–105.
96. Marcacci report, data on file, 2006.
97. Marlovits S, Zeller P, Singer P, et al. Cartilage repair: generations of autologous chondrocyte transplantation. *Eur J Radiol.* 2006;57:24–31.
98. Marlovits and Nehrer report, data on file, 2004.
99. Ferruzzi A, Buda R, Faldini C, et al. Autologous chondrocyte implantation in the knee joint: open compared with arthroscopic technique. Comparison at a minimum follow-up of five years. *J Bone Joint Surg Am.* 2008;90–101.
100. Kon E, Gobbi A, Filardo G, et al. Arthroscopic second-generation autologous chondrocyte implantation compared with microfracture for chondral lesions of the knee: prospective nonrandomized study at 5 years. *Am J Sports Med.* 2009;33–41.
101. Gobbi A, Kon E, Berruto M, et al. Patellofemoral full-thickness chondral defects treated with second-generation autologous chondrocyte implantation: results at 5 years' follow-up. *Am J Sports Med.* 2009;1083–1092.
102. Dell'Accio F, De Bari C, Luyten F. Molecular markers predictive of the capacity of expanded human articular chondrocytes to form stable cartilage in vivo. *Arthritis Rheum.* 2001;44:1608–1619.
103. Dell'Accio F, De Bari C, Luyten F. Microenvironment and phenotypic stability specify tissue formation by human articular cartilage-derived cells in vivo. *Exp Cell Res.* 2003;287:16–27.
104. Nehrer S, Chiari C, Domayer S, et al. Results of chondrocyte implantation with a fibrin-hyaluronan matrix: a preliminary study. *Clin Orthop Relat Res.* 2008;466:1849–1855.
105. Domayer SE, Welsch GH, Nehrer S, et al. T2 mapping and dGEMRIC after autologous chondrocyte implantation with a fibrin-based scaffold in the knee: Preliminary results. *Eur J Radiol.* 2010;73:636–642.
106. Rahfoth B, Weisser J, Sternkopf F, et al. Transplantation of allograft chondrocytes embedded in agarose gel into cartilage defects of rabbits. *Osteoarthr Cartil.* 1998;6:50–65.
107. De Vos P, De Haan BJ, Wolters GH, et al. Improved biocompatibility but limited graft survival after purification of alginate for microencapsulation of pancreatic islets. *Diabetologia.* 1997;40:262–270.
108. Wong M. Alginates in tissue engineering. *Methods Mol Biol.* 2004;238:77–86.
109. Hutmacher DW, Ng KW, Kaps C, et al. Elastic cartilage engineering using novel scaffold architectures in combination with a biomimetic cell carrier. *Biomaterials.* 2003;24:4445–4458.
110. Selmi TA, Verdonk P, Barnouin L, Neyret P. Surgical technique: Autologous chondrocyte transplantation in combination with an alginate-agarose based hydrogel (CARTIPATCH). *Tech Knee Surg.* (In press).
111. Selmi TA, Barnouin L, Bussiere C, Neyret P. CARTIPATCH. In: Zanasi S, Brittberg M, Marcacci M, eds. Basic science, clinical repair and reconstruction of articular cartilage defects: current status and prospects. 2006:431–438.
112. Selmi TA, Verdonk P, Chambat P, et al. Autologous chondrocyte implantation in a novel alginate-agarose hydrogel: outcome at 2 years. *J Bone Joint Surg Br.* 2008;90:597–604.
113. Mizuno S, Tateishi T, Ushida T, et al. Hydrostatic fluid pressure enhances matrix synthesis and accumulation by bovine chondrocytes in three-dimensional culture. *J Cell Physiol.* 2002;193:319–327.
114. Mizuno S, Glowacki J. Low oxygen tension enhances chondroinduction by demineralized bone matrix in human dermal fibroblasts in vitro. *Cells Tissues Organs.* 2005;180:151–158.
115. Glowacki J, Mizuno S. Collagen scaffolds for tissue engineering. *Biopolymers.* 2008;89:338–344.
116. Smith R, Rusk S, Ellison B, et al. In vitro stimulation of articular chondrocyte mRNA and extracellular matrix synthesis by hydrostatic pressure. *J Orthop Res.* 1996;14:53–60.
117. Smith RL, Lin J, Trindade MC, et al. Time-dependent effects of intermittent hydrostatic pressure on articular chondrocyte type II collagen and aggrecan mRNA expression. *J Rehabil Res Dev.* 2000;37:53–61.
118. Ikenoue T, Trindade MC, Lee M, et al. Mechanoregulation of human articular chondrocyte aggrecan and type II collagen expression by intermittent hydrostatic pressure in vitro. *J Orthop Res.* 2003;21:110–116.
119. Smith RL, Carter D, Schurman D. Pressure and shear differentially alter human articular chondrocyte metabolism: a review. *Clin Orthop Relat Res.* 2004;(suppl 427):S89–S95.
120. Wernike E, Li Z, Alini M, et al. Effect of reduced oxygen tension and long-term mechanical stimulation on chondrocyte-polymer constructs. *Cell Tissue Res.* 2008;331:473–483.
121. Kawanishi M, Oura A, Furukawa K, et al. Redifferentiation of dedifferentiated bovine articular chondrocytes enhanced by cyclic hydrostatic pressure under a gas-controlled system. *Tissue Eng.* 2007;13:957–964.

122. Domm C, Schünke M, Steinhagen J, et al. Influence of various alginate brands on the redifferentiation of dedifferentiated bovine articular chondrocytes in alginate bead culture under high and low oxygen tension. *Tissue Eng*. 2004;10(11–12):1796–1805.
123. Kurz B, Domm C, Jin M, et al. Tissue engineering of articular cartilage under the influence of collagen I/III membranes and low oxygen tension. *Tissue Eng*. 2004;10(7–8):1277–1286.
124. Williams 3rd RJ, Harnly HW. Microfracture: indications, technique, and results. *Instr Course Lect*. 2007;56:419–428.
125. Mithoefer K, Williams 3rd RJ, Warren RF, et al. Chondral resurfacing of articular cartilage defects in the knee with the microfracture technique. Surgical technique. *J Bone Joint Surg Am*. 2006;88(suppl 1 Pt 2):294–304.
126. Reinold MM, Wilk KE, Macrina LC, et al. Current concepts in the rehabilitation following articular cartilage repair procedures in the knee. *J Orthop Sports Phys Ther*. 2006;36(10):774–794.
127. Mithoefer K, Williams III R, Warren R, et al. The microfracture technique for the treatment of articular cartilage lesions in the knee. A prospective cohort study. *J Bone Joint Surg Am*. 2005;87:1911–1920.
128. Steadman JR, Rodkey WG, Briggs KK. Microfracture to treat full-thickness chondral defects: surgical technique, rehabilitation, and outcomes. *J Knee Surg*. 2002;15:170–176.
129. Steadman JR, Rodkey WG, Rodrigo JJ. Microfracture: surgical technique and rehabilitation to treat chondral defects. *Clin Orthop Relat Res*. 2001;391(suppl):S362–S369.
130. Potter HG, Foo LF. Magnetic resonance imaging of articular cartilage: trauma, degeneration, and repair. *Am J Sports Med*. 2006;34:661–677.

PART 4

EARLY INTERVENTION IN OSTEOARTHRITIS

Patellofemoral Arthroplasty

Tom Minas, MD, MS

INTRODUCTION
INDICATIONS
SURGICAL TECHNIQUE
RESULTS
CONCLUSIONS

INTRODUCTION

Anterior knee pain is a common symptom complex affecting young active adults. It represents a spectrum of disease ranging from intact articular surfaces with soft tissue imbalance and obvious patellofemoral maltracking with focal articular cartilage loss to end-stage bone-on-bone osteoarthritis. Treatment options range from conservative methods of physical therapy and patellar taping, intraarticular viscosupplementation, arthroscopic debridement and patellar lateral release, proximal soft tissue and/or distal tibial tubercle realignment procedures, and the addition of cartilage repair procedures, when indicated, to patellofemoral arthroplasty or total knee arthroplasty. A stepwise approach from conservative nonoperative measures to more invasive measures usually is followed clinically.

Isolated patellofemoral arthritis occurs in approximately 5% to 10% of patients undergoing prosthetic replacement. A radiographic study of 206 patients attending an outpatient orthopedic clinic with arthritis of the knee revealed that 9.2% of the patients had isolated patellofemoral arthritis.[1]

Complete loss of the patellofemoral radiographic joint space as noted by tangential skyline radiographic and lateral x-ray films of the knee is a contraindication to isolated osteotomy alone or in combination with cartilage repair. If the tibiofemoral joint remains intact with neutral alignment, isolated patellofemoral arthroplasty is possible.

Ideally, the goals of a patellofemoral prosthesis include alleviation of patellofemoral symptoms and improved functionality. The prosthetic design should be conservative and joint preserving. The trochlea implant should remove minimal bone stock and allow mismatch of sizes between the trochlea and patella with minimal incongruity. A trochlea design should allow for deep flexion prior to the patella prosthesis disengaging the trochlea prosthesis so that the native tibiofemoral cartilage is not abraded by the polyethylene patella (Figure 15–1).[2] Implant characteristics should include a design based on existing total knee arthroplasty models such that implant failure or progression of tibiofemoral arthritis would allow easy conversion to total knee arthroplasty while retaining the existing patella prosthesis.

Argenson et al[3] proposed a useful clinical categorization of osteoarthritis of the patellofemoral joint: (1) secondary to dysplasia, (2) osteoarthritis involving primarily the patellofemoral joint, and (3) posttraumatic osteoarthritis in the patellofemoral joint secondary to patellar fracture. The group with dysplasia was the youngest group of patients in the series. They generally had a chronic history of patellar maltracking. Realignment surgery was frequent prior to prosthetic reconstruction. The long-term results of the first group, the dysplastic group, was the best in the series. This is not unexpected because these patients generally had normal tibiofemoral alignment and did not have a propensity to osteoarthritis because their arthritic condition was secondary to dysplasia of the trochlea and with abnormal shear forces and secondary osteoarthritis. The second group, the osteoarthritic group, was the most unpredictable. These patients generally did well in the first 5 years; however, progression of tibiofemoral joint arthritis was the source of joint failure.

INDICATIONS

Indications for patellofemoral arthroplasty include end-stage patellofemoral osteoarthritis secondary to patellofemoral dysplasia, osteoarthritis, and patellar fracture as noted by Argenson et al.[3] Contraindications to the procedure include patella infera and inflammatory arthritis. Relative contraindications include age approaching that for total knee arthroplasty (i.e., 60s), crystal arthropathy, and tibiofemoral malalignment (Figure 15–2).

Patellofemoral replacement is used as a transition operation for patients prior to total knee arthroplasty. The younger the patient with end-stage patellofemoral arthritis, the more likely a patellofemoral prosthesis, including osteochondral graft transfer to early damage in the tibiofemoral joint (Figure 15–3) or excepting mild malalignment of the tibiofemoral joint (Figure 15–4), will be used rather than total knee arthroplasty with subsequent early failure of part of the joint. Conversion to total knee arthroplasty in a young patient has not always been necessary if isolated unicompartmental replacement could be performed in addition to leaving the existing patellofemoral replacement (Figure 15–5). In my experience, patients are in their 40s and early 50s when patellofemoral arthroplasty is performed. When patients present with patellofemoral dysplasia, they frequently have a longstanding history of recurrent instability and prior surgeries, frequently including tibial tubercle realignment osteotomy. Some patients undergo

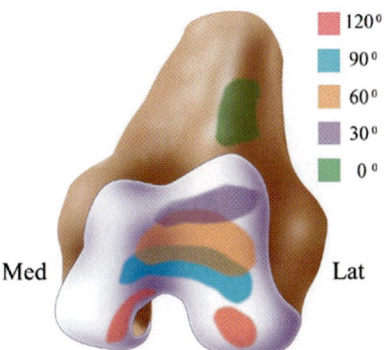

Figure 15-1 Diagrammatic representation of the articular surface contact areas in the trochlea between zero and 120 degrees. (From Aglietti P, Insall JN, Walker PS, et al: A new patella prosthesis. *Clin Orthop Relat Res* 1975;107:175.) At 120 degrees, the patella comes into the femoral weight-bearing surfaces. A trochlea prosthetic design should cover all of the trochlea to the sulcus terminalis of the medial and lateral anterior weight-bearing surfaces. Polyethylene on the patella surface is very abrasive to the articular cartilage and will erode any uncovered trochlea surface, potentially causing further pain and failure of a patellofemoral procedure.

The prosthesis itself generally did not fail. The third group, with posttraumatic patellar fracture, also did well as long as they did not have patella infera. Patella infera with a polyethylene resurfacing patella results in premature abrasive changes to the articular surface of the tibiofemoral joint and failure of the joint.

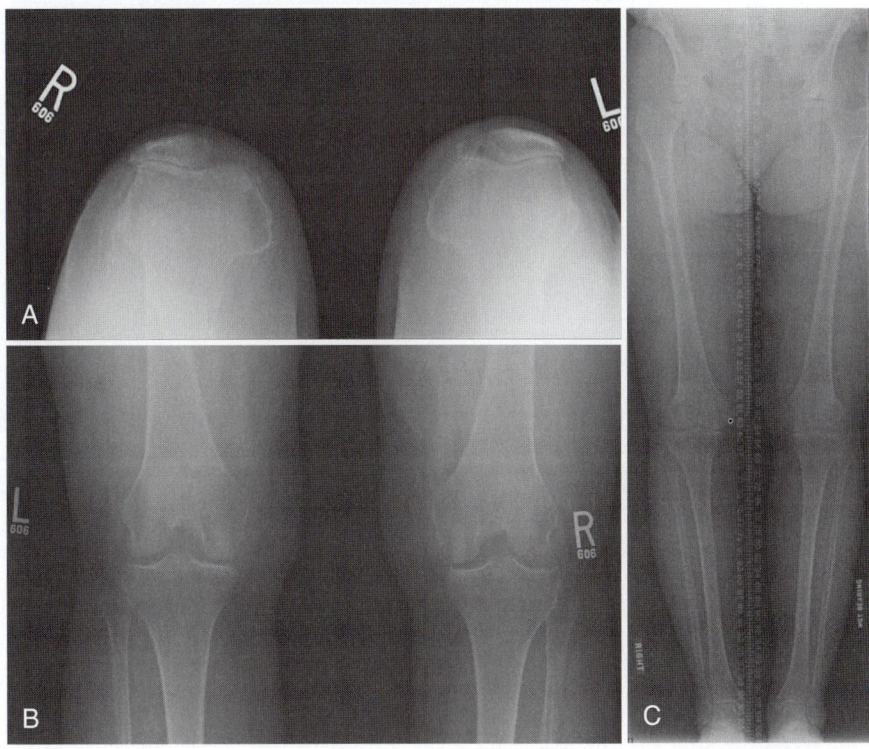

Figure 15-2 *A*, Skyline x-ray film of a 60-year-old man with end-stage patellofemoral osteoarthritis. *B*, Standing anteroposterior radiographs demonstrate medial compartment joint space narrowing. *C*, Long alignment x-ray film demonstrates mechanical axis falling into the medial compartment. This patient would be more suited for a total knee replacement because of presence of varus alignment, early medial joint space narrowing, end-stage patellofemoral arthritis, and age approaching that at which total knee arthroplasty usually is performed. Patellofemoral replacement in this situation usually fails due to progression of disease in the medial compartment.

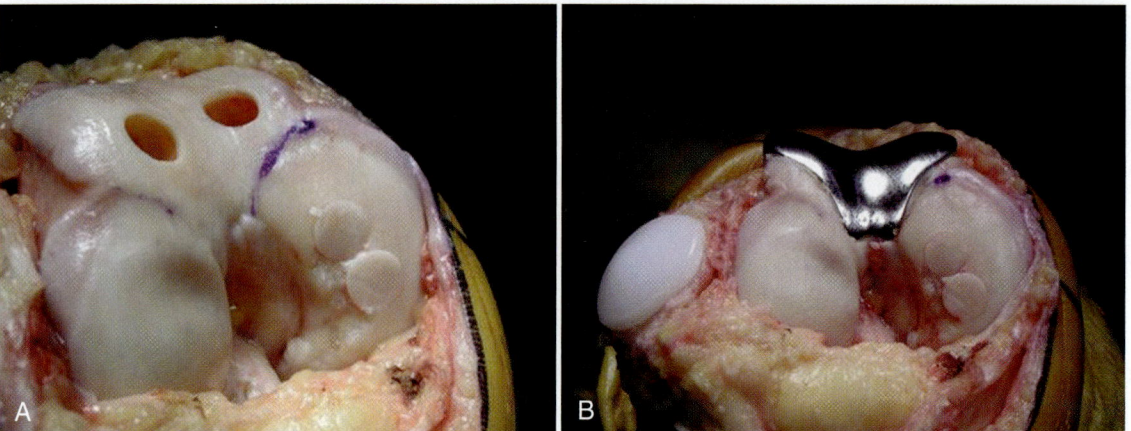

Figure 15–3 *A,* A 38-year-old woman undergoing patellofemoral replacement surgery. She has end-stage superior lateral patellofemoral osteoarthritis with subluxation. The distal end of the trochlea remains intact. The sulcus terminalis of the medial and lateral weight-bearing surfaces is marked with a blue marking pen. Medial femoral condyle Outerbridge grade IV wear measures approximately 20 mm in length. Rather than performing total knee replacement in this 38-year-old woman, two osteochondral plugs, 10 mm in diameter each, are harvested from the remaining healthy distal trochlea cartilage and transplanted to the medial femoral condyles as shown. *B,* Final appearance of a patellofemoral replacement (Avon Stryker Howmedica) positioned over the trochlea and osteochondral donor sites. Osteochondral graft transfer is intact. Such hybrid procedures (combination of prosthesis and biologic repair) are more common in younger patients in order to preserve the joint.

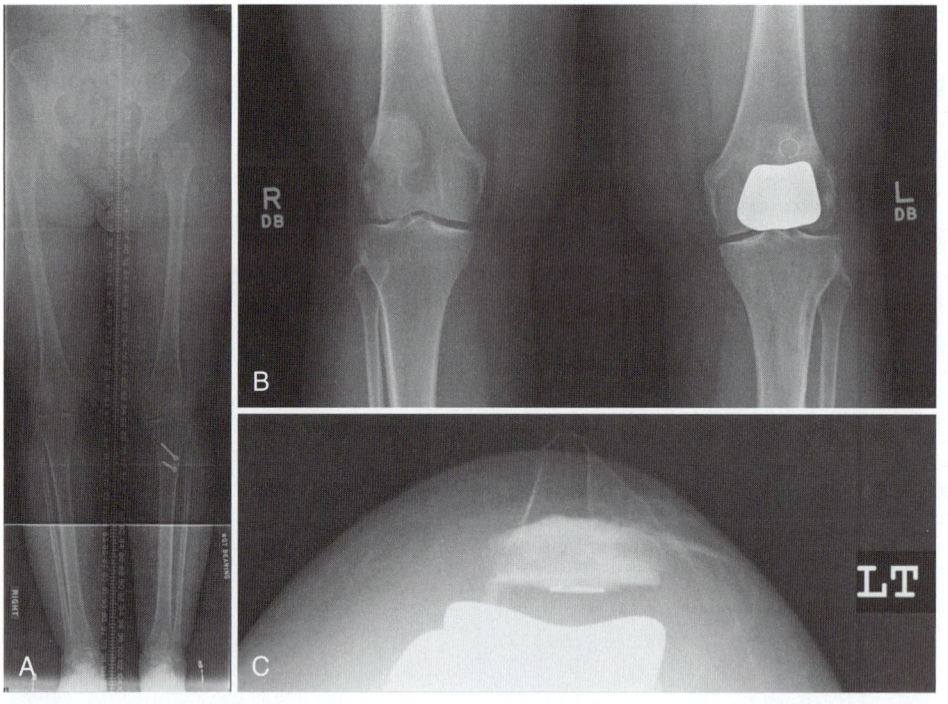

Figure 15–4 *A,* Long alignment x-ray film of a 40-year-old woman who has undergone previous tibial tubercle osteotomy for patellofemoral instability and arthrosis. Although the medial joint compartment remains intact, the mechanical axis falls to the center of the medial compartment. *B,* Standing anteroposterior x-ray film 1 year postoperative demonstrating intact tibiofemoral joint space and patellofemoral prosthesis. *C,* Skyline x-ray film 1 year postoperative shows well-functioning patellofemoral prosthesis.

tibial tubercle osteotomy at the time of patellofemoral replacement in order to maintain stability of the implant (Figure 15–6).

Preoperative planning frequently requires computed tomographic (CT) arthrogram or high-resolution magnetic resonance imaging scan to rule out articular damage to the tibiofemoral joint (Figure 15–7). Patellofemoral lateral maltracking may be assessed by CT scan with the quadriceps in the relaxed and contracted state in full extension (see Chapter 10). If the patella undergoes subluxation, then tibial tubercle osteotomy at the time of replacement usually is required. This is an additional test to the clinical examination when there is a question of maltracking, especially if the evaluation is difficult because the patient is obese. The CT scan also allows the sizing of custom implants with the DePuy system.

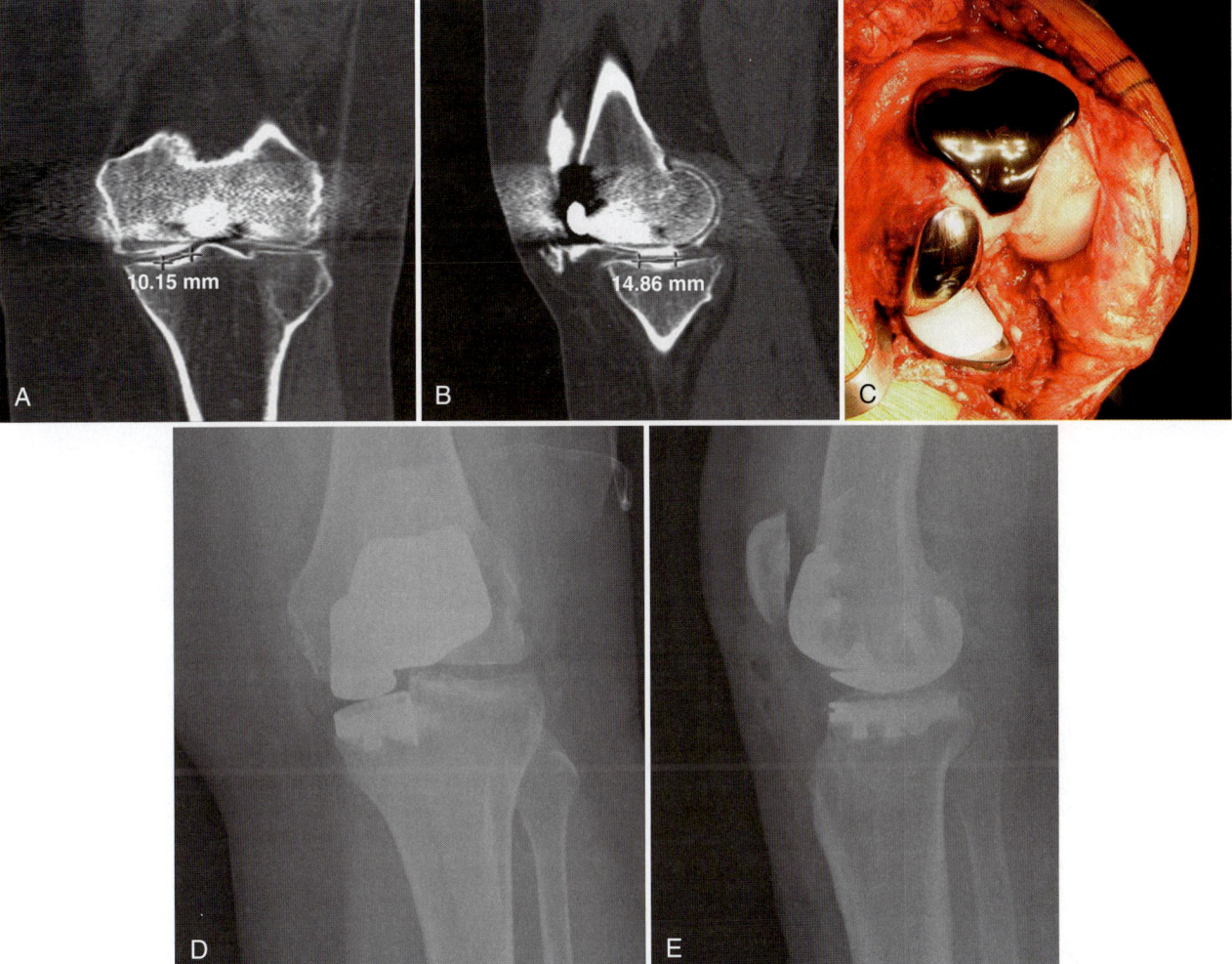

Figure 15–5 Four years after patellofemoral replacement, the same patient shown in Figure 15–4 develops sudden onset of medially based pain, catching, and effusions. *A,* Coronal computed tomographic (CT) scan arthrogram demonstrates a 10-mm–diameter, full-thickness grade 4 cartilage defect that has developed on the medial femoral condyle. *B,* Sagittal CT scan arthrogram demonstrates 15-mm-long, full-thickness cartilage loss. *C,* Based on the patient's age of 44 years, medial unicompartmental replacement is performed to treat the medial compartment chondrosis linked to the existing patellofemoral replacement rather than conversion to total knee arthroplasty. *D,* Postoperative anteroposterior x-ray film showing medial and patellofemoral replacements. *E,* Postoperative lateral x-ray film showing medial and patellofemoral replacements.

Several new patellofemoral replacements have become available since approval by the U.S. Food and Drug Administration in 2001. I have experience with the DePuy low-contact stress (LCS) patellar prosthesis (Figure 15–8), the DePuy custom Sigma patellofemoral prosthesis (Figure 15–9), and the Avon Howmedica Stryker prosthesis (see Figures 15–3, 15–4, 15–6, and 15–10). This chapter reviews my clinical experience with these implants.

SURGICAL TECHNIQUE

Once the decision for patellofemoral replacement has been made, the surgical technique is relatively straightforward. A medial parapatellar arthrotomy with eversion of the patella gives the best exposure. Most of the patella replacements are onset patellas that require a straightforward surgical technique. This may be performed at the onset of the procedure.

The trochlea varies among implant systems. The Stryker Howmedica Avon patellofemoral replacement and the Smith & Nephew Competitor patellofemoral replacement are onset trochleas. The technical aspects for performing a well-placed onset trochlea implant rely on the anterior femoral cut and distal transitioning to the implant cartilage interface. The anterior cut is externally rotated to match the transepicondylar axis, minimally flexed so that it does not notch the anterior femoral cortex, and positioned distally as close as possible to the intercondylar notch. This maximizes patellar tracking, allowing for easy distal transitioning to the native cartilage junction and maximal flexion of the patella before

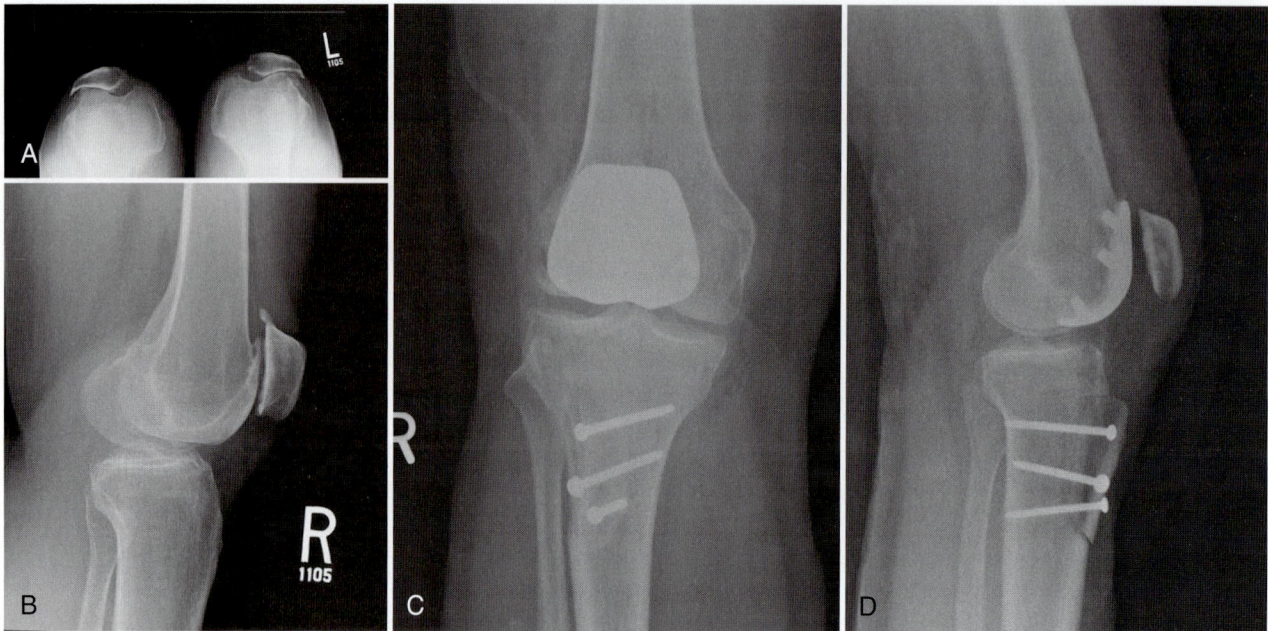

Figure 15–6 *A*, Skyline x-ray film of both knees of a 48-year-old woman who has experienced recurrent patellar instability with pain since adolescence. *B*, Lateral x-ray film demonstrates loss of articular cartilage in the patellofemoral joint with a convex barrel-shaped trochlea. *C*, At the time of surgery, a markedly laterally placed tibial tubercle was noted. A tubercle osteotomy was performed with the procedure to centralize the extensor mechanism and correct the maltracking of the prosthesis. Anteroposterior x-ray film shows lag screw fixation to the tibial tubercle osteotomy. *D*, Lateral postoperative x-ray film shows tibial tubercle osteotomy and patellofemoral replacement. Unlike total knee replacement in which patellar tracking can be managed with rotation of the tibial base plate component to decrease the quadriceps angle at the tibial tubercle, a patellofemoral replacement relies on the soft tissue balancing of the patella and the final tracking along with the quadriceps angle. The surgeon must be prepared to perform a tibial tubercle osteotomy when performing patellofemoral replacements for dysplastic disease.

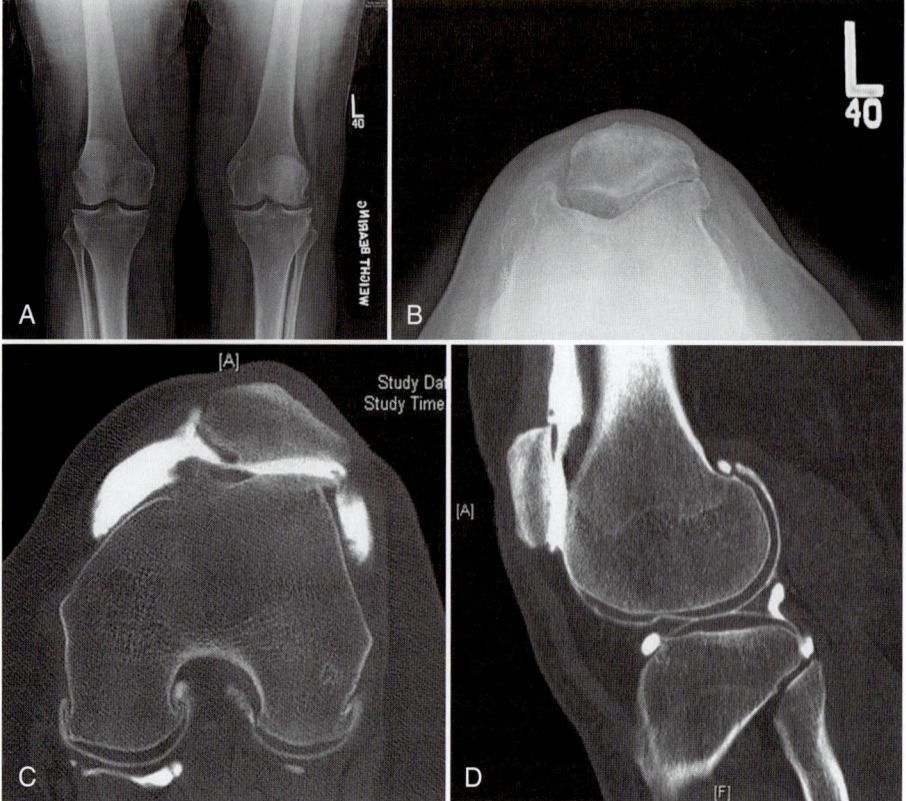

Figure 15–7 *A*, Standing anteroposterior radiographs in a 45-year-old woman with chronic anterior knee pain demonstrate well-preserved tibiofemoral joint. *B*, Skyline x-ray film demonstrates preserved cartilage space with peripheral osteophyte formation. The status of the articular cartilage is uncertain. *C*, Computed tomographic (CT) arthrogram axial cut demonstrates complete loss of articular cartilage to the entire median ridge and lateral patellar and trochlea facets. *D*, CT arthrogram sagittal cut demonstrates intact tibiofemoral articular surface and near complete loss of articular cartilage to the patella except for a small remnant of cartilage on the superior patella pole. Not enough articular cartilage remains for either Fulkerson osteotomy in isolation or in combination with autologous chondrocyte implantation.

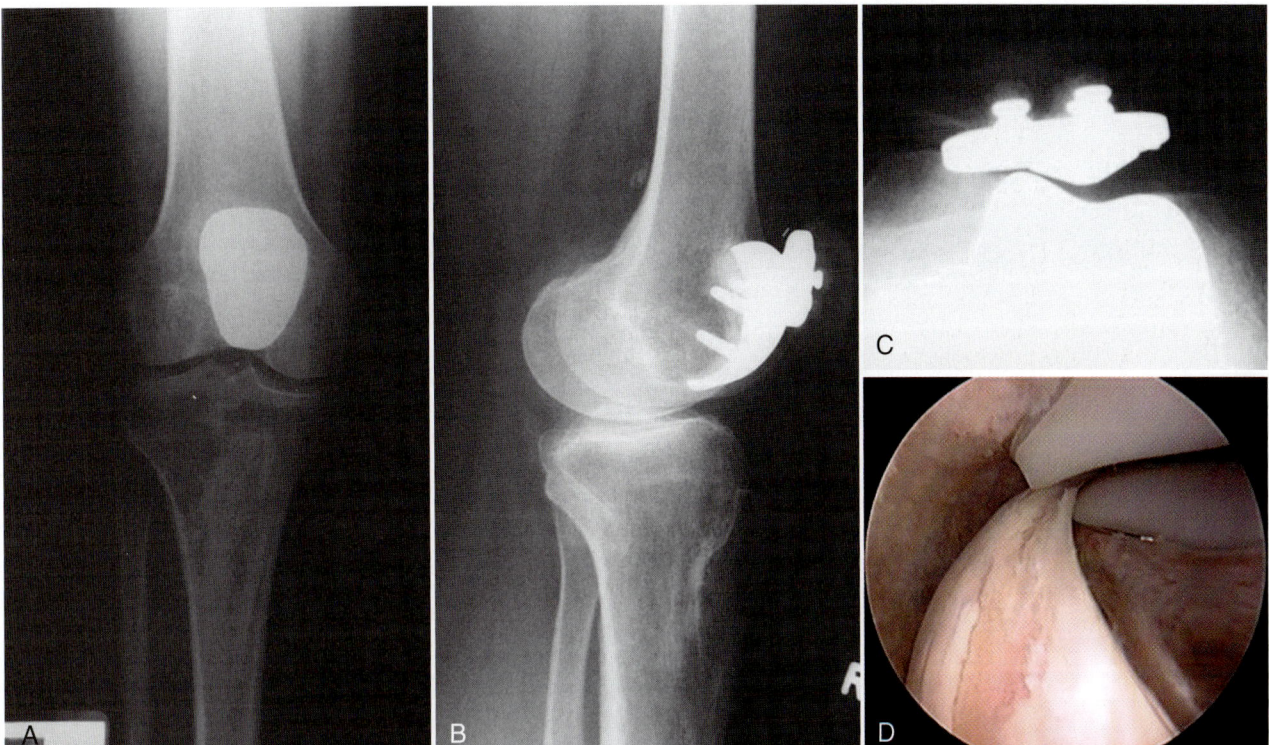

Figure 15-8 *A,* Postoperative anteroposterior x-ray film of an LCS (DePuy) mobile bearing patellofemoral replacement. This procedure was performed after prior failure of a tibial tubercle osteotomy. *B,* Lateral x-ray film of the same LCS mobile bearing implant. *C,* Skyline x-ray film demonstrates patellar tilt and mild subluxation with overhanging onto the native trochlea surface. *D,* Arthroscopic appearance viewed from an inferior lateral arthroscopic portal. The polyethylene patellar margin has completely eroded away the articular cartilage, which is uncovered by the trochlea prosthesis distally. Because of the patient's persistent pain and joint effusions, this was converted to a total knee replacement. This case illustrates the importance of good trochlea prosthetic coverage in a patellofemoral replacement design.

disengaging the trochlea into the native tibiofemoral cartilage, respectively. Transitioning the implant cartilage junction distally is critical to ensure a smooth flush transition. This will allow the patella to track well without mechanical catching as the patella disengages or reengages the trochlea prosthesis.

If maltracking continues after the medial capsular tissues are closed, a tibial tubercle osteotomy to medialize the tubercle under the tibial spines is performed and held with two anterior to posterior cortical lag screws to the posterior cortex.

If the need for a tubercle osteotomy is expected from the onset based on a very laterally positioned tibial tubercle, then a tibial tubercle osteotomy with lateral subvastus arthrotomy can be performed, leaving the entire medial sleeve intact (see Figure 15–6).

Inset trochleas (DePuy Sigma, LCS, and others) have the advantage of requiring much less bone removal; however, they must be implanted absolutely flush to the articular surface or their edges may abrade adjacent soft tissue or distally create a patellar "clunk" if the transition is not perfect, as with onset trochlea implant designs.

At the end of the procedure, I visualize the degree of flexion before the patella disengages into the native tibiofemoral cartilage. This is usually 110 degrees. However, if patella infera is present at the onset, patellar disengagement may occur as early as 80 to 90 degrees. After surgery, I inform patients of the level of flexion at which the patella will disengage. I then instruct them to avoid deep flexion in a kneeling or crouching position for life to prevent premature failure of the procedure due to tibiofemoral cartilage loss.

RESULTS

Between 2001 and 2006, 38 patients (41 knees) underwent patellofemoral arthroplasty. The LCS rotating metal-backed patellofemoral arthroplasty was performed in 9 knees (7 patients), the Avon patellofemoral arthroplasty in 8 knees (7 patients), and the Sigma custom patellofemoral replacement in 44 knees (38 patients).[4]

Patient recovery from patellofemoral arthroplasty was generally much easier than recovery from total knee arthroplasty. Blood transfusion was not required.

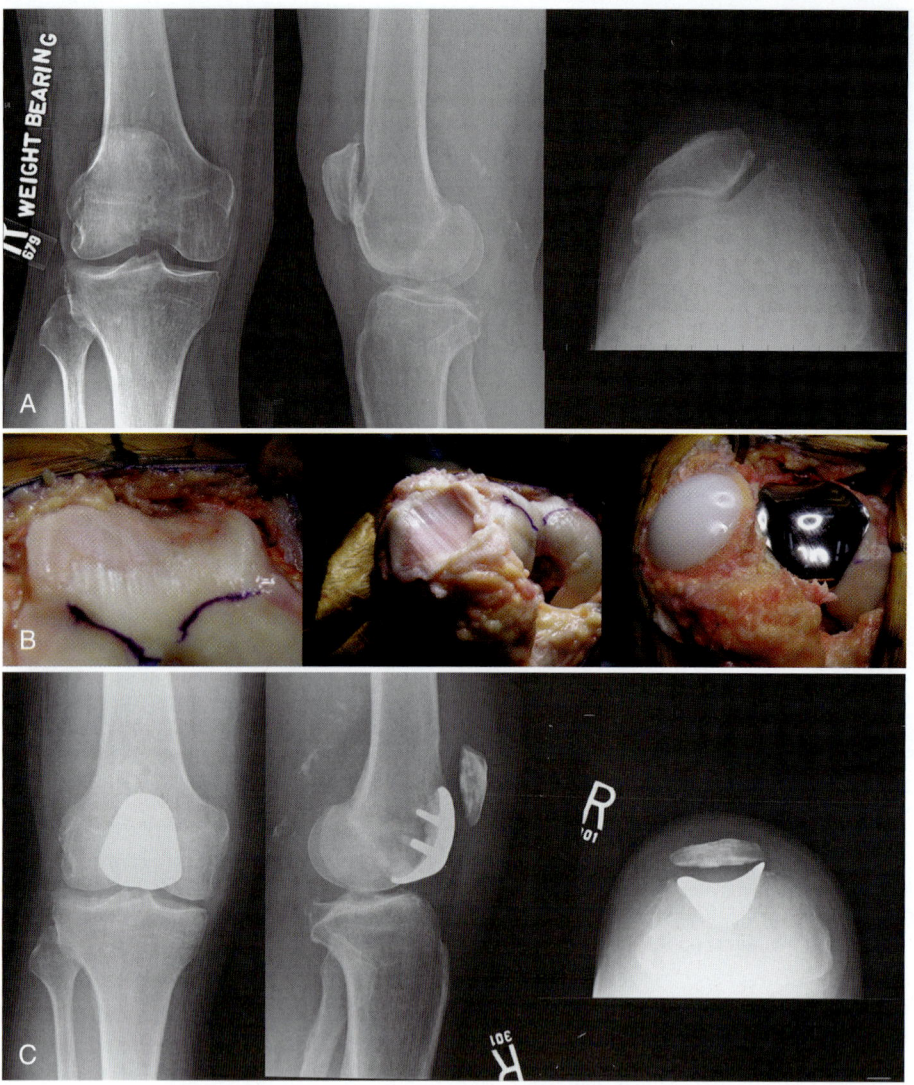

Figure 15-9 *A*, Standing anteroposterior, lateral, and skyline x-ray film of a 60-year-old physician with long-standing patellofemoral pain secondary to dysplasia. *B*, Intraoperative appearance of the dysplastic patella, trochlea, and intraoperative DePuy Sigma patellofemoral arthroplasty. *C*, Postoperative anteroposterior, lateral, and skyline x-ray film.

Immediate full weight bearing was allowed except when a concomitant tibial tubercle osteotomy had been performed. When tibial tubercle osteotomy was performed, 50% weight bearing for 6 weeks was instituted, but open chain quadriceps extensions were not allowed until osteotomy union occurred.

At the end of 5 years, 9 (22%) of 41 knees had failed, 7 due to progression of disease in the tibiofemoral joint and 2 due to LCS implants that produced painful clunks as the rotating platform prosthesis "spun out" through flexion and extension. The LCS metal-backed rotating patellas were relatively constrained in a narrow longitudinal prosthetic trochlea. As the patella captured the proximal trochlea and disengaged it distally, rotation of the polyethylene on the metal-backed patella was palpable and painful to the patient. Alternatively, the trochlea component was narrow distally, so if mild lateral maltracking occurred and the patient frequently used the knee in deep flexion, then abrasive cartilage loss to the exposed trochlea occurred, leading to clinical failure (see Figure 15-8). This implant was highly congruent with a deep V shape. Any mismatch in size was not tolerable, so a small trochlea would fit only with a small patella, which frequently would not cover the entire resected patellar surface. Because perfect tracking was not easy to obtain, this implant was abandoned early.

The Avon prosthesis has a shallow and forgiving trochlea groove. The patella prosthesis is asymmetric and easy to implant. It is an onset implant and requires an anterior femoral cut. I have found this implant to be both familiar and easy to implant. If the quadriceps angle was increased, a tubercle osteotomy was performed at the same setting. Failures occurred in patients who were either heavy or in their 60s with progression of disease in the tibiofemoral joint. No implant failures occurred; however, three knees developed progression of disease in the tibiofemoral joint and were converted to total knee arthroplasty.

The DePuy custom Sigma implant (see Figure 15-9), which I developed, is a 3-mm-thick trochlea implant

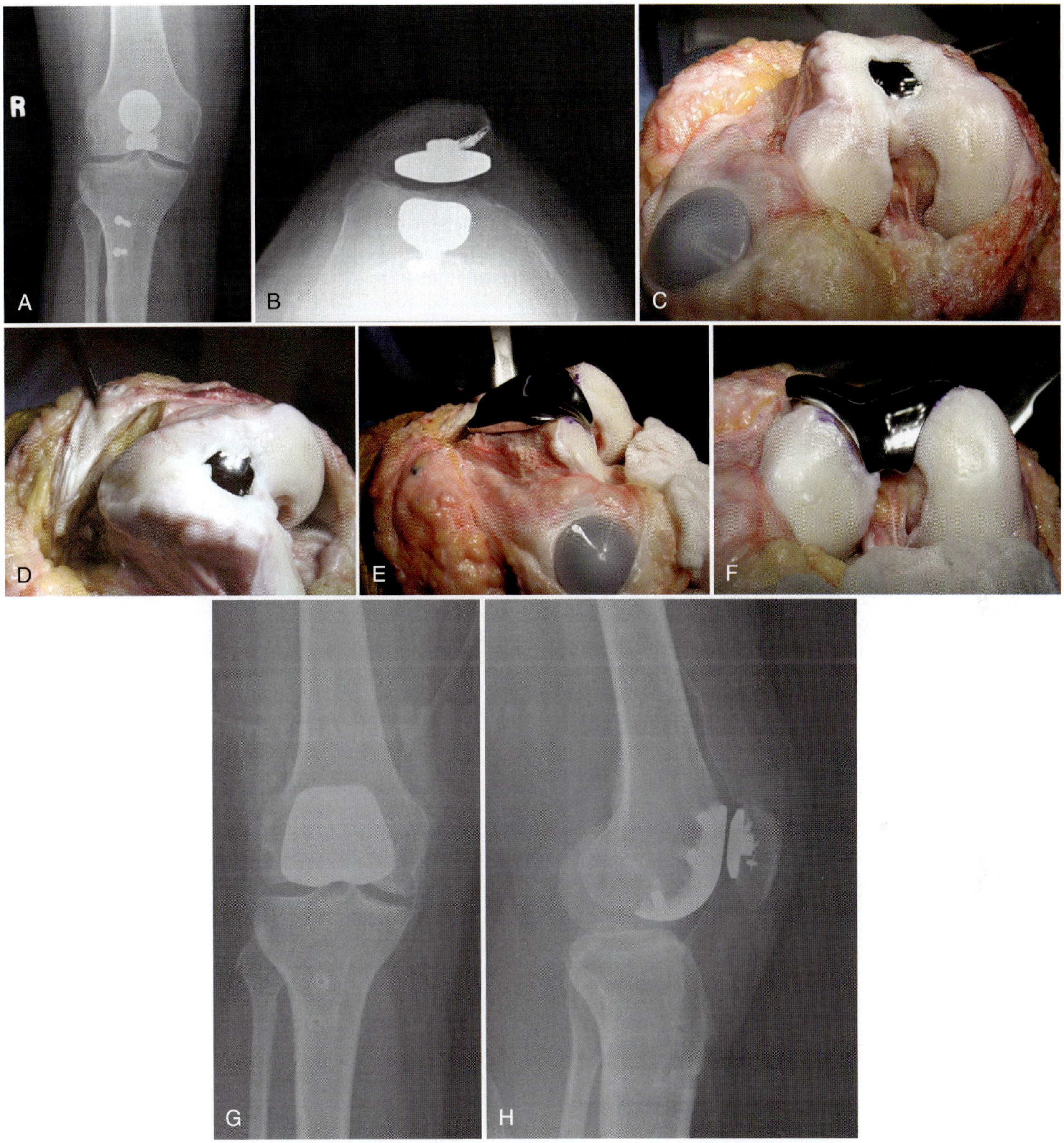

Patellofemoral Arthroplasty **CHAPTER 15** 259

Figure 15-10 Case demonstrating an inadequate patellofemoral design for an inappropriate indication. A 32-year-old woman had undergone prior tibial tubercle realignment osteotomy, which failed. Review of previous x-ray films showed the patellofemoral cartilage space was intact. Because of persistent pain, she underwent patellofemoral replacement. *A,* Anteroposterior x-ray film following patellofemoral replacement and prior tibial tubercle osteotomy. A metal-backed patella was used. *B,* Skyline x-ray film demonstrates an under-resurfaced trochlea and a metal-backed patellar prosthesis with tilt. *C,* Frontal view of the patellofemoral replacement, a markedly undersized trochlea implant. Erosive changes to the surrounding trochlea cartilage from the polyethylene abrasive patella are seen. *D,* Lateral view of the trochlea with implant in place shows a dysplastic trochlea with poorly formed entrance and trochlear spur. *E,* Lateral view after removal of the trochlea implant and resurfacing with an Avon patellofemoral replacement. *F,* Frontal view demonstrating that the prosthesis covers the entire trochlea to the sulcus terminalis on the medial and lateral femoral condyle surfaces (marked with blue marking pen). *G,* Postoperative anteroposterior x-ray film. *H,* Postoperative lateral x-ray film. Rather than resurfacing the patella and potentially losing bone stock, a full-thickness lateral patellar release was performed to alleviate the patellar tilt and the soft tissues were balanced to allow appropriate tracking.

that is inset. Trochlea sizing is performed by CT scan, then the implant is manufactured individually. A standard Sigma polyethylene patella is congruent with the trochlea, and size mismatch is allowed. As with all inset trochlea implants, preparation of the bony bed with a high-speed bur after outlining the trial implant must result in an absolutely flush distal prosthesis–cartilage border and is somewhat demanding. Minimal bone resection and easy conversion to total knee arthroplasty are clear advantages. Three knees developed progression of disease in the tibiofemoral joint and required conversion to total knee arthroplasty.

CONCLUSIONS

Based on my early experience, patellofemoral replacement is a reproducible procedure for improving function and alleviating anterior knee pain due to end-stage patellofemoral disease in patients with longstanding patellofemoral dysplasia and instability. The procedure removes minimal bone stock and is easy to convert to total knee replacement. Patellofemoral replacement for patellar fracture is also very reproducible as long as patella infera has not developed.

Implant designs are critical. The trochlea component should cover the entire trochlea surface into the sulcus terminalis of the medial and lateral weight-bearing surfaces. Other designs that have limited trochlea coverage frequently experience abrasive changes to the exposed trochlea cartilage with progressive loss of cartilage and increasing pain and failure of the procedure (Figure 15–10).

When patients are heavy, have mild tibiofemoral malalignment, or approach total knee arthroplasty age (in their 60s), patellofemoral arthroplasty becomes less predictable because of deterioration of the tibiofemoral joint in a variable manner that necessitates conversion to total knee arthroplasty, which probably is a more appropriate first-line treatment.

REFERENCES

1. Davies A, Vince A, Shepstone L, et al. The radiologic prevalence of patellofemoral osteoarthritis. *Clin Orthop Relat Res*. 2002;402: 206–212.
2. Aglietti P, Insall JN, Walker PS, et al. A new patella prosthesis. *Clin Orthop Relat Res*. 1975;107:175.
3. Argenson J, Flecher X, Parratte S, et al. Patellofemoral arthroplasty: an update. *Clin Orthop Relat Res*. 2005;440:50–53.
4. Minas T. Patellofemoral replacement: the third compartment. *Orthopedics*. 2008;31(9).

Chapter 16

Patient-Specific Unicompartmental and Bicompartmental Resurfacing Arthroplasty

Tom Minas, MD, MS

INTRODUCTION
IMAGING TECHNOLOGY
SURGICAL TECHNIQUE
  Patient Positioning and Preparation
  Cartilage Removal
  Balancing of the Knee
  Axial and Sagittal Tibial Cuts
  Femoral Preparation
  Balancing Verification and Tibial Preparation
  Trialing and Cementing of Implant
  Bicompartmental Resurfacing and iDuo Replacements
SUMMARY

INTRODUCTION

Total knee arthroplasty has become one of the most common surgical procedures due to its clinical success and longevity. In the United States, more than 500,000 primary total knee replacements were performed in 2006.[1] This volume is expected to grow to 3.48 million by 2030.[2]

In the early 2000s, the average age of patients undergoing knee replacements was between 67 and 68 years. Numerous studies and anecdotal experience from surgeons have reported a rise in the incidence of primary osteoarthritis (OA) in younger patients. Factors such as an aging baby boomer population with more active lifestyles, the rise of sports-related injuries in younger populations as a precursor to osteoarthritis, and a more demanding patient base unwilling to modify their activity levels appear to be potential causes of the increase in younger patients seen by surgeons.

In younger patients with moderate OA, a different set of considerations enters into the calculation for the appropriate treatment approach. Early intervention patients often are more active, have a higher potential for revision later in life, and exhibit patterns of OA that may be more localized. The ability to provide a joint-preserving option that can bridge the patient to a traditional total knee replacement is appealing.

In this chapter, I describe my experience with an imaging-based approach to partial knee resurfacing as a treatment for early intervention patients. I briefly describe the technology and then the surgical technique using patient-specific custom instruments.

IMAGING TECHNOLOGY

The process for building patient-specific implants and instruments begins with a preoperative computed tomographic (CT) scan performed on commonly available machines (Figure 16–1). The scan, which includes partial views of the hip and ankle, is converted into a virtual three-dimensional model of the patient's knee. The partial views of the hip and ankle are used to align the implant and cut guides in relation to the patient's anatomic and mechanical axes.

Design engineers at the manufacturer ConforMIS (Burlington, MA) use computer-aided design software to perform virtual osteophyte removal and to identify key anatomic landmarks. The proprietary software then generates a matching surface topography for the femur from the scan data and an outline of the tibia at the expected resection level.

The surface topography is used as the undersurface of the femoral implant, allowing the component to

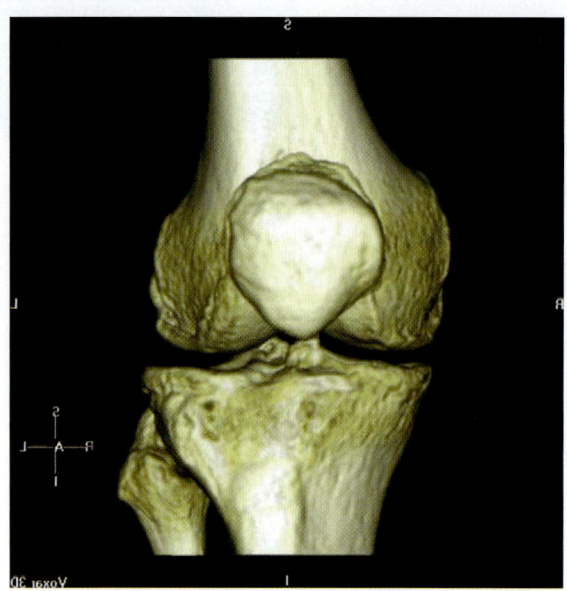

Figure 16-1 Three-dimensional image of the knee taken by a multidetector computed tomographic scanner

rest on the subchondral bone with close conformity to the patient's native anatomy. The articulating surface follows the anatomy but with an engineered curve in the coronal plane to minimize contact stress with the tibial surface. The femoral implant thickness is 3.5 mm, representing the native cartilage that is lost. Therefore, it is a resurfacing implant and exactly restores the joint line. The tibial implant is designed to match the outline of the cortical shell on the resected tibia. The custom nature of the implant design allows for complete cortical rim coverage in each patient. The tibial thickness is 9 mm: 7 mm polyethylene and 2 mm metal base plate.

One of the more unusual aspects of surgery using patient-specific implants is the instrumentation set, which consists of a small number of guides that are generated for one-time use with each implant. The cut guides are matched to the patient's anatomy using the same process as the implants, thus eliminating intraoperative sizing and allowing for tactile feedback to help establish positioning. The instruments are prenavigated using the scan data so that all cuts and drill holes are set with respect to the axis (Figure 16–2).

The design algorithms have been developed for a unicompartmental and a bicompartmental option. The unicompartmental option is well known in orthopedics, but the bicompartmental option is relatively novel. It allows for treatment of the patellofemoral joint in addition to one of the tibiofemoral compartments, and it provides a different option for treating OA in younger patients. Both implants can be designed for either the medial or the lateral compartment. Because the prosthetic trochlea surface is precisely that of the patient, the patella can be left unresurfaced and will have good congruence to the trochlea.

These implants and instruments are manufactured using processes that are designed to be cost competitive at single-unit or low-volume production. The implants are made of standard orthopedic materials, such as cobalt-chromium-molybdenum alloy and ultra-high-molecular-weight polyethylene (UHMWPE), but the cutting guides are made of disposable, engineered materials such as plastic or nylon. The production process takes 4 to 6 weeks for completion.

SURGICAL TECHNIQUE

The surgical technique described here uses a medial unicompartmental replacement to illustrate the differences of a custom implant with custom disposable jigs. The bicompartmental implant uses a surgical technique very similar to that for the unicompartmental implant except for patellofemoral preparation and fixation.

Patient Positioning and Preparation

The patient is positioned supine on the table with the leg resting on a foot support at 90 degrees of flexion. After a standard short midline skin incision, a medial or lateral parapatellar arthrotomy is performed. My preference is to dissect the medial (or lateral) sleeve subperiosteally around the tibia to the posteromedial corner to allow easy visibility of the tibial tray and polyethylene placement.

To begin the procedure, all femoral osteophytes must be removed completely, including those in the intercondylar notch. Removal of the tibial osteophytes is performed later with the tibial resection. The manufacturer provides images to assist in performing intraoperative osteophyte removal in order to replicate the virtual osteophyte removal performed in the design stage.

Cartilage Removal

In extension, the sulcus terminalis (the leading weight-bearing femoral surface that engages the anterior tibia) is marked with a marking pen, where the leading anterior tibial surface makes contact with the femur. The femoral cutting block, which is shaped to fit the condyle and represents the size and geometry of the femoral implant, is placed on the femoral condyle. In most cases the anterior edge of the femoral cutting block seats about 2 to 3 mm inferior to the sulcus terminalis. The round anterior silhouette of the femoral cutting block is marked on the femoral condyle.

The implant is designed to the surface of the subchondral bone with a thickness of approximately 3.5 mm.

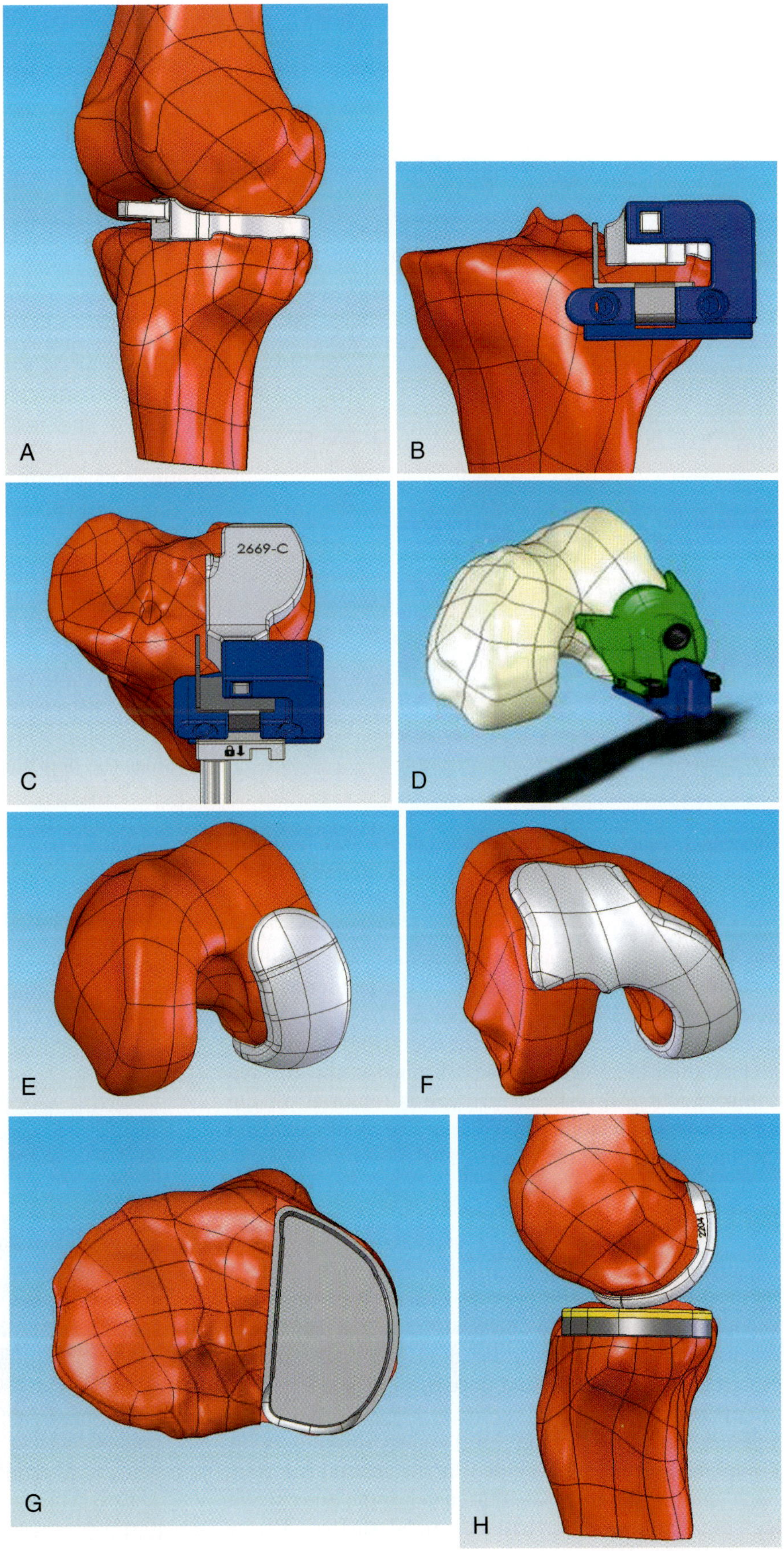

Patient-Specific Unicompartmental and Bicompartmental Resurfacing Arthroplasty   CHAPTER 16   263

Figure 16-2 Computer-assisted design (CAD) image of a patient-specific disposable instrument set based on exact patient specific anatomy of axial, sagittal, and coronal alignments to perform a unicompartmental or bicompartmental resurfacing arthroplasty. *A*, Virtual image after osteophyte removal on the femur and placement of a patient-specific balancing chip to tension the collateral ligaments in flexion and extension. *B*, Tibial cutting jig referenced from the balancing chip to determine the sagittal cut on the tibial spine, the axial cut alignment perpendicular to the ankle, and the tibial sagittal slope built and based on the native osteochondral junction. *C*, View from above with the tibial cutting jig dovetailed to an external tibial alignment guide for secondary confirmation of perpendicular ankle alignment and added stability when the jig is pinned into place prior to cutting. *D*, Virtual placement of the femoral alignment guide with L-guide to reference off the tibial spacer block once the tibia is cut. *E*, Virtual placement of a medial femoral component. *F*, Virtual placement of a medial bicompartmental patellofemoral component. *G*, Virtual design and placement of the exact tibial base plate. *H*, Final appearance of medial unicompartmental resurfacing arthroplasty that is virtually aligned, instrumented, and manufactured specifically for the patient.

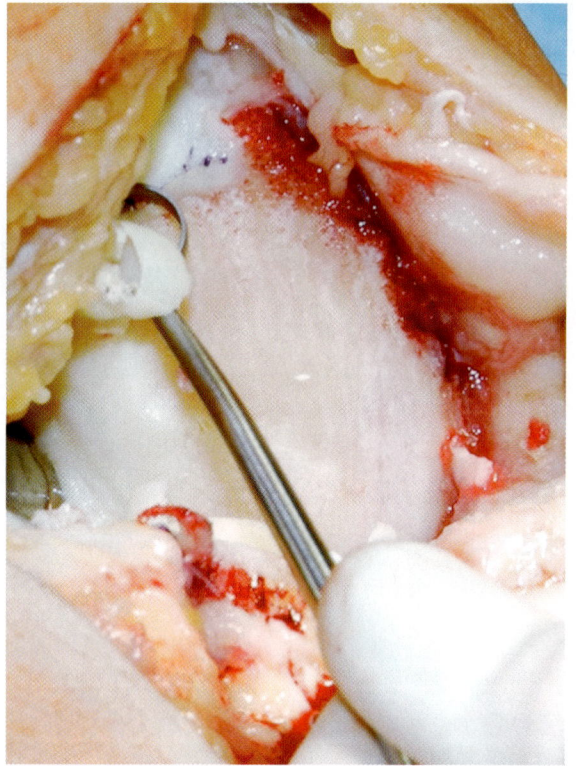

Figure 16-3 Cartilage removal on the femoral condyle using a sharp ring curette posterior to the sulcus terminalis, which is marked in *blue*.

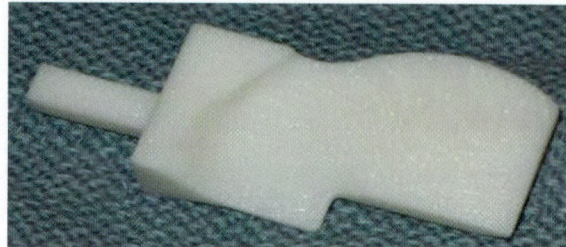

Figure 16-4 Balancing navigation chip.

Because it resurfaces the bone plate, all cartilage posterior to the sulcus terminalis, including the posterior condyle, must be removed. This is facilitated using a 10-mm blade, curved elevator, osteotome, and sharp ring curette (Figure 16–3). Complete removal of cartilage is critical for accurate balancing and placement of the femoral cutting guide.

Once cartilage removal on the femur has been completed, a full meniscectomy is performed in the affected compartment. All residual cartilage is removed off the tibial plateau, including the edge of the tibial spine and the anterior edge of the tibia.

Balancing of the Knee

Balancing is performed after osteophyte and cartilage removal but before any bone resection. With this balancing approach using prenavigated jigs, ligament releases are not recommended, and both the anterior cruciate ligament (ACL) and posterior cruciate ligament are preserved.

Four balancing "chips" of varying thicknesses in 1-mm increments are included in the instrument tray. Each chip has an underside that matches the exact shape and topography of the patient's tibial surface. When inserted into the compartment, the chip will self-seat into a stable position due to its conformity with the anatomic landmarks on the tibia. Accurate placement is dependent on avoidance of soft tissue impingement on the balancing chip.

Each chip is inserted in turn, from thinnest to thickest, with the knee in flexion and then taken through range of motion. The top surface of this chip is flat to allow referencing off the distal femoral condylar surface during balancing (Figure 16–4). Select the chip that provides optimal ligament tensioning (Figure 16–5). An opening under valgus stress of about 1 mm is recommended medially in extension and 90 degrees of flexion and about 1 to 3 mm under varus stress laterally in extension and about 3 to 5 mm in 90 degrees of flexion.

The selected navigation chip connects to a tibial cutting block. The thickness of the balancing chip determines the depth of the tibial resection. The prenavigated guides are designed to deliver a horizontal cut that replicates the balancing provided by the chip once the tibial component is implanted.

Axial and Sagittal Tibial Cuts

The tibial jig is referenced exactly to the shape of the anterior tibial cortex and includes data on the tibial

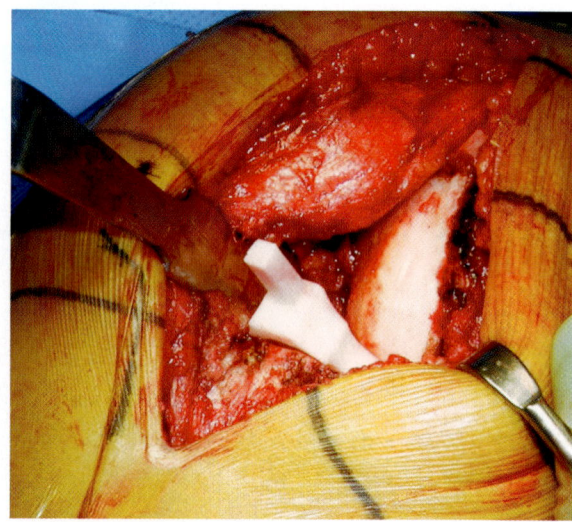

Figure 16-5 Balancing navigation chip in place, with equal tension in flexion and extension.

Patient-Specific Unicompartmental and Bicompartmental Resurfacing Arthroplasty CHAPTER 16 265

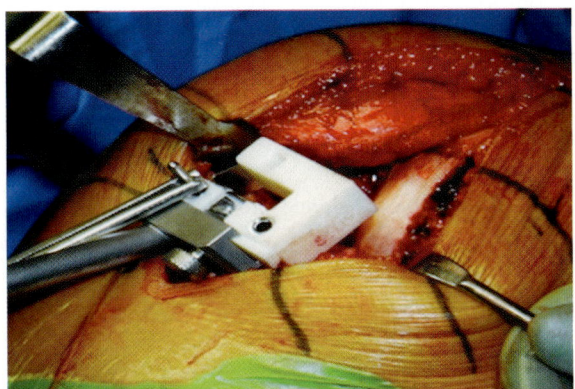

Figure 16-6 Tibial cutting jig attached to the navigation chip and alignment guide.

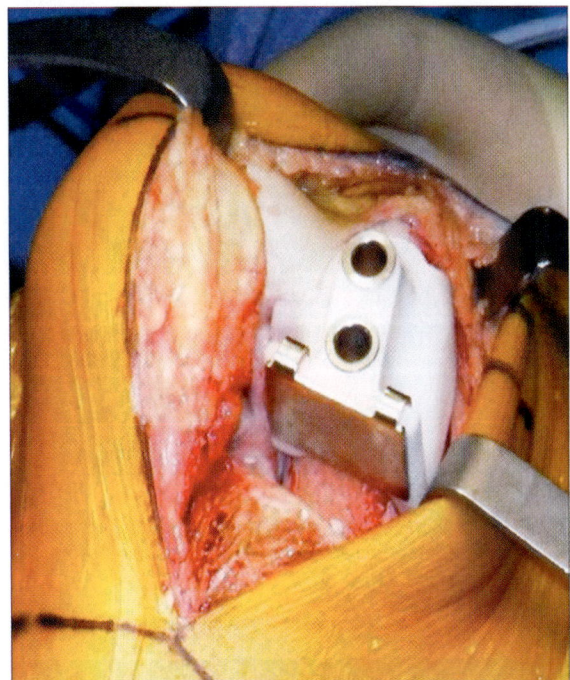

Figure 16-7 Femoral jig captured uniquely to the femoral geometry after removal of osteophytes and cartilage.

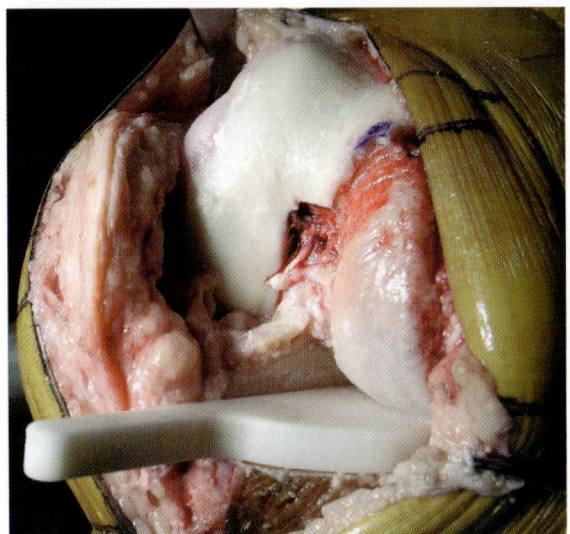

Figure 16-8 Placement of 9-mm tibial template after tibial cut demonstrating precise sizing to the tibial cortical margin. At 90 degrees of flexion, the native femoral condyle (after cartilage removal) rests easily on the template surface.

sagittal slope. It is perpendicular to the axis of the ankle center. For confirmation of axis and stability, it may be connected to an extramedullary alignment guide by sliding the dovetail feature of the tibial jig onto the top of the alignment guide. The balancing chip is left in place and the tibial cutting guide connected to it, which ensures a balanced flexion and extension gap (Figure 16-6).

Verification and confirmation of the position of the tibial cutting block in all three planes are necessary. The horizontal cut (90 degrees relative to the tibial mechanical axis), the sagittal cut, and the posterior slope are determined in this step.

The sagittal tibial cut is performed with a reciprocating saw, usually at the top of the tibial spine (to maximize the medial–lateral size of the tibial base plate as designed) using the tibial jig. The reciprocating saw blade can be left in place to protect the ACL insertion while performing the axial cut. A few fibers of the ACL usually require release. The axial tibial cut is made referencing off the tibial jig.

Femoral Preparation

The femoral jig is designed to conform to the femur in only one location to aid in proper positioning (Figure 16-7). Additional cartilage or osteophytes that were missed initially are now revisited until the femoral jig fit is snug and secure.

Two design features are considered for the femoral component. First, the peg holes are drilled in 15 degrees of flexion relative to the sagittal anatomic femoral axis. This prevents pistoning and loosening of the implant. Second, only one bone resection is required on the femur: a 3- to 4-mm resection of the posterior condyle (including the thickness of the saw blade). Thus, this is a resurfacing implant and possibly an easy revision to total knee replacement in the future if necessary.

To ensure a well-balanced compartment, the tibial spacer is applied to the tibia (Figure 16-8) and linked to the femoral jig via an L-guide (Figure 16-9) at 90 degrees of flexion so that the surfaces are parallel and no edge loading will occur. This also ensures that the flexion space is not too tight. The femoral cutting block is drilled and pinned in place, and the posterior femoral condyle resection is performed with an oscillating saw (Figure 16-10).

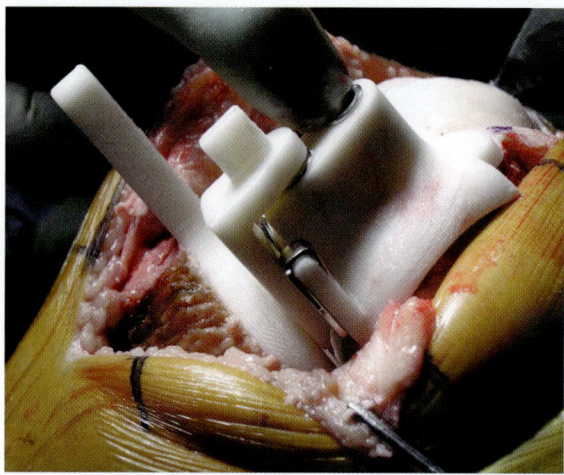

Figure 16-9 Femoral jig with L-guide linked to the tibial spacer block at 90 degrees of flexion to confer stability, parallelism of components, and flexion balance prior to drill lugs and posterior cut.

Balancing Verification and Tibial Preparation

A femoral trial component and a tibial balancing block are used to assess balancing. With the femoral trial in place, the 9-mm spacer block is inserted and the implants allow evaluation of balance in flexion and extension (Figure 16–11). A joint play of 1 mm is recommended for the medial iUni in extension and flexion. For lateral iUnis, I recommend 1 to 2 mm in extension and 2 to 4 mm in 90 degrees of flexion. If the knee is too tight, an additional 1 to 2 mm is resected from the tibia. If the knee is too loose, the thicker 11-mm spacer block is used to evaluate balance in flexion and extension.

At this stage, the procedure is essentially completed as the cuts and balancing have been confirmed. The tibial template is placed on the tibia and both holes are drilled, pinning the anterior hole only to accommodate instruments for the upcoming fin hole preparation (Figure 16–12). The fin hole is made using a 5-mm osteotome. The tibial implant is designed to match the

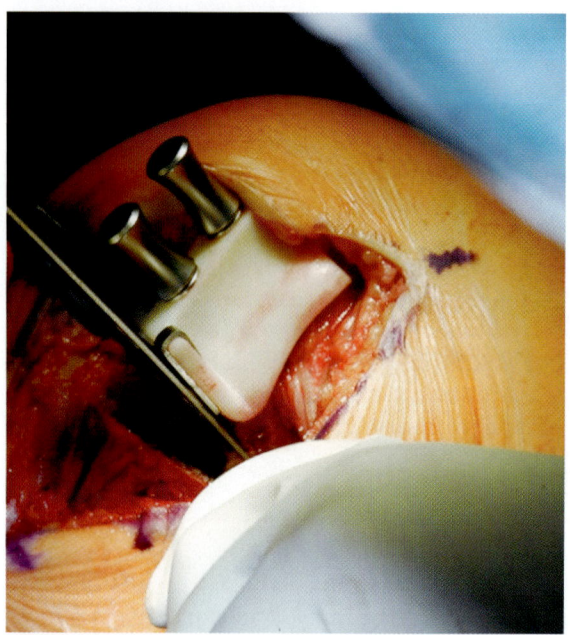

Figure 16-10 Posterior femoral cut removes 3 to 4 mm of bone only.

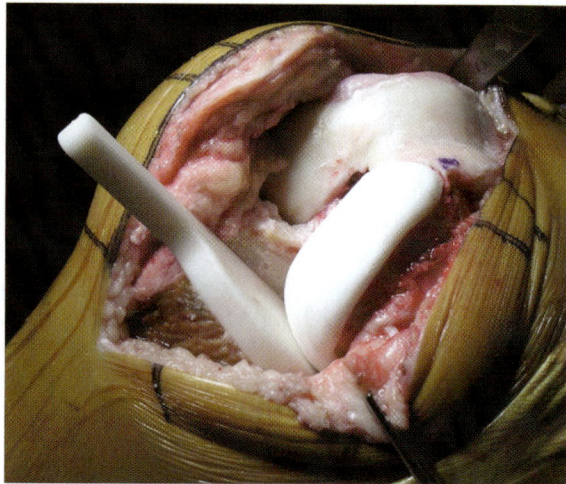

Figure 16-11 A 9-mm tibial template balanced precisely with femoral trial component in flexion and extension.

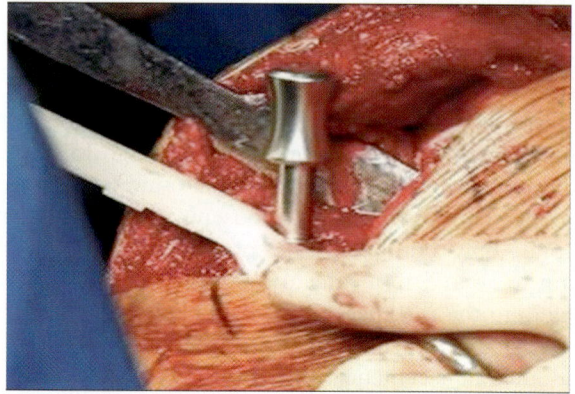

Figure 16-12 Tibial template drill lug placement and keel punch performed.

To complete femoral preparation, an anterior recess is prepared using a 5-mm bur to ensure a smooth anterior transition for the patella in deep flexion and allow the component to sit securely on the subchondral bone to which it was designed based on the CT scan data. The most anterior edge of the component submerges 3.5 mm below the subchondral bone plate. The taper starts 10 mm distal to it. The transition from the subchondral bone to the anterior edge of the posterior cut must be rounded using a bur. Verify smoothing of the edge and the placement and depth of recess with the femoral trial.

patient anatomy exactly and should cover the entire tibia cortex without overhang or undercoverage. The outline of the tibial template provides visual confirmation of the match.

Trialing and Cementing of Implant

Multiple 1.5- to 2-mm cement holes are drilled to enhance cement interdigitation with the femoral subchondral bone surface (Figure 16–13) and then pulse lavaged and dried. The metal implants are used as trials with trial plastic inserts in the tibial base plate to confirm optimal balancing (Figure 16–14). Two different thicknesses are provided, 7 and 9 mm. Combined with the 2-mm thickness of the tibial tray, the 7- and 9-mm trials will correspond to the 9- and 11-mm spacer blocks used to confirm proper balance (see Figure 16–11).

The tibial tray is cemented first, removing all extruded cement. The real insert is snapped into place. The femoral component is then cemented into place with a valgus–hyperflexion maneuver and impacted into place. The knee is brought into full extension in order to remove any excess cement, checking around the back of the tibia with curved curettes, and then the cement is allowed to cure in a few degrees of flexion (10–15 degrees). Wound closure of the arthrotomy is recommended in flexion and in multiple layers.

Bicompartmental Resurfacing and iDuo Replacements

The technique for bicompartmental replacement (iDuo) is identical to that for unicompartmental replacement except that femoral preparation includes the trochlea to the opposite sulcus terminalis of the opposite compartment. This opposite sulcus transition to native cartilage is ensured by the computer-aided design of the implant being tapered into the bone by 3.5 mm over the final 1 cm as the implant transitions. It is referenced off the native trochlea subchondral bone, intercondylar notch, and femoral condyle to ensure this important junction transition. Both a medial iDuo (Figure 16–15) and a lateral iDuo (Figure 16–16) are available. The patella may be resurfaced or left alone as desired because the trochlea is exactly congruent to the patient's patella.

In addition to a medial iUni, a lateral iUni (Figure 16–17) is available with the specific advantage of the implant being individualized for that compartment. The lateral compartment is unique in that the tibial bearing surface is more like a square compared to the rectangular medial compartment. The femur laterally is shorter in the anteroposterior dimension, and patellofemoral impingement is always a risk. "Off-the-shelf" implants are designed only for the medial compartment, so they pose many surgical challenges to correct placement of lateral unicompartmental implants.

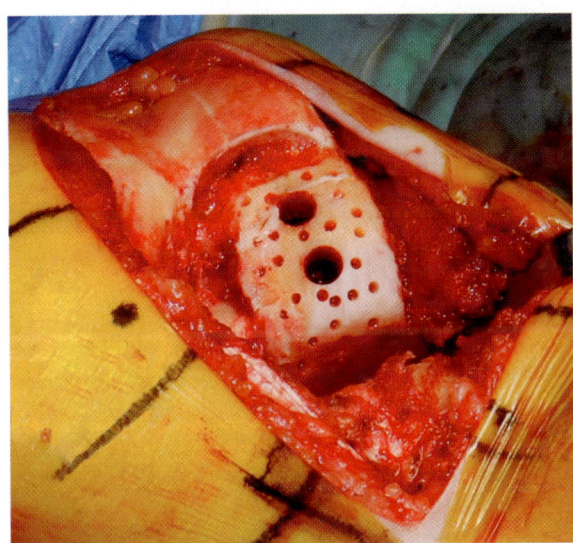

Figure 16–13 Appearance of femoral condyle with 2-mm drill holes to enhance cement interdigitation to subchondral bone. The leading edge of the femoral implant is deepened 3.5 mm anteriorly and at the junction using a bur. The posterior femoral cut is rounded with a bur.

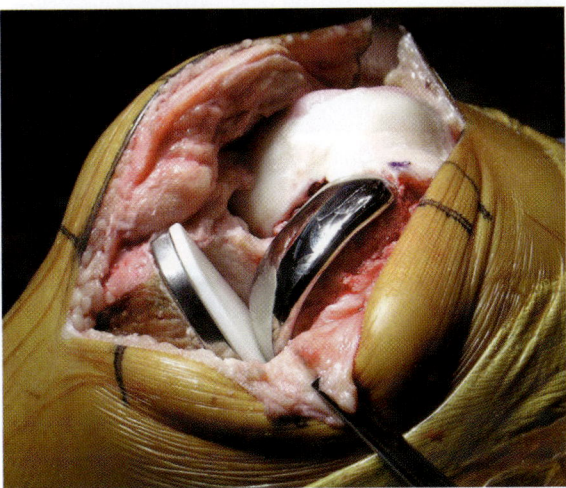

Figure 16–14 Final appearance of components trialed with a plastic tibial insert prior to final cementing.

SUMMARY

Baby boomers wish to remain active. However, until now total knee replacement was the only option available when advanced arthritic change developed. Unicompartmental replacements had the advantage of preserving the cruciate ligaments, thus producing a kinematically more normal knee, but were designed for the medial compartment alone. They still required intramedullary

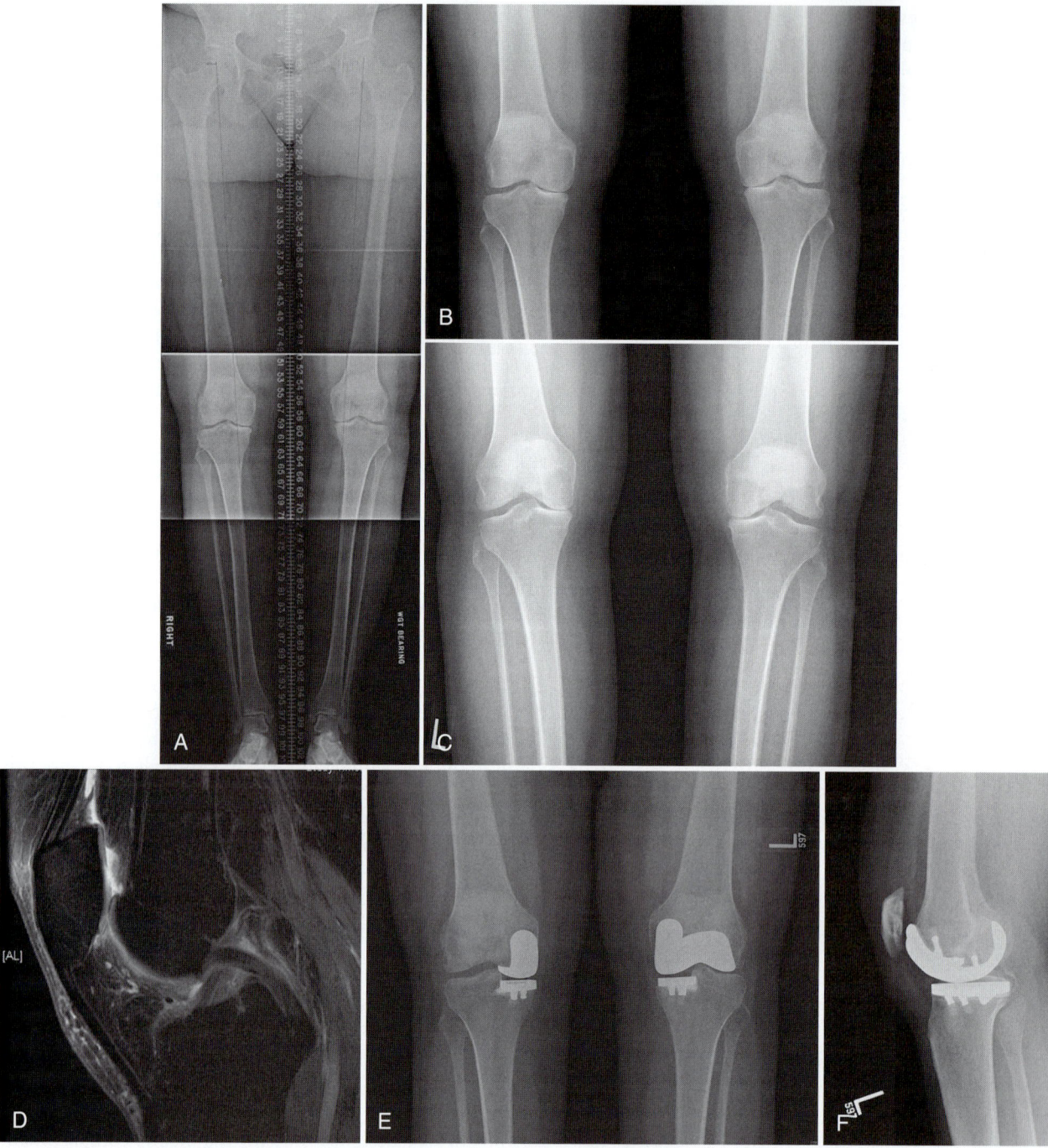

Figure 16–15 Case of a 48-year-old woman with bilateral knee pain and marked limitation in activities of daily living. Her pain was medially based on the right and medial and anterior on the left. *A,* Long alignment x-ray film demonstrating varus malalignment. *B,* Bilateral standing anteroposterior x-ray film. *C,* Bilateral standing posteroanterior x-ray film demonstrating severe bone-on-bone medial compartment disease. *D,* Magnetic resonance imaging with fat suppression demonstrates near complete cartilage loss on the patella of the left knee. *E,* The patient underwent simultaneous bilateral knee arthroplasty surgery via subvastus approach. Patient-specific medial unicompartmental replacement was performed on the right and bicompartmental medial on the left. Standing anteroposterior x-ray film. *F,* Lateral x-ray film of the left bicompartmental replacement. *G,* Lateral x-ray film of the right unicompartmental replacement.

Continued

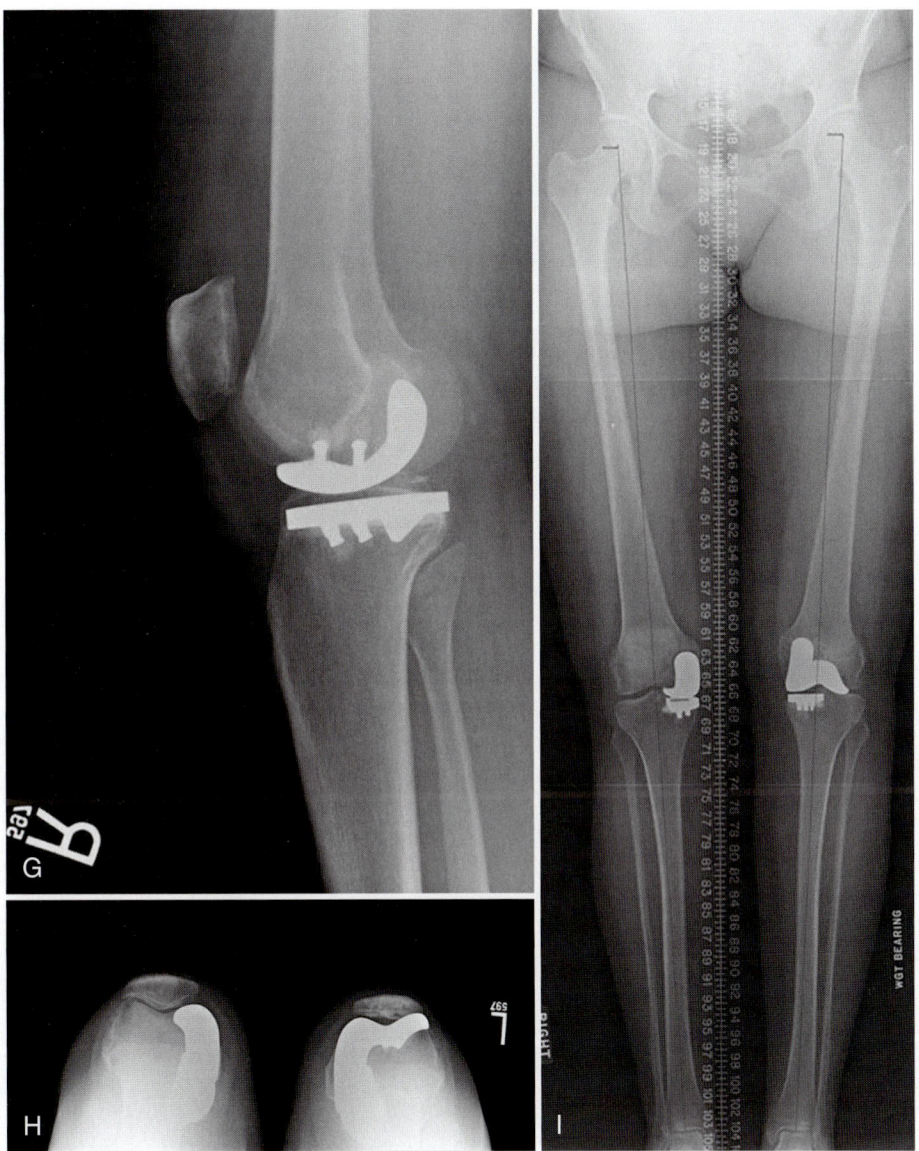

Figure 16-15—cont'd *H*, Postoperative bilateral skyline x-ray film. *I*, Postoperative long-leg alignment x-ray films demonstrating restoration of neutral mechanical axis with partial knee resurfacing implant technology, unicompartmental on the right knee and bicompartmental on the left knee.

instrumentation with inaccurate component fits and axial alignments encountered by the inexperienced surgeon.

Intraoperative computer-assisted navigation has enhanced the accuracy of placement of implants, mainly for outliers with larger deformities. Intraoperative navigation requires a learning curve, increased surgical time, and a large capital outlay by the institution for the equipment.

Gender-specific knee replacement surgery has caught the attention of the public as well as the orthopedic surgeon with regard to the accuracy of implant sizes developed based on gender.

Combining twenty-first–century technology for three-dimensional surface imaging and rapid computer-assisted manufacturing has allowed virtual prenavigation, instrument manufacture (disposable patient-specific jigs), and component manufacture at a cost-competitive rate.

The concepts are exciting. Only time will tell whether this technology will keep the promise of bone-preserving, durable results with enhanced recovery for patients. It would allow earlier treatment while maintaining the possibility of patients still undergoing primary total knee replacement in case of disease progression or implant failure in the future.

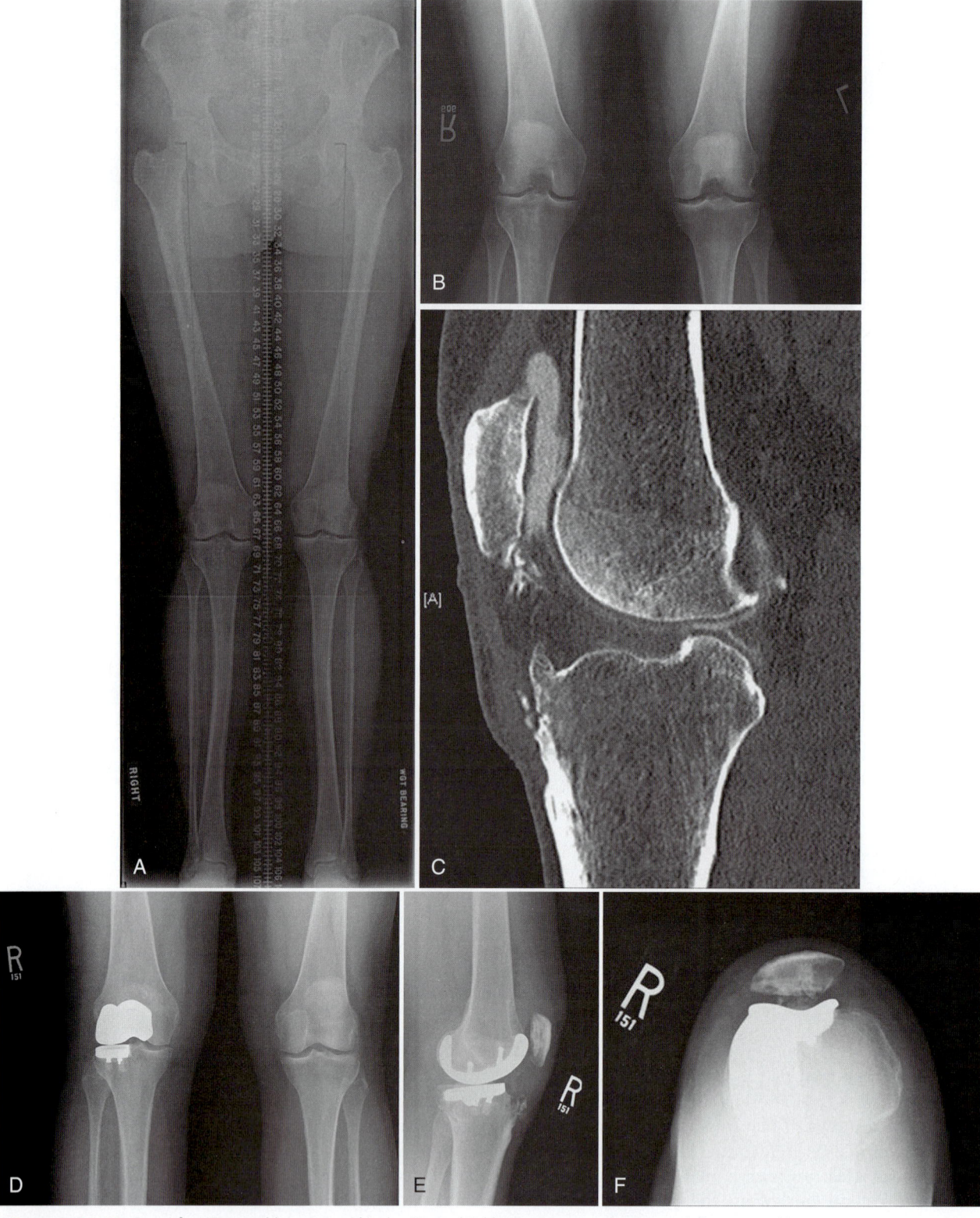

Figure 16-16 Case of a 58-year-old woman with prior Osgood-Schlatter disease and valgus malalignment with lateral and anterior knee pain. *A,* Long alignment x-ray film demonstrating valgus malalignment and lateral joint space narrowing. *B,* Standing posteroanterior x-ray film demonstrates posterior lateral cartilage loss with resultant joint space narrowing on the tibiofemoral joint. *C,* Computed tomographic arthrogram used for manufacture of the implants and jigs is useful for assessing the articular surfaces. Note loss of cartilage in the patella lateral tibiofemoral compartment but the well-maintained medial tibiofemoral compartment menisci and cruciate ligaments. *D,* Postoperative anteroposterior x-ray film after lateral patellofemoral bicompartmental resurfacing arthroplasty. *E,* Postoperative lateral x-ray film. *F,* Postoperative skyline x-ray film.

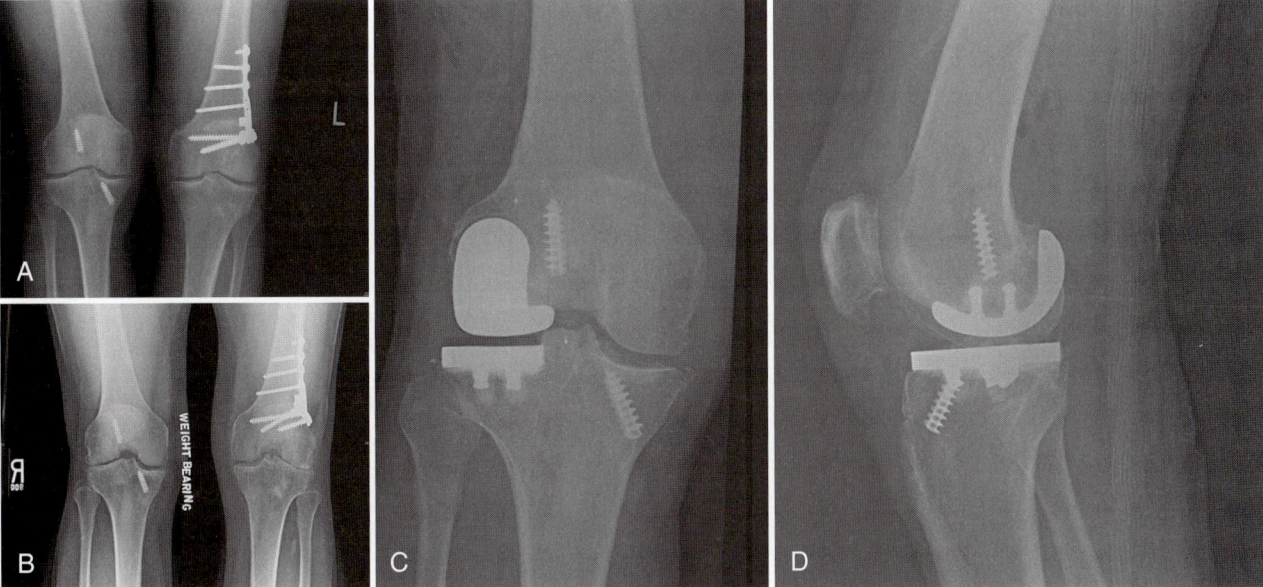

Figure 16-17 Case of a 52-year-old man who had undergone distal femoral varus-producing osteotomy to the left knee 5 years earlier for lateral compartment osteoarthritis. He now presents with identical symptoms and disease but would prefer a unicompartmental replacement because of the speed of recovery with the technique and his lessened clinical demands. *A,* Standing anteroposterior x-ray film of both knees. *B,* Standing posteroanterior x-ray film of both knees demonstrates lateral tibiofemoral cartilage loss with loss of joint space bilaterally. *C,* Postoperative anteroposterior x-ray film after patient-specific lateral unicompartmental replacement. Note complete coverage of the lateral tibial plateau and femoral condyle. *D,* Postoperative lateral x-ray film demonstrates complete coverage of both surfaces without patellofemoral impingement on the femur or overhang on the tibia. Patellofemoral impingement and tibial overhang are possible adverse outcomes of an "off-the-shelf" implant, which is designed specifically for the medial compartment but is transferred to the lateral side.

REFERENCES

1. Kurtz SM, Lau E, Ong K, Zhao K, Kelly M, Bozic KJ. Future young patient demand for primary and revision joint replacement: National projections from 2010 to 2030. *Clin Orthop Relat Res.* 2009;467:2606–2612.

2. Kurtz S, Ong K, Lau E, Mowat F. Projections of primary and revision hip and knee arthroplasty in the United States from 2005 to 2030. *J Bone Joint Surg Am.* 2007;89:780–785.

Index

Note: Page numbers followed by *b* indicate boxes, followed by *f* indicate figures and followed by *t* indicate tables.

A

Abrasion arthroplasty, 36
ACI. *See* Autologous chondrocyte implantation (ACI)
Acromegaly, 2
Adhesions, intra-articular
  autologous chondrocyte implantation-related, 93–94, 94*f*
  identification of, 32–34
Adolescent minced allograft cartilage, 59–61, 215–218, 229–231
Adolescents, autologous chondrocyte implantation in, 102–104
Agarose, 242
Age factors
  in anterior cruciate ligament injuries, 123
  in knee replacement, 261
  in osteoarthritis, 5–6
Alginate, 242
Allogeneic cells, 19–20
American Association of Tissue Banks (AATB), 54
Anabolic activities, of chondrocytes, 8–9, 16
Animal models, of cartilage repair procedures, 12–14, 14*f*
  of autologous chondrocyte implantation, 13, 15*f*, 17*f*
  of osteochondral grafts, 14*f*
  in translational research, 15–20
Anterior cruciate ligament deficiency
  radiographic assessment of, 24*f*
  tibial osteotomy treatment of, 143–145, 145*f*
  untreated, 3
Anterior cruciate ligament injuries, 3
  age factors in, 123
  as osteoarthritis cause, 3, 10
Anterior cruciate ligament reconstruction
  with autologous chondrocyte implantation, 85–89, 89*f*, 90*f*
  with microfracture, 50
  osteochondral bone plug failure following, 213–214
  rehabilitation following, 89
Anterior tibial artery, aberrant, 129, 130*f*
Antigenicity, cartilage, 9
Anti-human leukocyte (HLA) antigens, 55
Anxiety, in joint preservation surgery patients, 32
Arterial injuries, osteotomy-related, 129–130, 130*f*
Arthrofibrosis, autologous chondrocyte implantation-related, 93–94
Arthro Kinetics, 239, 240
Arthroplasty
  abrasion, 36
  bicompartmental, in younger patients, 22
  patellofemoral, 252–260
    contraindications to, 253
    conversion to total knee arthroplasty, 252
    with DePuy low-contact stress (LCS) patellar prosthesis, 254, 255, 257, 257*f*, 258
    with DePuy Sigma custom patellofemoral prosthesis, 257, 258–260, 258*f*
    indications for, 253–255

Arthroplasty (*Continued*)
  patellofemoral prostheses for, 178–180, 179*f*, 255–257, 258–260, 258*f*
  results of, 257–260
  with Smith & Nephew Competitor patellofemoral prosthesis, 255–257
  with Stryker Howmedica Avon patellofemoral prosthesis, 255–257, 258
  surgical technique of, 255–257
  patient-specific resurfacing, 261–271
    axial and sagittal tibial cuts in, 264–265, 265*f*
    balancing of the knee in, 264, 264*f*
    balancing verification in, 266–267
    bicompartmental, 262, 267, 268*f*, 270*f*, 271*f*
    cartilage removal in, 262–264
    femoral preparation in, 265–266, 265*f*, 266*f*
    with iDuo implants, 267, 268*f*
    imaging technology in, 261–262
    with iUni implants, 266, 267, 271*f*
    patient positioning and preparation for, 262
    surgical technique of, 262–267
    tibial preparation in, 266–267, 266*f*
    trialing and cementing of implant, 267, 267*f*
    unicompartmental, 262–267
  total knee, 252
    annual number performed, 10, 261
    average age of patients, 261
    contraindication in younger patients, 22
    development of, 122–123
    disadvantages of, 122–123
    as osteonecrosis treatment, 185–186
    patellofemoral arthroplasty prior to, 252, 253–254
    present *versus* future numbers of, 6
    in smokers, 32
    versus tibial osteotomy, 123, 122–123
  unicompartmental
    patient-specific, 262–267
    preoperative magnetic resonance imaging for, 27–28
    in younger patients, 22
Arthrotomy
  lateral
    for autologous chondrocyte implantation, 72*f*
    for osteochondral allograft transplantation, 55–57
    parapatellar, for autologous chondrocyte implantation, 76–77, 78*f*
    subvastus, in end-stage patellofemoral osteoarthritis, 209–211
  medial
    for autologous chondrocyte implantation, 72*f*
    for osteochondral allograft transplantation, 55–57
    parapatellar, 157, 157*f*
    subvastus, 154*f*, 157
Articular cartilage
  components of, 11
  mechanical properties of, 9–11
  porosity of, 9

Articular cartilage (*Continued*)
  surface layer of, 9–10
  viscoelasticity of, 9, 35*f*
Articular cartilage defects, 2–7
  asymptomatic, 4, 35, 38*f*
  Outerbridge grades of, 34, 37*f*
  patellar lateral maltracking-related, 4
  prevalence of, 34
  progression to osteoarthritis, 4, 5*f*, 35, 36, 1–7
    background factors in, 5*f*, 6
  repair of
    animal models of, 12–14, 14*f*
    evidence-based treatment algorithm for, 42, 43–45, 43*f*, 44*f*, 45*t*
    failed, 12*t*
    of full-thickness defects, 11
    goal of, 10–11
    guidelines for, 42
    obstacles to, 11
    potential for, 11
    tissue engineering research in, 16–18
    translational research in, 15–20
  size of, 4, 34, 34*f*
  tibial, obesity-related, 5
  tibiofemoral malalignment-related, 4
  trauma-related, 4, 34
  treatment options for, 35–38
  untreated, 36
Athletic participation
  as articular cartilage injury cause, 2, 34
  following autologous chondrocyte implantation, 103, 104, 105, 105*f*
  following Hyalograft C autograft treatment, 234–235
  as osteoarthritis cause, 2–3
  as patellofemoral articular defect cause, 161
Arthroscopic lateral release, of isolated patellar tilt, 166–167
Autologous chondrocyte-engineered scaffold, 222–223, 223*f*
Autologous chondrocyte implantation (ACI), 14*f*, 65–120
  in adolescents, 102–104
  advanced techniques in, 76–92
    after marrow stimulation techniques, 90–91, 113–115, 114*t*, 115*t*, 117–118
    for anterior cruciate ligament reconstruction, 85–89, 89*f*, 90*f*
    bone grafts, 82–84
    exposures, 76–92
    failed, 12*t*
    with high tibial osteotomy, 77–80
    meniscal allografts, 89–90
    for osteoarthritis, 91–92
    for osteochondritis dissecans, 82–84, 86*f*
    patellar debridement and transplantation, 81–82, 83*f*
    for posterior exposure/in patella or trochlear injuries, 80–82
    for posterior femoral lesions, 76–77
    for sclerotic subchondral bone, 91–92

273

Autologous chondrocyte implantation (ACI) (*Continued*)
    single-stage sandwich technique, 82–84, 86*f*, 87*f*
    subchondral bone alterations and, 90–92
    for tibial plateau lesions, 77*f*, 76–77
    trochlear debridement and transplantation, 81, 83*f*
    for uncontained defects, 91–92
    vastus medialis oblique advancement, 82
  after care/rehabilitation following, 92–93
  animal models of, 13, 15*f*, 17*f*
  with anteromedialization tibial tubercle osteotomy, 168–169
  arthroscopic assessment for, 68–69, 68*f*
  articular cartilage debridement in, 72–73, 73*f*
  with bone grafts, 82–84
  cartilage biopsy for, 66*f*, 67, 68–69
  cell culturing process for, 41–42
  with Chondro-Glide scaffolds, 224, 225
  classic technique of, 66*f*
  clinical cost effectiveness of, 116–117
  clinical outcomes of, 39*t*, 41, 67, 100–116
  closure and suturing techniques in, 66*f*
  collagen-covered, 36
    outcome studies of, 39*t*, 41
  complex, 67
  complications of, 93–100
  contraindications to, 67
  cost effectiveness of, 107*f*
  as deep contained osteochondral defect treatment, 190–191
  disadvantages of, 229–230, 231–232
  for end-stage patellofemoral osteoarthritis, 209–211, 210*f*
  failed, 100, 100*f*, 102*f*
    fresh osteochondral allografting following, 58, 59*f*
  for failed osteochondral graft plug salvage, 215, 216*f*
  FDA approval of, 36, 65–67
  following debridement, 48
  following lateral meniscectomy, 211–213, 212*f*
  graft failure in, 100, 100*f*, 102*f*
  historical perspective on, 65–67
  incisional approach in, 66*f*
  indications for, 45, 67
  for lateral defects, 71–72
  magnetic resonance imaging of, 26*f*, 26*t*
  matrix-induced, 231–233
    background of, 231–232
    Chondro-Gide scaffold use with, 224–225
    clinical outcomes of, 232–233, 233*f*
    commercial availability of, 232
    manufacturing process for, 232
  with medial arthrotomy, 66*f*
  membrane-associated, 36
    clinical outcomes of, 39*t*, 41
  with meniscal allograft transplantation, 198, 198*f*
  number of times performed, 65
  "off-label" use of, 65–67
  osteoarthritis development after, 2–3
  as osteochondritis dissecans treatment, 182, 185
  overview of, 36
  in the patellofemoral joint, 105–109, 117, 174–175
  in patients older than 45 years, 109–110, 117
  in patients with early osteoarthritis, 91–92, 110–113
  periosteal grafts
    clinical outcomes of, 41
    comparison with type I-III collagen membrane, 115–116, 116*t*
    hypertrophy of, 115–116, 116*t*
  periosteal patch use in, 66*f*
  periosteal substitute for, 106*f*
  periosteum or collagen membrane fixation in, 75–76
  periosteum procurement in, 73–75, 74*f*
  periosteum watertight integrity testing in, 76
  regulation of, 65–67
  rehabilitation after, 14*t*
  salvage, 67

Autologous chondrocyte implantation (ACI) (*Continued*)
    sandwich technique, after OBI plug failure, 213–214, 214*f*
    sclerotic bone/intralesional osteophytes take down in, 73, 74*f*
    second-generation cell-based, 231–242
      CaReS cartilage regeneration system, 239–240
      Cartipatch, 241–242, 242*f*
      ChondroCelect, 235–239
      Hyalograft C autografts, 233–235
      matrix-induced autologous chondrocyte implantation (MACI), 231–233
    simple, 67
    in soccer players, 104–105, 104*t*, 105*f*
    sports participation following, 103, 104–105, 104*t*, 105*f*
    subchondral bone plate in, 72–73, 74*f*
    surgical implantation of chondrocytes, 71–76
    suturing techniques for, 75–76, 75*f*
    third-generation, 243–245
    type I-III collagen membrane use in, 115–116, 116*t*, 118
    for unicondylar injuries, 71
    with varus-producing osteotomy, 207–209, 208*f*
    wound closure in, 76
Autologous chondrocyte transplantation. *See* Autologous chondrocyte implantation
Autologous matrix-induced chondrogenesis registry, 225
Autologous osteochondral grafts
  as deep contained osteochondral defect treatment, 186–190
  as osteochondritis dissecans treatment, 182, 185*f*
Autologous perichondral grafts, ossification of, 13*f*
Autologous procedures, for cartilage repair or restoration
  one-stage therapies, 229–231
  two-stage therapies, 229–230
Avascular necrosis (osteonecrosis), 2, 185–186
  autologous osteochondral bone graft treatment for, 186–191
  idiopathic, 186
  radiographic stages of, 185–186
  secondary, 185
  spontaneous, 185

B

Baby boomers, 122–123
Background factors
  in autologous chondrocyte implantation, 70–71
  in cartilage repair, 42
  in osteoarthritis, 2
Bacterial infections, osteochondral allograft-associated, 55
Barotrauma, as osteonecrosis cause, 185
Basketball players, patellofemoral cartilage defect prevalence in, 160–161
Bicompartmental arthroplasty
  patient-specific resurfacing, 262, 267, 268*f*, 270*f*, 271*f*
  in younger patients, 22
BioCart II, 240–241
Biologics License Application, 245
Biopsy, of cartilage, for autologous chondrocyte implantation, 68–69, 68*f*, 69*f*
Bioresorbable materials, 19
BioSyntech, 221
Blood clots, BST-CarGel-stabilized, 219–221
Blunt trauma, as chondral lesion cause, 10
Body mass index (BMI), 5, 31–32
Bone, as cartilage repair tissue, 11
Bone-bridge technique, 193, 194, 194*f*, 196, 197*f*
Bone bruises, 3, 10
Bone formation, marrow stimulation techniques-related, 36
Bone grafts. *See also* Osteochondral allografts
  combined with autologous chondrocyte implantation, 82–84
Bone-plug technique, 193, 194
Bone scans, patellofemoral, 166

C

CAIS (Cartilage Autograft Implantation System), 230–231, 230*f*, 231*f*
Calcium sulfate, 227
CaReS cartilage regeneration system, 239–240
Carticel, 231–232
Cartilage. *See also* Articular cartilage; Hyaline cartilage
  structure and function of, 8–9
Cartilage Autograft Implantation System (CAIS), 230–231, 230*f*, 231*f*
Cartilage fibrils, 8–9
Catabolic activities, of chondrocytes, 8–9, 16
Cell death, in cartilage, 10
Centers for Disease Control and Prevention (CDC), 122–123
Chitosan, 219–220. *See also* BST-CarGel
Chondral defects and injury, 2–7. *See also* Articular cartilage defects
  focal, 34
  incidence of, 10
Chondrocalcin, 9
ChondroCelect, 235–239
  clinical development of, 238–239, 239*f*
  ectopic cartilage formation assay (ECFA) of, 236–237, 236*f*
  gene marker assay of, 236–237, 237*f*
  manufacturing process for, 237
  preclinical studies of, 237–238, 238*f*
Chondrocytes
  as anabolic/catabolic cells, 8–9, 16
  deep freezing of, 55
  density of, 8, 11
  differentiation in vitro, 18–19
Chondrocytes. *See also* Autologous chondrocyte implantation
Chondro-Gide, 224–225
  use in autologous chondrocyte implantation, 224
  use in autologous matrix-induced chondrogenesis, 224–225
Chondrolysis, 9
Chondromalacia, 160, 164*f*
  grade II Outerbridge, 166–167
  trochlear dysplasia-related, 175
Chondrons, 8–9
Chondroplasty, technique of, 49
Cincinnati Rating Scale, 100, 102*f*
Collagen
  methylated, as autologous chondrocyte implant component, 243
  type I, 11, 36
    as fibrocartilage component, 11
    as Kensey Nash CRD device component, 225–226
  type II, 11
    as fibrocartilage component, 11
    synthesis and secretion of, 8–9
  type I/III membrane, for matrix-induced autologous chondrocyte implantation, 231–232
  type IX, synthesis of, 8–9
  type XI, synthesis of, 8–9
Collagen membrane, type I-III, for autologous chondrocyte implantation, 115–116, 116*t*
Comparative studies, of joint preservation techniques, 41–42
Compartment overload syndrome, 193
Complex cases, in cartilage repair, 200–218
  autologous chondrocyte implantation
    for end-stage patellofemoral osteoarthritis, 209–211, 210*f*
    for failed osteochondral graft plugs, 213–214, 214*f*, 215, 216*f*
    sandwich technique, 213–214, 214*f*
    with varus-producing osteotomy, 207–209, 208*f*
  extraarticular supracondylar femoral reverse dome osteotomy, 203–206, 205*f*
  intraarticular osteotomy after tibial plateau fracture, 203, 204*f*
  lateral meniscectomy cascade with valgus knee, 211–213, 212*f*

Complex cases, in cartilage repair (*Continued*)
  medial subvastus approach to the knee, 200–203, 202*f*
  revision lateral tibial plateau allograft, 206–207, 207*f*
Computed tomography (CT)
  for patellofemoral disorders assessment, 163–166, 163*f*
  for patient-specific resurfacing arthroplasty, 261–262, 262*f*
  prior to patellofemoral arthroplasty, 254
Computer-assisted design
  of resurfacing arthroplasty disposable instrument set, 262, 262*f*
  of resurfacing arthroplasty implants, 261–262, 262*f*, 264*f*
Computer-assisted navigation, use in implant placement, 261, 262, 263*f*, 264, 269
ConforMIS, 261
Continuous passive motion machine programs
  for autologous chondrocyte implantation patients, 92, 102–103
  for meniscal allograft transplantation patients, 198
  for microfracture patients, 51
  for osteochondral autograft transfer patients, 51
Corticosteroids, as osteonecrosis cause, 185
C-properide, 9
"Crossing sign,", 175–176, 176*t*
Culture media, for fresh osteochondral allografts, 54
Cysts
  Baker, 209
  osteochondral, 191
  subchondral, 71, 91, 185*f*, 220–221
Cytokines, immunomodulatory, 9

D
Debridement, arthroscopic, 36, 252
  in cartilage regeneration transplantation, 240*f*
  indications for, 48
  of meniscus, 50
  of osteonecrosis, 185–186
  technique of, 49
  of zone of calcified cartilage, 49–50, 50*f*
Decision making, regarding joint preservation surgery
  patient characteristics and, 31–32
  patient history and, 31
Decompression, core, as osteonecrosis treatment, 185–186
Delayed gadolinium-enhanced magnetic resonance imaging of cartilage (dGEMTIC), 25–27, 28*f*
Demineralized bone matrix, 172–173, 173*f*
DeNovo Engineered Tissue Graft, 245, 245*f*
DeNovo natural tissue (NT) graft, 231, 231*f*
Depression, in joint preservation surgery patients, 32
DePuy low-contact stress (LCS) patellar prosthesis, 254, 255, 257, 257*f*, 258
DePuy Sigma custom patellofemoral replacement, 257, 258–260, 258*f*
Dowel technique, of osteochondral allograft transplantation, 55–57, 56*f*, 57–58
Drilling, 36
Dysplasia
  of the joints, 2
  patellofemoral, as indication for patellofemoral arthroplasty, 252–254
  trochlear, 160, 161, 174–178
    assessment for, in patellar instability, 174–175
    Dejour classification grades of, 175–176, 176*f*, 176*t*
    of the distal femur, 175
    imaging of, 23, 25*f*, 165*f*
    moderate, 175*f*
    patellofemoral tracking-associated, 215–218, 217*f*
    patterns of, 164*f*
    recurrent patellar instability associated with, 175–176
    trochleoplasty of, 174–175

E
Ectopic cartilage formation assay (ECFA), 236–237, 236*f*
Ehlers-Danos syndrome, 2
Elmslie-Trillat operation, Fulkerson osteotomy modification of, 168, 169*f*
Emerging technologies, 219–249
  marrow stimulation technique augmentation, 219–221, 220*b*, 221*f*
  minced cartilage, 229–231, 230*f*, 231*f*
  scaffolds, 222–229, 222*f*, 223*f*, 224*f*, 225*f*, 226*f*, 227*f*, 228*f*, 229*f*
    Chondro-Gide, 224–225
    Kensey Nash Corporation Cartilage Repair Device, 225–227
    TruFit CB scaffold, for cartilage repair, 227–229, 227*f*, 228*f*, 229*f*
  second-generation cell-based autologous chondrocyte implantation, 231–242, 232*f*, 233*f*, 234*f*, 235*t*, 236*f*
Engineered tissue grafts. *See* Tissue engineering
European Medicines Agency (EMEA), 232
European Union Advanced Therapy Medicinal Products regulation, 232
Evidence-based treatment algorithm, for articular cartilage repair, 42, 43–45, 43*f*, 44*f*, 45*t*
Extracellular matrix (ECM), cartilage-specific, 243–245

F
Fat pad, infrapatellar, arthrofibrosis of, 4
Femoral articular surface, autologous chondrocyte implantation on, 67
Femoral condyle injuries
  autologous chondrocyte implantation treatment of, 67
  BST-CarGel treatment of, 221
  incidence of, 67
  in lateral condyles, 3
  in medial condyles, 3
    chondral lesions, 2
    high-grade chondral lesions, 34
    TruFit implant repair of, 229*f*
  microfracture treatment of, 221
Femoral implants, patient-specific computer-assisted design of, 261–262, 262*f*, 263*f*
Fibrocartilage
  as cartilage repair tissue, 11, 12*f*
  composition of, 11
  produced by marrow stimulation techniques, 36
Food and Drug Administration (FDA)
  autologous chondrocyte implantation approval by, 36, 65–67
  osteochondral allograft regulations of, 54
  patellofemoral prostheses approval by, 255
Framingham Osteoarthritis Study, 5–6
Fresh osteochondral allografts, 54–64
  chondrocyte viability in, 54
  comparison with
    fresh-frozen allografts, 55
    osteochondral autografts, 38
  contraindications to, 55
  definition of, 54
  disadvantages of, 38
  disease transmission risk associated with, 55
  donor-recipient size matching for, 55
  graft procurement and storage, 54–55
  immunology of, 55
  indications for, 38, 55
  results of, 63–64
  surgical transplantation techniques for, 55–57
    dowel technique, 55–57, 56*f*, 57–58
    shell technique, 55–57, 57*f*
    "snowman" technique, 57–58
Fulkerson Classification, of patellar chondral defects, 106*f*, 171*f*

G
Gait abnormalities, patellofemoral malalignment-related, 162
Gait training, for patellofemoral disorder patients, 162–163
Gastric bypass surgery, 31–32

Gaucher disease, 2
Geistlich Surgery, AMIC registry of, 225
Gene marker assay, 236–237, 237*f*
Gene therapy, 19
Genetic factors, in osteoarthritis, 2
Genzyme Biosurgery, 231–232
Golgi bodies, 8–9
Good Laboratory Practices, 41–42
Good Laboratory Standards, 65–67
Good Manufacturing Practices, 41–42, 240
Good Manufacturing Standards, 65–67

H
Health Canada, Special Access Program, 220–221
Hemochromatosis, 2
Hemophilia, 2
Hepatitis testing, 55
Histogenics Corporation, 243
Hoffa fat pad, contracture of, 32–34
Horizontal mattress stitch, 82
Human immunodeficiency virus (HIV) infection, 38
Human immunodeficiency virus (HIV) infection testing, 55
HYAFF 11, 233
Hyaline cartilage
  as cartilage repair tissue, 11
  immunoprivileged status of, 55
Hyaline-like cartilage, 34
Hyalograft C autograft, 233–235
  clinical development of, 233–235, 234*f*, 235*t*
  preclinical studies of, 233
Hydrogels, 19

I
Iliotibial band
  in femoral varus osteotomy, 146
  in open meniscal allograft transplantation, 195, 196*f*
Imaging, 22–30. *See also* Computed tomography (CT); Magnetic resonance imaging (MRI)
  for patient-specific resurfacing arthroplasty, 261–262
  preoperative, 32–34
Infectious disease transmission, in osteochondral allografts, 55
Informed consent, for osteochondral allograft procedures, 55
Intercondylar notch, as articular cartilage harvest site, 69*f*, 70*f*
Interleukins, 9
International Cartilage Repair Society, 31–32, 67
  Histological Scoring system of, 221
International Knee Documentation Committee (IKDC) score
  for Hyalograft C autografts, 233–235
  for NeoCart System, 244
  for TruFit CB scaffolds, 228–229
Internet, as medical information source, 31, 32*f*

J
Joints, lubricating barrier between, 9–10
J-sign, 32, 162, 163

K
Kensey Nash Corporation Cartilage Repair Device, 225–227
  implant description, 225–226, 225*f*
  preclinical studies of, 226–227, 226*f*
"Kissing lesions,", 91, 91*f*, 128*f*, 220–221
Knee
  computed tomography-based three-dimensional models of, 261, 262*f*
  lateral compartment of, meniscectomy-related changes in, 4
  medial compartment of, meniscectomy-related changes in, 3–4
  medial pivot of, 3–4
Knee Injury and Osteoarthritis Outcome Score (KOOS)
  for ChondroCelect, 238, 239*f*
  for TruFit CB scaffolds, 228–229, 228*f*
Knee pain, anterior, 252
  patellofemoral articular defects-related, 161

Knee Society Score (KSS), 100
Kurosaka point, in tibial valgus-producing osteotomy, 128f

L

Lateral collateral ligament, meniscal allograft transplantation-related injury to, 195
Lateral compartment, of the knee, meniscectomy-related changes in, 4
Lavage, arthroscopic, 36
Leg-length discrepancy
  in autologous chondrocyte implantation patients, 70
  open wedge osteotomy correction of, 128–129
  varus-producing osteotomy correction of, 146, 147
Ligamentous instability assessment, for autologous chondrocyte implantation, 70
Long-distance running, relationship to osteoarthritis development, 2–3
Loose bodies, 32–34, 36
Loose flaps, debridement of, 49–50, 49f

M

Magnetic resonance arthrography, 25, 28f
  delayed gadolinium-enhanced magnetic resonance imaging of cartilage (dGEMTIC) technique of, 25–27, 28f
Magnetic resonance imaging (MRI), of articular cartilage defects, 23–29
  of asymptomatic defects, 35, 38f
  diagnostic, preoperative, 32–34
  limitations of, 27
  of patellofemoral disorders, 164f
MaioRegen, 222–224, 222f, 223f
Malpractice cases, osteotomy-related, 129
Marrow stimulation techniques, 36, 229–230
  action mechanism of, 36
  autologous chondrocyte implantation following, 90–91, 113–115
  BST-CarGel augmentation of, 219–221
    background to, 219–220
    clinical experience with, 220–221
    mode of action of, 219–220, 220b
    nonclinical studies of, 220, 220b
Matrix metalloproteinases, 8–9
Medial compartment, meniscectomy-related changes in, 3–4
Medial pivot, 3–4
Medial subperiosteal flap, 172, 172f, 173f
Medial subvastus approach, 200–203, 202f
Medical Outcomes Study 36-Item Health Survey (SF-36), 31–32, 67, 100, 221
Meniscal allograft transplantation, 193–199
  arthroscopic techniques in, 195, 196–198
  with autologous chondrocyte implantation, 89–90, 198, 198f
  bone-bridge technique, 193, 194, 194f, 196, 197f
  bone-plug technique, 193, 194
  completion meniscectomy in, 195, 196f
  contraindications to, 193
  graft fixation in, 196, 197f
  graft placement in, 196
  graft preparation for, 194
  indications for, 193
  lateral, 211–213
  open lateral, 195, 196f
  with osteotomy, 89
  patient positioning for, 195
  planning for, 193–194
  posterolateral approach in, 195
  posteromedial approach in, 195
  preoperative magnetic resonance imaging for, 28
  preoperative measurements for, 193–194, 194f
  special instrumentation for, 194
  surgical anatomy of, 195
  surgical approach in, 195
  tibial slot preparation in, 195–196, 197f
Meniscal injury, 3–4
Meniscectomy, 3
  completion, in meniscal allograft transplantation, 195, 196f
  lateral compartment degeneration after, 3–4
  subtotal
    contact stress after, 193
    as meniscal allograft indication, 193
  total
    contact stress occurring after, 193
    lateral compartment changes after, 4
    medial compartment changes after, 3–4
    as meniscal allograft indication, 193
  valgus knee after, 211–213, 212f
Meniscus
  absence of, 3–4
  in autologous chondrocyte implantation, 68, 70, 72f
  debridement of, 50
Microfracture
  arthroscopic performance of, 49
  clinical outcomes of, 48
  clinical outcome studies of, 38–41, 39t
  comparison with
    BST-CarGel, 221
    ChondroCelect, 238–239
    Hyalograft C autograft, 234–235
    matrix-induced autologous chondrocyte implantation, 232
    NeoCart System, 245
  indications for, 45, 48
  osteoarthritis development after, 2–3
  planning for, 48
  surgical technique of, 49–51
Microfracture holes
  clot formation in, 50, 51f
  placement of, 50, 50f
Minced allograft adolescent cartilage, 59–61, 215–218, 229–231
MOCART (Magnetic resonance Observation of Cartilage Repair Tissue) score, 223–224, 238–239
Mosaicplasty, 36–38
  clinical outcome studies of, 39t, 41

N

Narcotic use, 32
National Basketball Association players, patellofemoral cartilage defect prevalence in, 160–161
NeoCart System, 243–245
  clinical trials of, 244–245, 244f, 245f
  description of, 243
  preclinical animal studies of, 243–244
  procedure, 243, 243f
Neuropathic arthropathy, 2

O

Obese patients, patellofemoral arthroplasty in, 254
Obesity
  body mass index (BMI) measure of, 5, 31–32
  implication for joint preservation surgery, 31–32
  as osteoarthritis risk factor, 2–3, 5, 31–32
Ochronosis, 2
Ossification, of autologous perichondral graft, 13f
Osteoarthritis
  Ahlback stages of, 123
  asymptomatic, 5–6
  definition of, 10
  economic burden of, 6
  economic cost of, 6, 10
  etiology of, 2
  genetic factors in, 2
  lateral tibiofemoral, radiographic assessment of, 23, 24f
  medial, radiographic assessment of, 22–23, 23f
  meniscal tissue loss-related, 193
  natural history of, 10
  patellofemoral
    clinical classification of, 252–253
    end-stage, 253f
    prevalence of, 252
  prevalence of, 5–6, 122–123
  radiographic findings in, 5–6, 22–23, 23f
  traumatic, 2
  tricompartmental, 23f

Osteochondral allografts, 36–38, 229–230. *See also* Fresh osteochondral allografts
  clinical outcome studies of, 41
  fresh-frozen, 55
  as osteochondritis dissecans treatment, 182, 185
  as osteonecrosis treatment, 186
Osteochondral autograft transfer (OAT), 36–38, 136f, 229–230
  arthroscopic approach in, 51
  clinical outcome studies of, 39t, 41
  indications for, 38–41, 48
  open approach in, 51
  osteochondral plug harvest for, 51, 51f, 52f
  osteochondral plug placement, 51, 52f, 53f
  planning for, 48
  surgical technique, 36–38, 51
Osteochondral defects. *See also* Osteochondritis dissecans
  avascular necrosis (osteonecrosis)
    idiopathic, 186, 189f
    radiographic stages of, 185–186
  deep contained, 186–190
    autologous osteochondral graft treatment of, 186–190, 189f, 190–191
  repair of, 11
Osteochondral grafts
  in animal models, 14f
  donor site complications of, 215
  failed, salvage procedure for, 215, 216f
Osteochondral shell allograft resurfacing, 18–19
Osteochondral units, 35f
Osteochondritis dissecans, 2, 181–185
  adult form of, 182, 183f, 191
  age factors in, 2, 34
  autologous chondrocyte implantation treatment of, 67, 71, 82–84, 182, 185
    in adolescents, 103
    after care/rehabilitation, 92–93
    bone grafts for, 82–84
    in posterolateral lesions, 80, 81f
  autologous osteochondral graft treatment of, 182, 185f, 191
  BST-CarGel treatment of, 220–221
  classification of, 181
  closing wedge osteotomy treatment of, 157f
  cystic degeneration in, 182, 182f
  etiology of, 181
  fragmented lesions in, 182, 191
  fresh osteochondral allograft treatment of, 55
  management of, 181–185
  optimal treatment of, 182, 183f, 185
  osteochondral allograft treatment of, 182, 185
  progression to osteoarthritis, 182f
Osteophytes, intralesional, takedown of, 73, 74f
Osteotomy. *See also* Tibial osteotomy; Tibial tubercle osteotomy
  extraarticular supracondylar femoral reverse dome, 203–206, 205f
  intra-articular, after tibial plateau fracture, 203, 204f
  with meniscal allograft transplantation, 89
  modified retrotubercular, 132–135
  valgus tibial, 3
  varus, with autologous chondrocyte implantation, 207–209, 208f
  varus femoral, 146–159
    angular correction calculation in, 147–148, 148f
    closing wedge: classic technique, 147, 148f, 152–156, 154f, 155f, 159
    distal closing wedge, 152–156, 157f
    goal of, 147
    indications for, 146–147
    opening wedge, 146, 149f, 150f, 151f, 159, 148–151
    planning for, 147–148
    reverse dome, 146–147, 151–152, 152f, 153f, 159
Outerbridge grades, of articular cartilage defects, 34, 37f

Index

P

Paget disease, 2
Pain
 osteoarthritis-related, 10
 post-autologous chondrocyte implantation, 100
Pain management, postoperative, 32
Pannus, 9
Patella
 angular degrees of flexion of, 161f
 dislocation of, articular injury patterns in, 161, 161f
 Fulkerson classification wear patterns in, 106f, 171f
 height of, measurement of, 163–166
 high-grade chondral lesions of, 34
 minced juvenile articular cartilage reconstruction of, 63f
 mobility assessment of, 162
 posttraumatic fractures of, 252–253
Patella alta, 160
 measurement of, 163–166
Patella baja, 4
Patella infera
 as contraindication to patellofemoral arthroplasty, 252–253
 measurement of, 163–166
Patellar facets
 as chondrocyte harvest site, 68–69
 lateral, arthritic changes in, 4
Patellar malalignment/maltracking.
 See also Patellofemoral malalignment/maltracking
 autologous chondrocyte implantation for, 79–82
 deep contained osteochondral defect-associated, 190–191
 dysplasia associated with, 252–253
 lateral, 4
  with valgus malalignment, 166, 167f
 physical examination of, 162
 with trochlear or patellar chondral injury, 79–82
Patellar subluxation, patellar tilt-associated, 167–169, 168f, 178–180
 with chondrosis, 167–169
Patellar taping, 252
Patellar tilt
 isolated, arthroscopic lateral release of, 166–167
 patellar subluxation associated with, 167–169, 168f, 178–180
 with chondrosis, 167–169
Patellofemoral alignment assessment, for autologous chondrocyte implantation, 70
Patellofemoral disorders
 autologous chondrocyte implantation treatment of, 67, 105–109, 108t
 arthroscopic assessment for, 68f
 history of, 161
 imaging studies of, 163–166
 osteoarthritis, clinical categorization of, 252–253
 pathomechanics of, 166
 physical examination of, 162
 physical therapy for, 162–163
 prevalence of, 160–161
 treatment algorithm for, 161f, 166
 trochlear dysplasia, imaging of, 23, 25f
Patellofemoral instability, minced juvenile articular cartilage treatment of, 63f
Patellofemoral joint, in valgus knee malalignment, 146
Patellofemoral malalignment/maltracking, 4
 as anterior knee pain cause, 252
 lateral
  imaging assessment of, 254
  subchondral bone in, 164f
  tibial tubercle to trochlear groove (TT-TG) distance in, 163–166, 165f
Patellofemoral prostheses, design of, 252
Patellofemoral tracking, in presence of trochlea dysplasia, 215–218, 217f
Patient evaluation, for joint preservation surgery, 31–46
Patient satisfaction survey, of autologous chondrocyte implantation patients, 100, 102f

Periosteal grafts
 delamination of, 97–100, 98f
 hypertrophy of, 94–97, 95f
 neochondrogenesis in, 13
Periosteal resurfacing, 15f
Peroneal nerve injury, meniscal allograft transplantation-related, 195
Physical examination, preoperative, 32
Physical therapy
 for chronic patellofemoral pain, 160
 for patellofemoral disorders, 162–163
Polyethylene glycols, as autologous chondrocyte implant component, 243
Polygraft, as scaffold material, 227
Polylactic acid, as Kensey Nash CRD device component, 225–226
Popliteal tendon injury, meniscal allograft transplantation-related, 195
Posterior cruciate ligament injury/insufficiency, 3
 asymptomatic, 3
 tibial osteotomy treatment of, 143, 143f
Postoperative management, patient-related issues in, 32
Precursor cells, 18–19
Procollagen II, 9
Progenitor cells, 18–19
Proteoglycans
 loss of, 9–10
 metabolism of, 8–9

Q

Quadriceps, strengthening exercises for, 162–163
Quadriceps (Q) angle, 162f
 abnormally increased, 160, 161
  in combined patellar subluxation and tilt, 167–168
 as lateral patellar maltracking cause, 174–175
 examination and measurement of, 162
 in patellofemoral defects, 162
Quadriceps wasting, 162

R

Ringer's solution, lactated, 54
Running, impact on osteoarthritis, 2–3

S

Sandwich technique
 in autologous chondrocyte implantation, 82–84, 86f, 87f
 in osteochondritis dissecans treatment, 185
 use following OBI plug failure, 213–214, 214f
Scaffold-guided regenerative medicine, 219–220
Scaffolds, 222–229
 autologous chondrocyte-engineered, 222–223, 223f
 CAIS (Cartilage Autograft Implantation System), 230
 Chondro-Gide, 224–225
  use in autologous chondrocyte implantation, 224
  use in autologous matrix-induced chondrogenesis, 224–225
 Hyalograft C autograft, 233–235
  clinical development of, 233–235, 234f, 235t
  preclinical studies of, 233
 Kensey Nash Corporation Cartilage Repair Device
  implant description, 225–226, 225f
  preclinical studies of, 226–227, 226f
 MaioRegen, 222–224, 222f, 223f
 "smart,", 19–20
 three-dimensional, 19
 TruFit CB, 227–229, 227f, 228f, 229f
  clinical case series of, 228–229
  preclinical study of, 227–228
  properties of, 227
Self-referral, of patients, 31, 32f
Serologic testing, of osteochondral allografts, 55
Shell graft technique, of osteochondral allograft transplantation, 55–57, 57f
Sigma custom patellofemoral replacement, 257, 258–260, 258f
Smith & Nephew Competitor patellofemoral replacement, 255–257

Smoking cessation, preoperative, 32
"Snowman" technique, of osteochondral allograft transplantation, 57–58
Soccer players, autologous chondrocyte implantation in, 104–105, 104t, 105f
Sports participation. *See* Athletic participation
Stryker Howmedica Avon patellofemoral replacement, 255–257, 258
Subchondral bone
 in lateral patellar maltracking, 164f
 marrow-stimulated, 90–91
 sclerotic, as autologous bone grafting indication, 185f
Subchondral bone plate
 microfracture of, 50, 50f
 as pain source, 10
Sulcus terminalis, as osteochondral plug harvest site, 51, 52f
SUMMIT (Superiority of MACI vs. Microfracture Treatment), 232
Surgeon-patient relationship, 31
 5Es of, 31, 33f

T

TBF Tissue Engineering Company, 241–242
Technical skills, in cartilage repair techniques, 42
Tibia, proximal medial, as periosteum procurement site, 73–75
Tibial alignment guide, external, 58–59
Tibial osteotomy, 123f, 121–145. *See also* Tibial tubercle osteotomy
 age factors in, 122–123
 anatomic considerations in, 129–130
 angular correction in, 124–126, 128f
 closing wedge
  aberrant anterior tibial artery in, 129, 130f
  Coventry, 128–129, 130–132
  indications for, 129
  postoperative radiographic assessment of, 135f
  in the sagittal plane, 143
  surgical technique in, 130–132, 131f, 133f
 contraindications to, 128
 indications for, 122, 123
 opening wedge
  with anteromedialization tibial tubercle osteotomy, 136f, 140
  versus closing wedge osteotomy, 127
  in the sagittal plane, 143
  surgical technique of, 132–139, 135f, 136f, 138f
  valgus, 128–129
 as osteonecrosis treatment, 185–186
 patient-related issues in, 124, 124f, 128
 postoperative care, 129
 procedural planning of, 124–126
 purpose of, 122
 realignment, with cartilage repair, 126
 reverse dome, 129
 reverse dome valgus
  postoperative care following, 141–143
  surgical technique of, 140–143, 141f, 142f
  in the sagittal plane, 143, 143f, 145f
 surgical setup for, 129
 technique-related issues in, 123
 technique selection for, 127–129
 versus total knee arthroplasty, 122–123
 tubercle realignment in, 253–254, 254f, 256f
 valgus, 3
  as osteonecrosis treatment, 186, 189f, 191
  preoperative imaging evaluation for, 27–28, 125f
  reverse dome, 141–143, 141f, 145f
 varus
  in lateral compartment osteoarthritis, 122
  in medial compartment osteoarthritis, 122
  proximal, 122
Tibial plateau, lateral, collapse of, 58–59, 62f
Tibial plateau allografts, revision lateral, 206–207, 207f
Tibial plateau fractures
 fresh osteochondral allograft treatment of, 55, 57f
 intra-articular osteotomy treatment of, 203, 204f
Tibial plateau slot, in meniscal allograft transplantation, 195–196, 197f

Tibial tubercle, surgical exposure of, 171*f*
Tibial tubercle osteotomy
    anteromedialization
        with autologous chondrocyte implantation, 168–169
        for combined patellar tilt and subluxation, 167–168, 169*f*
        with opening wedge high tibial valgus osteotomy, 136*f*, 140
    anteromedialization-Fulkerson, 136*f*, 168, 169*f*
        modification of, 169
        surgical technique of, 169–174, 170*f*, 171*f*, 172*f*
    with autologous chondrocyte implantation, 71–72, 76–80, 80–82, 83*f*, 84*f*
    with closing wedge femoral osteotomy, 157*f*
    contraindication to, 178–180
    as end-stage patellofemoral osteoarthritis treatment, 209–211
    with minced allograft adolescent cartilage, 215–218, 217*f*
Tibial tubercle to trochlear groove (TT-TG) distance, 163–166, 165*f*, 209
Tibiofemoral alignment, normal, 124, 125*f*
Tibiofemoral axis, 124–125
Tibiofemoral malalignment, 4
    as contraindication to patellofemoral arthroplasty, 253
TIGACT01 study, 238–239
TiGenix, 235
Tissue banking, of osteochondral allografts, 54–55
Tissue engineering, 16–18, 20*f*, 245, 245*f*
    DeNovo Engineered Tissue Graft, 245, 245*f*
    future directions in, 19–20
    hydrostatic pressure culture system for, 16–17, 18*f*
Total knee arthroplasty
    annual number performed, 10, 261
    average age of patients, 261
    contraindication in younger patients, 22
    development of, 122–123
    disadvantages of, 122–123
    patellofemoral arthroplasty prior to, 252, 253–254
    present *versus* future numbers of, 6
    in smokers, 32
    versus tibial osteotomy, 123, 122–123
Transitional tissue, as cartilage repair tissue, 11
Transplantation antigens, 9

Trauma
    as articular cartilage defect cause, 4, 34
    blunt, as articular cartilage defect cause, 10
    as osteoarthritis cause, 2
β-Tricalcium phosphate, 225–226
Trochlea
    bony reconstruction of, 177–178, 179*f*
    as chondrocyte harvest site, 68–69, 69*f*
    dysplasia of, 82, 106, 160, 161, 174–178
        assessment for, in patellar instability, 174–175
        Dejour classification grades of, 175–176, 176*f*, 176*t*
        of the distal femur, 175
        imaging of, 23, 25*f*, 165*f*
        moderate, 175*f*
        patellofemoral tracking-associated, 215–218, 217*f*
        patterns of, 164*f*
        recurrent patellar instability associated with, 175–176
        trochleoplasty of, 174–175
Trochlear implants
    design of, 252, 253*f*
    onset, 255–257
Trochlear lesions, autologous chondrocyte implantation treatment of, 68–69, 70, 80–82
    aftercare/rehabilitation following, 92, 93
    arthroscopic assessment for, 68–69
Trochlear ridge
    defects, of scaffold treatment of, 226, 226*f*
    as osteochondral plug harvest site, 51, 52*f*
"Trochlea spur,", 175–176, 175*f*
Trochleoplasty
    Dejour, 179*f*
    interposition soft tissue, 176–177
    with minced allograft adolescent cartilage, 215–218, 217*f*
    Peterson interposition, 177–178, 178*f*
    synovial interposition, 176–177, 177*f*
    for trochlear dysplasia, 82
TruFit CB scaffold, for cartilage repair, 227–229, 227*f*, 228*f*, 229*f*
    clinical case series of, 228–229
    preclinical study of, 227–228
    properties of, 227
TruFit osteochondral plugs, 45, 209–211, 210*f*
    failure of, 213–214, 214*f*

U

Unicompartmental arthroplasty
    patient-specific, 262–267
    preoperative magnetic resonance imaging for, 27–28
    in younger patients, 22

V

Valgus knee
    femoral varus osteotomy for, 146–159
    following lateral meniscectomy, 211–213, 212*f*
    with patellofemoral dysplasia and lateral maltracking, 166, 167*f*
Varus knee
    autologous chondrocyte implantation treatment of, 66*f*, 77–79, 79*f*
    deep contained osteochondral defect-associated, 190–191
    with medial femoral condyle lesions, 78–79, 79*f*
    with patellar injury, 78–79
    with trochlear injury, 78–79
Vastus medialis obliquus (VMO) advancement, 173, 174–175, 174*f*
    in autologous chondrocyte implantation, 82
    as patellofemoral malalignment cause, 4
Viral disease transmission, in osteochondral allografts, 38, 55
Viscoelasticity, of articular cartilage, 9

W

Water, as articular cartilage component, 9–10
Weight-bearing, after autologous chondrocyte implantation, 92–93
Weight training, after autologous chondrocyte implantation, 93
Western Ontario MacMaster (WOMAC) osteoarthritis index, 100, 220–221

X

Xenogeneic cells, 19–20
X-rays
    of osteoarthritis, 22–23
    of patellofemoral disorders, 163
    standing anteroposterior (AP)
        of lateral tibiofemoral osteoarthritis, 23, 24*f*
        of medial osteoarthritis, 22–23, 23*f*
    supine anterioposterior (AP), 22

Z

Zimmer Technologies, 245